New Frontiers in Chronic Kidney Disease Research

New Frontiers in Chronic Kidney Disease Research

Edited by Dakota Beckett

hayle
medical

New York

Hayle Medical,
750 Third Avenue, 9th Floor,
New York, NY 10017, USA

Visit us on the World Wide Web at:
www.haylemedical.com

This book contains information obtained from authentic and highly regarded sources. Copyright for all individual chapters remain with the respective authors as indicated. All chapters are published with permission under the Creative Commons Attribution License or equivalent. A wide variety of references are listed. Permission and sources are indicated; for detailed attributions, please refer to the permissions page and list of contributors. Reasonable efforts have been made to publish reliable data and information, but the authors, editors and publisher cannot assume any responsibility for the validity of all materials or the consequences of their use.

ISBN: 978-1-63241-661-2

Trademark Notice: Registered trademark of products or corporate names are used only for explanation and identification without intent to infringe.

Cataloging-in-Publication Data

New frontiers in chronic kidney disease research / edited by Dakota Beckett.
      p. cm.
Includes bibliographical references and index.
ISBN 978-1-63241-661-2
1. Kidneys--Diseases. 2. Chronic diseases. 3. Nephrology. I. Beckett, Dakota.
RC902 .N49 2019
616.61--dc23

Table of Contents

Permissions

List of Contributors

Index

Preface

This book has been an outcome of determined endeavour from a group of educationists in the field. The primary objective was to involve a broad spectrum of professionals from diverse cultural background involved in the field for developing new researches. The book not only targets students but also scholars pursuing higher research for further enhancement of the theoretical and practical applications of the subject.

Chronic kidney disease is a severe kidney disease in which the functioning of kidney stops gradually over a period of months or years. Its signs and symptoms include loss of appetite, tiredness, vomiting and swelling in the legs. In some cases, the risk factors may even include anemia, high blood pressure, bone disease and cardiovascular disease. Various clinical conditions may be associated with chronic kidney disease and decrease of kidney function, such as uremia, anemia, cardiac arrhythmias, pulmonary edema, etc. Uremia is a condition in which there are very high levels of urea present in the blood. It often leads to kidney failure. The topics included in this book on chronic kidney disease are of utmost significance and bound to provide incredible insights to readers. It aims to shed light on some of its unexplored aspects and the recent researches in this field. This book is a vital tool for all researching or studying about chronic kidney disease as it gives incredible insights into emerging trends and concepts.

It was an honour to edit such a profound book and also a challenging task to compile and examine all the relevant data for accuracy and originality. I wish to acknowledge the efforts of the contributors for submitting such brilliant and diverse chapters in the field and for endlessly working for the completion of the book. Last, but not the least; I thank my family for being a constant source of support in all my research endeavours.

Editor

Spontaneous BOLD Signal Fluctuations in Young Healthy Subjects and Elderly Patients with Chronic Kidney Disease

Hesamoddin Jahanian[1]*, Wendy W. Ni[1,2], Thomas Christen[1], Michael E. Moseley[1], Manjula Kurella Tamura[3], Greg Zaharchuk[1]

1 Department of Radiology, Stanford University, Stanford, California, United States of America, 2 Department of Electrical Engineering, Stanford University, Stanford, California, Untied States of America, 3 Geriatric Research and Education Clinical Center, Palo Alto Veterans Affairs Health Care System and Division of Nephrology, Stanford University, Stanford, California, United States of America

Abstract

Spontaneous fluctuations in blood oxygenation level-dependent (BOLD) images are the basis of resting-state fMRI and frequently used for functional connectivity studies. However, there may be intrinsic information in the amplitudes of these fluctuations. We investigated the possibility of using the amplitude of spontaneous BOLD signal fluctuations as a biomarker for cerebral vasomotor reactivity. We compared the coefficient of variation (CV) of the time series (defined as the temporal standard deviation of the time series divided by the mean signal intensity) in two populations: 1) Ten young healthy adults and 2) Ten hypertensive elderly subjects with chronic kidney disease (CKD). We found a statistically significant increase ($P<0.01$) in the CV values for the CKD patients compared with the young healthy adults in both gray matter (GM) and white matter (WM). The difference was independent of the exact segmentation method, became more significant after correcting for physiological signals using RETROICOR, and mainly arose from very low frequency components of the BOLD signal fluctuation ($f<0.025$ Hz). Furthermore, there was a strong relationship between WM and GM signal fluctuation CV's ($R^2 = 0.87$) in individuals, with a ratio of about 1:3. These results suggest that amplitude of the spontaneous BOLD signal fluctuations may be used to assess the cerebrovascular reactivity mechanisms and provide valuable information about variations with age and different disease states.

Editor: Yoko Hoshi, Tokyo Metropolitan Institute of Medical Science, Japan

Funding: This work is supported by NIH grants 1R01NS066506, 2R01NS047607, R01DK092241. However, NIH had no role in study design, data collection and analysis, decision to publish, or preparation of the manuscript.

Competing Interests: The authors have declared that no competing interests exist.

* E-mail· hesamj@stanford.edu

Introduction

Blood oxygenation level dependent (BOLD) is a complex signal arising from a combination of changes in cerebral blood volume (CBV), cerebral blood flow (CBF), and oxygen extraction fraction (OEF), leading to a change in the concentration of deoxyhemoglobin. Low frequency ($f<0.1$ Hz) spontaneous fluctuations in the BOLD signal have been observed in resting-state time series measurements [1]. These fluctuations appear to be correlated in functionally connected brain regions and form the basis of resting-state fMRI studies [2–4]. It has been shown that these fluctuations correlate with infraslow local field potential fluctuations at the recording sites with a delay comparable to the hemodynamic response [5]. Although the precise physiological origin of these signal fluctuations is not yet clear, they likely arise from oscillations in metabolic-linked brain physiology, arterial vasomotion, and hemodynamics [1,6,7], originating from myogenic and neurogenic sources [8]. They may also be sensitive to disease states. For example, previous research suggests that the amplitude of BOLD signal fluctuation changes in ischemic lesions [6,9,10]. In another study, Makedonov et al. recently showed that the BOLD signal in

white matter can be used as a biomarker for aging and small vessel disease [11].

We view the spontaneous BOLD signal fluctuations as the response of the brain to the internal challenges to the cerebrovascular system, including heartbeat, inhalation, and baseline neuronal activity. We hypothesize that the response of the brain to these tiny challenges, as expressed by the normalized amplitude of the BOLD fluctuations, may provide information about cerebral perfusion, blood volume, oxygenation, and cerebrovascular autoregulatory mechanisms, in addition to neuronal activity. Consequently, these signals may yield insight into factors modulating the cerebrovasculature, such as aging and disease. To test this hypothesis, we compared the magnitude of spontaneous BOLD fluctuations in two groups who might be expected to have large differences in vasomotor reactivity [12–15]: young healthy adults and hypertensive elderly subjects with chronic kidney disease (CKD).

Methods

Ethics Statement

This prospective study was approved by the Stanford University's internal review board and was Health Insurance Portability and Accountability Act (HIPAA) compliant. Written informed consent was obtained prior to all human studies. The Stanford University's internal review board approved the consent procedure.

Patient Population

Ten subjects (8 men and 2 women, age mean±std = 72±7 years; age [min max] = [56 83]) with hypertension and chronic kidney disease (CKD), defined as baseline estimated glomerular filtration rate (eGFR) <65 ml/min/1.73 m² were recruited. Patients with diabetes or prior history of stroke were excluded from the study. Ten healthy sex-matched young volunteers (8 men and 2 women, age mean±std = 28±4 years; age [min max] = [24 35]) with no history of renal disease or hypertension were recruited in the study as a control group. Demographic information can be found in Table 1.

MR Protocol

Subjects were scanned at 3T (MR750, GE Healthcare, Waukesha, WI) using an 8-channel head coil. Resting-state BOLD signals were measured using a 2D gradient echo planar imaging (GRE-EPI) sequence (FOV = 22 cm, matrix = 64×64, slice thickness/slice spacing = 3.5/0 mm, number of slices = 35 covering the whole brain, TR/TE = 2 s/25 ms, flip angle = 75°, Number of time points = 180, imaging time: 6 min). A 3D T1-weighted image was also acquired for anatomic reference using an IR-SPGR sequence covering the entire brain (TR/TE/TI = 8.18/3.2/900 ms, matrix = 256×256, in-plane resolution = 0.94×0.94 mm, slice thickness = 1 mm, 176 sagittal slices). Cardiac and respiratory functions were monitored using the scanner's built-in photo-plethysmograph and respiratory belt.

Post-processing

After reconstruction, EPI images were corrected for movement using least-squares minimization. The 3D T1-weighted image was co-registered to the EPI images and normalized to the Montreal Neurological Institute (MNI) template. Using the obtained transfer matrix, EPI images were also registered to the standard MNI space. These processing steps were carried out using the FSL software package (http://www.fmrib.ox.ac.uk/fsl). To further reduce any movement-related signal fluctuations, 6 rigid-body movement parameter time-courses (estimated in the motion correction step) were removed from the data by linear regression. Baseline scanner drifts were estimated and removed from the EPI images by first-order polynomial detrending. The coefficient of variation (CV) of signal fluctuation, defined as the temporal standard deviation of the EPI signal amplitudes normalized by the mean signal intensity, for each voxel was then calculated. To calculate the mean CV in GM and WM, we performed 3 different analyses to evaluate the sensitivity of the results to the segmentation process:

a) Partial Volume Estimation (PVE) Method: GM and WM partial volume maps were estimated from the T1-weighted structural images in each voxel. Each voxel was assigned a value between 0 and 1 that represents the proportion of GM or WM present in that given voxel [16] using the automated segmentation tool of FSL (FAST). Mean CV in GM and WM were calculated using Eq. 1:

$$Mean\ CV(tissue) = \frac{\sum_n [PVE_{tissue}(n).CV(n)]}{\sum_n PVE_{tissue}(n)} \qquad (Eq.1)$$

where PVE is the partial volume estimated for a particular tissue type and n is the number of voxels in the brain.

b) Strict Threshold Method: GM and WM masks were generated from the GM and WM PVE maps including only voxels with a partial volume threshold of >0.8. Only voxels that had PVE levels above this threshold were included in the analysis.

c) Standard Template Method: After placing the images into MNI atlas space using FSL, ICBM152 nonlinear GM and WM

Table 1. Demographic information of the CKD and Control cohorts along with quantitative CV values calculated using different segmentation analysis approaches.

	Control	CKD
Gender	8 M/2 F	8 M/2 F
Age, years (Range)	28±4 (24–35)	72±7 (56–83)
eGFR (ml/min)	-	49.4±11.7
Blood pressure (systolic), mmHg	-	142±15
Blood pressure (diastolic), mmHg	-	74±10
CV×10⁻³ (Method a, PVE), GM	4.7±0.6	7.7±1.7
CV×10⁻³ (Method a, PVE), WM	3.2±0.4	4.5±0.8
CV×10⁻³ (Method b, Strict Threshold), GM	4.6±0.6	7.9±1.8
CV×10⁻³ (Method b, Strict Threshold), WM	3.0±0.4	4.2±0.7
CV ×10⁻³ (Method c, Standard Template), GM	4.3±0.5	5.5±1.3
CV×10⁻³ (Method c, Standard Template), WM	2.9±0.3	3.6±0.8
CV×10⁻³ (Method b with RETROICOR), GM	4.4±0.7	7.8±1.8
CV×10⁻³ (Method b with RETROICOR), WM	2.8±0.4	4.1±0.7

Methods a, b, and c refer to partial volume estimation (PVE), strict threshold and standard template methods, respectively. All values reported as mean±SD unless otherwise noted. Estimated glomerular filtration rate (eGFR) and systolic/diastolic blood pressures were measured within 90 days from the date of imaging.

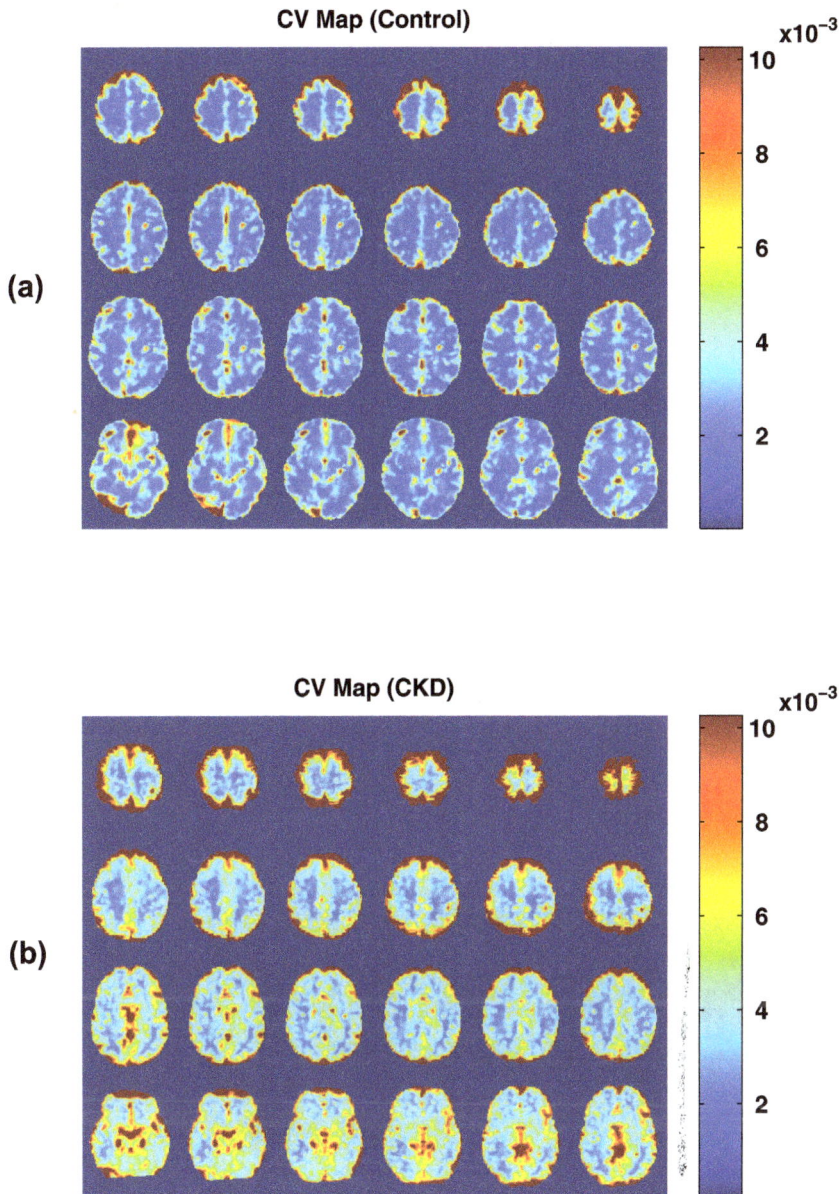

Figure 1. Coefficient of variation (CV) maps calculated for a representative (a) CKD patient and (b) young healthy control. No temporal filtration was applied.

standard templates (McConnell Brain Imaging Centre, Montreal Neurological Institute, McGill University) were used for the GM and WM regions-of-interest.

Given that resting-state fMRI data is often post-processed using low-pass filtering to minimize the effects of cardiac and respiratory variation, we examined the effect of different types of filtering. First, we studied the signal without any filtering, assuming there may be important and potentially useful information in the higher frequency bands. We also examined the results using three different band-pass filters (0.01–0.014 Hz, 0.014–0.025 Hz and 0.025–0.1 Hz) to estimate the contribution of these frequency bands to the BOLD signal fluctuations. These bands were chosen based on manual inspection of the frequency spectrum of the BOLD time series to capture the fast initial decay of the signal in the frequency domain.

Pulsatility of blood flow in the brain and respiration-induced magnetic field changes or motion can cause appreciable modulation of the BOLD signal [17]. To evaluate the contribution of these effects on the CV of signal fluctuations, we performed a separate analysis after removing the physiological motion effects from reconstructed images utilizing the RETROICOR method [17], based on the recorded cardiac and respiratory time-courses. RETROICOR fits a low-order Fourier model to the BOLD time series based on the time of each image acquisition relative to the phase of the cardiac and respiratory cycles for each slice. These effects are subsequently removed from of the BOLD time series using regression. Since RETROICOR is based on the assumption of quasi-periodic variation of physiological noise, cardiac and respiratory time-courses were also inspected for any sign of arrhythmia.

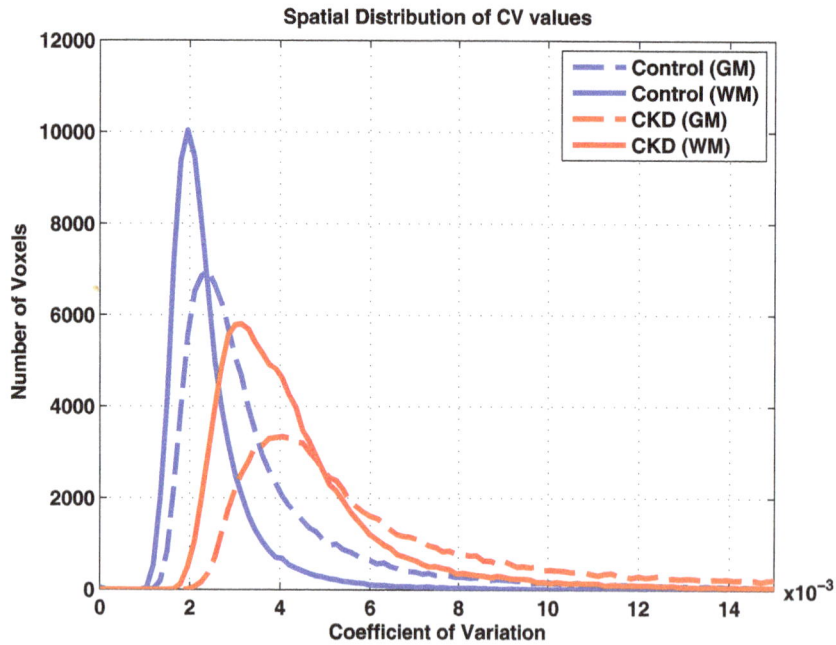

Figure 2. CV histograms in GM (dotted lines) and WM (solid lines) for a representative CKD patient (red) and young healthy control (blue), corresponding to the CV maps shown in Figure 1. GM and WM ROIs were defined using the strict threshold approach.

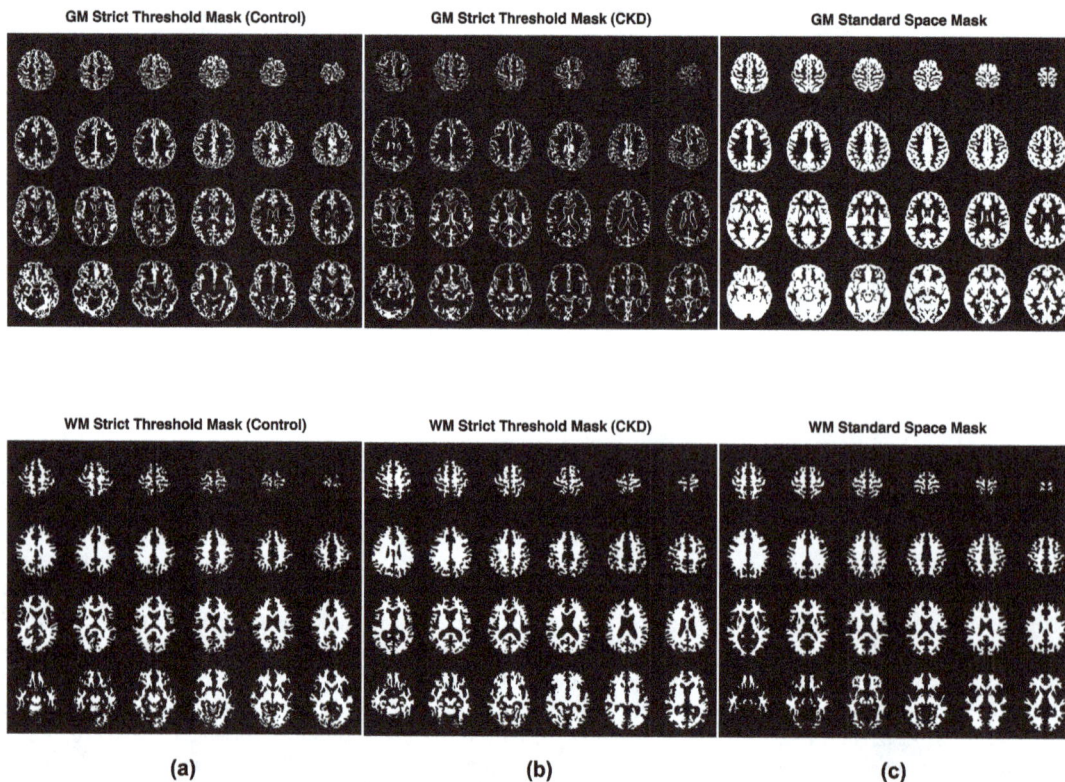

Figure 3. GM (top rows) and WM (bottom rows) masks used for calculating mean CV in these two tissue types: The GM and WM threshold masks derived from partial volume estimation (PVE) maps (PVE threshold>0.8) for representative (a) control and (b) CKD subjects. ICBM152 standard GM and WM template masks are shown in column (c), and were, of course, independent of the cohort group.

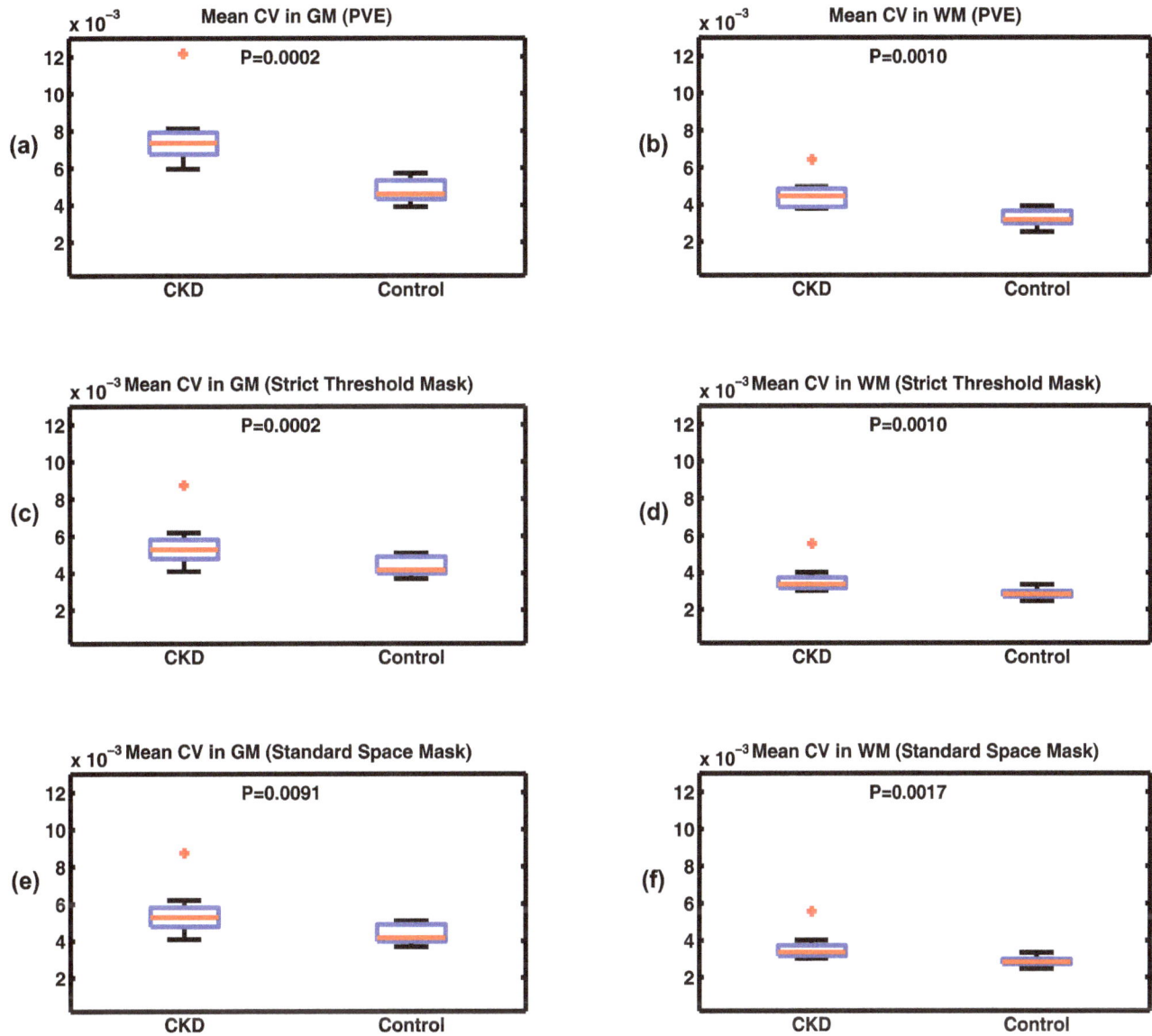

Figure 4. Mean CV of BOLD signal fluctuations in GM (left columns) and WM (right columns) for young healthy control and elderly CKD populations using different approaches: (a–b) PVE, (c–d) strict threshold masks, and (e–f) ICBM152 standard template masks. Mean CV is significantly higher in the CKD group in both tissue types using all approaches. The difference is more significant using PVE and the strict threshold masking approaches compared to the standard template approach.

Although the effect of motion upon the CV is corrected for by the initial step of motion correction and also by regressing the motion parameters, we also compared the estimated average displacement from the 6 rigid-body movement parameters for each subject before correction.

Statistical Analysis

To evaluate the statistical significance of the analyses we performed a Wilcoxon test, a nonparametric test for equality of population medians of two independent cohorts. The null hypothesis was that CV values in control and CKD cohorts are independent random samples with equal median. The alternative hypothesis was that the medians of these two random variables were not equal. A threshold of $p<0.05$ was considered significant.

Results

Figures 1 and 2 show CV maps and the histogram of the CV values obtained in representative control and CKD subjects. Contrast between GM and WM can be seen in both cohorts; however, the average CV in both GM and WM is higher in CKD subjects compared to that of the control population. For each subject, mean CV values in GM and WM were calculated using the 3 different methods for GM/WM segmentation. Figure 3 shows the GM and WM threshold masks for the subjects shown in Figure 1 using the different approaches described earlier.

Mean CV in GM and WM masks, calculated using these 3 methods for all subjects, is presented as Figure 4. There is significantly higher mean CV of fluctuations in the elderly CKD cohort in both GM and WM for all segmentation approaches. The results of PVE and strict threshold masking approaches (methods a

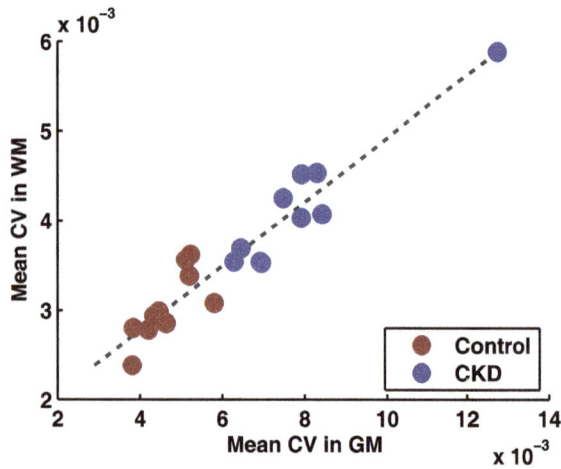

Figure 5. Scatterplot of mean CV in GM and WM for CKD (red) and Control (blue) populations. The dotted line represents a linear fit of the data ($y = 0.36 \times +0.0014$, $R^2 = 0.87$).

and b) are similar and are more significantly different compared to the standard template approach (method c). For all the subsequent analyses we quote values based on the strict threshold segmentation approach (method b). Table 1 summarizes the quantitative CV values in the two cohorts using the different segmentation methods.

The relationship between individual CV values in GM and WM for all subjects is presented in Figure 5. There is a strong linear relationship between CV values in GM and WM in both

populations, with the elderly CKD patients lying largely above the young normal subjects. The slope of a linear fit to the data was 0.36 ($y = 0.36 \times +0.0014$, $R^2 = 0.87$).

The results of the effects of the three different band-pass filters (0.01–0.014 Hz, 0.014–0.025 Hz and 0.025–0.1 Hz) on the mean CV in GM and WM are shown in Figure 6. It can be seen that the changes in the BOLD signal fluctuations mainly arise from very low frequency components (<0.025 Hz). Lower frequency components showed higher contribution to the overall signal fluctuation.

In a separate analysis of the data, we calculated the CV's in GM and WM after applying the RETROICOR technique to remove the effects of cardiac and respiratory motion (Figure 7). After applying RETROICOR, the difference in CVs in GM and WM became slightly larger between the two cohorts, though the increase itself due to RETROICOR was not significant. The quantitative CV values for this analysis are also summarized in Table 1. Differences in mean head displacement before correction in the two cohorts is shown as Figure 8. Although the movement in the elderly CKD patients before correction is higher (mean difference = 0.07 mm), it is not statistically different from the normal young subjects (P = 0.07). We expect this difference to be even less significant after the two-step motion correction used in this study. To evaluate the sensitivity of our measurements to non-rigid movements in the brain caused by heartbeat and respiration, we also calculated mean CV in the WM area in voxels immediately adjacent to the lateral ventricles. For this analysis, the region of interest (ROI) was manually drawn on the T1 weighted images in the MNI space (Figure 9a). Mean CV values calculated within the ROI in control and CKD cohorts are presented in Figure 9b. Average CV values obtained within the

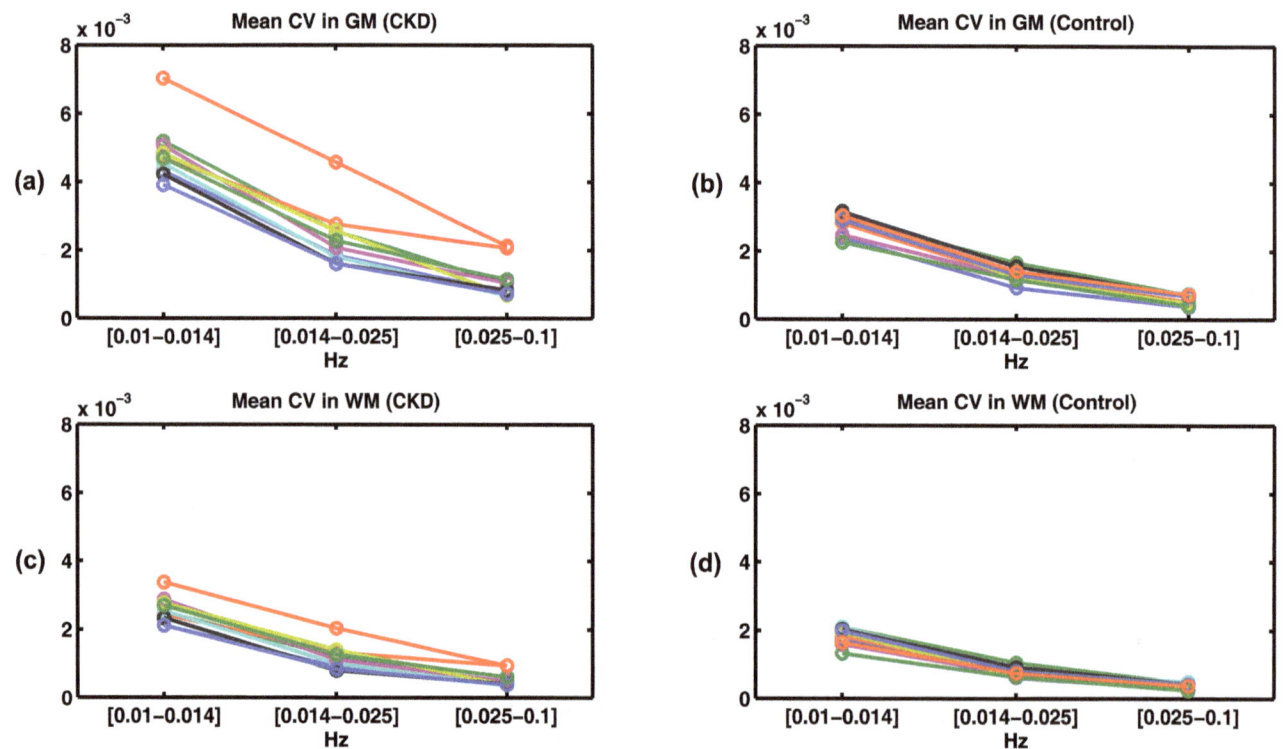

Figure 6. Mean CV of signal fluctuation in GM (a,b) and WM (c,d) in different frequency intervals ([0.01–0.014] Hz, [0.014–0.025] Hz and [0.025–0.1] Hz) for CKD (a,c) and control (b,d) cohorts. Lower frequency components have a larger contribution to the BOLD signal fluctuations.

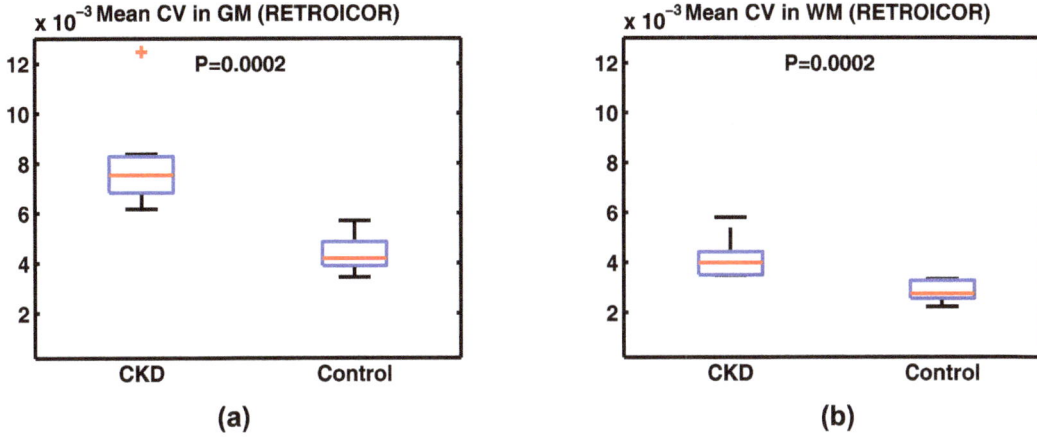

Figure 7. Mean CV of signal fluctuations in (a) GM and (b) WM for young healthy control and CKD populations after applying RETROICOR. Results are not significantly different from those achieved without RETROICOR (Figure 3c–d).

ROI in control and CKD cohorts were 3.0×10^{-3} and 3.5×10^{-3}, respectively. These values were similar to those measured in WM using the standard template method (2.9×10^{-3} and 3.6×10^{-3}). The difference between the two cohorts, however, was less significant within this ROI ($P = 0.064$) compared to that of the whole WM ($P = 0.0017$). This indicates that the reported difference of the CVs between the two cohorts does not arise from non-rigid body movements in the brain.

Discussion

In this study we compared the mean CV values in GM and WM between young normal and elderly, hypertensive CKD patients. Our results indicate a statistically significant increase in BOLD signal fluctuations in the CKD cohort and also between GM and WM within each cohort. We also investigated the origin of the fluctuations employing different analysis schemes. Using different GM/WM masking approaches, we evaluated the sensitivity of the results to the particular segmentation method. Using the strict threshold mask, there were different numbers of GM and WM voxels for different subjects; however, since the number of voxels was large (>2000) for all subjects, we believe that the difference in the number of voxels did not affect our estimation of the mean CVs. The fact that the strict threshold and PVE masking approaches generated very similar results also supports this assumption. The linear registration algorithm for transferring the

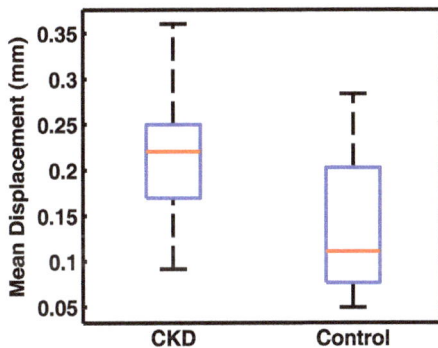

Figure 8. Mean head displacement (mm) before correction during the scan for CKD and control cohorts (p = 0.07).

data from the imaging space to the standard atlas was imperfect, particularly for the CKD patients, due to their larger CSF compartment. Therefore, the results of using the standard templates were slightly different from the PVE and strict threshold masking approaches. Another factor that can potentially affect the accuracy of the WM/GM segmentation in this study is the presence of white matter hyperintensities (WMHs), which are often associated with aging and can be segmented as GM using the segmentation tools [11]. In this study, the segmentation results were inspected manually and we observed no significant segmentation error. Due to large number of voxels in GM and WM, however, we do not expect minor segmentation errors to significantly affect the calculation of mean CVs. Particularly; the segmentation method C ("Standard Template Method") that used a standard template would not erroneously misclassify WMHs as gray matter. The fact that all methods used for calculating mean CVs in GM/WM demonstrated a significant difference between the two cohorts indicates that these results are somewhat independent of the precise segmentation strategy employed.

It is interesting that the WM to GM signal fluctuation lie on a line (Figure 5). The slope is close to the ratio of GM and WM cerebral blood volume (CBV) reported in the literature [18,19]. This may suggest that CBV is a major contributor to the fluctuations of the BOLD signal. However, it is interesting to note that most prior studies suggest that CBV decreases with age [19], suggesting that other hemodynamic factors such as changes in OEF or neuronal activity may also play a role in these findings. OEF is thought to increase with age [19], thus potentially offsetting the effects of CBV changes, if any. Grady et al. [20] demonstrated that there is an age-related decline in the ability to suspend non-task-related (i.e., resting state) brain activity and engage areas for carrying out memory tasks. This could be due to increased resting-state brain activation in the older population and can also be a contributing factor in higher BOLD signal fluctuations seen in the elderly CKD population. Since neuronal activity mainly arises from the GM, the presence of a significant difference of the CV values in WM as well as GM, suggests that the difference in the CV of the spontaneous BOLD signal fluctuation mainly originates from a difference in the vascular reactivity rather than neuronal activity. Differences in the baseline neuronal activity, however, might be the cause of a more significant difference in the CV values in GM compared to that of WM.

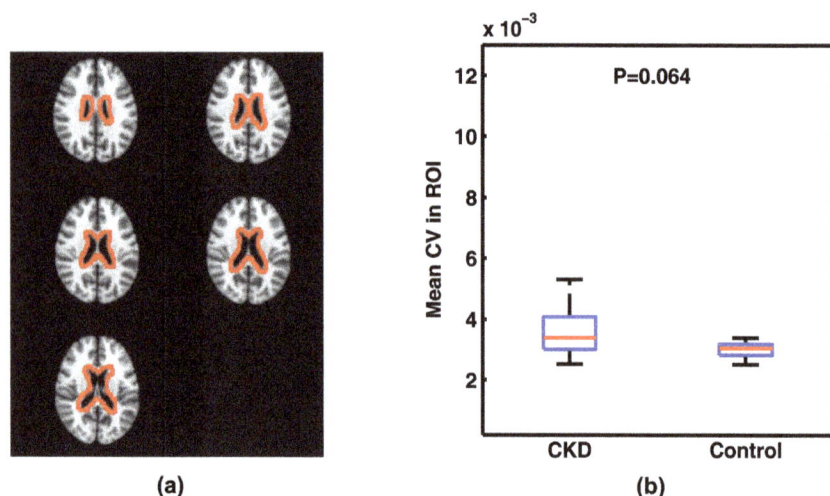

Figure 9. Mean CV measured in an area possibly susceptible to non-rigid body movements in the brain (interface between the lateral ventricles and brain parenchyma). (a): The ROI used for calculations. (b): Mean CV values calculated in the ROI.

To investigate the possibility of the difference of the CVs originating from physiological motion or respiration-induced magnetic field changes, we used RETROICOR to reduce the effects of these confounding components [17]. Using RETRO-ICOR resulted in more pronounced signal differences between the two cohorts. This change, however, was not large, suggesting that recording the respiratory and cardiac physiological signals may not be necessary in other similar applications and analyses. Although rigid body movements were used as a regressor in our analyses, motion correction algorithms cannot completely correct for non-rigid body movements of the brain due to heartbeat and respiration. But since these movements mainly appear at the CSF boundaries on the surface of the brain (note the high CV values on the surface in Figure 1), they are largely eliminated from the analysis for calculating CVs in GM and WM. In addition these voxels represent a very small fraction of voxels included in the analysis.

Our analysis indicated that most of the BOLD signal fluctuations originated from very low frequency components ($f < 0.025$ Hz). Using a reflected light imaging technique, it has been suggested that cerebral vasomotion demonstrates a 0.1 Hz oscillation [8]. The discrepancies can be explained by the difference in the point spread function of BOLD imaging as compared to that of the reflected light imaging as well as contributions from sources other than vasomotion, such as neuronal modulation. The long TR (2 s) used in this study does not allow for a true frequency analysis of the BOLD signal fluctuation power spectrum, due to the aliasing of the cardiac variations. Since the TR was considerably longer than the cardiac period (~0.9 s), one possibility is that the low-frequency fluctuations may in fact reflect the aliased response to cardiac fluctuations. Although, considering the frequency of the cardiac waveforms in our experiment (1.13+/−0.13 Hz) and the sampling frequency (0.5 Hz) lower frequency components ($f < 0.025$) probably do not result from an aliasing of the cardiac peak frequency or its first 2 harmonics. With a shorter TR (~400 ms), it would be possible to differentiate and compare the spontaneous neural activity, respiration, and cardiac response components between two populations, which are largely aliased into the low frequency band using longer TRs. Shorter TR scans would result in lower SNR images and limited number of slices resulting in partial brain coverage. Approaches to counter these problems include multi-band imaging [21] and the use of higher magnetic fields, such as 7 T [22]. Higher BOLD signal fluctuation in the elderly CKD population could be due to higher baseline concentrations of deoxyhemoglobin, difference in vascular compliance, increased instability of autoregulatory mechanisms, increased neuronal metabolic activity, and/or CSF contamination due to atrophy in these patients. Baseline oxygenation differences could be assessed using MR-based oxygenation methods [23] or PET [19]. Given that the differences between the cohorts are seen in both WM and GM, it is unlikely that differences in CSF partial volume are solely responsible.

A major limitation of this study is that we are not able to distinguish the possibly separate effects of aging, hypertension, and CKD on the signal fluctuations. The two cohorts were chosen based on the expectation that there would be a potentially large difference in arterial vasomotor function, based on prior work [12–15,24]. Further studies on healthy elderly populations, elderly hypertensive populations without CKD, and younger hypertensive patients will be required to assess the relative contributions of these various factors. However, these initial results suggest that spontaneous BOLD signal fluctuation amplitude may represent a unique source of contrast that is sensitive to cerebrovascular compensatory mechanisms.

Author Contributions

Conceived and designed the experiments: HJ WN TC MM MT GZ. Performed the experiments: HJ. Analyzed the data: HJ WN. Contributed reagents/materials/analysis tools: HJ. Wrote the paper: HJ WN TC MM MT GZ.

References

1. Kruger G, Glover GH (2001) Physiological noise in oxygenation-sensitive magnetic resonance imaging. Magn Reson Med 46: 631–637.

2. Biswal B, Yetkin FZ, Haughton VM, Hyde JS (1995) Functional connectivity in the motor cortex of resting human brain using echo-planar MRI. Magn Reson Med 34: 537–541.

3. Fox MD, Raichle ME (2007) Spontaneous fluctuations in brain activity observed with functional magnetic resonance imaging. Nat Rev Neurosci 8: 700–711.

4. Rogers BP, Morgan VL, Newton AT, Gore JC (2007) Assessing functional connectivity in the human brain by fMRI. Magn Reson Imaging 25: 1347–1357.

5. Pan WJ, Thompson GJ, Magnuson ME, Jaeger D, Keilholz S (2013) Infraslow LFP correlates to resting-state fMRI BOLD signals. Neuroimage 74: 288–297.

6. Wang HH, Menezes NM, Zhu MW, Ay H, Koroshetz WJ, et al. (2008) Physiological noise in MR images: an indicator of the tissue response to ischemia? J Magn Reson Imaging 27: 866–871.

7. Wise RG, Ide K, Poulin MJ, Tracey I (2004) Resting fluctuations in arterial carbon dioxide induce significant low frequency variations in BOLD signal. Neuroimage 21: 1652–1664.

8. Mayhew JE, Askew S, Zheng Y, Porrill J, Westby GW, et al. (1996) Cerebral vasomotion: a 0.1-Hz oscillation in reflected light imaging of neural activity. Neuroimage 4: 183–193.

9. Liu Y, D'Arceuil H, He J, Duggan M, Gonzalez G, et al. (2007) MRI of spontaneous fluctuations after acute cerebral ischemia in nonhuman primates. J Magn Reson Imaging 26: 1112–1116.

10. Yao QL, Zhang HY, Nie BB, Fang F, Jiao Y, et al. (2012) MRI assessment of amplitude of low-frequency fluctuation in rat brains with acute cerebral ischemic stroke. Neurosci Lett 509: 22–26.

11. Makedonov I, Black SE, Macintosh BJ (2013) BOLD fMRI in the white matter as a marker of aging and small vessel disease. PLoS One 8: e67652.

12. Chang KV, Wu CH, Wang TG, Hsiao MY, Yeh TS, et al. (2011) Pulsed wave Doppler ultrasonography for the assessment of peripheral vasomotor response in an elderly population. J Clin Ultrasound 39: 383–389.

13. Kozera GM, Dubaniewicz M, Zdrojewski T, Madej-Dmochowska A, Mielczarek M, et al. (2010) Cerebral vasomotor reactivity and extent of white matter lesions in middle-aged men with arterial hypertension: a pilot study. Am J Hypertens 23: 1198–1203.

14. Lux S, Mirzazade S, Kuzmanovic B, Plewan T, Eickhoff SB, et al. (2010) Differential activation of memory-relevant brain regions during a dialysis cycle. Kidney Int 78: 794–802.

15. Kimoto E, Shoji T, Shinohara K, Hatsuda S, Mori K, et al. (2006) Regional arterial stiffness in patients with type 2 diabetes and chronic kidney disease. J Am Soc Nephrol 17: 2245–2252.

16. Zhang Y, Brady M, Smith S (2001) Segmentation of brain MR images through a hidden Markov random field model and the expectation-maximization algorithm. IEEE Trans Med Imaging 20: 45–57.

17. Glover GH, Li TQ, Ress D (2000) Image-based method for retrospective correction of physiological motion effects in fMRI: RETROICOR. Magn Reson Med 44: 162–167.

18. Markus HS, Lythgoe DJ, Ostegaard L, O'Sullivan M, Williams SC (2000) Reduced cerebral blood flow in white matter in ischaemic leukoaraiosis demonstrated using quantitative exogenous contrast based perfusion MRI. J Neurol Neurosurg Psychiatry 69: 48–53.

19. Leenders KL, Perani D, Lammertsma AA, Heather JD, Buckingham P, et al. (1990) Cerebral blood flow, blood volume and oxygen utilization. Normal values and effect of age. Brain 113 (Pt 1): 27–47.

20. Grady CL, Springer MV, Hongwanishkul D, McIntosh AR, Winocur G (2006) Age-related changes in brain activity across the adult lifespan. J Cogn Neurosci 18: 227–241.

21. Moeller S, Yacoub E, Olman CA, Auerbach E, Strupp J, et al. (2010) Multiband multislice GE-EPI at 7 tesla, with 16-fold acceleration using partial parallel imaging with application to high spatial and temporal whole-brain fMRI. Magn Reson Med 63: 1144–1153.

22. Yacoub E, Shmuel A, Pfeuffer J, Van De Moortele PF, Adriany G, et al. (2001) Imaging brain function in humans at 7 Tesla. Magn Reson Med 45: 588–594.

23. Jain V, Langham MC, Floyd TF, Jain G, Magland JF, et al. (2011) Rapid magnetic resonance measurement of global cerebral metabolic rate of oxygen consumption in humans during rest and hypercapnia. J Cereb Blood Flow Metab 31: 1504–1512.

24. Fazekas G, Fazekas F, Schmidt R, Flooh E, Valetitsch H, et al. (1996) Pattern of cerebral blood flow and cognition in patients undergoing chronic haemodialysis treatment. Nucl Med Commun 17: 603–608.

2

Reduction of Circulating Endothelial Progenitor Cell Level Is Associated with Contrast-Induced Nephropathy in Patients Undergoing Percutaneous Coronary and Peripheral Interventions

Chia-Hung Chiang[1,2,5,6], Po-Hsun Huang[2,5,6]*, Chun-Chih Chiu[2,6], Chien-Yi Hsu[2,6], Hsin-Bang Leu[2,4,5,6], Chin-Chou Huang[2,3,6,7], Jaw-Wen Chen[2,3,6,7], Shing-Jong Lin[2,3,5,6]

1 Division of Cardiology, Department of Medicine, Taipei Veterans General Hospital, Hsinchu Branch, Hsinchu, Taiwan, 2 Division of Cardiology, Taipei Veterans General Hospital, Taipei, Taiwan, 3 Department of Medical Research and Education, Taipei Veterans General Hospital, Taipei, Taiwan, 4 Healthcare and Management Center, Taipei Veterans General Hospital, Taipei, Taiwan, 5 Institute of Clinical Medicine, National Yang-Ming University, Taipei, Taiwan, 6 Cardiovascular Research Center, National Yang-Ming University, Taipei, Taiwan, 7 Institute and Department of Pharmacology, National Yang-Ming University, Taipei, Taiwan

Abstract

Objectives: Reduced number and impaired function of circulating endothelial progenitor cells (EPCs) in patients with chronic kidney disease have been reported. However, there is little data about the association between circulating EPC levels and risk of contrast-induced nephropathy (CIN). The aim of this study was to investigate the relationship between circulating EPCs and CIN in patients after angiography.

Methods and Results: A total of 77 consecutive patients undergoing elective percutaneous coronary intervention (PCI) and percutaneous transluminal angioplasty (PTA) were enrolled. Flow cytometry with quantification of EPC markers (defined as $CD34^+$, $CD34^+KDR^+$, and $CD34^+KDR^+CD133^+$) in peripheral blood samples was used to assess EPC number before the procedure. CIN was defined as an absolute increase ≥ 0.5 mg/dl or a relative increase $\geq 25\%$ in the serum creatinine level at 48 hours after the procedure. Eighteen (24%) of the study subjects developed CIN. Circulating EPC levels were significantly lower in patients who developed CIN than in those without CIN ($CD34^+KDR^+$, 4.11 ± 2.59 vs. 9.25 ± 6.30 cells/10^5 events, P< 0.001). The incidence of CIN was significantly greater in patients in the lowest EPC tertile ($CD34^+KDR^+$; from lowest to highest, 52%, 15%, and 4%, P<0.001). Using univariate logistic regression, circulating EPC number ($CD34^+KDR^+$) was a significant negative predictor for development of CIN (odds ratio 0.69, 95% CI 0.54–0.87, P = 0.002). Over a two-year follow-up, patients with CIN had a higher incidence of major adverse cardiovascular events including myocardial infarction, stroke, revascularization of treated vessels, and death (66.7% vs. 25.4%, P = 0.004) than did patients without CIN.

Conclusions: Decreased EPC level is associated with a greater risk of CIN, which may explain part of the pathophysiology of CIN and the poor prognosis in CIN patients.

Editor: Zoran Ivanovic, French Blood Institute, France

Funding: This study was supported in part by research grants from the NSC 97-2314-B-075-039, NSC 98-2314-B-075-035, and UST-UCSD International Center of Excellence in Advanced Bio-engineering NSC-99-2911-I-009-101 from the National Science Council; VGH-V98B1-003 and VGH-V100E2-002 from Taipei Veterans General Hospital, and also a grant from the Ministry of Education "Aim for the Top University" Plan. The funders had no role in study design, data collection and analysis, decision to publish, or preparation of the manuscript.

Competing Interests: The authors have declared that no competing interests exist.

* E-mail: huangbs@vghtpe.gov.tw

Introduction

Contrast-induced nephropathy (CIN) remains a serious clinical problem in the use of iodinated contrast media [1,2]. Increasing use of contrast media in interventional procedures has led to a parallel increase in the incidence of CIN, despite the use of newer and less nephrotoxic contrast agents in high-risk patients in recent years. The reported incidence of CIN varies widely across the literature [1,3]. Its development has been associated with increased in-hospital and long-term morbidity and mortality, prolonged hospitalization, and long-term renal impairment [4]. Proposed pathophysiologic mechanisms through which contrast

administration may potentiate renal injury include oxidative stress, free radical damage, and endothelial dysfunction [5,6]. However, the actual pathogenesis of CIN and the pathophysiologic mechanisms underlying the evolution from CIN to atherosclerosis and cardiovascular events remain to be determined.

Vascular endothelium is a highly active organ that affects vascular tone, smooth muscle cell proliferation, monocyte adhesion, and platelet aggregation [7,8]. Endothelial dysfunction plays a critical role in the clinical manifestations of established atherosclerotic lesions. Clinical studies have demonstrated that endothelial dysfunction is present in the early stages of renal insufficiency, and that it is associated with a greater decline in renal function [9,10]. Recent insight suggests that the injured endothelial monolayer is regenerated by circulating bone marrow derived-endothelial progenitor cells (EPCs), and levels of circulating EPCs reflect endothelial repair capacity. An altered status of circulating EPCs represents a marker of endothelial dysfunction and vascular health, and the level of circulating EPCs could be used as a surrogate index of cumulative cardiovascular risk [11,12]. A reduced number of circulating EPCs independently predicts atherosclerotic disease progression and future cardiovascular events [13]. Furthermore, previous reports have indicated reduced number and impaired function of EPCs in chronic renal insufficiency [9]. However, there is currently little data about the association between circulating EPC levels and risk of CIN. To clarify this issue, we tested the hypothesis that decreased circulating EPC levels may be associated with increased risk of CIN and subsequent major cardiovascular events in patients undergoing cardiovascular interventional procedures.

Methods

Study Participants

We initially screened a total of 311 consecutive patients who were admitted to the ward at the Division of Cardiology, Taipei-Veterans General Hospital between October 2009 and January 2010. Patients, who were older than 18 years of age, with normal to subnormal GFR, and scheduled for elective cardiovascular procedures including percutaneous coronary intervention (PCI) and percutaneous transluminal angioplasty (PTA), were eligible for this study. Exclusion criteria were as follows: hemodynamically significant valvular disorders, uncontrolled hypertension, baseline serum creatinine levels of more than 7 mg/dL, preexisting dialysis, autoimmune disease, chronic or acute infectious disease, emergency catheterization, recent exposure to radiographic contrast within 10 days, medication with non-steroidal anti-inflammatory drugs or metformin up to 7 days before entering the study, anemia (hemoglobin level <12 g/dl), overt congestive heart failure, recent acute kidney injury, having another planned contrast-enhanced procedure within the following 72 hours, and allergy to radiographic contrast. On the basis of these screening criteria, we enrolled 77 patients in the current study (48 patients receiving PCI, 29 patients receiving PTA). Medical history, including information about conventional cardiovascular risk factors (smoking, hypertension, diabetes mellitus, hyperlipidemia, peripheral artery disease, coronary artery disease, and chronic kidney disease), previous cardiovascular events (myocardial infarction and cerebrovascular disease), and current drug treatment was obtained during a personal interview and from medical files. This study was approved by the Taipei Veterans General Hospital research ethics committee. All patients gave written informed consent and research was conducted according to the principles expressed in the *Declaration of Helsinki*.

Study Treatment and Cardiovascular Procedures

All patients received a periprocedural intravenous infusion (volume expansion) of 1 ml/kg/h with 0.45% saline for 24 hours (12 hours before and 12 hours after exposure to contrast medium). On the day before the procedure, the estimated glomerular filtration rate (eGFR) was assessed using the modified formula of Levey *et al* [14]. Chronic kidney disease was defined as an eGFR <60 ml/min/1.73 m^2, based on the recommendations of the National Kidney Foundation [15]. CIN was defined as an absolute increase $\geqq$0.5 mg/dl or a relative increase $\geqq$25% in the serum creatinine level within 48 hours after the procedure.

The performance of angiography, PCI and PTA was left to the discretion of the cardiologists responsible for the patient and the interventional cardiologist on the basis of current guidelines. Cardiologists performing cardiovascular procedures were blinded to EPC levels of study subjects. A nonionic iso-osmolar contrast agent (Iodixanol, Visipaque) was used in all patients. During hospitalization, medications were changed as required by the clinical situation. All study subjects also underwent a complete echocardiographic study, including tissue Doppler imaging, upon enrollment in this study.

Laboratory Investigations

Venous blood was drawn in the morning after overnight fasting. Plasma liver function tests and other biochemical blood measurements, including assessments of fasting blood glucose, uric acid, creatinine, total cholesterol, high-density lipoprotein cholesterol (HDL-C), and triglyceride levels were performed by standard laboratory procedures. The high-sensitivity C-reactive protein (hsCRP) levels in plasma were assessed using latex-enhanced immunonephelometric assay (Dade Behring, Marburg, Germany). Serum levels of matrix metalloproteinase-2 (MMP-2) and matrix metalloproteinase-9 (MMP-9) were determined using commercially available enzyme-linked immunoassays. Study subjects were also tested for Cystatin C and nitric oxide (NO) levels. Total NO assay was performed by spectrophotometry at 540 nm using an NO assay kit according to the manufacturer's instructions. The assay was based on nitrate and nitrite determinations.

Assay of Circulating EPCs

Assessment of the circulating EPCs by flow cytometry was performed by researchers masked to the clinical data [16]. A volume of 1000 μL of peripheral blood was incubated for 30 min in the dark with monoclonal antibodies against human kinase insert domain receptor (KDR) (R&D, Minneapolis, MN, USA), followed by allophycocyanin (APC)-conjugated secondary antibody, with the fluorescein isothiocyanate (FITC)-labeled monoclonal antibodies against human CD45 (Becton Dickinson, Franklin Lakes, NJ, USA), with the phycoerythrin (PE)-conjugated monoclonal antibody against human CD133 (Miltenyi Biotec, Germany), and with FITC-conjugated monoclonal antibodies against human CD34 (Becton Dickinson Pharmingen, USA). After incubation, the cells were lysed, washed with phosphate-buffered saline (PBS), and fixed in 2% paraformaldehyde before analysis. Each analysis included 100,000 events. The numbers of circulating EPCs were gated with monocytes and defined as CD34$^+$, CD34$^+$KDR$^+$, and CD34$^+$KDR$^+$CD133$^+$ (**Figure 1**). To assess the reproducibility of EPC measurements, circulating EPCs were measured from 2 separate blood samples in 10 subjects, and there was a strong correlation between the 2 measurements (r = 0.90, P<0.001).

Assessment of Major Cardiovascular Events

All subjects included in this study were followed up for a maximum of 2 years or until death. The primary endpoint of the current study was the development of major adverse cardiovascular events (MACE), including the composite of all-cause death, cardiovascular death, nonfatal myocardial infarction, stroke, and revascularization of treated vessels. Cardiovascular death was defined as death from cardiac causes, cardiac arrest, myocardial infarction, and stroke. Stroke was diagnosed based on the presence of a neurologic deficit confirmed by computed tomography or magnetic resonance imaging. No study subjects dropped out of the study, and all occurrences of adverse events were recorded.

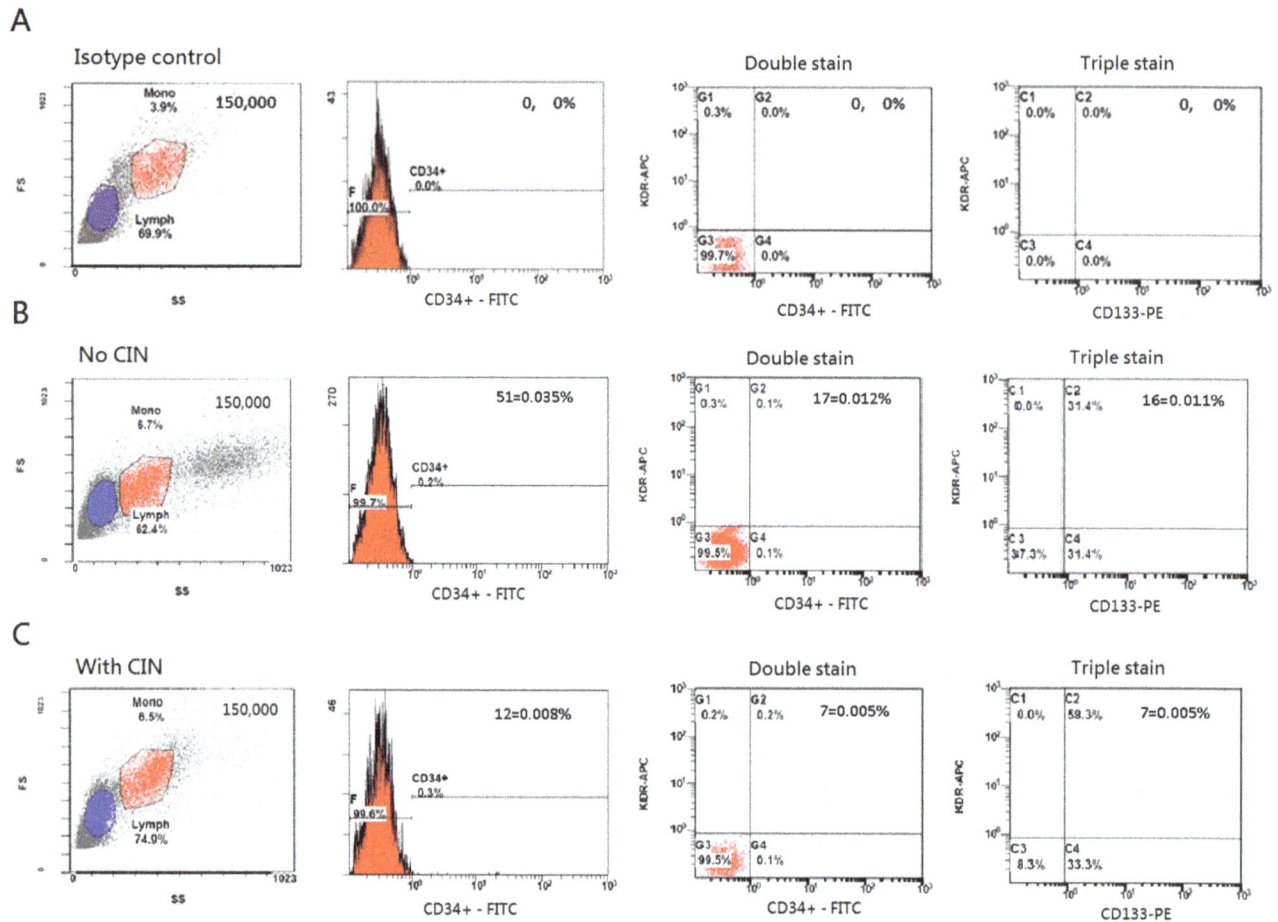

Figure 1. Representative flow cytometry analysis for quantifying the number of circulating endothelial progenitor cells in study subjects: (A) isotype control, (B) patients without CIN (C) patients with CIN. The numbers of circulating EPCs were gated with monocytes and defined as CD34+CD45low, CD34+KDR+CD45low, and CD34+KDR+CD133+CD45low. CIN, contrast-induced nephropathy.

Outcome data were collected by serial contact with the patients or their families until March 31, 2012.

Statistical Analysis

Data were expressed as the mean ± standard deviation (SD) or median with interquartile range for numeric variables and as the number (percent) for categorical variables. Comparisons of continuous variables between 2 or more groups were performed by Student's t test and ANOVA, respectively; post-hoc comparisons were performed by Tukey's honest significant difference test. Subgroup comparisons of categorical variables were assessed by the chi-squared test or Fisher's exact test. To examine the effects of various factors on development of CIN, the following factors were considered as variables for univariate and multivariate logistic regression analyses: EPC number (CD34+KDR+), age, gender, hypertension, diabetes, chronic kidney disease, heart failure, and contrast volume. To assess the risk of developing MACE during the 2 year follow-up period, the Kaplan-Meier method was employed for patients stratified by EPC levels. Data were analyzed using SPSS software (version 17, SPSS, Chicago, Illinois, USA). A P value of <0.05 was considered to indicate statistical significance.

Results

Clinical and Laboratory Data

A total of 77 subjects (mean age: 69±15 years; male subjects, 63 [82%]) were enrolled in the study. Of the 77 study subjects, 48 received PCI and 29 received PTA. Eighteen patients developed CIN after the procedures, giving an overall CIN incidence of 24% in the current study, with three of the CIN patients requiring dialysis. All patients were divided into two groups; those who developed CIN and those who did not. **Table 1** summarizes the demographic and clinical characteristics of study subjects. Baseline demographics and characteristics were comparable between these two groups. Baseline metabolic profiles and medication use are presented in **Table 2**. There was no significant difference between the two groups in regard to the baseline creatinine levels, metabolic profiles, and medication use. No significant differences were noted in angiographic and procedural characteristics of study subjects undergoing PCI and PTA between the two groups, except that CIN patients had higher post-procedural creatinine levels than those without CIN (CIN vs. non-CIN, 1.9±1.4 vs. 1.1±0.3, P = 0.019; **Table 3**).

Circulating EPC Levels and Other Biomarkers

As shown in **Table 4** and **Figure 2**, there were decreased circulating CD34+ cells in CIN patients compared to non-CIN

Table 1. Baseline characteristics of study subjects with and without contrast-induced nephropathy (CIN).

	No CIN	With CIN	P value
	n = 59	n = 18	
Age (years)	67.3±15.3	72.6±13.8	0.190
Men, n (%)	48 (81.4%)	15 (83.3%)	0.849
Hypertension, n (%)	43 (72.9%)	16 (88.9%)	0.213
Diabetes mellitus, n (%)	31 (52.5%)	11 (61.1%)	0.596
Coronary artery disease, n (%)	52 (88%)	17 (94%)	0.672
Peripheral artery disease, n (%)	4 (14.8%)	14 (31.1%)	0.132
Chronic kidney disease, n (%)	36 (61.0%)	10 (55.6%)	0.785
Hyperlipidemia, n (%)	36 (61.0%)	10 (55.6%)	0.785
Current smoker, n (%)	28 (47.5%)	9 (50.0%)	0.851
Previous myocardial infarction, n (%)	22 (37.3)	9 (50.0%)	0.414
Previous cerebrovascular disease, n (%)	11 (18.6%)	3 (16.7%)	0.849
Heart failure, n (%)	15 (25.4%)	5 (27.8%)	0.842
Atrial fibrillation, n (%)	14 (23.7%)	3 (16.7%)	0.748

Values are mean ± standard deviation (SD) or number (%).
CAD, coronary artery disease; PCI: percutaneous coronary intervention.

Table 2. Baseline metabolic profiles and medications of subjects with/without contrast-induced nephropathy (CIN).

	No CIN	With CIN	P value
	n = 59	n = 18	
Cholesterol (mg/dL)	172±46	160±23	0.173
LDL-C (mg/dL)	109±39	96±26	0.252
HDL-C (mg/dL)	45±21	37±11	0.171
Triglyceride (mg/dL)	117±70	111±70	0.754
Creatinine (mg/dL)	1.1±0.4	1.4±1.2	0.365
eGFR, ml/min/1.73 m^2	68±27	65±32	0.692
ALT (U/L)	33±35	30±33	0.731
Fasting glucose (mg/dL)	143±67	152±62	0.632
Body mass index (kg/m^2)	26.0±4.2	25.0±4.1	0.360
Medication, n (%)			
Aspirin	52 (88.1%)	14 (77.8%)	0.272
Clopidogrel	42 (71.2%)	10 (55.6%)	0.256
Cilostazol	21 (35.6%)	7 (38.9%)	0.787
ACEI	9 (15.3%)	4 (22.2%)	0.488
ARB	23 (39.0%)	5 (27.8%)	0.576
CCB	25 (42.3%)	8 (44.4%)	0.876
Beta blocker	19 (32.2%)	8 (44.4%)	0.402
Diuretics	15 (25.4%)	4 (22.2%)	0.783
Insulin	5 (8.5%)	3 (16.7%)	0.381
Statins	31(52.5%)	6 (33.3%)	0.185
Nitrates	31 (52.5%)	7 (38.9%)	0.421

Values are presented as mean ± standard deviation (SD) or number (%).
LDL-C: low-density lipoprotein cholesterol; HDL-C: high-density lipoprotein cholesterol; ALT: alanine aminotransferase; γGT: gamma-glutamyl-transferase; ACEI: angiotensin-converting enzyme inhibitor; ARB: angiotensin receptor blocker; CCB: calcium channel blocker.

Table 3. Angiographic and procedural characteristics of study subjects undergoing coronary artery intervention (PCI) and percutaneous transluminal angioplasty (PTA).

	No CIN	With CIN	P value
	n = 59	n = 18	
Undergoing PCI, n (%)	36 (61.0)	12(66.7)	0.784
Undergoing PTA, n (%)	23 (39.0)	6 (20.7)	0.784
Pre-procedural creatinine (mg/dL)	1.1±0.4	1.4±1.2	0.365
*Post-procedural creatinine (mg/dL)	1.1±0.3	1.9±1.4	0.019
SYNTAX score in CAD patients	16.6±11.5	18.0±9.9	0.648
CAD with left main disease, n (%)	8 (13.6)	5 (27.8)	0.169
Treated coronary artery, n (%)			
Left anterior descending	24 (40.7)	5 (27.8)	0.410
Left circumflex	8 (13.6)	3 (16.7)	0.712
Right coronary	14 (23.7)	5 (27.8)	0.760
Complexity of CAD, n (%)			
Multivessel disease	22 (37.3)	9 (50.0)	0.414
Bifurcation lesion	11 (18.6)	5 (27.8)	0.508
Chronic total occlusion	5 (8.4)	2 (11.1)	0.663
Number of treated segments per CAD patient	1.6±1.5	1.5±1.7	0.824
Number of stent deployments per CAD patient	1.3±1.6	1.4±2.2	0.796
Deployment of coronary BMS, n (%)	14 (23.7)	3 (16.7)	0.748
Deployment of coronary DES, n (%)	24 (40.7)	6 (33.3)	0.783
ABI in PAD patients	0.55±0.31	0.61±0.21	0.571
Treated peripheral arteries, n (%)			
Common iliac artery	2 (3.4)	1 (5.6)	0.556
Superficial femoral artery	17 (28.8)	4 (22.2)	0.765
Below -knee arteries	16 (27.1)	4 (22.2)	0.768
Contrast volume (mL)	210±136	242±136	0.190

Values are mean ± standard deviation (SD) or number (%).
CIN, contrast-induced nephropathy; ABI, ankle-brachial index; CAD, coronary artery disease; BMS, bare-metal stent; DES, drug-eluting stent.
*Post-procedural creatinine: 48 hours after the procedures.

patients (CIN vs. non-CIN, CD34$^+$: 0.011±0.007 vs. 0.035±0.033%, P = 0.004). Additionally, the EPC markers defined as CD34$^+$KDR$^+$ and CD34$^+$KDR$^+$CD133$^+$ were significantly decreased in CIN patients compared to non-CIN patients (CIN vs. non-CIN, CD34$^+$KDR$^+$: 0.003±0.001 vs. 0.012±0.010%, P<0.001; CD34$^+$KDR$^+$CD133$^+$: 0.003±0.002 vs. 0.010±0.010%, P<0.001). Furthermore, CIN patients had significantly enhanced Cystatin C levels (CIN vs. non-CIN, 1.4±0.8 vs. 0.9±0.3 mg/dl, P = 0.046) and reduced NO levels (CIN vs. non-CIN, 33±24 vs. 51±29 μmol/l, P = 0.031). However, no significant difference was noted in plasma levels of hsCRP between the two groups.

Independent Correlates of Development of CIN

In order to identify the independent predictors for development of CIN, univariate and multivariate logistic regression analyses were performed. As shown in **Table 5**, in univariate analysis, EPC number (CD34$^+$KDR$^+$, cells/10^5 events) was noted to be a significant negative predictor for development of CIN (crude odds ratio [95% CI]: 0.49 [0.34–0.72], P<0.001). In multivariate analysis, regardless of adjusting for other confounders like age, gender (male), hypertension, diabetes, chronic kidney disease,

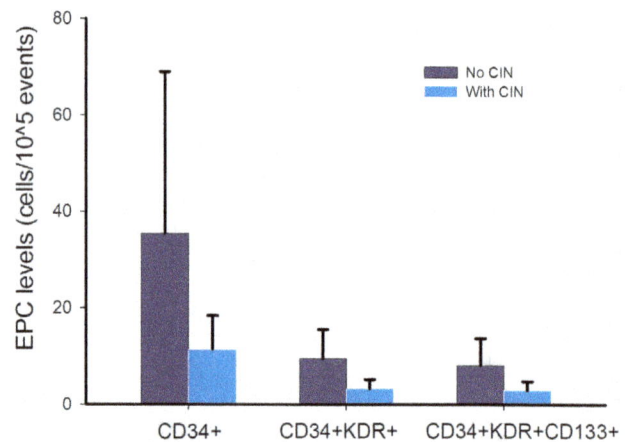

Figure 2. EPC levels (cells/10^5 events) in patients with and without development of contrast-induced nephropathy (CIN) (values presented as means ± standard deviation).

Table 4. Circulating endothelial progenitor cell (EPC) levels and other markers.

	No CIN	With CIN	P value
	n = 59	n = 18	
EPC levels (%)			
CD34+	0.035±0.033	0.011±0.007	0.004
CD34+KDR+	0.012±0.010	0.003±0.001	0.001
CD34+KDR+CD133+	0.010±0.010	0.003±0.002	<0.001
EPC levels (cells/10^5 events)			
CD34+	35.5±33.6	11.4±7.0	0.004
CD34+KDR+	9.5±6.1	3.3±1.9	<0.001
CD34+KDR+CD133+	8.1±5.6	3.1±1.8	<0.001
hsCRP (mg/L)	0.4 (0.2–1.1)	0.9 (0.2–3.3)	0.191
Nitric oxide (μmol/L)	51±29	33±24	0.031
Cystatin C (mg/dL)	0.9±0.3	1.4±0.8	0.046
MMP-2 (ng/mL)	151±45	159±45	0.545
MMP-9 (ng/mL)	55±37	44±19	0.314

Values are mean ± SD or median (interquartile range).
CIN, contrast-induced nephropathy; hsCRP: high-sensitivity C-reactive protein; MMP: matrix metalloproteinase.

heart failure, or contrast volume, EPC number was still inversely associated with risk of CIN (P<0.001).

Incidence of Cardiovascular Events, All-cause Deaths, and CIN

Table 6 illustrates the incidence of clinical outcomes in patients with and without CIN. Among the patients who developed CIN, the MACE rate was 67% compared with only 25% in patients who did not develop CIN during the maximum 2 years of follow-up period. Seven deaths occurred, with three of them considered to be cardiovascular deaths (two fatal myocardial infarction, one stroke-related death). Furthermore, CIN patients had significantly higher incidence of stroke and fatal/nonfatal myocardial infarction than patients without CIN.

We further determined the relationship between circulating EPC level and incidence of CIN and future cardiovascular events after cardiovascular interventional procedures. All study subjects were divided into 3 groups according to circulating EPC levels (high-EPC level [first EPC tertile], CD34+KDR+ $\geqq 9$ cells/10^5

events; intermediate-EPC level [second EPC tertile], CD34+KDR+ = 5–8 cells/10^5 events; low-EPC level [third EPC tertile], CD34+KDR+ $\leqq 4$ cells/10^5 events), and the incidence of CIN by tertiles of EPC levels is illustrated in **Figure 3A**. Patients with low-EPC levels had higher incidence of CIN compared to those with high-EPC levels and intermediate-EPC levels. Furthermore, as shown in **Figure 3B and 3C**, patients with low-EPC levels had more MACE during the follow-up period than the other two groups (High-EPC vs. Intermediate-EPC vs. Low-EPC: 19.2% vs. 26.9% vs. 60.0%, P = 0.005). Cumulative MACE-free survival in patients with and without CIN is shown in **Figure 4**. CIN patients had significantly lower cumulative event-free survival of MACE, fatal and nonfatal myocardial infarction, and revascularization of treated vessels compared to patients without CIN during the 2 year follow-up period.

Discussion

This is the first study to show that decreased circulating EPC level is associated with a greater risk of CIN in patients undergoing

Table 5. Association between endothelial progenitor cell (EPC) levels and development of contrast-induced nephropathy (CIN).

EPCs (CD34+KDR+, cells/10^5 events)	OR (95% CI)	P value
Univariate analysis	0.49 (0.34–0.72)	<0.001
Multivariate analysis		
Adjusted for age	0.48 (0.33–0.72)	<0.001
Adjusted for gender (male)	0.47 (0.31–0.71)	<0.001
Adjusted for hypertension	0.47 (0.32–0.71)	<0.001
Adjusted for diabetes	0.48 (0.33–0.71)	<0.001
Adjusted for chronic kidney disease	0.41 (0.26–0.67)	<0.001
Adjusted for heart failure	0.49 (0.33–0.72)	<0.001
Adjusted for contrast volume (mL)	0.40 (0.24–0.66)	<0.001

OR: odds ratio; CI: confidence interval.

Table 6. The incidence of clinical outcomes in patients with/without contrast-induced nephropathy (CIN).

Clinical outcomes, n (%)	No CIN n = 59	With CIN n = 18	P value
Stroke	3 (5.1)	4 (22)	0.048
Myocardial infarction	3 (5.1)	4 (22)	0.048
Revascularization of treated vessel	11 (18.6)	8 (44.4)	0.057
Cardiovascular death	1 (1.7)	2 (11.1)	0.135
All-cause death	4 (6.8)	3 (16.7)	0.202
Total number of MACE	15 (25.4)	12 (66.7)	0.004

MACE, major cardiovascular events including stroke, fatal/nonfatal myocardial infarction, revascularization of treated vessel, cardiovascular death, and all-cause death.

percutaneous interventional procedures. Furthermore, patients with decreased circulating EPC number as well as CIN have increased cardiovascular events after percutaneous coronary or peripheral interventions. These findings suggest that reduced circulating EPC levels, reflecting attenuated endothelial repair capacity, may contribute to atherosclerotic disease progression and increased risk of cardiovascular events in patients who have developed CIN after interventional procedures. Measurement of EPC levels might be useful for screening high CIN risk population before undergoing percutaneous interventions.

CIN, characterized by the development of acute renal failure after exposure to radiocontrast agents, is a common cause of hospital-acquired acute renal injury [17]. Although CIN is generally benign in most instances, it is associated with extended length of hospital stays, increased health care costs, and higher risk of death [4]. As well as an increased risk of death, contrast-induced acute kidney injury is also associated with other adverse outcomes including late cardiovascular events after percutaneous interventions. CIN is generally defined as an increase in serum creatinine concentration of >0.5 mg/dL or 25% above baseline within 48 hours after contrast administration [3]. The risk factors that may predispose patients to CIN after cardiovascular interventional procedures include advanced age, diabetes mellitus, dehydration, and pre-existing renal disease. Several strategies, including volume expansion, using iso-osmolar contrast, and limiting the amount of administered contrast media, have become well established methods for prevention of CIN.

Although the exact mechanisms of CIN have yet to be fully elucidated, several causes have been described. Most likely, a combination of various mechanisms is responsible for the development of CIN. A reduction in renal perfusion caused by a direct effect of contrast media on the kidney, and toxic effects on the tubular cells are generally accepted as the main factors in the pathophysiology of CIN. Accumulating evidence suggests that the acute renal failure caused by the radiocontrast agents seems to be a consequence of an imbalance between vasoconstrictor factors and vasodilator agents like the prostaglandins or NO [18]. The role of NO in renal hemodynamics regulation has been reported in many studies. A decreased NO synthesis, or a lack of response of the endothelium to vasodilators, have been suggested as possible mechanisms for the ischemic or the nephrotoxic ARF [19,20]. Our study is consistent with previous reports showing that decreased NO concentrations may predispose to CIN after percutaneous interventions. Schwartz *et al.* observed that the administration of radiocontrast agents to rats resulted in a significant decrease in urinary guanosine $3',5'$-cyclic monophosphate, as well as NO_2^- and NO_3^- excretion, and this decrease was significantly attenuated by administration of L-arginine [21]. These results indicate that NO plays a major role in the pathogenesis of acute renal failure induced by radiocontrast agents.

Convincing evidence suggests that atherosclerosis is associated with endothelial dysfunction at the early stage of the disease process. Intact endothelium and maintenance of endothelial

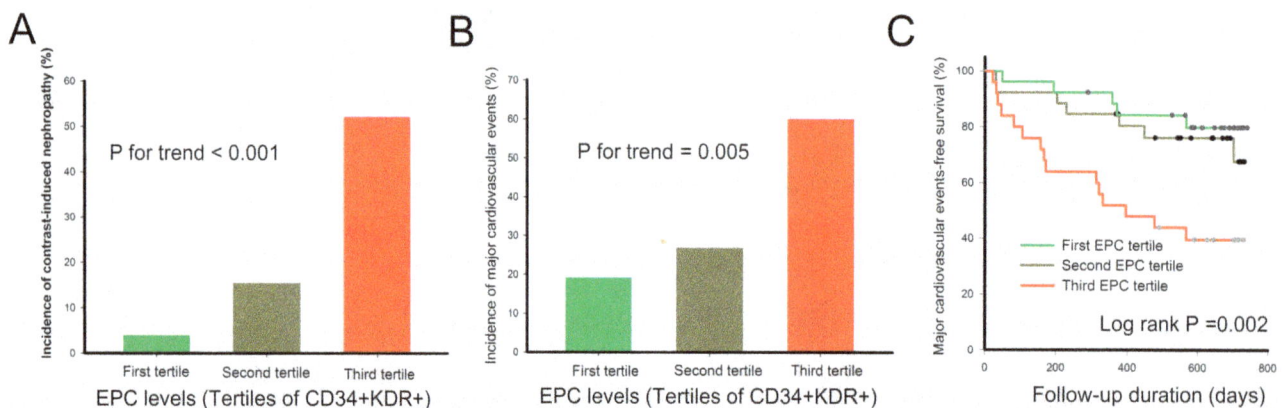

Figure 3. Association between tertiles of EPC level, and incidence of contrast-induced nephropathy (A), major cardiovascular events (MACE) (B), and MACE-free survival (C). First tertile: EPC (CD34$^+$KDR$^+$ $\geq$9 cells/10^5 events); Second tertile: EPC (CD34$^+$KDR$^+$ = 5–8 cells/10^5 events); Third tertile: EPC (CD34$^+$KDR$^+$ $\leq$ 4 cells/10^5 events).

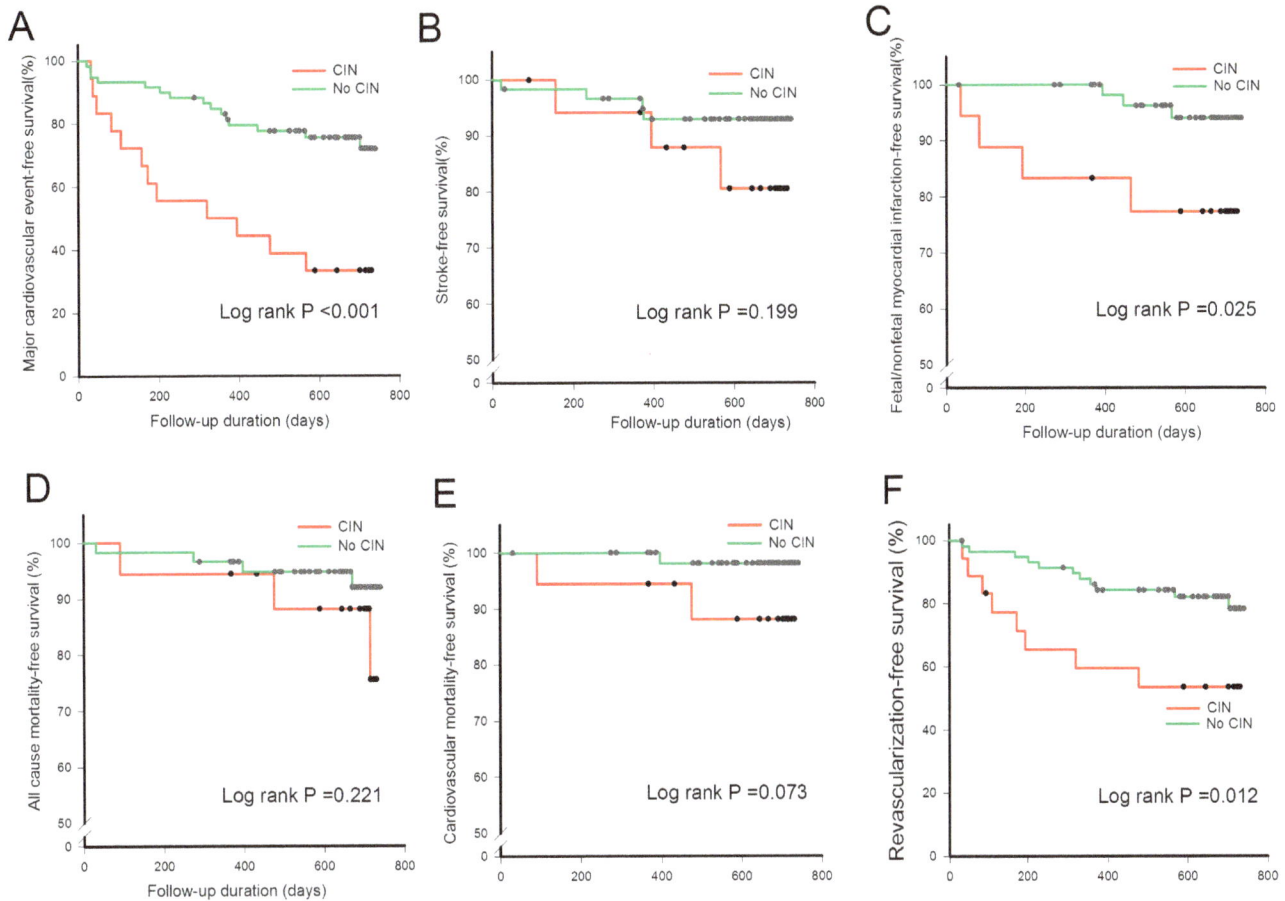

Figure 4. Association between contrast-induced nephropathy and major cardiovascular events (MACE), (A) MACE including stroke, fatal/nonfatal myocardial infarction, death and revascularization of treated vessels; (B) Stroke; (C) fatal/nonfatal myocardial infarction; (D) all-cause mortality; (E) cardiovascular death; (F) revascularization of treated vessels.

integrity play a pivotal role in preventing the development of atherosclerotic vascular disease. Recent insight suggests that the injured endothelial monolayer is regenerated by bone marrow-derived EPC, and circulating EPCs correlate with important clinical outcomes in vascular health [13]. They contribute to angiogenesis and organ repair in both animal and human models of ischemic injury [22,23]. With regard to renal injury, they appear to home in on, and incorporate into sites of active neovascularization in the kidney [7,24]. Pastchan *et al.* have demonstrated that, in mice models, renal ischemia rapidly mobilizes EPCs, which transiently home in on the spleen and subsequently accumulate in the medullopapillary region of the kidney [25]. They also proved that EPC-enriched cells from the medullopapillary parenchyma afforded partial renoprotection after renal ischemia, implying an important role of the recruited EPCs in the functional rescue of renal ischemia. It appears that bone marrow-derived EPCs may play a critical role in improving kidney function after ischemic or nephrotoxic injury in experimental models.

EPCs represent a very minor cell population in whole blood, and the choice of markers and controls is very important. However, there is still confusion about the definition used for EPC, and the circulating putative EPC identified in this study may include a monocyte subpopulation that may well have pro-angiogenic properties. However, in attempting an identification of EPC, a major limiting factor is that no simple definition of EPC

exists at the present time, while various methods to define EPC have been reported. Therefore, we used $CD34^+$, $CD34^+KDR^+$, $CD34^+KDR^+CD133^+$ markers to identify circulating EPCs in the current study [26]. Our data showed reduced circulating EPC levels were associated with development of CIN, and subsequent cardiovascular events after percutaneous interventions. Recent evidence indicates that mobilization and differentiation of EPCs are modified by NO, and that bone marrow-expressed eNOS is essential for the mobilization of stem cells and progenitor cells in vivo [27]. Therefore, decreased NO concentrations in CIN patients may modulate EPC behaviors and result in impaired vascular repair capacity, which suggests a pivotal role of EPC in modulation of CIN, and that a reduced number of these cells gives rise to the poor prognosis in CIN patients. These findings further provide pathophysiological insights into CIN development and raise the possibility that circulating EPCs may be a target for preventive interventions in selected individuals.

Some limitations of this study should be addressed. First, the sample size of this study was relatively small and may limit the interpretation of the study result. Due to the limited number of CIN patients, we were only able to adjust for 2 covariates in multivariate analysis to avoid over-fitting the problem. To draw a more definite conclusion, a larger population and longer follow-up duration would be required. Second, the EPC results showed relatively large standard deviations; however, these are not unusual for this kind of study. Third, we did not evaluate EPC function or clinical endothelial functions, such as adhesion, proliferation, migratory ability, and endothelium-dependent flow-mediated dilatation. However, we did check the nitric oxide levels in study subjects. Furthermore, a previous study has shown that EPC and endothelial functions exhibited changes in a similar pattern with respect to EPC number [28]. Finally, we did not recheck EPC levels after development of CIN in study subjects and had no idea if there was any distinct pattern of EPC mobilization in CIN patients.

In conclusion, circulating EPCs are decreased in patients who develop CIN, and a reduced number of circulating EPCs is significantly associated with MACE in CIN patients. Our findings may partially explain the pathophysiology of CIN and the poor prognosis in CIN patients. Furthermore, measurement of EPC number might be useful in identifying high CIN risk and high cardiovascular risk population.

Author Contributions

Conceived and designed the experiments: CHC PHH. Performed the experiments: CHC PHH CCC. Analyzed the data: CHC PHH CCC CYH. Contributed reagents/materials/analysis tools: CHC HBL CCH JWC SJL. Wrote the paper: CHC PHH.

References

1. Parfrey PS, Griffiths SM, Barrett BJ, Paul MD, Genge M, et al. (1989) Contrast material-induced renal failure in patients with diabetes mellitus, renal insufficiency, or both. A prospective controlled study. N Engl J Med 320: 143–149.

2. Rihal CS, Textor SC, Grill DE, Berger PB, Ting HH, et al. (2002) Incidence and prognostic importance of acute renal failure after percutaneous coronary intervention. Circulation 105: 2259–2264.

3. McCullough PA, Sandberg KR (2003) Epidemiology of contrast-induced nephropathy. Rev Cardiovasc Med 4 [Suppl 5]: S3–9.

4. Tepel M, Aspelin P, Lameire N (2006) Contrast-induced nephropathy: a clinical and evidence-based approach. Circulation 113: 1799–1806.

5. Heyman SN, Rosen S, Khamaisi M, Idee JM, Rosenberger C (2010) Reactive oxygen species and the pathogenesis of radiocontrast-induced nephropathy. Invest Radiol 45: 188–195.

6. Wong PC, Li Z, Guo J, Zhang A (2012) Pathophysiology of contrast-induced nephropathy. Int J Cardiol 158: 186–192.

7. Rehman J, Li J, Orschell CM, March KL (2003) Peripheral blood "endothelial progenitor cells" are derived from monocyte/macrophages and secrete angiogenic growth factors. Circulation 107: 1164–1169.

8. Bahlmann FH, DeGroot K, Duckert T, Niemczyk E, Bahlmann E, et al. (2003) Endothelial progenitor cell proliferation and differentiation is regulated by erythropoietin. Kidney Int 64: 1648–1652.

9. Jie KE, Zaikova MA, Bergevoet MW, Westerweel PE, Rastmanesh M, et al. (2010) Progenitor cells and vascular function are impaired in patients with chronic kidney disease. Nephrol Dial Transplant 25: 1875–1882.

10. Perticone F, Maio R, Perticone M, Sciacqua A, Shehaj E, et al. (2010) Endothelial dysfunction and subsequent decline in glomerular filtration rate in hypertensive patients. Circulation 122: 379–384.

11. Chu K, Jung KH, Lee ST, Park HK, Sinn DI, et al. (2008) Circulating endothelial progenitor cells as a new marker of endothelial dysfunction or repair in acute stroke. Stroke 2008;39: 1441–1447.

12. Yip HK, Chang LT, Chang WN, Lu CH, Liou CW, et al. (2008) Level and value of circulating endothelial progenitor cells in patients after acute ischemic stroke. Stroke 39: 69–74.

13. Werner N, Kosiol S, Schiegl T, Ahlers P, Walenta K, et al. (2005) Circulating endothelial progenitor cells and cardiovascular outcomes. N Engl J Med 353: 999–1007.

14. Levey AS, Bosch JP, Lewis JB, Greene T, Rogers N, et al. (1999) A more accurate method to estimate glomerular filtration rate from serum creatinine: a new prediction equation. Modification of Diet in Renal Disease Study Group. Ann Intern Med 130: 461–470.

15. Eknoya G, Levin N (2002) K/DOQI clinical practice guidelines for chronic kidney disease: evaluation, classification, and stratification. Am J Kidney Dis. 39: S1–266.

16. Chiang CH, Huang PH, Chung FP, Chen ZY, Leu HB, et al. (2012) Decreased circulating endothelial progenitor cell levels and function in patients with nonalcoholic fatty liver disease. PLoS One 7: e31799.

17. McCullough PA (2008) Contrast-induced acute kidney injury. J Am Coll Cardiol 51: 1419–1428.

18. Vallance P, Chan N (2001) Endothelial function and nitric oxide: clinical relevance. Heart 85: 342–350.

19. Agmon Y, Peleg H, Greenfeld Z, Rosen S, Brezis M (1994) Nitric oxide and prostanoids protect the renal outer medulla from radiocontrast toxicity in the rat. J Clin Invest 1994;94: 1069–1075.

20. Ribeiro L, de Assuncao e Silva F, Kurihara RS, Schor N, Mieko E, et al. (2004) Evaluation of the nitric oxide production in rat renal artery smooth muscle cells culture exposed to radiocontrast agents. Kidney Int. 65: 589–596.

21. Schwartz D, Blum M, Peer G, Wollman Y, Maree A, et al. (1994) Role of nitric oxide (EDRF) in radiocontrast acute renal failure in rats. Am J Physiol 267: F374–379.

22. Zhang ZG, Zhang L, Jiang Q, Chopp M (2002) Bone marrow-derived endothelial progenitor cells participate in cerebral neovascularization after focal cerebral ischemia in the adult mouse. Circ Res 90: 284–288.

23. Tateishi-Yuyama E, Matsubara H, Murohara T (2002) Therapeutic angiogenesis for patients with limb ischaemia by autologous transplantation of bone-marrow cells: a pilot study and a randomised controlled trial. Lancet 360: 427–435.

24. Ricardo SD, Deane JA (2005) Adult stem cells in renal injury and repair. Nephrology (Carlton). 10: 276–282.

25. Patschan D, Krupincza K, Patschan S, Zhang Z, Hamby C, et al. (2006) Dynamics of mobilization and homing of endothelial progenitor cells after acute renal ischemia: modulation by ischemic preconditioning. Am J Physiol Renal Physiol 291: F176–185.

26. Iwami Y, Masuda H, Asahara T (2004) Endothelial progenitor cells: past, state of the art, and future. J Cell Mol Med 8: 488–97.

27. Ozuyaman B, Ebner P, Niesler U, Ziemann J, Kleinbongard P, et al. (2005) Nitric oxide differentially regulates proliferation and mobilization of endothelial progenitor cells but not of hematopoietic stem cells. Thromb Haemost 94: 770–772.

28. Jialal I, Devaraj S, Singh U, Huet BA (2010) Decreased number and impaired functionality of endothelial progenitor cells in subjects with metabolic syndrome: implications for increased cardiovascular risk. Atherosclerosis 211: 297–302.

3

Hypertriglyceridemic Waist Phenotype and Chronic Kidney Disease in a Chinese Population Aged 40 Years and Older

Yongqiang Li[1,9], Chaomin Zhou[1,9], Xiaofei Shao[1], Xinyu Liu[1], Jia Guo[1], Ying Zhang[1], Honglei Wang[1], Xiaohong Wang[1], Bin Li[1], Kangping Deng[1], Qin Liu[1], Harry Holthöfer[2], Hequn Zou[1]*

1 Department of Nephrology, Third Affiliated Hospital of Southern Medical University, Guangzhou, Guangdong, China, 2 National Centre for Sensor Research/BioAnalytical Sciences, Dublin City University, Dublin, Ireland

Abstract

Objective: To examine the relationship between the HW phenotype and risk for CKD in a community population aged 40 years and older.

Methods: A cross-sectional study was conducted in Zhuhai from June to October 2012. The participants were divided into three groups: Group 1, Waist circumference >90 cm in men or >85 cm in women and triglycerides ≥2 mmol/l; Group 3, Waist circumference ≤90 cm in men or ≤85 cm in women and triglycerides <2 mmol/l; Group 2, The remaining participants. The prevalence of the three subgroups and CKD were determined. The association between HW phenotype and CKD was then analyzed using SPSS (version 13.0).

Results: After adjusting for age and sex, Group 1 was associated with CKD (OR 3.08, 95% CI 2.01, 4.73, P<0.001), when compared with Group 3. Further adjustment for factors which were potential confounders and unlikely to be in the causal pathway between the HW phenotype and CKD, Group 1 was still significantly associated with CKD. The OR for CKD was 2.65 (95% CI 1.65, 4.26, P<0.001). When adjusted for diabetes and hypertension, the association of Group 1 and CKD was still significant (OR 2.09, 95% CI 1.26, 3.45, P = 0.004). Group 2 was associated with CKD (OR 1.81, 95% CI 1.29, 2.53, P = 0.001), when compared with Group 3. Further adjustment for factors which were potential confounders, Group 2 was still significantly associated with CKD. The OR for CKD was 1.75 (95% CI 1.22, 2.51, P = 0.002). When adjusted for diabetes and hypertension, the association between Group 2 and CKD still existed. The OR for CKD was 1.48 (95% CI 1.01, 2.16, P = 0.046).

Conclusion: Our results showed that HW phenotype was associated with CKD in the population aged 40 years and older.

Editor: Reury F.P. Bacurau, University of Sao Paulo, Brazil

Funding: This study was supported by the following Science Foundation: 1. EU FP7 Program, UroSense, 2011; 2. Guangdong Provincial Science and Technique Program (No. 2011B031800386), 2011. The funders had no role in study design, data collection and analysis, decision to publish, or preparation of the manuscript.

Competing Interests: The authors have declared that no competing interests exist.

* E-mail: hequnzou@hotmail.com

9 These authors contributed equally to this work.

Introduction

Chronic kidney disease (CKD) has become a worldwide public health concern with an increasing prevalence during the last decade in China [1]. Zhang et al [1] recently reported that the overall prevalence of CKD in China was 10.8%. Outcomes of CKD include progression to end-stage renal disease (ESRD) and lots of complications of reduced kidney function such as increased cardiovascular events and a loss of disability-adjusted life years [2,3]. CKD has become a big challenge to the health care system. The major renal replacement therapy is hemodialysis in China [4] with poor outcomes and high cost. In 2002, the annual incidence of hemodialysis in Beijing and Shanghai was 146.4 and 148.1 per million population, respectively [5]. The cost of renal dialysis alone is $14,300 per patient-year in China while the percapita disposable income was $1,210 in urban areas and $375 in rural areas [5]. It's a great burden to patients, society and country. The exorbitant cost of CKD, and its high mortality rate call for early detection and prevention of CKD. Pre-CKD has however obtained an increasing amount of attention [6]. Identifying high-risk subjects of CKD and taking appropriate intervention measures are indispensable.

The hypertriglyceridemic waist phenotype (HW phenotype) has obtained attention increasingly [7,8]. Isabelle Lemieux and his colleagues firstly proposed the HW phenotype in 2000 [9]. The HW phenotype was defined as an elevated waist circumference (>90 cm in men and >85 cm in women), along with an elevated plasma triglyceride concentration (>2.0 mmol/L (177 mg/dl). Several studies have shown that the HW phenotype is a simple but sensitive marker of cardiovascular risk [9,10]. A recent study suggests that the HW phenotype is a better predictor of cardiovascular disease than the metabolic syndrome in non-diabetic subjects [11]. A recent study showed that the HW phenotype is associated with worse carotid atherosclerosis in CKD patients [12].

To the best of our knowledge, the association between the HW phenotype and CKD has never been evaluated in a developing country such as China.To fill this gap in the research field, we conducted this cross-sectional study of community population aged 40 years and older to examin the relationship between the HW phenotype and CKD in the city of Zhuhai in Guangdong province, China. Data were collected from1753 community residents older than 40 years from June to October, 2012. Participants were selected using a multi-stage stratified random cluster sampling method.

Methods

Subjects

The Ethics Committee of The Third Affiliated Hospital of Southern Medical University, Guangzhou, approved this study. This study was performed fulfilling the principles of Helsinki Declaration and the International Guidelines for Ethical Review for Epidemiological Studies. Data was collected from1753 community residents older than 40 years from June to October, 2012. Participants were selected using a multi-stage stratified random cluster sampling method. Step 1, two communities were selected randomly from Wanzhai Town; step 2, in each of the two selected communities, 500 families were randomly sampled as the target family; and step 3, all the residents aged 40 years and older in the selected families were sampled. The exclusion criteria included: missing gender; age; education status; missing any item of lifestyle information (for example, smoking status, alcohol intake, and physical activity); not being in the fasting state for at least 10 hours; missing any item of waist measurement, blood pressure (BP), body mass index (BMI), blood glucose, serum high-density lipoprotein (HDL) cholesterol, and triglyceride (TG) levels information. Using this method, a total of 1753 participants from 2198 residents completed the survey, with a response rate of 79.8%. 173 participants were assigned to Group 1.541 participants were assigned to Group 2 and 820 participants belonged to Group 3 according to their waist circumferences and triglyceride levels.

Participants were recruited by mail and home visits. First, we informed participants by mail. Then we visited the families and got the filled questionnaires from the participants. All participants signed a letter of informed consent.

Data collection

Data on age, sex, personal history (coronary artery disease, hypertension, and diabetes) and details about lifestyle (current or past cigarette smoking, alcohol intake, diet habits, educational status, and physical activity) were obtained through questionnaires. The participants completed the questionnaires under the professional guidance of physicians, medical students or nurses. All of them had received intensive training.

Physical measures

Physical measures were conducted in the community clinics. A well-trained nurse measured body weight, height, waist circumference and blood pressure in the morning between 08:00 am and 11:00 am. Body height and weight were measured with a calibrated clinical scale and stadiometer. Body mass index (BMI) was calculated as weight (kg) divided by height squared (m2). Waist circumference was taken midway between the last rib and iliac crest with the participants standing with light garments and breathing out gently [14]. The waist circumference was measured

two times and the average of two measures was recorded to the nearest 0.1 cm. Blood pressure was measured three times with a calibrated mercury sphygmomanometer and the average value was calculated. BP was measured in the sitting position after resting for at least 5 minutes.

Laboratory values

Following an overnight fast of at least 10 hours, blood specimens were collected for plasma glucose, HDL cholesterol, LDL cholesterol, triglycerides, serum creatinine, highsensitivity C-reactive protein (CRP) and insulin. First morning urine samples were collected from all participants, except those women who were actively menstruating.

Individuals having urinary tract infection symptoms were also excluded from the urine test. All specimens were transported to the central laboratory in the Third Affiliated Hospital of Southern Medical University within 3 hours from collection sites and stored at 4°C until analysis. Methods we used to detect laboratory variables had been described in our previous paper [13].

Definition of HW phenotype

The HW phenotype was defined as elevated waist circumference (>90 cm in men and >85 cm in women), along with an elevated plasma triglyceride concentration (>2.0 mmol/L (177 mg/dl) [12].

Determination of CKD

The estimated glomerular filtration rate (eGFR) was estimated using a formula from the Chinese-Modification of Diet Renal Disease (C-MDRD) study: GFR (ml/min/1.73 m^2) = 175 × (Scr)$^{-1.234}$ × (Age)$^{-0.179}$ ×(if female, ×0.79) [15]. Reduced renal function was defined as an eGFR of less than 60 mL/min per 1.73 m^2. For practical purposes, albuminuria was defined as a spot urinary albumin-to-creatinine ratio (ACR) higher than 30 mg/g. CKD was defined as an eGFR of less than 60 ml/min per 1.73 m^2 or albuminuria.

Determination of Diabetes and Hypertension

A blood pressure (BP) of 130/85 mmHg or higher or receiving treatment for previously diagnosed for hypertension. A fasting blood glucose (FBG) of 5.6 mmol/l or higher or with previously diagnosed for type 2 diabetes.

Socioeconomic factors. The socioeconomic factors used in this study were defined on educational status. Education status was classified into three categories: (1) 0 years of schooling;(2) primary school or junior middle school; (3) high school or above.

Health behavior factors. Alcohol consumption was evaluated based on the frequency of alcohol intake as recorded on the health interview questionnaire. We divided the residents into three groups: (1) No drinking; (2) Current alcohol use; (3) former but no present drinking. For physical exercise, the participants were divided into two groups: (1) no physical activity; (2) physical activity. For smoking, they were divided into three groups: (1) former smokers who quit smoking prior to the survey; (2) current smoker; (3) non-smoker.

Statistical Analysis

Data were analyzed using SPSS (version 13.0). Continuous variables were shown as mean ± standard deviation if they had normal distribution. Median and interquartile range were used to show skewed distributed continuous variables. The categorical variables were presented as absolute and relative (%) values or proportion. A two-tailed p value <0.05 was considered significant.

We divided the participants into three groups according to their waist circumferences and triglyceride levels: Group 1, waist circumference >90 cm in men or >85 cm in women and triglycerides ≥2 mmol/l; Group 2, waist circumference <90 cm in men or <85 cm in women along with a plasma triglyceride concentration of ≥2.0 mmol/L/waist circumference ≥90 cm in men or ≥85 cm in women along with a plasma triglyceride concentration of <2.0 mmol/L; Group 3, waist circumference ≤90 cm in men or ≤85 cm in women and triglycerides <2 mmol/l.

Baseline characteristics within Group 1, Group 2 and Group 3 were examined using the chi-squared test for categorical variables and one-way ANOVA or Wilcoxon rank-sum test for continuous variables.

Mutiple logistic regression models were used to explore whether the HW phenotype is associated with CKD. The first model was adjusted for age and sex. Next, history of hypertension, history of coronary heart disease, history of stroke, history of malignancy, current smoker, current alcohol use, physical inactivity and education status were added into the model. Furthermore we examined whether the associations were independent of diabetes or hypertension. Diabetes and hypertension were added to the above covariates. Group 3 was considered as the reference group.

Results

Initially there were 1753 participants aged 40 years and older in our study and all participants were Han ethnic. 219 subjects were excluded because of missing data for serum creatinine, ACR, triglyceride or waist circumference. Finally, we included 1534 participants with mean age 57.21±10.97 years in the current study. 173 participants were assigned to Group 1. 541 participants were assigned to Group 2 and 820 participants belonged to Group 3 according to their waist circumferences and triglyceride levels.

Baseline characteristics of the participants based on HW phenotype

As shown in Table 1, patients in Group 1 had significantly higher serum uric acid, serum C-reactive protein, HOMA-index, BMI than those in Group 2 and Group 3 (P<0.001). Additionally, these values in Group 2 were significantly higher than those participants in Group 3 (P<0.001). Participants in Group 1 were older and had a higher prevalence of hypertension, diabetes, a higher diastolic blood pressure, higher levels of fasting glucose, ACR, and lower serum high-density lipoprotein than those in Group 2 and Group 3 (P<0.001). Current smoker status and current alcohol use statuses are more common in Group 1 than those in groups 2 and 3. There were no differences in educational status (high school or above) and history of coronary heart disease among the participants in the three groups.

Prevalence of CKD in the three subgroups

As shown in Fig. 1, there were 46/173 subjects (26.6%) with CKD in group 1. Participants in group 2 had a higher prevalence of CKD 90/541 (16.6%) than those in group 3, 77/820(9.4%) (p<0.001). Participants in group 1 had the highest prevalence of CKD among the three subgroups. (p<0.001).

Association of the HW phenotype with CKD

As shown in Table 2, Group 1 was associated with CKD (OR 3.08, 95% CI 2.01, 4.73, P<0.001) in model one, when compared with Group 3. Further adjustment for factors which were potential confounders and unlikely to be in the causal pathway between the HW phenotype and CKD had an impact on the odd ratios, Group

1 was still significantly associated with CKD. The odd ratio for CKD was 2.65 (95% CI 1.65, 4.26, P<0.001). When adjusted for diabetes and hypertension, the association of Group 1 and CKD was still significant (OR 2.09, 95% CI 1.26, 3.45, P=0.004). Group 2 was associated with CKD (OR 1.81, 95% CI 1.29, 2.53, P=0.001) in model one, when compared with Group 3. Further adjustment for history of hypertension, history of coronary heart disease, history of stroke, history of malignancy, current smoker, current alcohol use, physical inactivity, educational status, Group 2 was still significantly associated with CKD. The odd ratio for CKD was 1.75 (95% CI 1.22, 2.51, P=0.002). When adjusted for diabetes and hypertension, the association between Group 2 and CKD still existed. The odd ratio for CKD was 1.48 (95% CI 1.01, 2.16, P=0.046).

Discussion

In the present study, we found that population aged 40 years and older characterized by the presence of the HW phenotype were at a higher risk of CKD than those without this phenotype. The HW phenotype was positively associated with CKD. Meanwhile, This relationship was independent of age, sex, history of hypertension, history of coronary heart disease, history of stroke, history of malignancy, current smoker, current alcohol use, physical inactivity, educational status, diabetes and hypertension.

During recent years the HW phenotype has obtained an increasing amount of attention. Accumulating evidences show that the HW phenotype might be a simple, yet a significant marker of CAD [9,16]. The HW phenotype was associated with worse carotid atherosclerosis in CKD patients [12] and was positively associated with hyperglycemia [17]. To the best of our knowledge, this is the first study evaluating the relationship between the HW phenotype and CKD. In the present study, individuals with the HW phenotype were 2.09-fold as likely to have CKD as were those with both low waist circumference and low TG concentration.

Multiple potential mechanisms might be responsible for a higher risk of CKD in individuals showing a HW phenotype even after adjustment for life style, hypertension, diabetes and other potentially confounding factors. The HW phenotype is actually a marker of visceral obesity [18]. Visceral obesity or excess fatty acids accompanied with increased levels of triglyceride may result in accumulation of fat at ectopic tissues such as liver, pancreatic b-cells and the kidneys [11,19]. The ectopic accumulation of fat at these organs would result in steatohepatitis, insulin resistance, compression of the kidneys and therefore hypertension, diabetes, hyperuricemia and unfavorable renal hemodynamic pattern [20], which contribute to CKD. In another hand, there is a close correlation between hypertriglyceridemia and uric acid (UA) production. Production of UA in viscerally obesity subjects is higher [21]. Furthermore, the hypertriglyceridemic waist is reported to be an important factor increasing high-sensitivity C-reactive protein levels [22]. Both hyperuricemia and high levels of C-reactive protein contribute to CKD. Our results that partic-ipants with the HW phenotype had higher levels of fasting glucose, serum uric acid, VLDL-C, insulin, blood pressure and C-reactive protein and therfore higher risk of CKD might further support these mechanisms. These results were consistent with previous reports [9,23–25].

The increasing prevalence of CKD requests us to find out more efficient markers for monitoring the prevalence of CKD. Several studies have suggested that obesity and the metabolic syndrome are independent predictors of CKD [17,26–29]. Body mass index (BMI) was widely used as a marker of obesity. But fluid overload

Table 1. Baseline characteristics of the participants based on HW phenotype.

	Group1	Group2	Group3	
	n = 173	n = 541	n = 820	p
Age (years)	59.24±11.44	58.25±10.34	56.1±11.16	<0.001
Male (%)	86(49.7)	208(38.4)	274(33.4)	<0.001
Clinical Characteristics				
Hypertension history (%)	77 (44.5)	156 (28.8)	138 (16.8)	<0.001
Diabetes history (%)	19 (11.0)	51(9.4)	46(5.6)	0.007
Coronary heart disease history (%)	5 (2.9)	14 (2.6)	28 (3.4)	0.68
Current smoker (%)	33 (19.1)	61 (11.3)	91 (11.1)	0.011
Current alcohol use (%)	52 (30.1)	124 (22.9)	156 (19.0)	0.004
Educational status (≥high school)(%)	51 (29.5)	150(27.7)	269(32.8)	0.13
Systolic blood pressure (mm Hg)	137.15 ±18.27	135.37±18.48	126.63±19.71	<0.001
Diastolic blood pressure (mm Hg)	84.16±9.44	81.44±10.38	76.52±10.215	<0.001
Body mass index (kg/m 2)	26.63±2.69	25.23±3.07	21.86±2.65	<0.001
Waist circumference (cm)	95.57±5.91	90.38±8.98	77.79±6.55	<0.001
Laboratory values				
Fasting glucose (mmo/l)	5.58±1.58	5.31±1.37	4.88±0.96	<0.001
Serum C-reactive protein (mg/l)	95.57±5.91	90.38±8.98	77.79±6.55	<0.001
Serum triglyceride (mmol/L)	2.5 (2.32–3.33)	1.53 (1.13–2.26)	1.04 (0.78–1.33)	<0.001
Serum low density lipoprotein (mmol/l)	3.13±1.01	3.37±0.93	3.26±0.84	0.005
Serum high density lipoprotein (mmol/l)	1.38±0.28	1.45±0.28	1.63±0.34	<0.001
Very low density lipoprotein (mmol/l)	1.32±0.45	0.81±0.43	0.49±0.17	<0.001
HOMA-index (uU/ml.mmol/ml)	3.2 (2.34–4.64)	2.43 (1.69–3.45)	1.38 (0.99–1.93)	<0.001
Serum creatitine (umol/L)	80.84±17.38	75.03±18.46	71.81±15.87	<0.001
eGFR (mL/min/1.73 m 2)	88.27±16.37	95.17±20.91	99.34±21.67	<0.001
ACR (mg/g)	12 (6–23)	9 (6–17)	7 (5–13)	<0.001
Serum uric acid (umol/L)	421.12±97.47	375.09±97.91	325.46±86.14	<0.001

Note: Values expressed as absolute and relative (%) percent for categorical variables and mean ± SD for continuous variables. Note: Values expressed as absolute and relative (%) percent for categorical variables and Mean ± SD or median (25th to 75th percentiles) for continuous variables.
Abbreviations: ACR, albumin-creatinine ratio; eGFR: estimated Glomerular filtration rate; HOMA-IR: Homeostatic model assessment of insulin resistance;

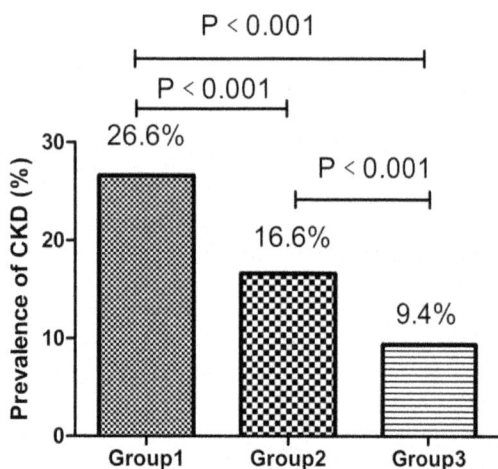

Figure 1. Prevalence of CKD in 1534 subjects based on HW phenotype.

and body fat distribution should be considered. In the present study, participants in all groups were non-obese according to their respective BMI. But they were at a high risk of CKD especially in those with the HW phenotype, which is a marker of visceral obesity. Chinese are known to have a predisposition to visceral fat accumulation despite having generally low BMI [30]. These results supported that BMI was not an ideal marker of obesity and was not as sensitive as the HW phenotype in capturing the risk of CKD. Though waist circumference is recommended to be a relatively ideal marker of obesity [31], it is rather difficult to identify subcutaneous and visceral adiposity. Several studies indicate that it is visceral obesity but not the subcutaneous adiposity that correlates with the metabolic abnormalities [32,33] and not all population with an elevated waist circumference are viscerally obese. Hence the waist circumference alone is not an ideal marker of obesity. Recent studies showed that the HW phenotype is a better marker of visceral obesity [18].

The metabolic syndrome and its components were also reported to be risk factors of CKD [34]. However, recent studies suggest that the HW phenotype predicts metabolic abnormalities better than the metabolic syndrome [9]. In Henry S Kahn's study, enlarged waist with elevated triacylglycerols alone identified more persons with greater concentrations of LDL cholesterol and

Table 2. Association of the hypertriglyceridemic waist phenotype with CKD.

	Model one[a]		Model two[b]		Model three[c]	
	OR (95% CI)	P value	OR (95% CI)	P value	OR (95% CI)	P value
Group 3	Reference		Reference		Reference	
Group 1	3.08(2.01–4.73)	<0.001	2.65(1.65–4.26)	<0.001	2.09(1.26–3.45)	0.004
Group 2	1.81(1.29–2.53)	0.001	1.75(1.22–2.51)	0.002	1.48(1.01–2.16)	0.046

a.Adjusted for age, sex.
b.Adjusted for age, sex, history of hypertension, history of coronary heart disease, history of stroke, history of malignancy, current smoker, current alcohol use, physical inactivity, educational status.
c. Adjusted for above + diabetes and hypertension.

apolipoprotein B than did metabolic syndrome alone [35]. In addition, the diagnosis of metabolic syndrome needs more laboratory data and therefore it's somewhat easier to evaluate the HW phenotype. Based on those advantages of the HW phenotype and the finding of our study that the HW phenotype was significantly associated with CKD, we advise that the HW phenotype might be a simple but sensitive marker for screening individuals who have higher CKD risk factors.

There are several limitations in the current study. Firstly, the cross-sectional nature of our study disabled us to make causal inferences. Prospective studies are needed to prove whether this phenotype could predict major outcomes such as CKD events or mortality. Secondly, all the indicators of CKD (eGFR and ACR) were obtained on the basis of single measurements without repeating tests. Thirdly, Cut-offs of 90 cm and 2.0 mmol/L in men of 85 cm and 2.0 mmol/L in women were advocated for the diagnosis of visceral obesity and metabolic syndrome in Europeans, these cut-offs need to be validated for Chinese population, in different Chinese ethnic groups, genders and across different age

groups. Fourthly, Participants were selected from the chosen families. Lifestyle and even potential genetic determinants might widely differ between participants from our selected families and non-related individuals from the general population, these issues might have a potential effect on the incidence of CKD in our study.

In summary, our study showed that the HW phenotype was associated with the presence of CKD in the population aged 40 years and older, from which we can speculate that the HW phenotype might be considered as a simple, yet sensitive marker for identifying adults at risk of CKD in the population aged 40 years and older.

Author Contributions

Conceived and designed the experiments: YL HZ CZ. Performed the experiments: KD QL. Analyzed the data: CZ YL. Wrote the paper: YL CZ HZ HH. Performed this epidemiological survey: XL JG YZ HW XW BL KD QL XS.

References

1. Zhang L, Wang F, Wang L, Wang W, Liu B, et al. (2012) Prevalence of chronic kidney disease in China: a cross-sectional survey. Lancet 379: 815–822.
2. Go AS, Chertow GM, Fan D, McCulloch CE, Hsu CY (2004) Chronic kidney disease and the risks of death, cardiovascular events, and hospitalization. N Engl J Med 351: 1296–1305.
3. Ayodele OE, Alebiosu CO (2010) Burden of chronic kidney disease: an international perspective. Advances in chronic kidney disease 17: 215–224.
4. Yao Q, Zhang W, Qian J (2008) Peritoneal dialysis in Shanghai. Peritoneal Dialysis International 28: S42–S45.
5. Wang H, Zhang L, Lv J (2005) Prevention of the progression of chronic kidney disease: practice in China. Kidney Int Suppl 67: S63–67.
6. Curhan GC (2010) Prediabetes, Prehypertension… Is It Time for Pre-CKD? Clinical Journal of the American Society of Nephrology 5: 557–559.
7. Blackburn P, Lemieux I, Lamarche B, Bergeron J, Perron P, et al. (2012) Hypertriglyceridemic waist: a simple clinical phenotype associated with coronary artery disease in women. Metabolism 61: 56–64.
8. Carlsson AC, Risérus U, Ärnlöv J (2014) Hypertriglyceridemic Waist Phenotype is Associated with Decreased Insulin Sensitivity and Incident Diabetes in Elderly Men. Obesity 22: 526–529
9. Lemieux I, Pascot A, Couillard C, Lamarche B, Tchernof A, et al. (2000) Hypertriglyceridemic waist: A marker of the atherogenic metabolic triad (hyperinsulinemia; hyperapolipoprotein B; small, dense LDL) in men? Circulation 102: 179–184.
10. Arsenault BJ, Lemieux I, Després J-P, Wareham NJ, Kastelein JJ, et al. (2010) The hypertriglyceridemic-waist phenotype and the risk of coronary artery disease: results from the EPIC-Norfolk prospective population study. Canadian Medical Association Journal 182: 1427–1432.
11. Després J-P, Lemieux I, Bergeron J, Pibarot P, Mathieu P, et al. (2008) Abdominal obesity and the metabolic syndrome: contribution to global cardiometabolic risk. Arterioscler Thromb Vasc Biol 28: 1039–1049.
12. Zhe X, Bai Y, Cheng Y, Xiao H, Wang D, et al. (2013) Hypertriglyceridemic Waist is Associated with Increased Carotid Atherosclerosis in Chronic Kidney Disease Patients. Nephron Clinical Practice 122: 146–152.

13. Li Y, Zhao L, Chen Y, Liu A, Liu X, et al. (2013) Association between Metabolic Syndrome and Chronic Kidney Disease in Perimenopausal Women. International journal of environmental research and public health 10: 3987–3997.
14. Irwin ML, Mayer-Davis EJ, Addy CL, Pate RR, Durstine JL, et al. (2000) Moderate-intensity physical activity and fasting insulin levels in women: the Cross-Cultural Activity Participation Study. Diabetes Care 23: 449–454.
15. Ma YC, Zuo L, Chen JH, Luo Q, Yu XQ, et al. (2006) Modified glomerular filtration rate estimating equation for Chinese patients with chronic kidney disease. J Am Soc Nephrol 17: 2937–2944.
16. LaMonte MJ, Ainsworth BE, DuBose KD, Grandjean PW, Davis PG, et al. (2003) The hypertriglyceridemic waist phenotype among women. Atherosclerosis 171: 123–130.
17. St-Pierre J, Lemieux I, Vohl M-C, Perron P, Després J-P, et al. (2002) Contribution of abdominal obesity and hypertriglyceridemia to impaired fasting glucose and coronary artery disease. The American journal of cardiology 90: 15–18.
18. Sam S, Haffner S, Davidson MH, D'Agostino RB, Sr., Feinstein S, et al. (2009) Hypertriglyceridemic waist phenotype predicts increased visceral fat in subjects with type 2 diabetes. Diabetes Care 32: 1916–1920.
19. Weinberg JM (2006) Lipotoxicity. Kidney Int 70: 1560–1566.
20. Kwakernaak AJ, Zelle DM, Bakker SJ, Navis G (2013) Central Body Fat Distribution Associates with Unfavorable Renal Hemodynamics Independent of Body Mass Index. Journal of the American Society of Nephrology 24: 987–994.
21. Matsubara K, Matsuzawa Y, Jiao S, Takama T, Kubo M, et al. (1989) Relationship between hypertriglyceridemia and uric acid production in primary gout. Metabolism 38: 698–701.
22. Rosolova H, Petrlova B, Simon J, Sifalda P, Sipova I (2008) High-sensitivity C-reactive protein and the hypertriglyceridemic waist in patients with type 2 diabetes and metabolic syndrome. Medical science monitor: international medical journal of experimental and clinical research 14: CR411–415.
23. Esmaillzadeh A, Mirmiran P, Azizi F (2006) Clustering of metabolic abnormalities in adolescents with the hypertriglyceridemic waist phenotype. Am J Clin Nutr 83: 36–46.

24. St-Pierre J, Lemieux I, Vohl MC, Perron P, Tremblay G, et al. (2002) Contribution of abdominal obesity and hypertriglyceridemia to impaired fasting glucose and coronary artery disease. Am J Cardiol 90: 15–18.

25. Gomez-Huelgas R, Bernal-Lopez MR, Villalobos A, Mancera-Romero J, Baca-Osorio AJ, et al. (2011) Hypertriglyceridemic waist: an alternative to the metabolic syndrome? Results of the IMAP Study (multidisciplinary intervention in primary care). Int J Obes (Lond) 35: 292–299.

26. Hallan S, de Mutsert R, Carlsen S, Dekker FW, Aasarød K, et al. (2006) Obesity, smoking, and physical inactivity as risk factors for CKD: are men more vulnerable? American journal of kidney diseases 47: 396–405.

27. Hsu CY, McCulloch CE, Iribarren C, Darbinian J, Go AS (2006) Body mass index and risk for end-stage renal disease. Ann Intern Med 144: 21–28.

28. Ejerblad E, Fored CM, Lindblad P, Fryzek J, McLaughlin JK, et al. (2006) Obesity and risk for chronic renal failure. J Am Soc Nephrol 17: 1695–1702.

29. Wahba IM, Mak RH (2007) Obesity and obesity-initiated metabolic syndrome: mechanistic links to chronic kidney disease. Clinical Journal of the American Society of Nephrology 2: 550–562.

30. Lear SA, Humphries KH, Kohli S, Chockalingam A, Frohlich JJ, et al. (2007) Visceral adipose tissue accumulation differs according to ethnic background: results of the Multicultural Community Health Assessment Trial (M-CHAT). Am J Clin Nutr 86: 353–359.

31. Lemieux I, Alméras N, Mauriege P, Blanchet C, Dewailly E, et al. (2002) Prevalence of hypertriglyceridemic waist in men who participated in the Quebec Health Survey: association with atherogenic and diabetogenic metabolic risk factors. The Canadian journal of cardiology 18: 725–732.

32. Ross R, Aru J, Freeman J, Hudson R, Janssen I (2002) Abdominal adiposity and insulin resistance in obese men. Am J Physiol Endocrinol Metab 282: E657–663.

33. Ross R, Freeman J, Hudson R, Janssen I (2002) Abdominal obesity, muscle composition, and insulin resistance in premenopausal women. J Clin Endocrinol Metab 87: 5044–5051.

34. Buchholz A, Bugaresti J (2005) A review of body mass index and waist circumference as markers of obesity and coronary heart disease risk in persons with chronic spinal cord injury. Spinal cord 43: 513–518.

35. Kahn HS, Valdez R (2003) Metabolic risks identified by the combination of enlarged waist and elevated triacylglycerol concentration. Am J Clin Nutr 78: 928–934.

4

Comparison of High vs. Normal/Low Protein Diets on Renal Function in Subjects without Chronic Kidney Disease

Lukas Schwingshackl*, Georg Hoffmann

University of Vienna, Faculty of Life Sciences, Department of Nutritional Sciences, Vienna, Austria

Abstract

Background: It was the aim of the present systematic review and meta-analysis to investigate the effects of high protein (HP) versus normal/low protein (LP/NP) diets on parameters of renal function in subjects without chronic kidney disease.

Methods: Queries of literature were performed using the electronic databases MEDLINE, EMBASE, and the Cochrane Trial Register until 27th February 2014. Study specific weighted mean differences (MD) were pooled using a random effect model by the Cochrane software package Review Manager 5.1.

Findings: 30 studies including 2160 subjects met the objectives and were included in the meta-analyses. HP regimens resulted in a significantly more pronounced increase in glomerular filtration rate [MD: 7.18 ml/min/1.73 m^2, 95% CI 4.45 to 9.91, p<0.001], serum urea [MD: 1.75 mmol/l, 95% CI 1.13 to 237, p<0.001], and urinary calcium excretion [MD: 25.43 mg/24h, 95% CI 13.62 to 37.24, p<0.001] when compared to the respective LP/NP protocol.

Conclusion: HP diets were associated with increased GFR, serum urea, urinary calcium excretion, and serum concentrations of uric acid. In the light of the high risk of kidney disease among obese, weight reduction programs recommending HP diets especially from animal sources should be handled with caution.

Editor: Jeff M. Sands, Emory University, United States of America

Funding: The authors have no support or funding to report.

Competing Interests: The authors have declared that no competing interests exist.

* E-mail: lukas.schwingshackl@univie.ac.at

Introduction

In face of the worldwide increase in prevalence of obesity, a large number of dietary measures aiming at weight reduction of weight management have been described. These diets differ mainly with respect to macronutrient composition, and among them, a high protein (HP) regimen has gained interest in recent years. However, there is inconsistent data regarding the potential beneficial or detrimental effects of HP diets on parameters of obesity as well as its associated risks. While HP protocols were reported to be advantageous when compared to their low/normal protein counterparts in short-term trials [1], no such benefits on outcome markers of obesity, cardiovascular disease or glycemic control could be reported in a recent meta-analysis investigating long-term interventions [2]. In 2002, the Institute of Medicine published an acceptable macronutrient distribution range (AMDR) for protein of 5–35% of daily calories (depending on age), with a special emphasis that there is insufficient data on the long-term safety of the upper limit of this range [3]. A major concern in relation to potential deleterious effects of HP diets is the increased risk of renal dysfunction [4,5]. High protein intake is regarded to be a trigger of renal hyperfiltration and may therefore cause renal damage [6]. In animal and human studies, HP consumption has been found to accelerate chronic kidney disease (CKD), raise albuminuria and diuresis, natriuresis, and kaliuresis [7]. Epidemiological data from the Nurses' Health study showed that high intake of non-dairy animal protein may accelerate renal dysfunction in women with an already established mild renal insufficiency (glomerular filtration rate (GFR) <80 ml/min/1.73 m^2), while HP intake was not associated with a decline in regular renal function in women (initial GFR values > 80 ml/min/1.73 m^2) [8]. In a long-term study in pigs, an HP diets (35% of total energy consumption, TEC) resulted in enlarged kidneys accompanied by histological damage as well as renal and glomerular volumes being 60–70% higher when compared to control animals (protein intake = 15% of TEC) [9]. Moreover, risk of kidney stone formation due to high urinary calcium excretion was increased in healthy subjects following an HP dietary protocol for 6 weeks [10]. In contrast to these findings, a 2-year trial in non-diabetic obese individuals reported that an HP diet was not associated with harmful effects on GFR, urinary albumin excretion, or fluid and electrolyte balance compared with a NP diet [11]. However, evidence indicates that obesity itself may accelerate the progression of CKD, induced by pathophysiological mechanism such glomerular hyperfiltration/hypertrophy caused by the raised metabolic needs of the obese individual [12]. In addition, due to the National Health and Nutrition Examination Survey III (NHANES) data, approximately 30% of the US population feature characteristics of reduced kidney function (GFR $= 60$–89 ml/min/1.73 m^2) increasing with age > 40 years [13]. Regarding the increased prevalence of overweight and obesity in this age group, HP diets might thus not represent a reasonable tool in weight management programs even for subjects without an established kidney dysfunction. Therefore, it was the aim of the present systematic review to examine the effects of HP versus LP/NP diets on parameters of renal function in adult subjects. To the best of our knowledge, this is the first meta-analysis performed to investigate the effects of HP diets on outcomes of renal function in subjects without CKD (GFR $\geq$ 60 ml/min/1.73 m^2).

Methods

Data Sources and Searches

Queries of literature were performed using the electronic databases MEDLINE (until 27th February 2014), EMBASE (until 27th February 2014), and the Cochrane Trial Register (until 27th February 2014) with restrictions to randomized controlled trials, but no restrictions to language and calendar date using the following search term: *("protein")* AND *("renal" OR "kidney" OR "glomerular filtration" OR "creatinine" OR "urea" OR "albumin" OR "calcium")*. Moreover, the reference lists from retrieved articles were checked to search for further relevant studies. This systematic review was planned, conducted, and reported in adherence to standards of quality for reporting meta-analyses [14]. Literature search was conducted independently by both authors, with disagreements resolved by consensus.

Study Selection

Studies were included in the meta-analysis if they met all of the following criteria: *(i)* randomized controlled or cross-over design; *(ii)* minimum intervention period of 1 week; *(iii)* comparing a HP dietary intervention with a NP/LP intervention (using a 5% difference in total energy intake, as defined previously by Santesso et al. 2012 [1]) that were designed for weight loss or not; *(iv)* age: $\geq$ 18 years; *(v)* sample size: healthy, overweight, obese, type 2 diabetes (T2D); *(vi)* assessment of the "outcome of interest" markers: GFR, serum creatinine, serum urea, urinary calcium excretion, urinary albumin excretion, serum uric acid, urinary pH; *(vii)* report of post-intervention mean values (if not available, change from baseline values were used) with standard deviation (or basic data to calculate these parameters: standard error, 95% confidence interval, p-values). If data of ongoing studies were published as updates, results of only the longest duration periods were included. Studies enrolling subjects with CKD (GFR $<$ 60 ml/min/1.73 m^2), type 1 diabetes, and macroalbuminuria were excluded. Trials were included if subjects had microalbuminuria, since data from the NHANES III indicated that 12% of the included population suffered from microalbminuria, whereas only 1.5% had macroalbuminuria [15].

Data Extraction and Quality Assessment

The risk of bias assessment tool by the Cochrane Collaboration was applied specifying the following bias domains: selection bias (random sequence generation, allocation concealment), performance/detection bias (blinding of participants and personnel/blinding of outcome assessment), attrition bias (incomplete data outcome), and reporting bias (selective reporting) [16] (Figure S1).

The following data were extracted from each study: the first author's last name, year of publication, study length, gender distribution and age, BMI, % diabetics, sample size, protein intake (% of total energy content, TEC or g $*$ kg body weight^{-1} $*$ d^{-1}), protein origin, calcium intake, energy content of HP and NP/LP diets, outcomes and post mean values or differences in mean of two time point values with corresponding standard deviation.

Data Synthesis and Analysis

For each outcome measure of interest, a meta-analysis was performed in order to determine the pooled effect of the intervention in terms of weighted mean differences (MDs) between the post-intervention (or change from baseline) values of the HP and NP/LP groups. Combining both the post-intervention values and difference in means in one meta-analysis is an accepted method described by the Cochrane Collaboration [17]. All data were analyzed using the REVIEW MANAGER software provided by the Cochrane Collaboration (http://ims.cochrane.org/revman). The random-effects model was used to estimate MDs with 95% confidence intervals (CIs). Forest plots were generated to illustrate the study-specific effect sizes along with a 95% CI. Heterogeneity between trial results was tested with a standard χ^2 test. The I^2 parameter was used to quantify any inconsistency: $I^2 = [(Q - d.f.)]/Q \times 100\%$, where Q is the χ^2 statistic and d.f. is its degrees of freedom. A value for I^2 greater than $\geq$ 75% was considered to indicate considerable heterogeneity [18]. Funnel plots were sketched to indicate potential publication bias (e.g. the tendency for studies yielding statistically significant results to be more likely to be submitted and accepted for publication). To evaluate substantial heterogeneity, several post hoc univariate random-effects meta-regressions were performed to examine the association between age, BMI, study length, and % protein intake as independent variables, and changes in GFR, creatinine, urea, and pH (were substantial heterogeneity could be detected) as depending variables, respectively. The p-*values* for differences in effects between the covariates were obtained using the *metareg* command of Stata 12.0 (Stata-Corp, College Station, TX. USA). Two sided p-*values* <0.05 were considered to be statistically significant. To determine the presence of publication bias, the symmetry of the funnel plots in which mean differences were plotted against their corresponding standard errors were assessed.

Results

Literature Search

A total of 30 trials (32 reports) extracted from 15734 articles met the inclusion criteria and were analyzed in the systematic review (References S1). The detailed steps of the meta-analysis article selection process are given as a flow chart in Figure S2. Although in accordance with the overall inclusion criteria, one trial was excluded due to inconsistencies in the mean GFR ($\leq$60 ml/min/1.73 m^2 in 45% of the study population), which was considered to increase the potential for selection bias (Figure S1) [19].

Characteristics of Studies and Participants

All studies included in this systematic review were RCTs with a duration ranging between 1 week and 24 months, published between 1993 and 2013, and enrolling a total of 2160 participants. All studies compared a HP diet to a NP/LP regimen. The mean age of participants varied between 22.3 and 67 years. Protein intakes in the HP groups were mostly of animal origin except for one trial, where wheat gluten protein was used [20]. General study characteristics are given in Table 1.

Table 1. Characteristics of the included studies in the meta-analyses.

References (References S1)	Sample size	Mean baseline BMI (kg/m²) / % diabetics	Mean age (yrs) / Female, %	Duration (weeks)	Study design	Protein (g * kg body weight⁻¹ * d⁻¹, % of TEC)	Protein sources in the HP group	Calcium (mg/d)	Daily energy (kcal)	Microalbuminuria	GFR- measurement
Brinkworth et al. 2004	58		50.2	68	RCT	HP: 30%	30 g skim milk powder, 60 g low-fat cheese, 200 g diet yogurt, 200 g lean meat or poultry, 250 ml low-fat milk	n.d	12-week energy restricted		According to [46,47] (ml/min)
	34	0%	78%			NP/LP: 15%		n.d	12-week energy restricted		
Brinkworth et al. 2010	68		51.5	52	RCT	HP: 35%	125 ml milk, 70 g cheddar cheese, 1 egg, 300 g (raw weight) beef, chicken or fish, 100 g (cooked) ham, tuna, beef, turkey, chicken, 40 g raw unsalted nuts	n.d	1433–1672		Modification in renal disease study equation was used [48] (ml/min/1.73 m²)
	33.5	0%	64%			NP/LP: 24%		n.d	1433–1672		
Cao et al. 2011	16		56.9	7	Crossover	HP: 1.6 g; 20%	500 ml milk, 80 g ham, 120 g roast beef, 120 g baked chicken, 50 g steamed peas	865	Isocaloric		
	26.8	0%	100%			NP/LP: 0.8 g; 10%		907	Isocaloric		
Ferrara et al. 2006	15		26.4	24	RCT	HP: 1.9 g	Beaf, pork, ham, poultry	n.d	n.d		
	23.5	0%	0%			NP/LP: 1.3 g		n.d	n.d		
Frank et al. 2009	24		24.1	1	crossover	HP: 2.4 g; 26.6%; 21.7% (animal protein)	Animal sources including milk and milk products	n.d	2743		Assessed on the basis of sinistrin clearence (ml/min)

Table 1. Cont.

References (References S1)	Sample size / Mean baseline BMI (kg/m^2) / % diabetics	Mean age (yrs), / Female, %	Duration (weeks)	Study design	Protein ($g * kg$ body weight$^{-1} * d^{-1}$, % of TEC)	Protein sources in the HP group	Calcium (mg/d)	Daily energy (kcal)	Microalbuminuria	GFR- measurement
	BMI 22.3; Female 0%; 0% diabetics				NP/LP: 1.2 g; 13.3%; 7.4% (animal protein)		n.d	2736		
Friedman et al. 2012	307; BMI 36.1; 0% diabetics	45.5; 68%	104	RCT	HP: LC diet; NP/LP: 15%	Unlimited protein consumption	n.d	n.d; 1200–1500		Calculated by dividing the 24-hr urinary creatinine excretion (mg/d) by 1440 (min/d) and then dividing aigan by the serum creatinine (mg/dll) x100. (ml/min)
Gross et al. 2002	28; BMI 26.3; 100% diabetics	57.3; 25%	4	Crossover	HP: 1.4 g; NP/LP: 0.66 g	Chicken	712; 732	n.d	x	Measured using the [51] Cr-EDTA single-injection technique ($ml/min/1.73\ m^2$)
Jenkins et al. 2001	20; 26; 0% diabetics	55.6; 25%	4	Crossover	HP: 27.4%; 20.1% (vegetable protein); NP/LP: 15.6%; 8.2% (vegetable protein)	80 g wheat gluten protein (bread)	n.d	2764; 2835		Not described (ml/min)
Jesudason et al. 2013	45; BMI 36; 100% diabetics	60.9; 22%	12	RCT	HP: 30%; NP/LP: 20%	90–120 g/d	n.d	1435–1674; 1435–1674	x	Calculated from serum creatinine using the Modification of diet and renal disease study formula [49] ($ml/min/1.73\ m^2$)

Table 1. Cont.

References (References S1)	Sample size / Mean baseline BMI (kg/m²) / % diabetics	Mean age (yrs), Female, %	Duration (weeks)	Study design	Protein (g * kg body weight⁻¹ * d⁻¹, % of TEC)	Protein sources in the HP group	Calcium (mg/d)	Daily energy (kcal)	Microalbuminuria	GFR- measurement
Johnston et al. 2004	20	19–54	6	RCT	HP: 31.5%	Egg beater scramble with 28 g ham and 28 g cheese, 1 l milk, 84 open faced turkey, 28 g provolone, chicken chow mien dinner, peas and beans	1828	1700		Not described (ml/s/m²)
	28.9	90%			NP/LP: 15%		1187	1700		
	0%									
Juraschek et al. 2013	164	53.5	6	Cross-over	HP: 25%, 12.5%	Food sources used for protein replacement primarily were vegetable-based	n.d	n.d		eGFR was calculated using the CKD Epidemiology Collaboration cystatin C equation [43] (ml/min/1.73 m²)
	30.2	45%			NP/LP: 15%, 5.4%		n.d	n.d		
	0%									
Krebs et al. 2012	419	57.8	104	RCT	HP: 30%	n.d	n.d	-500	x	
	36.6	60%			NP/LP: 15%		n.d	-500		
	100%									
Larsen et al. 2011	99	59.4	52	RCT	HP: 30%	A combination of lean meat, chicken and fish	n.d	12-week energy restricted	x	Not described (ml/min/1.73 m²)
	27–40	52%			LP/NP: 15%		n.d	12-week energy restricted		
	100%									
Leidy et al. 2007	46	50	12	RCT	HP: 1.4 g; 30%	180 g cooked pork, loin, ham, or Canadian bacon	n.d	-750		Calculated from serum creatinine using the Modification of diet and renal disease study formula [49] (ml/min/1.73 m²)
	30.6	100%			NP/LP: 0.8 g; 18%		n.d	-750		
	0%									

Table 1. Cont.

References (References S1)	Sample size / Mean baseline BMI (kg/m²) / % diabetics	Mean age (yrs) / Female, %	Duration (weeks)	Study design	Protein (g * kg body weight⁻¹ * d⁻¹, % of TEC)	Protein sources in the HP group	Calcium (mg/d)	Daily energy (kcal)	Microalbuminuria	GFR-measurement
Li et al. 2010	100	49.3	52	RCT	HP: 2.2 g, 30%	Formula 1, Herbalife Intl, Los Angeles	n.d	~500		Not described (ml/min)
	34.5	66%			NP/LP: 1.1 g, 15%		n.d	~500		
	0%									
Liu et al. 2013	50	47.9	12	RCT	HP: LC diet	Boiled eggs 2 (ad libitum for snacks, Lactalbumin (15 g), Duck leg (220 g)	n.d	ad libitum		
	26.7	100%			NP/LP: 18%			1500		
	0%									
Luger et al. 2013	44	62.4	12	RCT	HP: 30%	Received data sheets referring to protein-rich foods: major high-protein sources included: soy-based foods, milk products, fish and poultry	n.d	1272	x	Calculated from serum creatinine using the Modification of diet and renal disease study formula [49] (ml/min/1.73 m²)
	33.3	55%			NP/LP: 15%		n.d	1235		
	100%									
Luscombe-Marsh et al. 2005	73	20-65	16	RCT	HP: 40%	400 ml skim milk, 40 g skim milk powder, 40 g low-fat cheese, 300 g meat, poultry or fish, 20 g almonds, 200 g low-fat artificially sweetened yogurt	n.d	12-week energy restricted		(urine creatinine concentration in mmol/l x urine volume in ml/1140 min/ plasma creatinine concentration in µmol/l ×1000 ml x min) ×0.7. (ml/min)
	27-40	65%			NP/LP: 20%		n.d	12-week energy restricted		
	0%									
Noakes et al. 2005	100	49.5	12	RCT	HP: 34%	250 ml milk, 200 g low-fat yogurt, 300 g lean meat, poultry or fish	777	1342		Not described (ml/min)
	32.5	100%			NP/LP: 17%		594	134		
	0%									

Table 1. Cont.

References (References S1)	Sample size	Mean baseline BMI (kg/m^2)	% diabetics	Mean age (yrs)	Female, %	Duration (weeks)	Study design	Protein (g * kg body weight^{-1} * d^{-1}, % of TEC)	Protein sources in the HP group	Calcium (mg/d)	Daily energy (kcal)	Microalbuminuria	GFR- measurement
Nuttall et al. 2003;Gannon et al. 2003	12	n.d	100%	n.d	17%	5	Crossover	HP: 30%	1 l low-fat milk, 113 g beef, 255 g baked chicken, 113 g low-fat cheese, 227 g low-fat yogurt	n.d	2235	x	
								NP/LP: 15%		n.d	2266		
Nuttall et al. 2006	8	31	100%	63	0%	5	Crossover	HP: 30%	124 g egg substitute, 56 g cheddar cheese, 226 g roasted ham, 85 g swiss cheese, 253 split pea soup, 170 g tuna, 80 g peas, 56 g dry-roasted peanuts	n.d	Isocaloric	x	
								NP/LP: 15%		n.d	Isocaloric		
Pomerleau et al. 1993	20	33	100%	58	33%	3	Crossover	HP: 1.9 g; 22%;	Supplements (casein, gelatin, vegetable proteins, yeast, and soy)	883	2182	x	^{99m}Technicum-DTPA (diethylenetriamine pentaacetic acid) plasma clearance (ml/s/1.73 m^2)
								NP/LP: 0.8 g; 10%		930	2110		
Roughead et al. 2003	15	26.5	0%	60.5	100%	8	Crossover	HP: 1.62 g; 20%	Pork, turkey breast, beef round, ham, chicken breast	596	2296		Calculated from serum and urinary creatinine, which were measured using alkaline picric acid (ml/s)
								NP/LP: 0.94 g; 12%		617	2296		
Sargrad et al. 2005	12	34.5	100%	47.5	75%	8	RCT	HP: 30%	Chicken, fish, eggs, low-fat milk, cheeses, nuts	567	1275	n.d	
								NP/LP: 15%		521	1371		

Table 1. Cont.

References (References S1)	Sample size / Mean baseline BMI (kg/m²) / % diabetics	Mean age (yrs), Female, %	Duration (weeks)	Study design	Protein (g * kg body weight⁻¹ * d⁻¹, % of TEC)	Protein sources in the HP group	Calcium (mg/d)	Daily energy (kcal)	Microalbuminuria	GFR- measurement
Skov et al. 1999	50	39.6	24	RCT	HP: 25%	Dairy products and meat, the latter represented by both beef, pork, poultry, lamb	n.d	ad libitum		Measured using the ⁵¹Cr-EDTA single-injection technique (ml/min)
	30.4	76%			NP/LP: 12%		n.d	ad libitum		
	0%									
Stern et al. 2004	132	53.5	12	RCT	HP: LC diet	Unlimited: meat, fowl, fish, shellfish, eggs, 110 g hard cheese	n.d	−500		
	42.9	17%			NP/LP: 15%		n.d	no		
	41%									
Velázquez Lopez et al. 2008	41	67	4	RCT	HP: 1–1.2 g	n.d	n.d	isocaloric	x	Assessed using creatinine-clearance estimation by the Cockroft and Gault formula [50] (ml/min)
	26.82	65%			NP/LP: 0.6–0.8 g		n.d	Isocaloric		
	100%									
Wagner et al. 2007	22	30.8–60.2	1	Crossover	HP: 2 g	Meat, dairy products, and egg white powder	n.d	Isocaloric		Calculated from serum creatinine using the Modification of diet and renal disease study formula [49] (ml/min/1.73 m²)
	25.5	69%			NP/LP: 0.5 g		n.d	Isocaloric		
	0%									
Westman et al. 2008; Yancy et al. 2007	84	51.8	24	RCT	HP: VLC diet	Unlimited: meat, fowl, fish, shellfish, eggs, 120 g hard cheese; 60 g fresh cheese	n.d	ad libitum	x	
	38	78%			NP/LP: 15%		n.d	−500		
	100%									

Table 1. Cont.

References (References S1)	Sample size	Mean baseline BMI (kg/m²) / % diabetics	Mean age (yrs), Female, %	Duration (weeks)	Study design	Protein (g * kg body weight⁻¹ * d⁻¹, % of TEC)	Protein sources in the HP group	Calcium (mg/d)	Daily energy (kcal)	Microalbuminuria	GFR- measurement
Wycherley et al. 2012	68		50.8	52	RCT	HP: 35%	3 serves low-fat dairy, 300 g lean red meat, 100 deli-scliced meat/ canned fish	n.d	1680		According to [51] (ml/ min/1.73 m²)
	33	0%	0%			LP: 17%		n.d	1680		

BMI, Body-Mass-Index; CKD, chronic kidney disease; HP, high protein; n.d, no data; NP/LP, normal/low protein; RCT, randomized controlled trial; VLC, very-low carbohydrate.

Outcomes

The pooled estimates of effect size for the effects of HP as compared to NP/LP on outcomes of kidney function are summarized in Table 2. Changes in serum creatinine (Figure S3), urinary albumin excretion (Figure S5), uric acid (Figure S4), and urinary pH (Figure S7) were not significantly different following HP diets as compared to NP/LP diets and are given as Supplementary material.

HP diets were associated with a significantly more pronounced increase in GFR as compared to NP/LP protocols [MD: 7.18 ml/ min/1.73 m² (95% CI 4.45 to 9.91), p<0.001] (Figure 1). Serum urea [MD: 1.75 mmol/l (95% CI 1.13 to 2.37), p<0.001] (Figure 2) and urinary calcium excretion [MD: 25.43 mg/24h (95% CI 13.62 to 37.24), p<0.001] (Figure S6) were significantly more increased by HP diets in comparison to the NP/LP settings, respectively.

Sensitivity Analyses

Including RCTs investigating only subjects without T2D (18 trials) confirmed the results or the primary meta-analysis (Table S1). Furthermore, with the exception of urinary pH (only 1 trial) and urinary calcium excretion (5 trials), the main results could be confirmed when including only obese subjects (20 trials) (Table S2). Similar observations could be made for long-term trials (≥ 12 weeks, 17 trials) (Table S3). Sensitivity analysis including only T2D subjects resulted in similar observations (Table S4). Following exclusion of the trial by Jenkins et al. [20] (being the only RCT not using animal protein as a source for supplementations in HP protocols), HP diets resulted in a significantly more pronounced increase in uric acid as compared to NP/LP protocols.

Publication Bias

The funnel plots (with respect to effect size changes for markers of kidney health in response to HP diets, respectively) indicates little to moderate asymmetry, suggesting that publication bias cannot be completely excluded as a factor of influence on the present meta-analysis (Figure S8-S14). It remains possible that small studies yielding inconclusive data have not been published or failed to do so.

Heterogeneity

Considerable heterogeneity was found with respect to serum urea ($I^2 = 88\%$), urinary pH ($I^2 = 95\%$), and urinary calcium excretion ($I^2 = 90\%$) (Table 2). It was assumed that high heterogeneity might be explained by non-uniform study characteristics in the high protein groups such as variations in age, BMI, study length, and protein intake. To gain insight into these potential correlations, a random-effects meta-regression was performed to examine the associations between HP and NP/LP group parameters and changes in GFR, serum creatinine, serum urea, uric acid, urinary albumin, and urinary pH, respectively. A statistically significant dose-response relationship could be detected between protein intake and increases in serum urea (p = 0.023) No such correlations could be detected between the other study characteristics and parameters mentioned.

Discussion

It was the aim of the present meta-analysis to investigate the impact of HP vs. LP/NP diets on parameters of kidney function in subjects without an established CKD. The main findings suggest that subjects following an HP diet presented themselves with increased GFR, serum urea, and urinary calcium excretion, respectively. Further increases in serum concentrations of uric acid

Table 2. Pooled estimates of effect size (95% confidence intervals) expressed as weighted mean difference for the effects of HP vs. NP/LP diets on outcomes of renal function.

Outcomes	No. of Studies	Sample size	MD	95% CI	p-values	Inconsistency I^2
GFR (ml/min/1.73 m²)	21	1599	7.18	[4.45, 9.91]	<0.001	52%
Creatinine (μmol/l)	22	1764	−1.42	[−3.50, 0.65]	0.18	57%
Urea (mmol/l)	13	910	1.75	[1.13, 2.37]	<0.001	88%
Uric acid (μmol/l)	8	295	0.18	[−0.08, 0.44]	0.17	3%
Urinary pH	7	210	−0.39	[−0.82, 0.03]	0.07	95%
Urinary Albumin/Protein (mg/24h)	11	783	0.50	[−2.83, 3.82]	0.77	63%
Urinary calcium excretion (mg/24h)	10	708	25.43	[13.62, 37.24]	<0.001	90%

could be observed in those individuals following an HP regimen, when the trial by Jenkins et al. [20] was excluded from the analysis due to the fact, that it was the only study using vegetable protein exclusively as a supplement.

The choice of diet as a tool in weight management often includes variations in macronutrient composition differing from the regular recommendations of national as well as international authorities. Due to their proposed effects on thermogenesis and satiety, HP diets have gained increasing interest in recent years. The potential detrimental effects of HP diets on kidney function are still discussed controversially. In a long-term study in rats, feeding an HP diet (35% of TEC) resulted in a significant

reduction in body weight, however this was accompanied by 17% higher kidney weights, a 3-fold raise in proteinuria, larger glomeruli, and a 27% increase in creatinine clearance as compared to the NP (15% of TEC) feed rats, respectively [21]. Other detrimental effects of HP diets on kidney function include higher organ weight, and histologically detectable tissue damage [9]. Despite the limited transferability of results gained in animal experiments, pathophysiological side-effects of HP diets could appear in humans as well. At least in patients with established CKD, reducing protein intake decreases the occurrence of renal death by 32% when compared to higher/unrestricted protein intake [22]. Data of a meta-analysis investigating 17 cohort studies

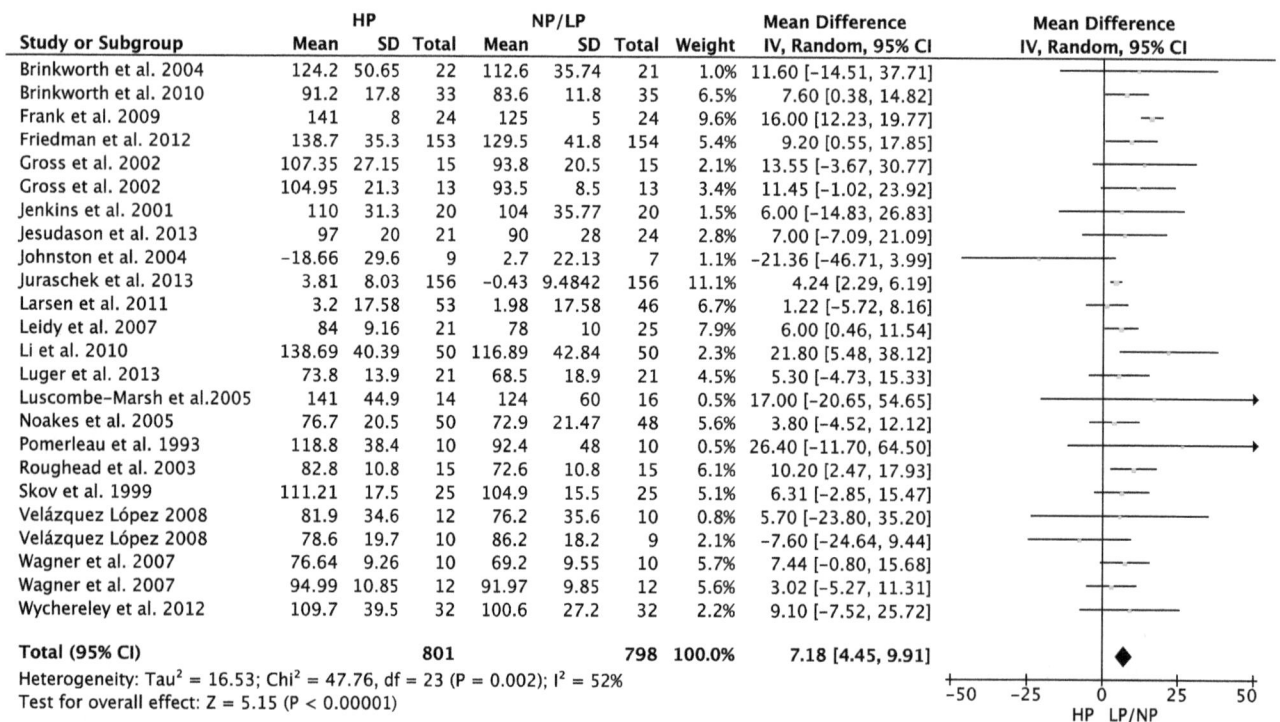

Study or Subgroup	HP Mean	HP SD	HP Total	NP/LP Mean	NP/LP SD	NP/LP Total	Weight	Mean Difference IV, Random, 95% CI
Brinkworth et al. 2004	124.2	50.65	22	112.6	35.74	21	1.0%	11.60 [−14.51, 37.71]
Brinkworth et al. 2010	91.2	17.8	33	83.6	11.8	35	6.5%	7.60 [0.38, 14.82]
Frank et al. 2009	141	8	24	125	5	24	9.6%	16.00 [12.23, 19.77]
Friedman et al. 2012	138.7	35.3	153	129.5	41.8	154	5.4%	9.20 [0.55, 17.85]
Gross et al. 2002	107.35	27.15	15	93.8	20.5	15	2.1%	13.55 [−3.67, 30.77]
Gross et al. 2002	104.95	21.3	13	93.5	8.5	13	3.4%	11.45 [−1.02, 23.92]
Jenkins et al. 2001	110	31.3	20	104	35.77	20	1.5%	6.00 [−14.83, 26.83]
Jesudason et al. 2013	97	20	21	90	28	24	2.8%	7.00 [−7.09, 21.09]
Johnston et al. 2004	−18.66	29.6	9	2.7	22.13	7	1.1%	−21.36 [−46.71, 3.99]
Juraschek et al. 2013	3.81	8.03	156	−0.43	9.4842	156	11.1%	4.24 [2.29, 6.19]
Larsen et al. 2011	3.2	17.58	53	1.98	17.58	46	6.7%	1.22 [−5.72, 8.16]
Leidy et al. 2007	84	9.16	21	78	10	25	7.9%	6.00 [0.46, 11.54]
Li et al. 2010	138.69	40.39	50	116.89	42.84	50	2.3%	21.80 [5.48, 38.12]
Luger et al. 2013	73.8	13.9	21	68.5	18.9	21	4.5%	5.30 [−4.73, 15.33]
Luscombe-Marsh et al.2005	141	44.9	14	124	60	16	0.5%	17.00 [−20.65, 54.65]
Noakes et al. 2005	76.7	20.5	50	72.9	21.47	48	5.6%	3.80 [−4.52, 12.12]
Pomerleau et al. 1993	118.8	38.4	10	92.4	48	10	0.5%	26.40 [−11.70, 64.50]
Roughead et al. 2003	82.8	10.8	15	72.6	10.8	15	6.1%	10.20 [2.47, 17.93]
Skov et al. 1999	111.21	17.5	25	104.9	15.5	25	5.1%	6.31 [−2.85, 15.47]
Velázquez López 2008	81.9	34.6	12	76.2	35.6	10	0.8%	5.70 [−23.80, 35.20]
Velázquez López 2008	78.6	19.7	10	86.2	18.2	9	2.1%	−7.60 [−24.64, 9.44]
Wagner et al. 2007	76.64	9.26	10	69.2	9.55	10	5.7%	7.44 [−0.80, 15.68]
Wagner et al. 2007	94.99	10.85	12	91.97	9.85	12	5.6%	3.02 [−5.27, 11.31]
Wychereley et al. 2012	109.7	39.5	32	100.6	27.2	32	2.2%	9.10 [−7.52, 25.72]
Total (95% CI)			**801**			**798**	**100.0%**	**7.18 [4.45, 9.91]**

Heterogeneity: Tau² = 16.53; Chi² = 47.76, df = 23 (P = 0.002); I² = 52%
Test for overall effect: Z = 5.15 (P < 0.00001)

Mean Difference IV, Random, 95% CI

−50 −25 0 25 50
HP LP/NP

Figure 1. Forest plot showing pooled MD with 95% CI for glomerular filtration rate (ml/min/1.73 m²) of 21 randomized controlled HP diet trails. For each high protein study, the shaded square represents the point estimate of the intervention effect. The horizontal line joins the lower and upper limits of the 95% CI of these effects. The area of the shaded square reflects the relative weight of the study in the respective meta-analysis. The diamond at the bottom of the graph represents the pooled MD with the 95% CI. HP, high protein; NP/LP, normal protein/low protein.

Study or Subgroup	HP Mean	SD	Total	NP/LP Mean	SD	Total	Weight	Mean Difference IV, Random, 95% CI	Mean Difference IV, Random, 95% CI
Frank et al. 2009	6.78	1.428	24	5	0.714	24	8.1%	1.78 [1.14, 2.42]	
Friedman et al. 2012	5.43	2.081	153	4.69	1.46	154	8.6%	0.74 [0.34, 1.14]	
Jenkins et al. 2001	8.54	2.1	20	6.16	1.38	20	7.0%	2.38 [1.28, 3.48]	
Johnston et al. 2004	0.82	1.5	9	-1.04	0.79	7	6.9%	1.86 [0.72, 3.00]	
Li et al. 2010	5.044	2.06	50	4.27	1.33	50	8.1%	0.77 [0.09, 1.45]	
Liu et al. 2013	6.6	1.5	25	5.7	0.97	24	8.0%	0.90 [0.20, 1.60]	
Noakes et al. 2005	6.2	1.41	50	5.1	1.38	48	8.3%	1.10 [0.55, 1.65]	
Pomerleau et al. 1993	7.2	3	10	4.5	1.4	10	4.5%	2.70 [0.65, 4.75]	
Sargard et al. 2005	5.71	2.62	6	6.43	3.5	6	2.3%	-0.72 [-4.22, 2.78]	
Skov et al. 1999	5.9	1.5	25	4.1	1	25	8.0%	1.80 [1.09, 2.51]	
Stern et al. 2004	6.1	1.8	44	5	1.8	43	7.9%	1.10 [0.34, 1.86]	
Wagner et al. 2007	7.56	1.099	10	3.07	0.44	10	7.9%	4.49 [3.76, 5.22]	
Wagner et al. 2007	5.38	1.22	12	2.29	0.46	12	7.9%	3.09 [2.35, 3.83]	
Yancy et al. 2007	6.21	1.71	27	4.89	1.93	12	6.5%	1.32 [0.05, 2.59]	
Total (95% CI)			**465**			**445**	**100.0%**	**1.75 [1.13, 2.37]**	

Heterogeneity: Tau² = 1.13; Chi² = 112.57, df = 13 (P < 0.00001); I² = 88%
Test for overall effect: Z = 5.52 (P < 0.00001)

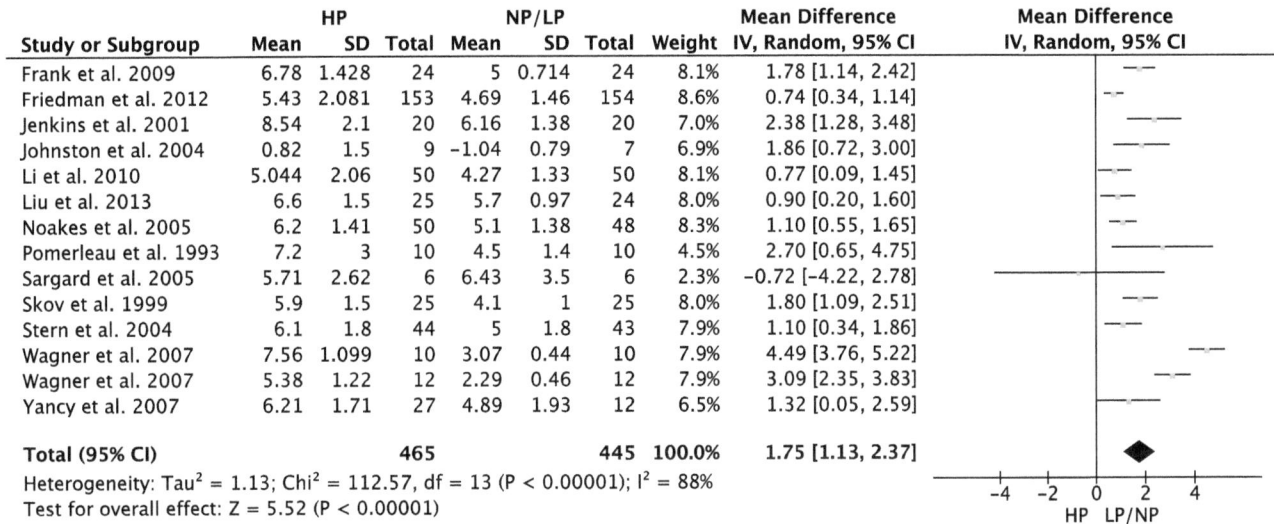

Figure 2. Forest plot showing pooled MD with 95% CI for serum urea (mmol/l) of 13 randomized controlled HP diet trails. For each high protein study, the shaded square represents the point estimate of the intervention effect. The horizontal line joins the lower and upper limits of the 95% CI of these effects. The area of the shaded square reflects the relative weight of the study in the respective meta-analysis. The diamond at the bottom of the graph represents the pooled MD with the 95% CI. HP, high protein; NP/LP, normal protein/low protein.

suggest that HP/lower carbohydrate intakes were associated with increased all-cause mortality [23].

Some 30 years ago, Brenner et al. [24] expressed the hypothesis that an increase in GFR and glomerular pressure might cause renal dysfunction and raise the risk for renal injury. Although this hypothesis could neither be validated nor refuted to date, one might argue that long-term HP intakes exert harmful effects on kidney function by causing renal hyperfiltration. Concerning the mechanism mediating the increased GFR, Frank et al. [25] hypothesized that protein load induces a vasodilatatory response leading to hyperemia. In a meta-analysis of 14 observational studies enrolling 105.872 participants, a GFR > 105 ml/min/1.73 m² was associated with an increased risk of all-cause mortality [26]. However, the authors of this study stated that their findings should be interpreted conservatively. Instead of being a pathophysiological reaction, HP-induced changes in kidney function such as the increase in GFR might as well represent a physiological adaptation process [27,28]. The capacity of the kidney to increase functional level with protein intake suggest a renal function reserve [29].

The raise in serum uric acid concentrations observed in the present meta-analysis in individuals following an HP diet was most likely probably caused by the higher intake of animal source foods rich in purines. Epidemiological data suggest that protein per se does not raise serum uric acid [30]. Among others, the Health Professionals Follow-up Study observed a 41% increase in the risk of first attack of gout when comparing the highest vs. lowest meat consumption quintile [31]. In addition to gout disorders, serum uric acid has been described as a modifiable risk factor for CVD and all-cause mortality in men and women [32,33]. From these data, one may conclude that the source of protein is of higher importance than its absolute amount. A 26-year follow up of the Nurses' Health Study (NHS) revealed that protein sources such as red meat and high-fat dairy products were significantly associated with an elevated risk of CHD, while higher intakes of poultry, fish, and nuts (although rich in protein as well) were correlated with a lower risk of CHD [34]. In contrast to these findings, Bernstein et al. [35] concluded that long-term consumption of high-protein diets may cause renal injury and accelerate the onset of CKD in persons with normal renal function independent of the fact, whether the protein food source is either predominantly animal or vegetable protein.

Reductions in urinary pH (p = 0.07) as observed in this meta-analysis for HP diets are regarded as an independent risk factor for nephrolithiasis [7]. In addition, HP intake raised urinary calcium excretion which is a common characteristic in patients with calcareous stones [36,37]. Impairment of calcium homeostasis might lead to a decrease in bone mineral density. However, clinical and epidemiological data do not support the concept that HP diets exert harmful effects on bone health.[1,38] Moreover, the differences observed in the present meta-analysis do not seem to be clinically relevant.

Two meta-analyses including observational studies showed that overweight, obesity and the metabolic syndrome increase the risk of kidney disease by 40 to 83% [39,40]. Considering that some two thirds the trials included in the present meta-analysis were enrolling obese subjects, it could be speculated that a high protein intake will add another detrimental factor to the increased risk of kidney dysfunction already established for this population. According to the recommendations of the American Diabetes Association, patients with T2D should not refer to HP diets as a means for weight loss due to the unknown long-term effects of protein intakes > 20% of TEC [41].

Limitations

Regarding the validity of the main outcome parameter GFR, the creatinine-based estimating equations used in the trials included in this systematic review are known to have some limitations with respect to precision as well as being affected by variations in protein intake, which might be further aggravated by the fact that the study population did not suffer from manifested chronic kidney disease. Thus, the GFR effects observed in the present meta-analysis have to be interpreted in a conservative manner, since increased creatinine values would translate into a lower estimated GFR [42]. A cross-sectional study by Inker et al. has shown that cystatin C might represent a more useful marker for estimating GFR especially when combined with creatinine [43]. Moreover, a post hoc analysis of the "Modification of Diet and Renal Disease" study (the origin of eGFR based on serum creatinine) has shown that dietary protein reduced the change in creatinine, but did not significantly affect cystatin C changes [44].

Other limitations of the present review include the limited number of studies and the heterogeneity of the study designs. Thus, this meta-analysis does not consider unpublished data. Examination of funnel plots showed little to moderate asymmetry suggesting that publication bias cannot be completely excluded as a confounder of the present meta-analysis (e.g. lack of published studies with inconclusive results) which may have had at least a moderate impact on the effect size estimates. A major limitation of nutritional intervention trials is the heterogeneity of various aspects and characteristics of the study protocols. Therefore, it is not surprising that the RCTs and crossover studies included in the present analyses varied regarding type(s) of diets used (energy restriction, isocaloric), definitions of HP and NP/LP diets, study population (i.e. age, sex, healthy, overweight, obese, type 2 diabetics), intervention time (1–108 weeks), as well as nutritional assessment. Following sensitivity analyses excluding only trials enrolling patients with T2D, the effect of HP diets on GFR remained the same as those observed in the conclusive analyses. With respect to other potential modulating variables, sensitivity analyses and meta-regressions failed to show any correlations between the findings of the meta-analyses and age, gender, BMI, and study duration and % protein intakes (data not shown). Only few studies provided information on the quality of their respective setup (e.g. method of randomization, follow-up protocol with reasons for withdrawal, see Figure S1 for Risk of bias assessment according to the Cochrane Collaboration) demanding a conservative interpretation of results. To estimate GFR heterogeneous equation were used (see Table 2). Moreover, the included trials varied with respect to dietary assessment methods to validate adherence of participants. In an HP dietary intervention study by Friedman et al. [11], significant increases in serum creatinine clearance were found after 3 and 12 months, but were not detectable anymore following a 24 month interval, indicating that adherence to the HP diet was not present at the end of the trial. In addition, Krebs et al. [45] could not measure significant differences in renal function at any time-point (6, 12, and 24 months) when comparing an HP with a LP regimen. Assessment of protein intakes revealed that the difference between the two groups did not exceed more than 2% of TEC suggesting a very low adherence to the dietary interventions. Therefore, adherence of individuals assigned to a HP diet might change over time. Although adherence is usually good in the short term, the long-term effects of HP vs. LP/NP diets are of higher interest. Augmentations of urinary calcium excretions found in the present meta-analysis in individuals following an HP diet might be interpreted as an adherence marker of HP diets. Some of the present meta-analyses were done using both post-intervention values and changes in mean difference, however, this was considered to be an acceptable procedure as described by the Cochrane Collaboration [17]. On the other hand, this meta-analysis has several strengths as well. All analyses were conducted following a stringent protocol, e.g. participants were randomly assigned to the intervention groups in all trials. Randomized controlled trials are considered to be the gold standard for evaluating the effects of an intervention and are subject to fewer biases as compared to observational studies. With a sample size of 2160 volunteers, the present meta-analysis provides the power to detect statistically significant mean differences as well as to assess publication bias.

In conclusion, HP diets were associated with increased GFR, serum urea, urinary calcium excretion, and serum concentrations of uric acid. Most of these changes could be interpreted as physiological adaptive mechanism induced by HP diet without any clinical relevance. However, considering of the fact that subclinical CKD is highly prevalent, and that obesity is associated with kidney disease, weight reduction programs recommending HP diets especially from animal sources should be handled with caution.

Supporting Information

Figure S1   Risk of bias assessment tool.

Figure S2   Flow chart.

Figure S3   Forest plot showing pooled MD with 95% CI for serum creatinine.

Figure S4   Forest plot showing pooled MD with 95% CI for serum uric acid.

Figure S5   Forest plot showing pooled MD with 95% CI for urinary albumin/protein excretion.

Figure S6   Forest plot showing pooled MD with 95% CI for urinary calcium excretion.

Figure S7   Forest plot showing pooled MD with 95% CI for urinary pH.

Figure S8   Funnel plot: glomerular filtration rate.

Figure S9   Funnel plot: serum creatinine.

Figure S10   Funnel plot: serum urea.

Figure S11   Funnel plot: serum uric acid.

Figure S12   Funnel plot: urinary pH.

Figure S13   Funnel plot: urinary albumin/protein excretion.

Figure S14   Funnel plot: urinary calcium excretion.

Table S1   Sensitivity analysis for subjects without T2D.

Table S2   Sensitivity analysis for obese subjects.

Table S3   Sensitivity analysis for long-term studies (≥12 weeks).

Table S4   Sensitivity analysis for T2D subjects.

Comparison of High vs. Normal/Low Protein Diets on Renal Function in Subjects without Chronic Kidney...

37

Checklist S1 PRISMA checklist.

Author Contributions

Conceived and designed the experiments: LS GH. Performed the experiments: LS GH. Analyzed the data: LS GH. Contributed reagents/materials/analysis tools: LS GH. Contributed to the writing of the manuscript: LS GH.

References

1. Santesso N, Akl EA, Bianchi M, Mente A, Mustafa R, et al. (2012) Effects of higher- versus lower-protein diets on health outcomes: a systematic review and meta-analysis. Eur J Clin Nutr 66: 780–788.

2. Schwingshackl L, Hoffmann G (2013) Long-term effects of low-fat diets either low or high in protein on cardiovascular and metabolic risk factors: a systematic review and meta-analysis. Nutr J 12: 48.

3. Food and Nutrition Board IoM (2002) Dietary reference intakes for energy, carbohydrates, fiber, fatty acids, cholesterol, protein, and amino acids (macronutrients). In: Washington DNAP, editor. pp. 207–264.

4. Adam-Perrot A, Clifton P, Brouns F (2006) Low-carbohydrate diets: nutritional and physiological aspects. Obes Rev 7: 49–58.

5. Crowe TC (2005) Safety of low-carbohydrate diets. Obes Rev 6: 235–245.

6. Brenner BM, Lawler EV, Mackenzie HS (1996) The hyperfiltration theory: a paradigm shift in nephrology. Kidney Int 49: 1774–1777.

7. Friedman AN (2004) High-protein diets: potential effects on the kidney in renal health and disease. Am J Kidney Dis 44: 950–962.

8. Knight EL, Stampfer MJ, Hankinson SE, Spiegelman D, Curhan GC (2003) The impact of protein intake on renal function decline in women with normal renal function or mild renal insufficiency. Ann Intern Med 138: 460–467.

9. Jia Y, Hwang SY, House JD, Ogborn MR, Weiler HA, et al. (2010) Long-term high intake of whole proteins results in renal damage in pigs. J Nutr 140: 1646–1652.

10. Reddy ST, Wang CY, Sakhaee K, Brinkley L, Pak CY (2002) Effect of low-carbohydrate high-protein diets on acid-base balance, stone-forming propensity, and calcium metabolism. Am J Kidney Dis 40: 265–274.

11. Friedman AN, Ogden LG, Foster GD, Klein S, Stein R, et al. (2012) Comparative effects of low-carbohydrate high-protein versus low-fat diets on the kidney. Clin J Am Soc Nephrol 7: 1103–1111.

12. Griffin KA, Kramer H, Bidani AK (2008) Adverse renal consequences of obesity. Am J Physiol Renal Physiol 294: F685–696.

13. Coresh J, Astor BC, Greene T, Eknoyan G, Levey AS (2003) Prevalence of chronic kidney disease and decreased kidney function in the adult US population: Third National Health and Nutrition Examination Survey. Am J Kidney Dis 41: 1–12.

14. Moher D, Liberati A, Tetzlaff J, Altman DG (2009) Preferred reporting items for systematic reviews and meta-analyses: the PRISMA statement. PLoS Med 6: e1000097.

15. Snyder JJ, Foley RN, Collins AJ (2009) Prevalence of CKD in the United States: a sensitivity analysis using the National Health and Nutrition Examination Survey (NHANES) 1999–2004. Am J Kidney Dis 53: 218–228.

16. Higgins JP, Altman DG, Gotzsche PC, Juni P, Moher D, et al. (2011) The Cochrane Collaboration's tool for assessing risk of bias in randomised trials. BMJ 343: d5928.

17. Higgins JP, Green S (updated March 2011) Cochrane Handbook of systematic reviews, Version 5.1.0

18. Higgins JP, Thompson SG, Deeks JJ, Altman DG (2003) Measuring inconsistency in meta-analyses. BMJ 327: 557–560.

19. Tirosh A, Golan R, Harman-Boehm I, Henkin Y, Schwarzfuchs D, et al. (2013) Renal Function Following Three Distinct Weight Loss Dietary Strategies During 2 Years of Randomized Controlled Trial. Diabetes Care.

20. Jenkins DJ, Kendall CW, Vidgen E, Augustin LS, van Erk M, et al. (2001) High-protein diets in hyperlipidemia: effect of wheat gluten on serum lipids, uric acid, and renal function. Am J Clin Nutr 74: 57–63.

21. Wakefield AP, House JD, Ogborn MR, Weiler HA, Aukema HM (2011) A diet with 35% of energy from protein leads to kidney damage in female Sprague-Dawley rats. Br J Nutr 106: 656–663.

22. Fouque D, Laville M (2009) Low protein diets for chronic kidney disease in non diabetic adults. Cochrane Database Syst Rev: CD001892.

23. Noto H, Goto A, Tsujimoto T, Noda M (2013) Low-carbohydrate diets and all-cause mortality: a systematic review and meta-analysis of observational studies. PLoS One 8: e55030.

24. Brenner BM, Meyer TW, Hostetter TH (1982) Dietary protein intake and the progressive nature of kidney disease: the role of hemodynamically mediated glomerular injury in the pathogenesis of progressive glomerular sclerosis in aging, renal ablation, and intrinsic renal disease. N Engl J Med 307: 652–659.

25. Frank H, Graf J, Amann-Gassner U, Bratke R, Daniel H, et al. (2009) Effect of short-term high-protein compared with normal-protein diets on renal hemodynamics and associated variables in healthy young men. Am J Clin Nutr 90: 1509–1516.

26. Matsushita K, van der Velde M, Astor BC, Woodward M, Levey AS, et al. (2010) Association of estimated glomerular filtration rate and albuminuria with all-cause and cardiovascular mortality in general population cohorts: a collaborative meta-analysis. Lancet 375: 2073–2081.

27. Martin WF, Armstrong LE, Rodriguez NR (2005) Dietary protein intake and renal function. Nutr Metab (Lond) 2: 25.

28. Fliser D, Ritz E, Franek E (1995) Renal reserve in the elderly. Semin Nephrol 15: 463–467.

29. Bosch JP, Saccaggi A, Lauer A, Ronco C, Belledonne M, et al. (1983) Renal functional reserve in humans. Effect of protein intake on glomerular filtration rate. Am J Med 75: 943–950.

30. Choi HK, Liu S, Curhan G (2005) Intake of purine-rich foods, protein, and dairy products and relationship to serum levels of uric acid: the Third National Health and Nutrition Examination Survey. Arthritis Rheum 52: 283–289.

31. Choi HK, Atkinson K, Karlson EW, Willett W, Curhan G (2004) Purine-rich foods, dairy and protein intake, and the risk of gout in men. N Engl J Med 350: 1093–1103.

32. Niskanen LK, Laaksonen DE, Nyyssonen K, Alfthan G, Lakka HM, et al. (2004) Uric acid level as a risk factor for cardiovascular and all-cause mortality in middle-aged men: a prospective cohort study. Arch Intern Med 164: 1546–1551.

33. Kim SY, Guevara JP, Kim KM, Choi HK, Heitjan DF, et al. (2010) Hyperuricemia and coronary heart disease: a systematic review and meta-analysis. Arthritis Care Res (Hoboken) 62: 170–180.

34. Bernstein AM, Sun Q, Hu FB, Stampfer MJ, Manson JE, et al. (2010) Major dietary protein sources and risk of coronary heart disease in women. Circulation 122: 876–883.

35. Bernstein AM, Treyzon L, Li Z (2007) Are high-protein, vegetable-based diets safe for kidney function? A review of the literature. J Am Diet Assoc 107: 644–650.

36. Parmar MS (2004) Kidney stones. BMJ 328: 1420–1424.

37. Cao JJ, Johnson LK, Hunt JR (2011) A diet high in meat protein and potential renal acid load increases fractional calcium absorption and urinary calcium excretion without affecting markers of bone resorption or formation in postmenopausal women. J Nutr 141: 391–397.

38. Calvez J, Poupin N, Chesneau C, Lassale C, Tome D (2012) Protein intake, calcium balance and health consequences. Eur J Clin Nutr 66: 281–295.

39. Wang Y, Chen X, Song Y, Caballero B, Cheskin LJ (2008) Association between obesity and kidney disease: a systematic review and meta-analysis. Kidney Int 73: 19–33.

40. Thomas G, Sehgal AR, Kashyap SR, Srinivas TR, Kirwan JP, et al. (2011) Metabolic syndrome and kidney disease: a systematic review and meta-analysis. Clin J Am Soc Nephrol 6: 2364–2373.

41. Bantle JP, Wylie-Rosett J, Albright AL, Apovian CM, Clark NG, et al. (2008) Nutrition recommendations and interventions for diabetes: a position statement of the American Diabetes Association. Diabetes Care 31 Suppl 1: S61–78.

42. Levey AS, Bosch JP, Lewis JB, Greene T, Rogers N, et al. (1999) A more accurate method to estimate glomerular filtration rate from serum creatinine: a new prediction equation. Modification of Diet in Renal Disease Study Group. Ann Intern Med 130: 461–470.

43. Inker LA, Schmid CH, Tighiouart H, Eckfeldt JH, Feldman HI, et al. (2012) Estimating glomerular filtration rate from serum creatinine and cystatin C. N Engl J Med 367: 20–29.

44. Tangri N, Stevens LA, Schmid CH, Zhang YL, Beck GJ, et al. (2011) Changes in dietary protein intake has no effect on serum cystatin C levels independent of the glomerular filtration rate. Kidney Int 79: 471–477.

45. Krebs JD, Elley CR, Parry-Strong A, Lunt H, Drury PL, et al. (2012) The Diabetes Excess Weight Loss (DEWL) Trial: a randomised controlled trial of high-protein versus high-carbohydrate diets over 2 years in type 2 diabetes. Diabetologia 55: 905–914.

46. Hallynck TH, Soep HH, Thomis JA, Boelaert J, Daneels R, et al. (1981) Should clearance be normalised to body surface or to lean body mass? Br J Clin Pharmacol 11: 523–526.

47. Skov AR, Toubro S, Bulow J, Krabbe K, Parving HH, et al. (1999) Changes in renal function during weight loss induced by high vs low-protein low-fat diets in overweight subjects. Int J Obes Relat Metab Disord 23: 1170–1177.

48. Gross JL, de Azevedo MJ, Silveiro SP, Canani LH, Caramori ML, et al. (2005) Diabetic nephropathy: diagnosis, prevention, and treatment. Diabetes Care 28: 164–176.

49. Levey AS, Greene T, Beck GJ, Caggiula AW, Kusek JW, et al. (1999) Dietary protein restriction and the progression of chronic renal disease: what have all of the results of the MDRD study shown? Modification of Diet in Renal Disease Study group. J Am Soc Nephrol 10: 2426–2439.

50. Kesteloot H, Joossens JV (1996) On the determinants of the creatinine clearance: a population study. J Hum Hypertens 10: 245–249.

51. Du Bois D, Du Bois EF (1989) A formula to estimate the approximate surface area if height and weight be known. 1916. Nutrition 5: 303–311; discussion 312–303.

5

Estimated Glomerular Filtration Rate Decline Is a Better Risk Factor for Outcomes of Systemic Disease-Related Nephropathy than for Outcomes of Primary Renal Diseases

Shuo-Chun Weng[1,2,3§]**, Der-Cherng Tarng**[3,4,5§]**, Chyong-Mei Chen**[6]**, Chi-Hung Cheng**[2,7]**, Ming-Ju Wu**[2,3,8,9]**, Cheng-Hsu Chen**[2,9]**, Tung-Min Yu**[2]**, Kuo-Hsiung Shu**[2,8]* **on behalf of the CKDBHPDH investigators**

1 Center for Geriatrics and Gerontology, Taichung Veterans General Hospital, Taichung, Taiwan, 2 Division of Nephrology, Department of Internal Medicine, Taichung Veterans General Hospital, Taichung, Taiwan, 3 Institute of Clinical Medicine, National Yang-Ming University, Taipei, Taiwan, 4 Department and Institute of Physiology, National Yang-Ming University, Taipei, Taiwan, 5 Division of Nephrology, Department of Medicine and Immunology Research Center, Taipei Veterans General Hospital, Taipei, Taiwan, 6 Department of Statistics and Informatics Science, Providence University, Taichung, Taiwan, 7 Department of Biotechnology, HungKuang University, Taichung, Taiwan, 8 School of Medicine, Chung Shan Medical University, Taichung, Taiwan, 9 School of Medicine, College of Medicine, China Medical University, Taichung, Taiwan

Abstract

Background: Currently, the contribution of kidney function decline in renal and patient outcomes is unclear. There are few data on the associations of different etiologies of estimated glomerular filtration rate (eGFR) decline with outcomes in multidisciplinary care. The purpose of this investigation was to establish whether eGFR decline in patients with disease is an important risk factor for developing end-stage renal disease (ESRD) and death.

Methods: From December 1, 2001 to December 31, 2011, 5097 adults with chronic kidney disease (CKD) received biochemical tests, physical examinations, a pathological examination, and a comprehensive questionnaire. We used linear regression models and multivariate Cox proportional hazards model to examine the outcome of eGFR decline in renal diseases with different etiologies.

Results: Mean age was 68.1 ± 16.1 (standard deviation, SD) years, and 63.3% patients were male. In the studied cohort, 58.2% of the patients had systemic disease-related nephropathy (SDRN), 29.4% had primary renal diseases (PRDs), and 12.4% had other etiologies. The eGFR decline in SDRN had a significant association with dialysis in the Cox proportional hazards model [crude hazard ratio (HR) = 1.07, 95% confidence interval (CI), 1.04 to 1.10; adjusted HR 1.05, 95% CI, 1.02 to 1.08]. Diabetic nephropathy (DN) had the most severe eGFR decline in CKD stages 3, 4, and 5, and all contributed to the initiation of dialysis and death regardless of whether DN with or without eGFR decline was considered to be the cause. Although hypertensive nephropathy (HN) was related to significant acceleration of eGFR decline, it did not lead to poor outcome. There were still discrepancies between eGFR decline and outcomes in PRDs, hypertensive nephropathy, and lupus nephritis.

Conclusions: eGFR decline and CKD staging provide an informative guide for physicians to make proper clinical judgments in the treatment of CKD, especially SDRN. Poor control of the underlying systemic disease will thus lead to more rapid progression of SDRN.

Editor: Valquiria Bueno, UNIFESP Federal University of São Paulo, Brazil

Funding: The authors are very grateful for the study grants provided by TCVGH, Taiwan, R.O.C. (TCVGH-1003606A, TCVGH-1013602A, TCVGH-1023601A, CGG-TCVGH1020101-4.4), and Taipei Veterans General Hospital (V97S5-004, V98S5-002, V99S5-002, V100E4-003, V101E4-001), and the Ministry of Education, Taiwan, Aim for the Top University Plan. The funders had no role in study design, data collection and analysis, decision to publish, or preparation of the manuscript.

Competing Interests: The authors have declared that no competing interests exist.

* E-mail: khshu@vghtc.gov.tw

§ These authors contributed equally to this work.

Introduction

The prediction of need for dialysis and risk of death in chronic kidney disease (CKD) patients has been shown to underestimate the importance of the rate of decline in renal function [1–4]. Although global guidelines have been proposed for estimating the need for preventive services for dialysis, in practice, they might not have been used for those purposes. Renal function is affected by both intrinsic mechanisms of renal disease (e.g., impaired auto-regulation [5–6], renal micro-inflammation [7–8], or limited renal functional reserve [9]) and extrinsic factors, such as hemodynamic changes, diabetes mellitus, hypertension, cardiovascular diseases

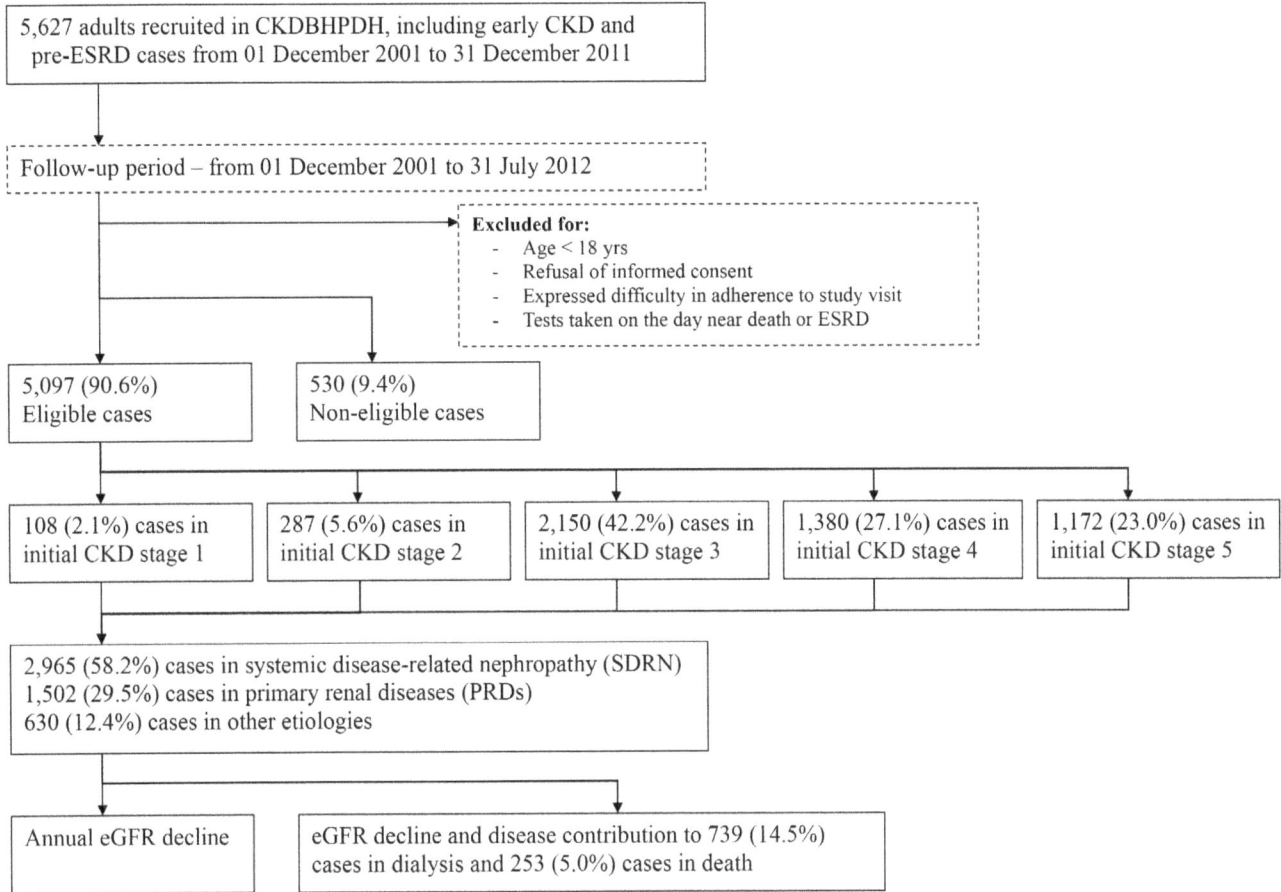

CKDBHPDH – case management care system of Chronic Kidney Disease Division of the Bureau of Health Promotion, Department of Health, R.O.C.

Figure 1. Study diagram of study cohort.

or medication [6]. Physiological decline in kidney occurs due to the aging process, with approximately 10% of eGFR and 10% of renal plasma flow lost per decade after age 40 [10].

Systemic disease-related nephropathy (SDRN) more specifically refers to renal manifestations of systemic disease. A huge variety of systemic conditions can affect the function of the kidneys, from acute illnesses (including, for example, prolonged hypotension) to drugs and more insidious illnesses [2,11,12]. The highest prevalence of secondary glomerular diseases was diabetic nephropathy (44.3%) in the United States and systemic lupus erythematous (54.3%) in China [11]. Primary renal diseases include most common forms of glomerulonephritis, tubulointerstitial diseases, and microvascular or infectious etiologies without diabetic nephropathy, hypertensive nephropathy, lupus nephritis, congestive heart failure, human immunodeficiency virus (HIV) infection, liver disease, and dysproteinemias [11,13,17,18]. It has been shown that extreme eGFR variation may occur in blacks with established CKD (from 1st percentile, -23.6 mL/min/ 1.73 m^2 per year to 99th percentile, 18.5 mL/min/1.73 m^2 per year), but annual change in eGFR was similar in all race groups with CKD (-3.7% to -4.3% per year) [3]. Biopsy-proved normo- and micro-albuminuric diabetic nephropathy ($-4.9 \sim -2.3$ ml/ min/1.73 m^2 per year) [14], and overt diabetic nephropathy (-3.8 ± 3.7 ml/min per 1.73 m^2 per year) were reported in an observational retrospective study [15]. Renal function rates in lupus nephritis (LN) stratified by average urine protein excretion

over time, i.e., 0–1, 1–2, and >2 g/day, respectively, were -1.15 ± 5.37, 0.32 ± 8.98, and -6.68 ± 14.6 ml/min per 1.73 m^2 per year [16]. For PRDs, the focal and segmental glomerulosclerosis (FSGS) displayed the highest incidence of ESRD (25.8%) and the fastest decline of eGFR (-4.6 ± 17.6 ml/min per 1.73 m^2 per year) [17]. The prognoses of SDRN and PRDs can be complicated by various modifiable risk factors, racial differences, glomerular hyperfiltration, interstitial fibrosis, tubular atrophy, and primitive etiologies [19]. However, relatively few studies have been conducted to establish whether the effects of different rates of eGFR decline, due to ordinary renal disease etiologies, on outcomes in the same cohort are dependent on SDRN and PRDs [14–20]. Therefore, in the present study, we investigated whether eGFR decline or diseases themselves have different pathological effects superimposed on physiological decline in the overall outcomes. Annual eGFR decline based on the coefficient of variation of the regression line is the most widely used method for estimation, and is used to show correlations with distinct histopathology and clinical diagnosis of CKD [1–6].

In this study, we investigated the effect of eGFR decline on the outcomes of different disease etiologies by conducting a prospective cohort study. The subjects were mostly middle-aged. We hypothesized that eGFR decline in patients with disease is an important risk factor for developing ESRD and death in cause-specific groups.

Materials and Methods

Study Population

Using administrative data from the Chronic Kidney Disease division of the Bureau of Health Promotion, Department of Health, R.O.C. (CKDBHPDH), we identified records of men and women aged older than 18 years with CKD from five counties and cities in central Taiwan from 2001 to 2011. Study participants were recruited and followed up in three major hospitals under the Veterans Affairs Commission, Taiwan, namely, Taichung Veterans General Hospital (VGHTC; main institute), VGHTC Puli branch, and VGHTC Chiayi Branch. The referral centers included more than 4 million residents and the in-charge area was 10,660 square kilometers. The cohort database enrolled early CKD and pre-ESRD patients who were followed-up for longer than 6 months, from December 1, 2001, to July 31, 2012 (Figure 1). Reasons for disenrollment included initiation of dialysis, transfer to another hospital, all-cause mortality, and loss of contact. This study was approved by the institutional review board of Taichung Veterans General Hospital (No.CE12252). Although informed consent was required, the multidisciplinary care did not interfere with clinical decisions related to patient care. Whether written informed consent was given by participants (or next of kin/caregiver in the case of children) for their clinical records to be used in this study, every consent was obtained before the patient records/information was anonymized and de-identified prior to analysis.

Study Design

Patients who had electronic medical records (visits for emergency department, outpatient clinic or hospitalization) in three hospitals were screened for potential recruitment. Screening for recruitment identified in previous units, the acute change in serum creatinine may have been affected by other factors during hospitalizations/emergency department presentations. We recruited the CKD cases under a relatively stable condition which may necessarily reflect their true eGFR change. To examine this question, we assembled a cohort with initial and subsequent eGFR using the 4-variable composite index (serum creatinine, age, race, and gender) – Modification of Diet in Renal Disease (MDRD) equation [1,21]. The enrolled participants were allocated to five CKD groups, from stage 1 to stage 5. The eGFR decline (ml/min/1.73 m^2 per year) with respect to time in different etiologies was analyzed by linear regression models. The coefficient of variation of the eGFR regression line accounts for the eGFR slope in repeated measurements [1–6]. This study considered three separate time intervals, 0–20, 20–40, and 40–60 months because the chosen cut-off points provided adequate statistical power for performing various subgroup analyses during the follow-up period. The cases with representative values of eGFR decline in each time interval excluded the cases that were censored when a value occurred outside the range of a measuring instrument. Such a situation can occur if an individual withdraws from the follow-up study, or if the individual is currently alive and on dialysis at the observational age.

A checklist providing information on socio-demographic characteristics, initial registration day, symptoms and signs of CKD, pre-existing comorbidity, current medication, and laboratory data requested from the Taiwan Society of Nephrology (TSN) for each patient, was completed by research nurses. Demographic information including age, sex, current smoking status, alcohol status, and malignancy were recorded. Diabetes mellitus, hypertension, and current medications were self-reported by the patients or retrieved from electronic records. Presence of cardiovascular diseases, i.e., coronary artery disease, stroke, congestive heart failure, arrhythmia, and peripheral arterial disease, was defined when identified in medical records. Body mass index (BMI) was calculated from the recorded height and weight. Serum creatinine was measured by the Jaffe method using a Beckman Synchron CX5 analyzer (USA) calibrated in accordance with the standards of the Chinese National Laboratory Accreditation program. Measurements of serum uric acid were obtained using the uricase method. Serum albumin was measured using bromocresol green (BCG) assay. Serum glycosylated hemoglobin A1c (HbA1c) was assessed by high-performance liquid chromatography (HPLC), and urine protein to creatinine ratio was measured by strip test. All biochemical laboratory tests were conducted by the Pathology and Laboratory Medicine Department of VGHTC. The time interval between the two eGFR tests or laboratory tests was required to be at least 3 months. Furthermore, we reviewed the medical records of clinical or pathological diagnoses of SDRN and PRDs partly with the assistance of our Clinical Informatics Research and Development Center. The primary outcome measures were incident ESRD warranting renal replacement therapy initiation and mortality due to eGFR decline based on etiological differences.

Statistical Analyses

Our primary goal was to investigate the contribution of eGFR decline to the outcome of CKD patients with SDRN or PRDs after adjusting for age, sex, traditional risk factors (proteinuria, angiotensin-converting-enzyme inhibitor, ACEI/angiotensin receptor blocker, ARB, diabetes mellitus, and hypertension), and antilipemic agents in different stages of CKD [6,19,22–30]. For continuous variables, descriptive results were summarized by mean ± standard deviation and differences were tested by one-way ANOVA if the normality assumption was satisfied, or by Kruskall-Wallis test when the normal assumption was violated. For categorical variables, analyses were conducted using the Pearson χ^2 test. Moreover, the P-value for trends was calculated using the Pearson correlation test when a variable was normal and using the Spearman's rank test for continuous non-normal variables. Normality of continuous variables was tested with the Kolmogorov-Smirnov method. If the overall test for homogeneity was rejected, we further conducted pairwise comparison for post-hoc analysis to determine significant differences in risk factors among the five CKD groups.

For each patient, the eGFR decline rate (ml/min/1.73 m^2) with respect to time in different etiologies was estimated by linear regression analysis for all outpatient measures of eGFR during different time intervals. If a patient had at least two outpatient eGFR measures in a specified interval, the eGFR decline for the corresponding etiology would be used.

We performed survival analysis to analyze the duration prior to events. Cox proportional hazards regression was used to determine the associations of eGFR decline in different CKD stages, except CKD stage 1 and 2, with initiation of chronic dialysis and all-cause mortality. Since early eGFR decline has less effect on the later outcome of CKD, this study investigated the contribution of eGFR decline in the last year of follow-up. Unadjusted rates were also reported because these represent actual etiological differences and the full burden of the diseases. Multivariate Cox proportional hazards model was conducted to assess the association of different eGFR decline rates as well as SDRN and PRDs with the primary endpoints, dialysis and death. A two-tailed P value <0.05 was considered statistically significant. Statistical analyses were implemented using **R** statistical software, version 2.15.3.

Table 1. Participants' characteristics by different initial CKD stages.

	Stage 1	Stage 2	Stage 3	Stage 4	Stage 5	P value[a]
No. of participants	108	287	2,150	1,380	1,172	
Age (years)	38.6±16.7	52.2±17.7	67.5±14.9	67.2±14.8	63.5±14.6	<0.001[b]
Male gender (%)	46.3	57.1	74.8	59.9	48.9	<0.001[c]
Smoking history (%)	17.6	23.7	40.7	35.0	26.9	0.001[c]
Alcohol history (%)	53.7	42.9	25.2	40.1	51.1	<0.001[c]
Diabetes mellitus (%)	13.9	18.5	34.1	42.3	34.0	<0.001[c]
Hypertension (%)	25.9	47.4	71.4	70.5	65.7	<0.001[c]
Cardiovascular disease (%)	2.8	1.7	8.4	9.5	6.2	0.337[c]
Malignancy (%)	0.0	2.1	6.0	7.4	5.1	0.080[c]
BMI (kg/m2)[†]						
Male, abnormal (%)	71.2	61.7	65.4	61.8	61.4	0.094[c]
Female, abnormal (%)	55.4	59.8	71.6	70.3	59.5	0.085[c]
Average initial eGFR, MDRD (ml/min, median [IQR])	104.5 (95.3–113.0)	71.6 (65.3–79.2)	39.9 (35.1–44.4)	23.1 (19.1–26.6)	9.2 (6.5–12.0)	<0.001[d]
Average initial eGFR, CKD-EPI (ml/min, median [IQR]) [††]	106.3 (100.2–117.0)	73.1 (66.3–81.7)	37.5 (32.9–42.6)	21.3 (17.6–21.2)	8.3 (5.8–10.8)	<0.001[d]
Urine PCR (mg/mmol, median [IQR])	2.9 (1.2–6.5)	1.5 (0.8–3.2)	0.5 (0.1–1.4)	1.0 (0.3–2.5)	1.5 (0.7–2.9)	<0.001[d]
Serum albumin <3.5g/dL, (%)	52.8	33.1	10.2	16.4	23.3	0.718[c]
Serum uric acid ≥7.2mg/dL, (%)	37.0	42.9	58.6	67.8	71.5	<0.001[c]
HbA1C						<0.001[c]
≥6.5 (%)	10.2	13.6	22.8	26.4	14.2	
<6.5 (%)	9.3	7.0	16.4	17.7	18.6	
NA (%)	80.5	79.4	60.8	55.9	67.2	
ACEI & ARB (%)	44.4	54.3	57	58.2	32.4	<0.001[c]
Insulin (%)	3.7	2.1	9.3	18.0	13.6	<0.001[c]
OAD (%)	13.0	16.0	31.3	38.0	24.7	0.105[c]
Antilipemic agents (%)	54.6	36.6	37.2	40.1	18.6	<0.001[c]
ESA (%)	0.9	0.7	2.2	12.9	47.9	<0.001[c]
Final status – Dialysis (%)	0.9	1.0	2.0	10.6	46.7	<0.001[c]
Final status – Death (%)	0.9	4.5	4.6	6.2	4.7	0.158[c]
Median follow-up in months (IQR)	20.3 (12.0–31.5)	27.5 (15.5–40.6)	27.7 (15.8–41.1)	25.7 (14.3–41.6)	16.0 (9.4–27.5)	<0.001[d]

Note: Data for categorical variables are given as percentage; data for continuous variables are given as mean ± standard deviation or median (interquartile range).
[†]The normal BMI value: male is 19.2–23.7 kg/m² and female is 18.3–22.7 kg/m² (Department of Health, Executive Yuan, Taiwan, R.O.C.). [Spindle 2009 health education advocacy plan survey summary report - The definition of body mass index in adults in Taiwan. February 2009 36(1) 23–26].
[a]For trend; [b]By one-way ANOVA test; [c]By Chi-square test; [d]By Kruskal-Wallis test.
Abbreviations: BMI, body mass index; MDRD, Modification of Diet in Renal Disease equation; CKD-EPI, Chronic Kidney Disease Epidemiology Collaboration formula; PCR, urine protein to urine creatinine ratio; eGFR, estimated glomerular filtration rate; NA, non-available; ACEI & ARB, angiotensin-converting enzyme inhibitors & angiotensin II receptor blockers; OAD, oral antidiabetics; ESA, erythropoiesis-stimulating agent.
[††]CKD-EPI formula, references:
1. Delanaye, P, Mariat, C. (2013) The applicability of eGFR equations to different populations. Nat. Rev. Nephrol 9: 513–522.
2. Levey AS, Stevens LA, Schmid CH, Zhang YL, Castro AF 3rd, et al. (2009) A new equation to estimate glomerular filtration rate. Ann Intern Med 150: 604–612.
3. Matsushita K, Mahmoodi BK, Woodward M, Emberson JR, Jafar TH, et al. (2012) Comparison of risk prediction using the CKD-EPI equation and the MDRD study equation for estimated glomerular filtration rate. JAMA. 307: 1941–1951.

Results

Baseline Demographics

Participants' characteristics were stratified by initial eGFR (Table 1). We also simulated the CKD cohort with the Chronic Kidney Disease Epidemiology Collaboration (CKD-EPI) formula which included variables such as age, sex, and serum creatinine, and concordance was found with a positive correlation between MDRD and CKD-EPI (Figure S1, Figure S2, Figure S3). Of the 5,097 patients included in the cohort, the mean age was 68.1±16.1 years. Patients with late-stage (stage 3, 4, 5) CKD were slightly older, more likely to have diabetes (CKD stage 3, 34.1%; stage 4, 42.3%; stage 5, 34.0%, P for trend <0.001),

hypertension (CKD stage 3, 71.4%; stage 4, 70.5%; stage 5, 65.7%, P for trend <0.001), and hyperuricemia (CKD stage 3, 58.6%; stage 4, 67.8%; stage 5, 71.5%, P for trend <0.001). There was a high rate of prescription of patients on insulin (CKD stage 3, 9.3%; stage 4, 18.0%; stage 5, 13.6%, P for trend <0.001) and using an erythropoiesis-stimulating agent (ESA) in late-stage CKD patients (CKD stage 3, 2.2%; stage 4, 12.9%; stage 5, 47.9%, P for trend <0.001). Those with early-stage (stage 1 and 2) CKD were younger and smoking was less prevalent, but were more likely to have significant proteinuria. There were no differences in the distributions of cardiovascular disease, malignancy, abnormal

Table 2. Diagnosed etiologies by different initial CKD stages.

	Stage 1	Stage 2	Stage 3	Stage 4	Stage 5	P value[a]
No. of participants	108	287	2,150	1,380	1,172	
Systemic disease-related nephropathy (n = 2,965, 58.2%)						
Diabetic nephropathy (%)	9.3	16.0	29.0	38.1	32.1	<0.001
Hypertensive nephropathy (%)	4.6	10.1	23.9	19.2	22.4	0.011
Lupus nephrophritis (%)	4.6	3.1	0.6	1.0	2.2	0.641
Others (%)[††]	0.0	2.8	5.6	5.4	3.4	0.034
Primary renal diseases (n = 1,502, 29.4%)						
IgA nephropathy (%)	14.8	11.5	3.1	3.4	1.6	<0.001
Membranous nephropathy (%)	16.7	11.5	1.5	0.8	0.6	<0.001
Focal segmental glomerulosclerosis (%)	3.7	3.8	1.8	1.8	1.3	0.012
Minimal change disease (%)	10.2	3.5	0.4	0.1	0.1	<0.001
Membranoproliferative glomerulonephritis (%)	0.0	0.7	0.2	0.4	0.1	0.524
Crescentic GN, RPGN (%)	0.0	0.0	0.1	0.2	0.6	0.002
Other renal parenchyma disease (%)*	33.3	26.5	21.6	18.0	20.7	0.001
Other etiology (n = 630, 12.4%)**						<0.001
	2.8	10.5	12.2	11.6	14.9	

[a]By Chi-square test.
[††]Other systemic disease-related nephropathy included amyloidosis, scleroderma, multiple myeloma, gouty nephropathy, liver cirrhosis, heart failure, eclampsia, metabolic diseases causing renal failure, and other systemic disease causing renal failure.
*Other renal parenchyma disease of the primary renal diseases including chronic pyelonephritis, unrecovered acute renal failure, chronic glomerulonephritis, post-infectious glomerulonephritis, chronic interstitial nephritis, rejection of kidney allograft.
**Other etiology included obstructive nephropathy, urinary tract diseases, renal vascular diseases, hereditary diseases, other causes of renal failure, and renal failure with unknown causes.

body mass index (BMI) by gender, serum albumin, oral antidiabetics (OADs), and final death status among the five groups.

After using pairwise comparison for post-hoc analysis, males were distributed equally in all CKD stages, except for 1,608 cases (74.8%) in CKD stage 3. With regard to lifestyle behaviors, never-smoking patients were more prevalent in early-stage CKD and the highest proportions of never-alcohol patients were observed in CKD stages 3 and 4. During follow-up, patients with CKD stages 4 or 5 were more likely to have dialysis (10.6% and 46.7%). But for the other rigorous outcome, all-cause mortality, there were no differences among the five groups. Furthermore, patients with CKD stage 5 had a shorter median follow-up in months (Table 1).

Systemic Disease-related Nephropathy (SDRN) and Primary Renal Disease (PRD) Based on Initial Clinical or Pathological Diagnosis

Most SDRN was diagnosed by clinical judgment (96.1%). SDRN was diagnosed by pathological report in 3.9% of cases, but almost all cases of lupus nephritis were diagnosed by pathology. For entry eGFRs, diabetic nephropathy (DN) and hypertensive nephropathy (HN) were largely found in patients with relatively late-stage CKD (DN, stage 3, 29.0%; stage 4, 38.1%; stage 5, 32.1%, P for trend <0.001; HN, stage 3, 23.9%; stage 4, 19.2%; stage 5, 22.4%, P for trend 0.011, Table 2). Patients with diagnosis of PRDs included 32.8% cases diagnosed by renal-biopsy report and 67.2% cases that were identified in a search of index hospitals in Taiwan's National Health Insurance Research Database (NHIRD). Several subgroups in PRDs had early-stage CKD, such as IgA nephropathy (IgAN) (stage 1, 14.8% and stage 2, 11.5% vs. other stages, P for trend <0.001), membranous nephropathy (MN) (stage 1, 16.7% and stage 2, 11.5% vs. other

stages, P for trend <0.001), FSGS (stage 1, 3.7% and stage 2, 3.8% vs. other stages, P for trend = 0.012), and minimal change disease (MCD) (stage 1, 10.2% and stage 2, 3.5% vs. other stages, P for trend <0.001). Crescentic glomerulonephritis (GN) and rapidly progressive glomerulonephritis (RPGN) were found to be more prevalent in late-stage CKD (3, 4, 5). For other renal parenchymal diseases, most patients with chronic interstitial nephritis or rejection of kidney allograft had CKD stage 1, 2, or 3. Other etiologies, including obstructive nephropathy, urinary tract diseases, renal vascular diseases, hereditary diseases, and unknown causes were less prevalent in CKD stage 1 (Table 2).

Different eGFR Decline Rates in Systemic or Primary Renal Etiology among Different Time Intervals

The data revealed the more skewed the linear regression line in disease etiology, the higher the variation in primitive eGFR. The importance of eGFR variation and decline can be seen in figure 2, which shows the serial eGFR changes in early-stage CKD (1 and 2) in SDRN during different time intervals was quite diverse. Rapid and significant eGFR decline was obvious in late-stage diabetic nephropathy (stage 3: -1.792 mL/min/1.73 m^2 per year during 0–20th month, $P<0.001$; stage 4: -1.29 mL/min/1.73 m^2 per year during 0–20th month, $P<0.001$, -0.867 mL/min/ 1.73 m^2 per year during 20–40th month, $P=0.033$, and -1.982 mL/min/1.73 m^2 per year during 40–60th month, $P=0.023$; stage 5: -1.208 mL/min/1.73 m^2 per year during 0–20th month, $P=0.008$ and -1.741 mL/min/1.73 m^2 per year during 20–40th month, $P<0.001$, Figure 2A). There were also significantly faster rates of eGFR decline in the later stages of hypertensive nephropathy (stage 4: -1.197 mL/min/1.73 m^2 per year during 20th –40th month, $P=0.006$, -2.601 mL/min/ 1.73 m^2 per year during 40th –60th month, $P=0.003$; stage 5:

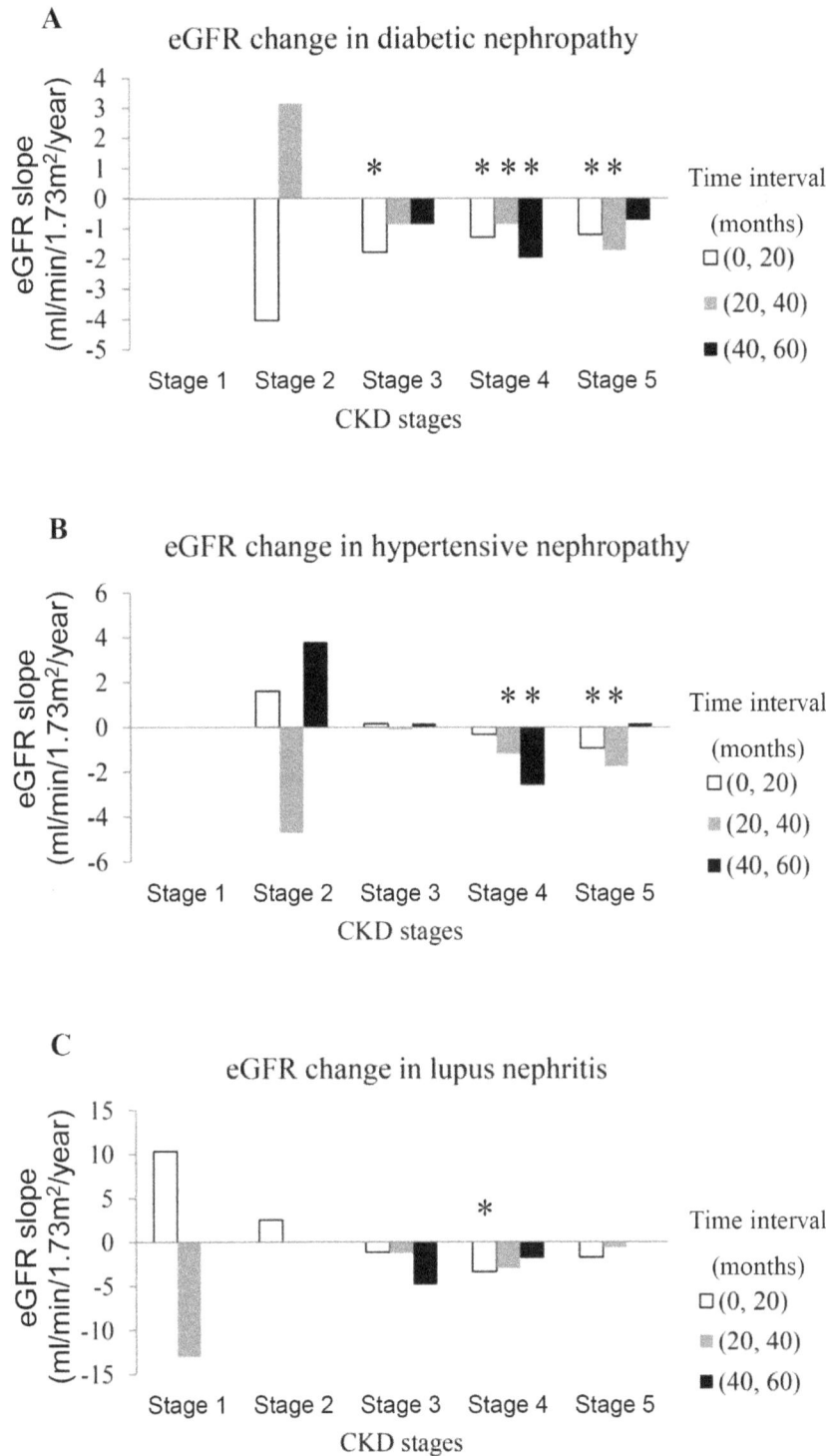

A   eGFR change in diabetic nephropathy

B   eGFR change in hypertensive nephropathy

C   eGFR change in lupus nephritis

Figure 2. eGFR decline in systemic disease-related nephropathy (Significant codes: *, <0.05 means the eGFR decline is a significant value during this time interval under lineal regression model).

-0.942 mL/min/1.73 m^2 per year during 0–20th, $P<0.001$, -1.761 mL/min/1.73 m^2 per year during 0–20th, $P<0.001$, Figure 2B). Lupus nephritis was not significantly associated with eGFR decline, except in CKD stage 4, with -3.384 mL/min/1.73 m^2 per year during 0–20th, $P=0.027$ (Figure 2C).

For PRDs, membranous nephropathy (MN) was associated with rapid eGFR decline in the early follow-up period (-4.210 mL/min/1.73 m^2 per year during 0–20th month). Minimal change disease was correlated with significantly elevated eGFR in the early follow-up period (7.551 mL/min/1.73 m^2 per year during 0–20th month). Focal segmental glomerulosclerosis (FSGS) was

Primary renal diseases

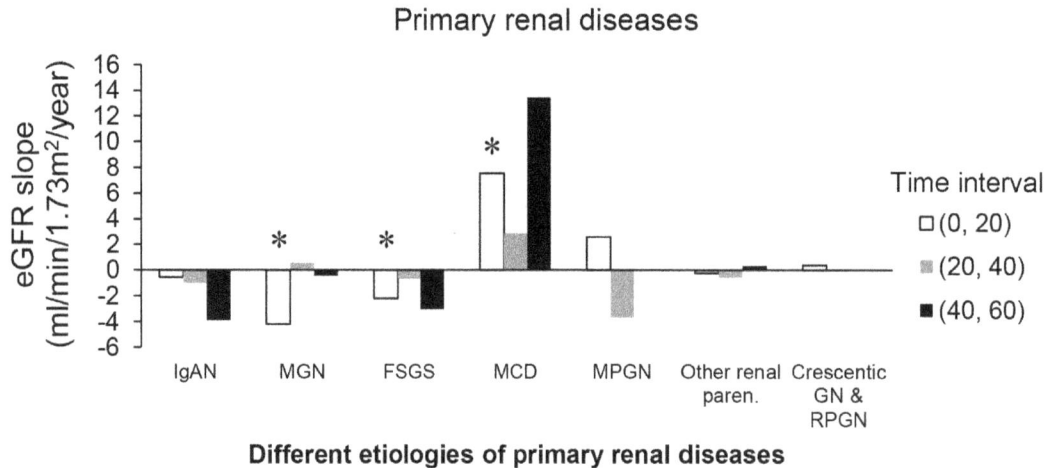

Figure 3. eGFR decline in primary renal diseases; IgAN, IgA nephropathy; MGN, membranous glomerulonephritis; FSGS, focal and segmental glomerulosclerosis; MCD, minimal change disease; MPGN, membranoproliferative glomerulonephritis; Other renal paren., other renal parenchymal disease; Crescentic GN& RPGN, crescentic glomerulonephritis and rapidly progressive glomerulonephritis (Significant codes: *, <0.05 means the eGFR decline is a significant value during this time interval under lineal regression model).

related to rapid eGFR decline in the early follow-up period (-2.203 mL/min/1.73 m² per year during 0–20th month) (Figure 3).

eGFR Decline Independently Predicted Poor Outcomes, Especially for SDRN in Maintenance of Dialysis

With regard to the primary endpoint, (434/2,723) 15.9% dialysis cases were stage 1–5 SDRN patients compared with (56/432) 13.0% dialysis cases who were stage 1–5 PRD ($P=0.113$) (Table 3). The crude eGFR decline and adjusted (age, gender, eGFR decline, proteinuria, ACEI/ARB, and antilipemic agents) risk of dialysis and all-cause mortality in those with SDRN and PRDs are listed in Table 3. Several disease types categorized as SDRN (e.g., multiple myeloma) that could potentially be successfully treated were excluded. In addition, PRDs (e.g., Crescentic GN or RPGN, obstructive nephropathy, acute

rejection in kidney transplant recipients, and pyelonephritis) with extreme values were excluded in the preliminary analysis.

SDRN individuals with eGFR decline (per 1 ml/min/1.73 m² per month) had a greater risk of initiating dialysis than that of PRDs (crude HR = 1.07, 95% CI = 1.04–1.10 and multivariate analysis, adjusted HR = 1.05, 95% CI = 1.02–1.08). That is to say, each unit of eGFR decline in SDRN increased the risk for dialysis by 5% after multivariate analysis. For the other outcome, (164/2,723) the mortality rate was 6.0% in stage 1–5 SDRN patients compared with (4/432) 0.9% in stage 1–5 PRDs ($P<0.001$), which was significantly different. However, there was no significant difference in the HR of eGFR decline to death between SDRN and PRD stages 1–5 in the analysis.

Table 4 presents an overall view of the average effects on outcomes (dialysis and all-cause mortality based on the most impactful CKD stages 3–5. eGFR declined independently and

Table 3. Association of eGFR decline with outcomes during study period by different disease etiologies.

	HR and 95% C.I. for dialysis	HR and 95% C.I. for death
	CKD stage 1–5	CKD stage 1–5
Systemic disease-related nephropathy, eGFR decline		
Number of events/Total numbers	434/2,723	164/2,723
Model 1	1.07 (1.04–1.10)***	0.95 (0.88–1.02)
Model 2	1.05 (1.02–1.08)***	0.99 (0.91–1.07)
Primary renal disease, eGFR decline		
Number of events/Total numbers	56/432	4/432
Model 1	1.01 (0.93–1.09)	1.02 (0.91–1.14)
Model 2	0.99 (0.92–1.08)	1.03 (0.75–1.43)

Model 1 is crude. Model 2 is adjusted for age, gender, eGFR decline, proteinuria, ACEI/ARB, and antilipemic agents.
Several disease types categorized as SDRN (e.g., multiple myeloma) that could potentially be successfully treated were excluded. In addition, PRDs (e.g., Crescentic GN or RPGN, obstructive nephropathy, acute rejection in kidney transplant recipients, and pyelonephritis) with extreme values were excluded in the preliminary analysis.
HR, hazard ratio; C.I., confidence interval.
Significant codes: *, <0.05; **, <0.01; ***, <0.001.

Table 4. Association of eGFR decline with dialysis and death in CKD stages 3~5 cohort using univariate and multivariate cox proportional hazards analysis.

CKD	HR and 95% C.I. for dialysis			HR and 95% C.I. for death		
	Stage 3	Stage 4	Stage 5	Stage 3	Stage 4	Stage 5
Average eGFR decline (ml/min)	−0.115	−0.143	−0.272	−0.115	−0.143	−0.272
Number of events/Total numbers	42/2,150	146/1,380	547/1,172	98/2,150	86/1,380	55/1,172
Model 1	1.40 (1.24–1.58)***	1.79 (1.52–2.12)***	1.61 (1.44–1.80)***	0.87 (0.77–0.98)*	1.39 (1.01–1.89)*	1.61 (0.70–3.71)
Model 2	1.50 (1.30–1.73)***	1.60 (1.37–1.88)***	1.69 (1.49–1.92)***	0.91 (0.79–1.04)	1.69 (1.23–2.33)**	1.82 (0.62–5.32)

Model 1 is crude. Model 2 is further adjusted for age, gender, proteinuria, ACEI/ARB, antilipemic agents, diseases with a relatively large subgroup of patients (diabetic nephropathy, hypertensive nephropathy, IgA nephropathy, and membranous nephropathy).
HR, hazard ratio; C.I., confidence interval
Significant codes: *, <0.05; **, <0.01; ***, <0.001.

significantly increased the risk of poor outcome of dialysis in patients with CKD stages 3, 4, and 5 (Table 3B). However, only in CKD stage 4 did eGFR decline have a positive association with death after univariate and multivariate analysis. The effect of eGFR decline on death in patients with CKD stage 3 was observed to be inversely correlated with risk of death (HR = 0.87, 95% C.I. = 0.77–0.98, Table 4).

Table 5 shows the associations of disease etiologies and eGFR decline with dialysis and all-cause mortality in the cohort with CKD stages 3, 4, and 5 using multivariate Cox proportional hazards analysis. Regarding SDRN, diabetic nephropathy (DN) had the greatest effect on initiation of dialysis (model 1: CKD stage 3: HR = 3.04, 95% C.I. = 1.66–5.58; CKD stage 5: HR = 1.29, 95% C.I. = 1.08–1.55). DN also had the greatest contribution to initiation of dialysis after adjustment for traditional risk factors (model 2: CKD stage 3: HR = 5.06, 95% C.I. = 2.63–9.71; CKD stage 4: HR = 2.02, 95% C.I. = 1.42–2.87; CKD stage 5: HR = 1.51, 95% C.I. = 1.26–1.82). Furthermore, when additive eGFR decline was added to the model, there was a strong association between CKD stages of DN and dialysis. We also found a correlation of DN with additive eGFR decline to all-cause mortality among CKD stages 3,4, and 5 with the application of the same statistical analysis. A small increase in the percentage of dialysis in patients with hypertensive nephropathy (HN) was found after adjusting for conventional risk factors with additive eGFR decline. However, in CKD stage 5 in the HN group, there was a lower mortality rate (model 1: CKD stage 5: HR = 0.62, 95% C.I. = 0.33–1.26; model 2: CKD stage 5: HR = 0.47, 95% C.I. = 0.23–0.97; model 3: CKD stage 5: HR = 0.47, 95% C.I. = 0.23–0.97) after adjusting for eGFR decline and traditional risk factors. Multiple post hoc comparisons showed a greater prevalence of ACEI/ARB usage in patients with stage 5 CKD in the HN group compared with usage rates in the other groups.

For PRDs, IgA nephropathy had a greater effect on initiation of dialysis (model 1: CKD stage 3: HR = 2.94, 95% C.I. = 1.14–7.42; CKD stage 5: HR = 1.81, 95% C.I. = 1.07–3.08). However, no worse effects for CKD progression were observed after adjusting for conventional risk factors as well as the additive eGFR decline factors. Those non-available data were small sample size (Table 4); 95% confidence interval of hazard ratio is wide, which is the reasons for the data being inadequate for appropriate analysis. There was a large diversity of other renal parenchymal diseases and thus the data were difficult to interpret.

Discussion

In this study, we found that eGFR decline independently predicted poor outcomes, especially the initiation of dialysis in systemic disease-related nephropathy (SDRN). For DN, each unit of eGFR decline had 5.20 times more risk for dialysis than that for other etiologies in CKD stage 3, 1.91 times more risk for dialysis than that for other etiologies in CKD stage 4, and 1.48 times more risk for dialysis than that for other etiologies in CKD stage 5 after multivariate analysis. The eGFR decline in primary renal diseases only makes a small contribution to the renal outcome and patients' outcome in a unified and integrated health care system. This risk was independent of traditional risk factors (age, diabetes mellitus, proteinuria, baseline eGFR, and hypertension), and was recently shown to be a non-traditional risk factor reflecting both intrinsic and extrinsic factors in the kidney [2,6,19]. In this multi-center study we attempted to better understand the association of eGFR decline with the renal outcome and all-cause mortality. We found eGFR decline had a major effect on risk of dialysis and all-cause mortality after univariate and multi-variate analysis with specific primary renal disease etiologies (Table 3 and 4). This study demonstrated that eGFR decline rate, defined as ml/min per 1.73 m^2 per year decrease, was associated with an increased risk for initiation of dialysis in SDRN, especially DN. Even after adjustment for age, the overall effect of eGFR decline beyond the normal aging process may be due to multiple co-morbidities, metabolic syndrome, and insulin resistance, which are risk factors for progression of CKD, and the rapid decline in renal function in the elderly [1].

One of the strengths of this study is that it is a long-term follow-up study spanning 10 years. In addition, a large sample size was analyzed which provided important information on the major etiologies of renal diseases. This study comprehensively examined long-term changes of eGFR in different renal diseases and showed associations of long-term outcomes with CKD. We explored the changes in eGFR over different time intervals in order to establish the relationships between longitudinal behavior of renal function and renal etiologies. Importantly, we investigated the contribution of eGFR decline (non-traditional risk factors) [2,6,19] in the final year of follow-up to the outcomes of CKD stages 3–5. Slopes were not calculated based on ordinary least squares as the renal outcome is technically problematic due to autocorrelation and heteroskedasticity. We did not adjust for baseline eGFR in slope models in order to avoid the so-called "horse-racing effect" [31].

Most predictors for ESRD and all-cause mortality found in ethnic Chinese cohorts showed similar findings in previous studies

Table 5. Associations of Disease Etiologies eGFR Decline with Dialysis and Death in CKD Stages 3~5 Cohort Using Multivariate Cox Proportional Hazards Analysis.

	HR and 95% C.I. for dialysis			HR and 95% C.I. for death		
CKD	Stage 3	Stage 4	Stage 5	Stage 3	Stage 4	Stage 5
Systemic disease-related nephropathy						
DM nephropathy						
Model 1	3.04 (1.66–5.58)***	1.37 (0.99–1.90)	1.29 (1.08–1.55)**	1.58 (1.05–2.39)*	1.35 (0.88 – 2.07)	2.42 (1.42 – 4.12)**
Model 2	5.06 (2.63–9.71)***	2.02 (1.42–2.87)***	1.51 (1.26–1.82)***	1.77 (1.17 – 2.69)**	1.62 (1.05 – 2.50)*	2.93 (1.70 – 5.03)***
Model 3	5.20 (2.72– 9.96)***	1.91 (1.34–2.70)***	1.48 (1.23–1.78)***	1.74 (1.15–2.65)**	1.59 (1.03–2.46)*	2.87 (1.66-4.95)***
Hypertensive nephropathy						
Model 1	0.24 (0.07–0.77)*	0.99 (0.66–1.50)	0.91 (0.74–1.12)	1.23 (0.80 – 1.91)	1.04 (0.61 – 1.77)	0.62 (0.33 – 1.26)
Model 2	0.32 (0.10–1.07)	1.14 (0.75–1.74)	0.98 (0.80–1.20)	0.92 (0.59 – 1.43)	0.68 (0.39 – 1.16)	0.47 (0.23 – 0.97)*
Model 3	0.36 (0.11–1.18)	1.18 (0.77–1.80)	0.97 (0.79–1.20)	0.90 (0.57–1.41)	0.68 (0.40–1.18)	0.47 (0.23–0.97)*
Lupus nephritis						
Model 1	–	2.78 (0.88–8.73)	1.49 (0.86–2.59)	–	–	–
Model 2	–	1.47 (0.46–4.72)	1.32 (0.75–2.31)	–	–	–
Model 3	–	1.60(0.50–5.16)	1.31(0.75–2.31)	–	–	–
Primary renal diseases						
IgA nephropathy						
Model 1	2.91 (1.14–7.42)*	1.68 (0.85–3.29)	1.81 (1.07–3.08)*	–	–	–
Model 2	1.48 (0.55–3.93)	0.93 (0.46–1.89)	1.25 (0.73–2.14)	–	–	–
Model 3	1.43 (0.54–3.82)	0.89 (0.44–1.82)	0.90 (0.52–1.57)	–	–	–
MGN						
Model 1	2.39 (0.58–9.92)	0.74 (0.10–5.31)	1.43 (0.53–3.82)	1.1 (0.27 – 4.47)	–	–
Model 2	2.74 (0.65–11.56)	1.13 (0.16–8.12)	1.25 (0.47–3.36)	2.42 (0.58 – 10.09)	–	–
Model 3	2.28 (0.54–9.67)	1.22 (0.17–8.82)	1.34 (0.50–3.61)	2.54 (0.61–10.65)	–	–
FSGS						
Model 1	–	1.66 (0.68–4.06)	1.29 (0.64–2.59)	0.40 (0.06 – 2.88)	–	–
Model 2	–	0.95 (0.38–2.38)	0.99 (0.49–2.01)	–	–	–
Model 3	–	0.82 (0.33–2.08)	0.98 (0.48–1.98)	–	–	–
MCD						
Models 1 & 2 & 3	–	–	–	–	–	–
MPGN						
Model 1	–	2.63 (0.65 – 10.65)	–	–	–	–
Model 2	–	1.80 (0.44 – 7.36)	–	–	–	–
Model 3	–	1.81 (0.44 – 7.40)	–	–	–	–
Crescentic GN & RPGN						
Model 1	–	–	1.34 (0.50–3.57)	–	–	–
Model 2	–	–	1.17 (0.44–3.14)	–	–	0.96 (0.51 – 1.81)
Model 3	–	–	1.21 (0.45–3.25)	–	–	–
Other renal parenchymal diseases						
Model 1	0.80 (0.37–1.73)	0.86 (0.56–1.32)	0.82 (0.66–1.00)	0.89 (0.54 – 1.45)	0.78 (0.44 – 1.38)	0.94 (0.50 – 1.76)
Model 2	0.57 (0.26–1.25)	0.73 (0.48–1.12)	0.75 (0.61–0.92)*	0.96 (0.58 – 1.58)	0.85 (0.48 – 1.50)	–
Model 3	0.55 (0.25 – 1.22)	0.73 (0.48–1.13)	0.78 (0.63–0.96)*	0.99 (0.60–1.64)	0.88 (0.49–1.55)	0.95 (0.50–1.79)

Model 1 is crude for disease itself. Model 2 is further adjusted for age, gender, proteinuria, ACEI/ARB, antilipemic agents. Model 3 is further adjusted for all the items in model 2+ eGFR decline.
Significant codes: *, <0.05; **, <0.01; ***, <0.001.

[32–36]. Taiwan is the only country to have achieved a hugely significant reduction in the incidence of ESRD in recent years, partly due to the inclusion of early CKD and pre-end-stage renal disease (ESRD) management programs in the National Health Insurance scheme [17,32]. Despite the successful reduction of CKD, it must be remembered that there is a growing burden of CKD. In part this is due to the growth of other non-communicable diseases (NCDs), most notably diabetes. However, the emergence of new epidemics of CKD in the developing world, some of which appear to have environmental causes, has also contributed to the overall burden. Rapid decline of eGFR is a clinical concern for physicians and patients. GFR decline with aging is a sign of normal senescence, not disease [10]. However, among patients with similar levels of eGFR, clinical outcomes vary substantially by age. The well-known reasons for risk of rapid GFR decline are aging, racial difference (young blacks), albuminuria, hypertension, diabetes, and variable primary renal diseases [19]. However, the discrepancy between eGFR decline and clinical outcomes in long-term observational studies has yet to be fully elucidated.

To the best of our knowledge, the present study is the first to investigate the importance of eGFR decline and its differing contributions to rigorous clinical endpoints. However, several equivocal findings could be partly explained by different behaviors of medical practice. In clinical practice, eGFR decline in DN was kept under control in stage 2–4 CKD, but the improvements in stage 4 CKD of DN were lost after 40 months of follow-up. The decline of eGFR could be seen in stage 5 CKD in DN, and the decreased eGFR decline in the last period (40–60 months) was due to the ceiling effect of the lowest value of the eGFR (Figure 2A). Efforts to retard eGFR decline in stage 1–3 CKD in HN were effective, but no benefit was found after stage 4–5 CKD (Figure 2B). For PRDs, IgA nephropathy, FSGS, and memrano-proliferative glomerulonephritis (MPGN) the decline rates were difficult to control (Figure 3). MN required more time to observe due to its chronic disease status and changes in eGFR were not obvious (Figure 3). In the episodic 12-month follow-up of eGFR decline, it was shown that multidisciplinary predialysis education (MPE) can be efficacious in motivated systemic-disease patients, especially for prolonging survival. Questions remain about its effectiveness (i.e., whether it works in everyday life) as it may be very hard to convince "non-compliant" patients. Skilled non-medical educators are often better than physicians at conveying information to patients, as they tend to have a more solid pedagogic and methodological background. There is no need for strong experimental, multidisciplinary care and non-randomized observational trials [36]. However, long-term follow-up studies are still worthwhile as they are capable of identifying potential risk factors.

In conclusion, eGFR decline was demonstrated to be superior to absolute GFR value as an indicator of kidney disease progression by the overall changes in kidney function over time. Diverse eGFR variations had better predictive values in systemic disease-related nephropathy than those in primary renal diseases. Diabetic nephropathy and hypertensive nephropathy were correlated with significantly greater eGFR decline in CKD stages 3, 4, and 5 compared with that of other disease etiologies. eGFR decline has a predictive value for dialysis and death in CKD stages 3, 4, and 5 in SDRN patients, especially DN. There were still discrepancies between eGFR decline and clinical outcomes in PRDs, hypertensive nephropathy, and lupus nephritis.

Supporting Information

Figure S1 Concordance was found with a positive correlation between MDRD and CKD-EPI.

Figure S2 The similar distribution of estimated GFR and eGFR-risk relationship were found between the CKD-EPI equation (red) and the MDRD Study equation (black) in our CKD cohort.

Figure S3 The positive correlation and distribution of eGFR between MDRD and CKD-EPI were shown by age categories (< and ≥65 years) in the CKD cohorts (female).

Acknowledgments

The authors thank the Clinical Informatics Research and Development Center and the Biostatistics Task Force of Taichung Veterans General Hospital (TCVGH), Taichung, Taiwan, R.O.C., for their help with the statistical analysis. This study was also conducted on behalf of the GREEnS Project, Tunghai University, Taiwan, and the CKDBHPDH investigators (Division of Nephrology, RN. Chia-Fang Hung, RN. Chia-Ying Tung, RN. Su-Chi Hung, RN. Tzu-Mei Lin, email: tmlin@vghtc.gov.tw), Taichung Veterans General Hospital, Taiwan, R.O.C.

Author Contributions

Conceived and designed the experiments: S-CW D-CT. Performed the experiments: K-HS C-H. Cheng C-H. Chen T-MY M-JW. Analyzed the data: S-CW C-MC. Wrote the paper: S-CW D-CT.

References

1. Cheng HT, Huang JW, Chiang CK, Yen CJ, Hung KY, et al. (2012) Metabolic syndrome and insulin resistance as risk factors for development of chronic kidney disease and rapid decline in renal function in elderly. J Clin Endocrinol Metab 97: 1268–1276.

2. Al-Aly Z, Balasubramanian S, McDonald JR, Scherrer JF, O'Hare AM (2012) Greater variability in kidney function is associated with an increased risk of death. Kidney Int 82: 1208–1214.

3. Derose SF, Rutkowski MP, Crooks PW, Shi JM, Wang JG, et al. (2013) Racial differences in estimated GFR decline, ESRD, and mortality in an integrated health system. Am J Kidney Dis 62: 236–244.

4. Peralta CA, Vittinghoff E, Bansal N, Jacobs D Jr, Muntner P, et al. (2013) Trajectories of kidney function decline in young black and white adults with preserved GFR: results from the Coronary Artery Risk Development in Young Adults (CARDIA) study. Am J Kidney Dis 62: 261–266.

5. Hansen HP, Hovind P, Jensen BR, Parving HH (2002) Diurnal variations of glomerular filtration rate and albuminuria in diabetic nephropathy. Kidney Int 61: 163–168.

6. Perkins RM, Tang X, Bengier AC, Kirchner HL, Bucaloiu ID (2012) Variability in estimated glomerular filtration rate is an independent risk factor for death among patients with stage 3 chronic kidney disease. Kidney Int 82: 1332–1338.

7. Kajitani N, Shikata K, Nakamura A, Nakatou T, Hiramatsu M, et al. (2010) Microinflammation is a common risk factor for progression of nephropathy and atherosclerosis in Japanese patients with type 2 diabetes. Diabetes Res Clin Pract 88: 171–176.

8. Shikata K Makino H (2013) Microinflammation in the pathogenesis of diabetic nephropathy. J Diabetes Investig 4: 142–149.

9. Hinchliffe SA, Lynch MR, Sargent PH, Howard CV, Van Velzen D (1992) The effect of intrauterine growth retardation on the development of renal nephrons. Br J Obstet Gynaecol 99: 296–301.

10. Jocelyn W, Sanjeevkumar RP (2009) Changes in Kidney Function. Hazzard's geriatric medicine and gerontology. 6th ed. Seattle, USA: McGraw-Hill; p.1009–1015.

11. Li LS, Liu ZH (2004) Epidemiologic data of renal diseases from a single unit in China: analysis based on 13,519 renal biopsies. Kidney Int 66: 920–923.

12. Sowers JR, Epstein M (1995) Diabetes mellitus and associated hypertension, vascular disease, and nephropathy. An update. Hypertension 26: 869–879.

13. Crook ED, Flack JM, Salem M, Salahudeen AK, Hall J (2002) Primary renal disease as a cardiovascular risk factor. Am J Med Sci 324: 138–145.

14. Moriya T, Tsuchiya A, Okizaki S, Hayashi A, Tanaka K, et al. (2012) Glomerular hyperfiltration and increased glomerular filtration surface are associated with renal function decline in normo- and microalbuminuric type 2 diabetes. Kidney Int 81: 486–493.

15. Mulec H, Blohmé G, Grände B, Björck S (1998) The effect of metabolic control on rate of decline in renal function in insulin-dependent diabetes mellitus with overt diabetic nephropathy. Nephrol Dial Transplant 13: 651–655.

16. Reich HN, Gladman DD, Urowitz MB, Bargman JM, Hladunewich MA, et al. (2011) Persistent proteinuria and dyslipidemia increase the risk of progressive chronic kidney disease in lupus erythematosus. Kidney Int 79: 914–920.

17. Chou YH, Lien YC, Hu FC, Lin WC, Kao CC, et al. (2012) Clinical outcomes and predictors for ESRD and mortality in primary GN. Clin J Am Soc Nephrol 7: 1401–1408.

18. Andreoli SP (1998) Renal manifestations of systemic diseases. Semin Nephrol 18: 270–279.

19. Al-Aly Z (2013) Prediction of renal endpoints in chronic kidney disease. Kidney Int 83: 189–191.

20. Mahajan A, Simoni J, Sheather SJ, Broglio KR, Rajab MH, et al. (2010) Daily oral sodium bicarbonate preserves glomerular filtration rate by slowing its decline in early hypertensive nephropathy. Kidney Int 78: 303–309.

21. Estimation of GFR. KDOQI Clinical Practice Guidelines for Chronic Kidney Disease: Evaluation, Classification, and Stratification (Guideline 4). National Kidney Foundation, Inc. http://www.kidney.org/professionals/kdoqi/guidelines_ckd/p5_lab_g4.htm. Accessed 2002.

22. Chang TI, Li S, Chen SC, Peralta CA, Shlipak MG, et al. (2013) Risk factors for ESRD in individuals with preserved estimated GFR with and without albuminuria: results from the Kidney Early Evaluation Program (KEEP) Am J Kidney Dis 61(4 Suppl 2): S4–S11.

23. Kuo HW, Tsai SS, Tiao MM, Yang CY (2007) Epidemiological features of CKD in Taiwan. Am J Kidney Dis 49: 46–55.

24. Chadban SJ, Briganti EM, Kerr PG, Dunstan DW, Welborn TA, et al. (2003) Prevalence of kidney damage in Australian adults: The AusDiab kidney study. J Am Soc Nephrol 14(7 Suppl 2): S131–138.

25. Hallan SI, Matsushita K, Sang Y, Mahmoodi BK, Black C, et al. (2012) Age and association of kidney measures with mortality and end-stage renal disease. JAMA 308: 2349–2360.

26. Gansevoort RT, Correa-Rotter R, Hemmelgarn BR, Jafar TH, Heerspink HJ, et al. (2013) Chronic kidney disease and cardiovascular risk: epidemiology, mechanisms, and prevention. Lancet 382: 339–352.

27. Mahmoodi BK, Matsushita K, Woodward M, Blankestijn PJ, Cirillo M, et al. (2012) Associations of kidney disease measures with mortality and end-stage renal disease in individuals with and without hypertension: a meta-analysis. Lancet 380: 1649–1661.

28. Nitsch D, Grams M, Sang Y, Black C, Cirillo M, et al. (2013) Associations of estimated glomerular filtration rate and albuminuria with mortality and renal failure by sex: a meta-analysis. BMJ 346: f324.

29. Hsu TW, Liu JS, Hung SC, Kuo KL, Chang YK, et al. (2013) Renoprotective Effect of Renin-Angiotensin-Aldosterone System Blockade in Patients With Predialysis Advanced Chronic Kidney Disease, Hypertension, and Anemia. JAMA Intern Med Dec 16. doi: 10.1001/jamainternmed.2013.12700 [Epub ahead of print].

30. Wen CP, David Cheng TY, Chan HT, Tsai MK, Chung WS, et al. (2010) Is high serum uric acid a risk marker or a target for treatment? Examination of its independent effect in a large cohort with low cardiovascular risk. Am J Kidney Dis 56: 273–288.

31. Glymour MM, Weuve J, Berkman LF, Kawachi I, Robins JM (2005) When is baseline adjustment useful in analyses of change? An example with education and cognitive change. Am J Epidemiol 162: 267–278.

32. Yang WC, Hwang SJ, Taiwan Society of Nephrology (2008) Incidence, prevalence and mortality trends of dialysis end-stage renal disease in Taiwan from 1990 to 2001: the impact of national health insurance. Nephrol Dial Transplant 23: 3977–3982.

33. Chiu YL, Chien KL, Lin SL, Chen YM, Tsai TJ, et al. (2008) Outcomes of stage 3–5 chronic kidney disease before end-stage renal disease at a single center in Taiwan. Nephron Clin Pract 109: c109–118.

34. Wu IW, Wang SY, Hsu KH, Lee CC, Sun CY, et al. (2009) Multidisciplinary predialysis education decreases the incidence of dialysis and reduces mortality–a controlled cohort study based on the NKF/DOQI guidelines. Nephrol Dial Transplant 24: 3426–3433.

35. Chen YR, Yang Y, Wang SC, Chiu PF, Chou WY, et al. (2013) Effectiveness of multidisciplinary care for chronic kidney disease in Taiwan: a 3-year prospective cohort study. Nephrol Dial Transplant 28: 671–682.

36. Van Biesen W, Verbeke F, Vanholder R (2009) We don't need no education …. (Pink Floyd, The Wall) Multidisciplinary predialysis education programmes: pass or fail? Nephrol Dial Transplant 24: 3277–3279.

6

SDF-1/CXCR4 Signaling Preserves Microvascular Integrity and Renal Function in Chronic Kidney Disease

Li-Hao Chen[1], Suzanne L. Advani[1], Kerri Thai[1], M. Golam Kabir[1], Manish M. Sood[2], Ian W. Gibson[3], Darren A. Yuen[1], Kim A. Connelly[1], Philip A. Marsden[1], Darren J. Kelly[4], Richard E. Gilbert[1], Andrew Advani[1]*

1 Keenan Research Centre for Biomedical Science and Li Ka Shing Knowledge Institute of St. Michael's Hospital, Toronto, Ontario, Canada, 2 Ottawa Hospital Research Institute, University of Ottawa, Ottawa, Ontario, Canada, 3 Health Sciences Centre, University of Manitoba, Winnipeg, Manitoba, Canada, 4 Department of Medicine, St. Vincent's Hospital, Melbourne, Victoria, Australia

Abstract

The progressive decline of renal function in chronic kidney disease (CKD) is characterized by both disruption of the microvascular architecture and the accumulation of fibrotic matrix. One angiogenic pathway recently identified as playing an essential role in renal vascular development is the stromal cell-derived factor-1α (SDF-1)/CXCR4 pathway. Because similar developmental processes may be recapitulated in the disease setting, we hypothesized that the SDF-1/CXCR4 system would regulate microvascular health in CKD. Expression of CXCR4 was observed to be increased in the kidneys of subtotally nephrectomized (SNx) rats and in biopsies from patients with secondary focal segmental glomerulosclerosis (FSGS), a rodent model and human correlate both characterized by aberration of the renal microvessels. A reno-protective role for local SDF-1/CXCR4 signaling was indicated by i) CXCR4-dependent glomerular eNOS activation following acute SDF-1 administration; and ii) acceleration of renal function decline, capillary loss and fibrosis in SNx rats treated with chronic CXCR4 blockade. In contrast to the upregulation of CXCR4, SDF-1 transcript levels were decreased in SNx rat kidneys as well as in renal fibroblasts exposed to the pro-fibrotic cytokine transforming growth factor β (TGF-β), the latter effect being attenuated by histone deacetylase inhibition. Increased renal SDF-1 expression was, however, observed following the treatment of SNx rats with the ACE inhibitor, perindopril. Collectively, these observations indicate that local SDF-1/CXCR4 signaling functions to preserve microvascular integrity and prevent renal fibrosis. Augmentation of this pathway, either purposefully or serendipitously with either novel or existing therapies, may attenuate renal decline in CKD.

Editor: Niels Olsen Saraiva Câmara, Universidade de Sao Paulo, Brazil

Funding: These studies were supported by grants from CIHR (grant MOP-97791) and the Canadian Diabetes Association (CDA, OG-3-10-2949-AA) to Dr. Advani. Mr. Chen was supported by a CIHR Frederick Banting and Charles Best Graduate Scholarship and a Banting and Best Diabetes Centre Graduate Studentship. Dr. Advani is a Canadian Diabetes Association Clinician Scientist and this work was supported, in part, by the Canadian Diabetes Association. Dr. Gilbert is a Canada Research Chair in Diabetes Complications. Dr. Yuen is a KRESCENT New Investigator and Canadian Diabetes Association Clinician Scientist. The funders had no role in study design, data collection and analysis, decision to publish, or preparation of the manuscript.

Competing Interests: REG and AA report having received funds through their institution from Servier to assist with patient care. KAC reports having received honoraria from Servier for CME talks.

* E-mail: advania@smh.ca

Introduction

The progressive decline of renal function in chronic kidney disease (CKD) is characterized by both fibrotic scarring of the kidney and obliteration of the renal microvessels, these two pathogenetic hallmarks commonly occurring in tandem and enjoying a reciprocal relationship. On the one hand, microvascular loss may occur as a result of the occlusive actions of accumulating matrix proteins, whereas on the other hand the same process may itself contribute to organ fibrosis and progressive renal decline by predisposing the kidney to hypoxic injury [1]. Coupled with an increasing appreciation for the pivotal role that angiogenic factors may play in renal development [2], homeostasis [3] and disease [4,5], preservation of the glomerular and peritubular capillary architecture is thus a desirable characteristic of both existing and novel renoprotective therapies [6].

One pathway that has recently emerged as playing an essential role in renal vascular development is the stromal cell-derived factor-1α (SDF-1)/CXCR4 pathway [7]. SDF-1 is a CXC chemokine and the principal ligand for its cognate receptor, CXCR4, a seven transmembrane domain G-protein coupled receptor and the most prevalent chemokine receptor found in endothelial cells [8]. While originally defined for its role in maintenance of the hematopoietic stem cell niche and B-cell lymphopoiesis [9], the near ubiquitous tissue distribution of SDF-1 and its rapid degradation in blood indicate the capacity for much broader intra-organ specific functions [10]. The fundamental nature of the SDF-1/CXCR4 relationship is attested to by the development of identical defects in vasculogenesis and organogenesis that occur in the absence of either gene [11]. However, as with other angiogenic pathways [4,5,12], the role that SDF-1/CXCR4 signaling may play in the adult kidney appears to be context-dependent. For instance, studies in acute kidney injury support a reno-protective function for SDF-1/CXCR4 [13], whereas CXCR4-mediated hyperproliferation may actually contribute to the development of certain glomerular diseases [14].

Although reactivation of ontogenetic pathways is a common response of cells, tissues and organisms to a variety of injurious insults [15], the function of the developmentally essential SDF-1/CXCR4 pathway in CKD is unclear. Accordingly, in the present study we sought to combine studies conducted in experimental animals, cultured cells and human biopsy tissue to define the role of SDF-1/CXCR4 signaling in CKD, focusing on the bidirectional relationship between renal fibrosis and microvascular loss.

Materials and Methods

Ethics statement

Human biopsy studies were approved by the Institutional Research Board of the Health Sciences Centre, University of Manitoba. All patients gave written informed consent and the study was performed in accordance with the Declaration of Helsinki. All animal work was conducted according to the Canadian Council on Animal Care Guidelines. The specific experimental protocol, ACC 166, was approved by the Animal Care Committee of St. Michael's Hospital.

Human studies

Localization of CXCR4 and SDF-1 was determined in kidney sections from patients who had undergone nephrectomy for tumor, with tissue removed from the opposite pole [16]. For gene expression studies, kidney tissue was obtained from patients with either secondary focal segmental glomerulosclerosis (FSGS) or time zero live kidney donors.

Animals

Study 1. Expression of CXCR4 and SDF-1 was determined in the kidneys of sham (n = 6) and subtotally nephrectomized (SNx) (n = 8) rats after 8 weeks. Subtotal (5/6) nephrectomy or sham surgery was performed, in female Fischer 344 rats (F344, Charles River, Montreal, Quebec) aged 8 weeks, as previously described [17].

Study 2. For the study of chronic CXCR4 antagonism, female F344 rats aged 8 weeks underwent sham or subtotal nephrectomy surgery. Two days later, animals were randomized to receive either vehicle (PBS) or AMD3100 (1 mg/kg/day, Cayman Chemical, Ann Arbor, MI) s.c. and were followed for 8 weeks (sham, PBS n = 18, AMD3100 n = 12; SNx, PBS n = 14, AMD3100 n = 15). Glomerular filtration rate (GFR) was determined by FITC-inulin clearance [18]. Urine protein excretion was determined after 24 h metabolic caging. Systolic blood pressure (SBP) was measured with a 2F micro-manometer (Model SPR-838 Millar Instruments, Houston, TX) and analysed using Chart Software v5.6 (AD Instruments, NSW, Australia).

Study 3. In Study 3, we examined the effect of acute SDF-1 administration on glomerular signaling. Eight week old female F344 rats were first randomized to receive either PBS or AMD3100 (1 mg/kg) s.c. Four hours later, recombinant rat SDF-1 (10 μg/kg [19]; PeproTech, Rocky Hill, NJ) or vehicle (PBS) was delivered to the kidneys via the abdominal aorta (n = 6/group). To achieve this, the abdominal aorta was dissected, the right kidney was removed and the descending aorta was ligated distal and transiently ligated proximal to the renal artery. Either PBS or SDF-1 was delivered via an 18 G angiocath, circulation into the left kidney was then restored for 30 min before flushing the kidney with heparin (100 U), followed by 1 mL of PBS, with perfusion-exsanguination facilitated by severance of the external jugular vein. The kidney was then removed and glomeruli isolated by differential sieving [20].

Study 4. To determine whether either CXCR4 or SDF-1 mRNA were altered with ACE inhibition, real-time PCR was performed on mRNA isolated from the kidneys of sham (n = 8) and SNx (n = 7) Sprague Dawley rats after 12 weeks or SNx rats treated with the ACE inhibitor perindopril (8 mg/L in drinking water) (n = 8). The clinical characteristics of these rats have been previously described [21].

Immunohistochemistry

Immunohistochemistry was performed as previously described [4,16,22] with antibodies in the following concentrations: SDF-1 1:25 (R&D Systems, Minneapolis, MN), CXCR4 1:50 (Abcam, Cambridge, MA), collagen IV 1:100 (Southern Biotech, Birmingham, AL) and JG-12 1:1000 (Bender Medsystems GbdH, Vienna, Austria). For quantitation of JG-12 and collagen IV immunostaining, kidney sections were scanned with the Aperio ScanScope system (Aperio Technologies Inc., Vista, CA) and analyzed using ImageScope (Aperio Technologies Inc.). Glomerular endothelial (JG-12) immunostaining was determined in 30 glomerular profiles from each rat kidney section [4,23]. For estimation of peritubular JG-12 and tubulointerstitial collagen IV, the proportional area of positive immunostaining (excluding glomeruli) was determined in 10 randomly selected cortical fields (x100 magnification).

Glomerulosclerosis Index

A minimum of 50 glomeruli were examined in PAS-stained kidney sections from each rat. The degree of sclerosis was subjectively graded on a scale of 0 to 4 as previously described [4].

Fluorescent microangiography

Fluorescent microangiography (FMA) was performed in n≥3 rats/group as previously described [18]. Briefly, the abdominal aorta was ligated proximal to the renal artery and distally at the level of the aortic bifurcation and 1 ml of heparinized saline followed by 1 ml of 3% KCl were delivered, before perfusion with 100 ml 0.9% saline. A pre-warmed (40°C) agarose-fluorescent microbead mixture (1% low melting point agarose [Sigma] and 10% 0.02 μm fluospheres [Invitrogen, Carlsbad, CA]) was then delivered via an 18G angiocath. After infusion, the rat was cooled on ice and the kidney removed and fixed in 10% NBF. Subsequently, 200 μm thick kidney cross-sections were washed in PBS overnight and embedded in 95% 2,2'-thiodiethanol (Sigma). Serial images were collected with a confocal microscope (Leica TCS SL, Leica, Richmond Hill, ON) across the z-stack (0.8141 μm steps) in 6 glomeruli/rat. Glomerular capillary volume was calculated using ImageJ version 1.39 (National Institutes of Health, Bethesda, MD). Three dimensional reconstructions were generated using Neurolucida (MBF Bioscience, Williston, VT).

Cell culture

In vitro experiments were conducted in NRK-49F renal fibroblasts (ATCC, Manassas, VA) and human umbilical vein endothelial cells (HUVECs) [4,23]. NRK-49F cells were treated with 10 ng/ml recombinant rat transforming growth factor β (TGF-β) (R&D Systems) for 24 h, with or without pre-treatment with the histone deacetylase (HDAC) inhibitor vorinostat (5 μM) (Exclusive Chemistry, Obninsk, Russia) for 4 h. HUVECs were pre-incubated with 20 μM LY294002 (LC Laboratories, Woburn, MA), 1 μM AMD3100 or vehicle (0.1% DMSO) for 30 min before the addition of recombinant human SDF-1 (100 ng/ml) (R&D Systems) (or 1% BSA) for 30 min.

Immunoblotting

Immunoblotting was performed as previously described [23] with antibodies in the following concentrations: phospho-eNOS

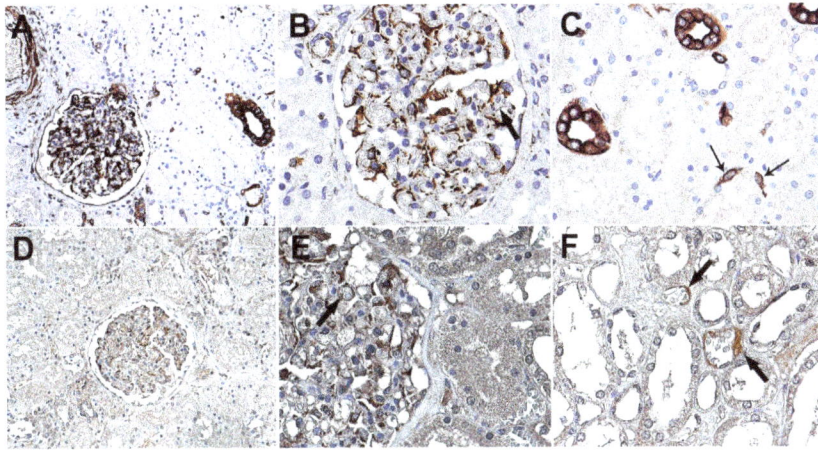

Figure 1. Immunostaining for SDF-1 (A–C) and CXCR4 (D–F) in adult human kidney. There is focal tubular (A and C) and glomerular podocyte staining for SDF-1. The thick arrows mark scattered positively staining glomerular and peritubular capillary endothelial cells; the thin arrows mark positively staining interstitial fibroblasts (C). (A and D) Original magnification x160. (B, C, E and F) Original magnification x400.

Ser1177 1:1000 (Cell Signaling, Danvers, MA), total eNOS 1:2500 (BD Transduction Laboratories, Lexington, KY). Densitometry was performed using Image J.

Real-time PCR

RNA was isolated from homogenized rat kidney tissue using TRIzol reagent (Life Technologies, Grand Island, NY). Total RNA (4 µg) was treated with RQ1 DNAse (1 U/µl) (Promega). For *in vitro* experiments, RNA isolation and DNase treatment of cultured cell extracts were performed using RNAspin Mini (GE Healthcare, Buckinghamshire, UK). DNase treated RNA (4 µg) was reverse-transcribed in a final volume of 25 µl using 0.5 µl AMV-RT (Roche Diagnostics, Laval, Quebec) in the manufacturer's buffer containing 1 mmol/L dNTPs, 0.5 µl RNase inhibitor (Roche) and 2 µg random hexamers (Amersham). Total RNA was extracted from human tissue using a Paradise Plus Reagent System (Arcturus, Mountain View, CA). SYBR green based real time PCR was performed on an ABI Prism 7900 HT Fast PCR System (Applied Biosystems, Foster City, CA) using the following primer sequences: rCXCR4, forward ATCATCTC-CAAGCTGTCACACTCC, reverse GTGATGGAGATCCAC-TTGTGCAC; rSDF-1, forward GCTCTGCATCAGTGACGG-TAAG, reverse TGGCGACATGGCTCTCAAA; rTGF-β, forward CACCCGCGTGCTAATGGT, reverse TGTGTGATGT-CTTTGGTTTTGTCA; rRPL13a, forward GATGAACACCA-ACCCGTCTC, reverse CACCATCCGCTTTTTCTTGT; r18S, forward ATGTGGTGTTGAGGAAAGCAGAC, reverse GGATCTTGTATTGTCGTGGGTTCTG; hCXCR4, forward TGACGGACAAGTACAGGCTGC, reverse CCAGAAGGGA-AGCGTGATGA; hSDF-1, forward AATTCTCAACACTC-CAAACTGTGC, reverse TGCACACTTGTCTGTTGTTGT-TC; hRPL32, forward CAACATTGGTTATGGAAGCAACA, reverse TGACGTTGTGGACCAGGAACT. Expression of the housekeeping genes did not differ between groups. Data analysis was performed using Applied Biosystems Comparative C_T method.

Statistics

Data are expressed as means ± SEM except numerical proteinuria data which are presented as geometric mean ×/÷ tolerance factor. Statistical significance was determined by one-way ANOVA with a Newman-Keuls post-hoc comparison or Student's t-test where appropriate. Statistical analyses were performed using GraphPad Prism 5 for Mac OS X (GraphPad Software Inc., San Diego, CA).

Results

CXCR4 and SDF-1 localization in the adult kidney

In our first experiments, we set out to define the sites of expression of SDF-1 and CXCR4 in the adult kidney. This initial immunostaining survey revealed constitutive expression of both SDF-1 and CXCR4 protein distributed prominently, although not exclusively, within the renal glomerulus (Figure 1). SDF-1 protein was notable within interstitial fibroblasts, podocytes, arteriolar smooth muscle and endothelial cells, epithelial cells of Bowman's capsule and scattered distal tubular cells, with weak, focal immunostaining within renal glomerular endothelial cells (Figure 1A-C). CXCR4 protein was present in glomerular podocytes and endothelial cells of the glomerular and peritubular capillaries (Figure 1D-F).

Altered expression of SDF-1/CXCR4 in subtotally nephrectomized rats

To elucidate the role of SDF-1/CXCR4 signaling in CKD we first determined gene expression of both receptor and ligand in the kidneys of rats that had undergone subtotal nephrectomy (SNx), a well-established model of progressive renal fibrosis. In these experiments, we observed an approximate two-fold increase in CXCR4 mRNA in the kidneys of SNx rats in comparison to sham-operated animals (Figure 2A). By way of contrast, SDF-1 mRNA was reduced in SNx kidneys (Figure 2B).

In exploring potential mechanisms that may mediate the downregulation of SDF-1 in SNx kidneys we considered the chemokine's prominent presence within interstitial fibroblasts and the sensitivity of these cells to the pro-fibrotic growth factor, TGF-β. TGF-β mRNA was increased >50% in the kidneys of SNx rats in comparison to sham animals (Figure 2C), whereas exposure of cultured NRK-49F renal fibroblasts to recombinant TGF-β resulted in an approximate 80% reduction in SDF-1 mRNA (Figure 2D). Consistent with an emerging recognition for the importance of post-translational protein acetylation in regulating the cellular response to TGF-β [24], SDF-1 downregulation was

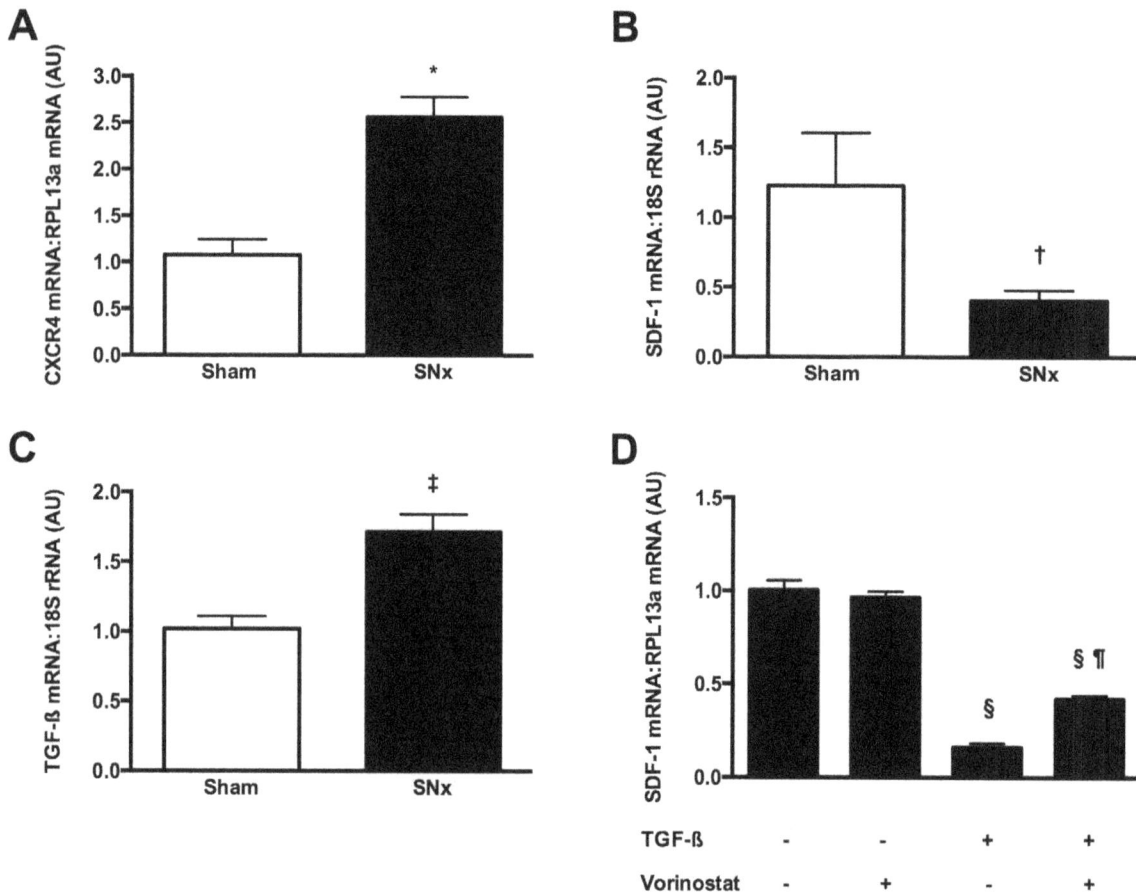

Figure 2. CXCR4 and SDF-1 mRNA in sham-operated and subtotally nephrectomized (SNx) rats. CXCR4 expression is increased in the kidneys of SNx rats (A), whereas SDF-1 is reduced (B). The kidneys of SNx rats also demonstrated an upregulation of the pro-fibrotic growth factor, transforming growth factor-β (TGF-β) (C). In cultured NRK-49F renal fibroblasts, recombinant TGF-β downregulated SDF-1 mRNA, with this effect being attenuated by HDAC inhibition with vorinostat (D). *$p < 0.001$ vs. sham, †$p < 0.05$ vs. sham, ‡$p < 0.01$ vs. sham, §$p < 0.001$ vs. control, ¶$p < 0.001$ vs. TGF-β.

attenuated by pre-treatment of fibroblasts with the histone deacetylase (HDAC) inhibitor, vorinostat (Figure 2D).

Chronic CXCR4 antagonism accelerates renal decline in subtotally nephrectomized rats

Having identified a dysregulation in SDF-1/CXCR4 expression in the kidneys of SNx rats, we next sought to determine the role of this pathway in the chronically ischemic kidney. Sham and SNx rats were therefore randomized to receive either vehicle (PBS) or the CXCR4 antagonist AMD3100 (1 mg/kg/day s.c.) for eight weeks. AMD3100 is a non-peptide, highly specific antagonist of CXCR4 (IC_{50} for calcium flux 572 ± 190 nM vs. >100 μM for CCR1, CCR2b, CXCR3, CCR4, CCR5 and CCR7 [25]) that binds to the receptor through three primary acid residues Asp^{171} (AspIV:20), Asp^{262} (AspVI:23) and Glu^{288} (GluVII:06) in an irreversible or slowly reversible manner [26]. At the end of the eight week study period, systolic blood pressure (SBP) and urine protein excretion were increased while GFR was decreased in SNx rats relative to sham animals (Table 1). Change in each of these parameters was augmented in SNx rats receiving AMD3100, with a rise in SBP and urine protein and decrease in GFR relative to vehicle-treated SNx rats (Table 1). AMD3100 had no effect on SBP, urine protein excretion or GFR in sham rats (Table 1).

Examination of kidney sections by light microscopy revealed that SNx surgery was associated with an expected increase in glomerulosclerosis (Figure 3A–E) and tubulointerstitial collagen IV deposition (Figure 3F–J), with both of these indicators of renal fibrosis being augmented with CXCR4 antagonism in SNx rats (Figure 3).

CXCR4 blockade accelerates capillary loss in subtotally nephrectomized rats

As CXCR4 was detectable in the endothelial cells of both the glomerular and peritubular capillaries we next sought to determine the effect of CXCR4 antagonism on both capillary density and capillary volume in sham and SNx rats. To assess the density of the glomerular and peritubular capillaries, kidney sections were immunostained with the monoclonal antibody JG-12 that binds to endothelial cells of capillaries but not lymphatics in rat kidneys [27]. Endothelial immunostaining was reduced in both the glomerular and peritubular compartments eight weeks after SNx surgery, with a further reduction in capillary density noted in kidney sections of AMD3100-treated SNx rats (Figure 4A–J). To determine whether glomerular capillary volume was also affected, we used the novel technique of fluorescent microangiography (FMA) that allows the generation of virtual three dimensional

Table 1. Functional characteristics of sham and subtotal nephrectomy (SNx) rats treated with vehicle or AMD3100.

	Body weight (g)	Left kidney weight (g)	Left kidney weight / body weight (%)	SBP (mmHg)	GFR (ml/min/kg)	Urine protein excretion (mg/day)
Sham + vehicle	186±3	0.56±0.01	0.300±0.005	113±2	5.36±0.25	1.71×/÷1.12
Sham + AMD3100	185±5	0.54±0.02	0.296±0.005	112±3	5.29±0.28	2.37×/÷1.08
SNx + vehicle	172±3*†	0.67±0.04‡§	0.400±0.031§¶	145±7‡§	3.22±0.32‡§	20.42×/÷1.52‡§
SNx + AMD3100	180±3	0.67±0.03‡§	0.378±0.016†‡	165±5‡§||	1.73±0.10‡§**	50.70×/÷1.26‡§||

SBP = systolic blood pressure.
*$p<0.05$ vs. sham + vehicle, †$p<0.05$ vs. sham + AMD3100, ‡$p<0.01$ vs. sham + vehicle, §$p<0.01$ vs. sham + AMD3100, ¶$p<0.001$ vs. sham + vehicle, ||$p<0.05$ vs. SNx + vehicle, **$p<0.01$ vs. SNx + vehicle.

glomerular microvascular casts following confocal optical sectioning [18]. Consistent with the hypertrophic response that accompanies renal mass ablation, glomerular volume was increased in vehicle-treated SNx rats in comparison to sham rats and this was also significantly reduced with CXCR4 blockade (Figure 4K-O).

Local SDF-1/CXCR4 signaling activates glomerular eNOS in the adult kidney

Since chronic CXCR4 antagonism accelerated renal decline and augmented capillary loss in SNx rats and since both the receptor and ligand were present in both the glomerular and tubulointerstitial compartments, we next sought to determine

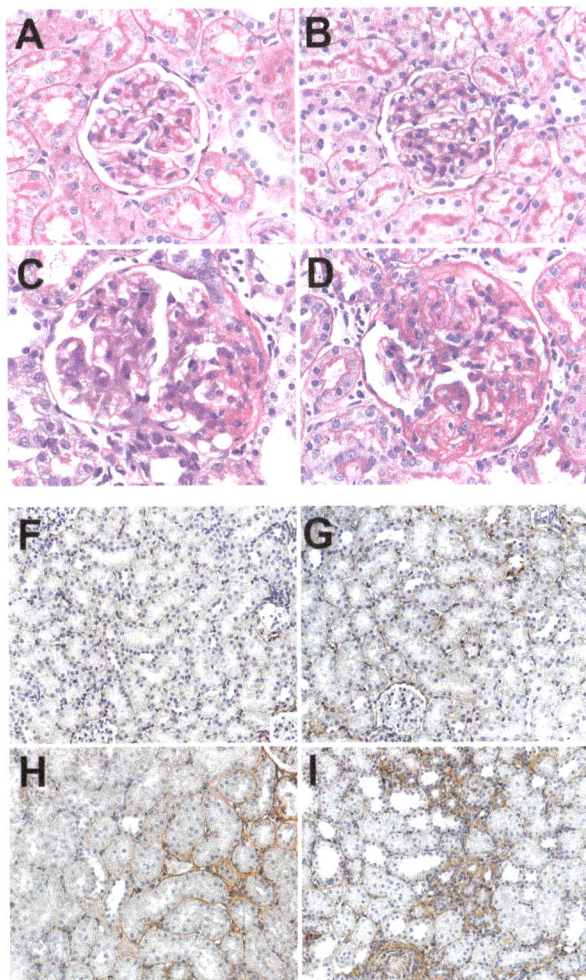

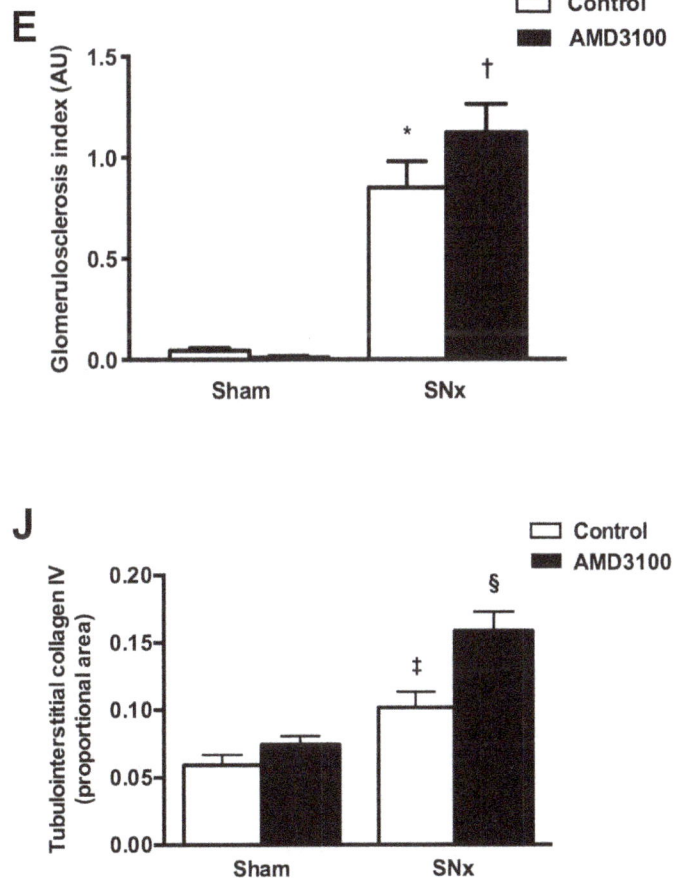

Figure 3. Effect of the CXCR4 antagonist, AMD3100 on glomerulosclerosis and renal fibrosis in subtotally nephrectomized (SNx) rats. PAS-stained kidney sections from sham (A and B) and SNx (C and D) rats treated with vehicle (A and C) or AMD3100 (B and D) for eight weeks. Original magnification x400. (E) Glomerulosclerosis index. Tubulointerstitial collagen IV immunostaining of kidney sections from sham (F and G) and SNx (H and I) rats treated with vehicle (F and H) or AMD3100 (G and I) for eight weeks. Original magnification x160. (J) Quantitation of tubulointerstitial collagen IV. AU = arbitrary units. *$p<0.001$ vs. sham, †$p<0.05$ vs. SNx + vehicle, ‡$p<0.05$ vs. sham, §$p<0.01$ vs. SNx + vehicle.

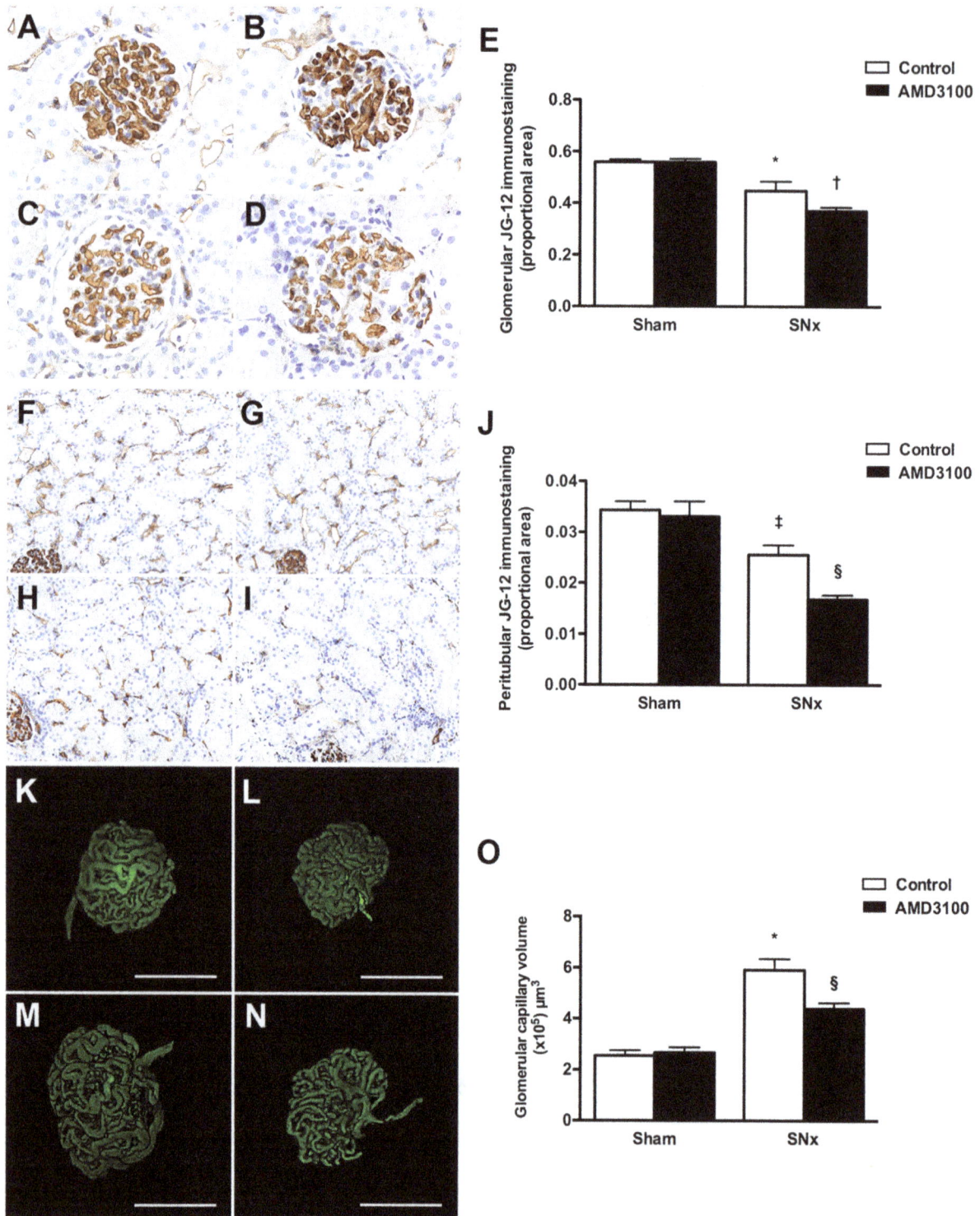

Figure 4. Effect of CXCR4 antagonism with AMD3100 on capillary loss in subtotally nephrectomized (SNx) rats. (A–D) Glomerular endothelial (JG-12) immunostaining of kidney sections from sham (A and B) and SNx (C and D) rats treated with vehicle (A and C) or AMD3100 (B and D) for eight weeks. Original magnification x400. (E) Quantitation of glomerular JG-12. (F–I) Peritubular JG-12 immunostaining of kidney sections from sham (F and G) and SNx (H and I) rats treated with vehicle (F and H) or AMD3100 (G and I). Original magnification x160. (J) Quantitation of peritubular JG-12. (K–N) Fluorescent microangiography (FMA) images of glomeruli from sham (K and L) and SNx (M and N) rats treated with vehicle (K and M) or AMD3100 (L and N) for eight weeks. (O) Glomerular capillary volume. *p<0.001 vs. sham, †p<0.05 vs. SNx + vehicle, ‡p<0.01 vs. sham, §p<0.01 vs. SNx + vehicle.

whether the SDF-1/CXCR4 axis may mediate local vascular signaling pathways in the adult kidney. One downstream regulator of the endothelial response to SDF-1, is endothelial nitric oxide synthase (eNOS) that may be activated by phosphorylation of its serine 1177 residue, through an Akt/phospho-inositide 3-kinase (PI3-kinase) dependent pathway [28]. To confirm the role of this pathway in endothelial eNOS activation, we first exposed cultured human umbilical vein endothelial cells (HUVECs) to recombinant SDF-1 with or without pre-treatment with either AMD3100 or the PI3-kinase antagonist, LY294002. Immunoblotting cell lysates confirmed that SDF-1 induced eNOS Ser1177 phosphorylation and that this was prevented by either CXCR4 or PI3-kinase inhibition (Figure 5A). To determine whether a similar signaling cascade is functional within the adult glomerulus, recombinant SDF-1 was next delivered to the kidneys of normal rats, via the abdominal aorta, with or without pre-treatment with AMD3100 (n = 6/group). Immunoblotting of glomeruli, isolated by differential sieving 30 min later, revealed that acute SDF-1 delivery induced an increase in eNOS Ser1177 phosphorylation and that this was antagonized by pre-treatment with AMD3100 (Figure 5B).

SDF-1/CXCR4 expression is altered in the biopsies of patients with secondary focal segmental glomerulosclerosis

Our experiments thus far had revealed that local SDF-1/CXCR4 signaling functions to preserve microvascular integrity and renal function in SNx rats, whereas the expression of both SDF-1 and CXCR4 is dysregulated following renal mass ablation, being characterized by downregulation of the former and upregulation of the latter. To determine whether the SDF-1/CXCR4 pathway is similarly dysregulated in human CKD, we

examined gene expression of both receptor and ligand in biopsies from patients with secondary focal segmental glomerulosclerosis (FSGS) and time zero live kidney donor controls. FSGS is a common cause of progressive proteinuric kidney disease that bears pathophysiological similarity to the kidney injury that follows experimental renal mass ablation [29]. Sufficient archival formalin-fixed paraffin-embedded biopsy tissue was available to determine CXCR4 and SDF-1 expression in six samples from patients with biopsy-proven and clinically correlated obesity-related secondary FSGS compared with ten samples from time-zero live kidney donors. The clinical characteristics of patients with FSGS are shown in Table 2. All patients were hypertensive with an elevated urine protein excretion and two subjects had concomitant diabetes mellitus. For kidney donors, all patients were normotensive, with normal renal function and none of the donors had diabetes. In these studies, CXCR4 mRNA was observed to be increased approximately 5-fold in the kidneys of patients with FSGS relative to controls (Figure 6A), while there was a doubling in SDF-1 mRNA (Figure 6B).

ACE inhibition augments renal SDF-1 expression in CKD

Although CXCR4 expression was consistently increased in both experimental and human CKD, SDF-1 mRNA was more variable, with a decrease in expression in SNx kidneys and an increase in FSGS biopsies. In considering potential mechanisms that may contribute to this apparent discordance, we recognized that five of the six FSGS patients were treated with ACE inhibitors (Table 2). To determine whether either SDF-1 or CXCR4 expression may be altered by ACE inhibition, we finally examined mRNA levels in a separate cohort of rats that had been treated with the ACE inhibitor perindopril, as previously described [21].

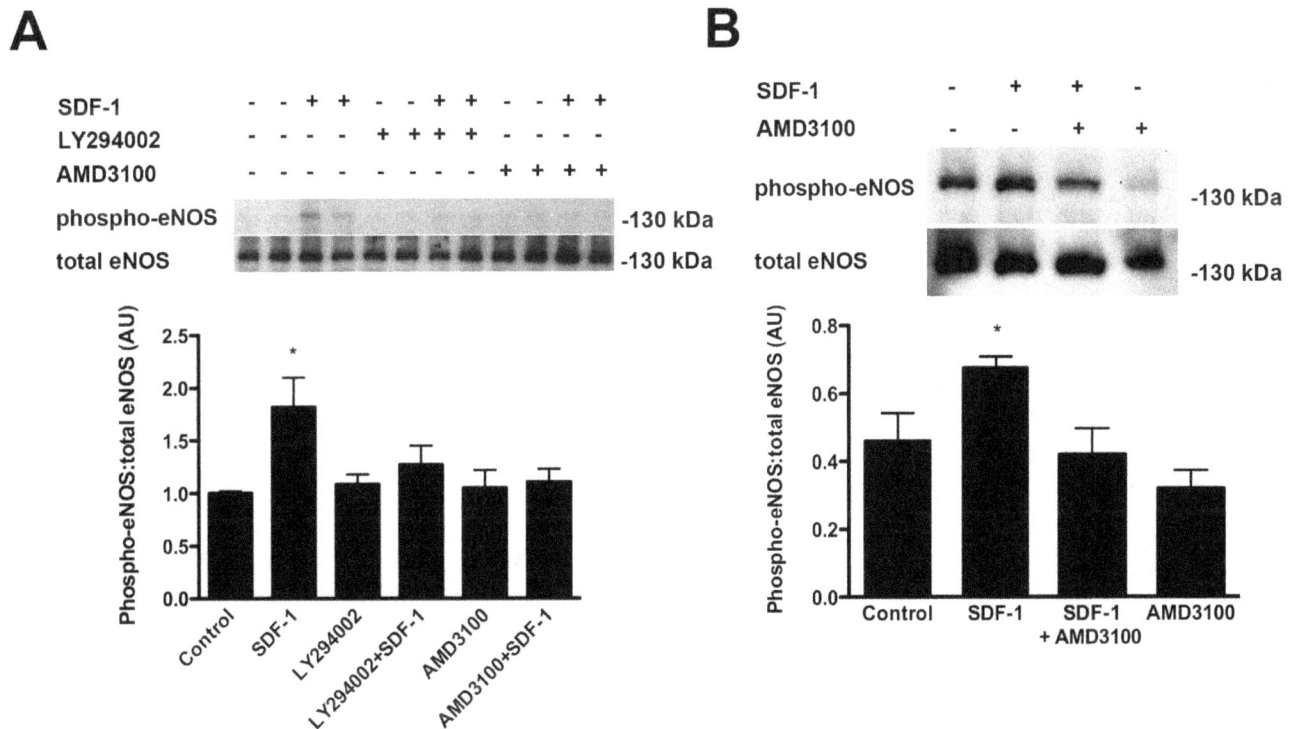

Figure 5. Phosphorylation of eNOS by SDF-1 at the activation site Ser1177. (A) Effect of SDF-1, the PI3-kinase inhibitor, LY294002 and the CXCR4 inhibitor, AMD3100 on eNOS Ser1177 phosphorylation in human umbilical vein endothelial cells (HUVECs). (B) Effect of acute SDF-1 administration on eNOS Ser1177 phosphorylation in sieved rat glomeruli following pre-treatment with PBS or the CXCR4 antagonist AMD3100. AU = arbitrary units. *p<0.05 vs. all other groups.

Table 2. Clinical characteristics of patients with secondary focal segmental glomerulosclerosis (FSGS).

Patient	Age (years)	Weight (kg)	Sex (M/F)	Hypertension (Y/N)	ACEi/ARB	Diabetes (Y/N)	Urine protein excretion	Serum creatinine (μmol/L)
1	13	102.6	M	Y	Enalapril 10 mg o.d.	N	Protein:creatinine ratio 400 mg/mmol	83
2	34	102.6	M	Y	Ramipril 10 mg o.d.	N	24 h urine protein excretion 1.87 g/24 h	300
3	55	106.6	M	Y	Ramipril 10 mg o.d.	Y	Protein:creatinine ratio 679 mg/mmol	108
4	34	104.5	F	Y	No	N	Protein:creatinine ratio 338mg/mmol	76
5	17	154.9	M	Y	Enalapril 10mg o.d.	Y	Protein:creatinine ratio 118mg/mmol	53
6	38	116	M	Y	Enalapril 20mg o.d.	N	Protein:creatinine ratio 120mg/mmol	98

These experiments revealed that CXCR4 mRNA was increased in SNx rats and, while reduced with perindopril-treatment, remained significantly elevated relative to sham rats (Figure 7A). Moreover, SDF-1 mRNA was markedly increased in the kidneys of perindopril-treated SNx rats when compared with either sham animals or SNx rats treated with vehicle, consistent with the change in gene expression observed in human FSGS biopsies (Figure 7B).

Discussion

Despite existing therapies and regardless of the underlying etiology, renal function continues to decline in the majority of people with CKD. Over recent years, the almost universal failure of novel anti-albuminuric therapies to meaningfully impact on clinical outcomes has encouraged investigators to direct their attention to pathogenetic processes that commonly occur during the later stages of CKD development. These pathogenetic processes include renal fibrosis and the associated disruption in the microvascular architecture, acting together and compounding the deleterious effects of one another in the relentless progression towards end-stage renal disease. In the present study, we identified a novel role for SDF-1/CXCR4 signaling in this reciprocal relationship, observing that local SDF-1/CXCR4 signaling preserves microvascular integrity and attenuates fibrogenesis, whereas the pro-fibrotic growth factor TGF-β, overelaborated in the CKD setting, downregulates SDF-1 expression. Augmentation of SDF-1/CXCR4 signaling by novel or existing agents, either purposefully or serendipitously, may thus slow the progression of renal decline in CKD.

SDF-1 signaling through CXCR4 promotes cell survival [30], migration [28], and proliferation [31], favoring neo-angiogenesis both through direct effects and through the creation of a permissive microenvironment that facilitates the actions of the angiogenic factor, vascular endothelial growth factor (VEGF) [32,33]. In the present study we observed that i) CXCR4 is expressed on the surface of endothelial cells in both the glomerular and peritubular compartments, ii) chronic CXCR4 blockade accelerates capillary loss in rats with CKD and iii) local SDF-1 delivery induces glomerular eNOS activation in a CXCR4-dependent manner. Moreover, accelerated disruption of the microvascular architecture with chronic CXCR4 blockade was associated with augmented renal decline and progressive renal fibrosis, analogous to the exacerbation of cardiac dysfunction with chronic CXCR4 blockade in the post-myocardial infarction setting [34]. Collectively, these observations highlight a hitherto unrecognized role for local SDF-1/CXCR4 signaling in preserving microvascular integrity and preventing coincident renal fibrosis in CKD.

In light of the detrimental effects observed with chronic CXCR4 blockade, the consistent upregulation of CXCR4 in the kidneys of SNx rats and in biopsies from patients with secondary FSGS is likely indicative of a compensatory response. CXCR4 upregulation has previously been described as a feature of a hypoxia-related glomerulopathy in patients with hypertensive nephrosclerosis [35]. Although both CXCR4 and SDF-1 are recognized as being hypoxia-responsive genes [36], their expression patterns were not indistinguishable in rat and human CKD. Whereas CXCR4 was consistently upregulated in both rats and humans with CKD, SDF-1 expression was more variable, the chemokine being notably downregulated in SNx kidneys of both female and male rats. In considering plausible mediators for SDF-1 downregulation in rats with CKD, we recognized the reciprocal relationship between fibrogenesis and capillary loss and hypoth-

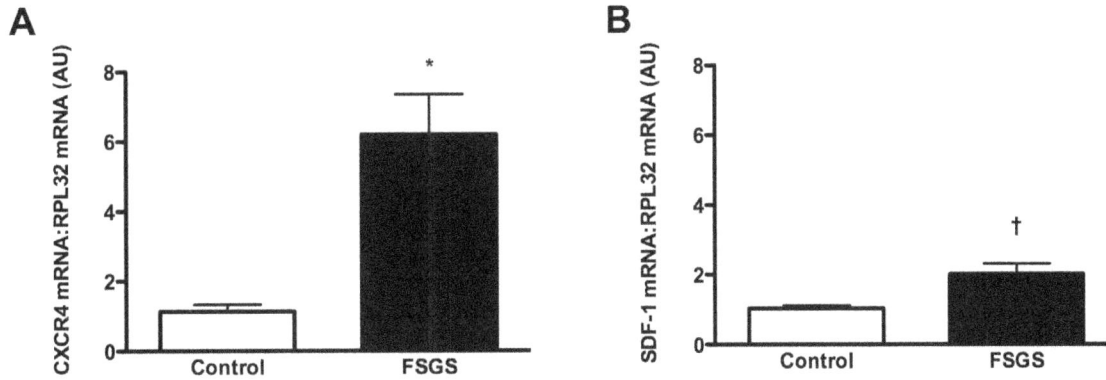

Figure 6. Real-time PCR for CXCR4 (A) and SDF-1 (B) mRNA in biopsies from time zero live kidney donors (Control, n = 10) and patients with secondary focal segmental glomerulosclerosis (FSGS, n = 6). AU = arbitrary units. *p<0.001, †p<0.01.

esized that decreased SDF-1 expression may occur as a consequence of the fibrotic process itself. TGF-β is a pro-sclerotic cytokine implicated in the fibrogenic response of many organs, including the kidney. Consistent with previous studies in oral myofibroblasts [37] and mimicking the changes in gene expression observed in the kidneys of SNx rats, exposure of cultured renal fibroblasts to recombinant TGF-β resulted in a marked downregulation in SDF-1 expression.

The post-translational modification of proteins, by the addition or removal of functional groups, is a common mechanism for controlling protein behaviour, perhaps most readily appreciated when considering the essential role that (de)phosphorylation plays in cellular homeostasis. More recently, post-translational protein modification through the addition or removal of acetyl groups has been recognized to rival phosphorylation in its diversity of substrates and the functional pathways affected [38]. (De)acetylation of proteins on lysine residues is regulated by the opposing actions of groups of enzymes called histone acetyltransferases and histone deacetylases (HDACs). In recent times, increasing evidence has begun to emerge for a pivotal role for HDACs in mediating both the progression of renal fibrosis and the response to TGF-β itself. For instance, work from our own group showed that HDAC inhibition attenuated glomerular matrix accumulation in diabetic mice [23], whereas acetylation may alter the cellular

response to TGF-β through affecting Smad 2/3 activity [39], Smad7 stability [39] and/or the actions of downstream transcription factors [40] among other processes. Confirming that TGF-β mediated SDF-1 downregulation is under the regulatory control of protein acetylation, the decrement in SDF-1 transcript levels induced by TGF-β was attenuated by pre-treatment of cells with the HDAC inhibitor, vorinostat.

One of the challenges restricting the translation of promising experimental observations to the clinic is the limited ability of rodent models to recapitulate human disease. For instance, we observed that whereas SDF-1 expression was downregulated in SNx rats, the opposite effect occurred in biopsies from patients with secondary FSGS. This superficial discordance encouraged us to consider the differences between the human disease and experimental model. To account for the confounding effects of medication usage among patients, we therefore examined SDF-1 expression patterns in historical samples from SNx rats that had or had not been treated with the ACE inhibitor, perindopril [21]. In contrast to vehicle treatment, ACE inhibition, previously shown to decrease the overelaboration of TGF-β in SNx rats [41], resulted in a marked upregulation in SDF-1. Augmentation of SDF-1 activity may thus represent a novel mechanism by which renin angiotensin system blockade preserves the renal vasculature [42].

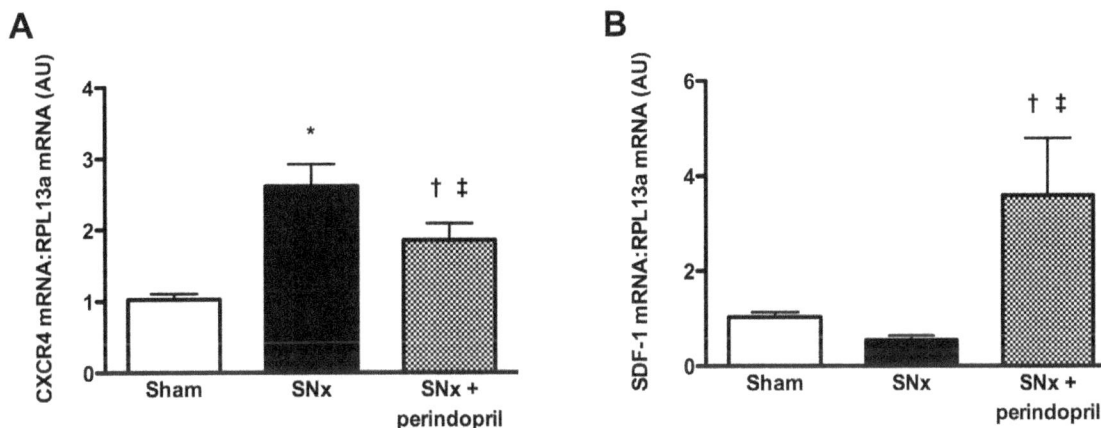

Figure 7. Real-time PCR for CXCR4 (A) and SDF-1 (B) mRNA in kidneys from sham rats, subtotally nephrectomized (SNx) rats and SNx rats treated with perindopril. *p<0.001 vs. sham, †p<0.05 vs. sham, ‡p<0.05 vs. SNx.

Although SDF-1/CXCR4 interaction was originally considered a monogamous relationship, more recent evidence suggests that this is not the case. CXCR4 also acts as a receptor for the HIV envelope receptor glycoprotein gp120 [43] and for the small protein ubiquitin [44], while SDF-1 may also bind to CXCR7. The renal actions of CXCR7 are complex with reports that the receptor signals in "renal multipotent progenitors" [45] while also functioning as a scavenger protein for SDF-1 [46]. Similarly, under some alternative conditions renal SDF-1/CXCR4 may play a potentially detrimental role through promoting podocyte proliferation [14], inflammatory cell recruitment [47] or, in the case of Shiga-toxin induced injury, endothelial phenotypic switch [48]. Thus, as with other angiogenic mediators [4,5], the role of renal SDF-1/CXCR4 is likely to be contextual, varying according to stage of development and the underlying injurious insult. The collective *in vitro*, acute and chronic *in vivo* and human correlative studies herein described indicate a reno-protective function for this pathway in CKD.

In summary, SDF-1/CXCR4 signaling is not only important for renal vascular development but the same system also plays a pivotal role in preserving microvascular integrity in CKD. Augmentation of this pathway by novel or existing therapies may attenuate renal fibrosis and slow the progression of renal decline in CKD.

Acknowledgments

The authors thank Ms. Bridgit Bowskill, Ms. Bailey Stead, Ms. Christine Kuliszewski, Ms. Krystina Vecchio and Ms. Katrina Zefkic for their excellent technical assistance.

Author Contributions

Conceived and designed the experiments: LHC DAY KAC PAM REG AA. Performed the experiments: LHC SLA KT MGK. Analyzed the data: LHC SLA KT MGK AA. Contributed reagents/materials/analysis tools: MMS IWG DJK. Wrote the paper: AA.

References

1. Fine LG, Orphanides C, Norman JT (1998) Progressive renal disease: the chronic hypoxia hypothesis. Kidney Int Suppl 65: S74–78.
2. Eremina V, Sood M, Haigh J, Nagy A, Lajoie G, et al. (2003) Glomerular-specific alterations of VEGF-A expression lead to distinct congenital and acquired renal diseases. J Clin Invest 111: 707–716.
3. Eremina V, Jefferson JA, Kowalewska J, Hochster H, Haas M, et al. (2008) VEGF inhibition and renal thrombotic microangiopathy. N Engl J Med 358: 1129–1136.
4. Advani A, Kelly DJ, Advani SL, Cox AJ, Thai K, et al. (2007) Role of VEGF in maintaining renal structure and function under normotensive and hypertensive conditions. Proc Natl Acad Sci U S A 104: 14448–14453.
5. Jeansson M, Gawlik A, Anderson G, Li C, Kerjaschki D, et al. (2011) Angiopoietin-1 is essential in mouse vasculature during development and in response to injury. J Clin Invest 121: 2278–2289.
6. Fogo AB (2005) New capillary growth: a contributor to regression of sclerosis? Curr Opin Nephrol Hypertens 14: 201–203.
7. Takabatake Y, Sugiyama T, Kohara H, Matsusaka T, Kurihara H, et al. (2009) The CXCL12 (SDF-1)/CXCR4 axis is essential for the development of renal vasculature. J Am Soc Nephrol 20: 1714–1723.
8. Gupta SK, Lysko PG, Pillarisetti K, Ohlstein E, Stadel JM (1998) Chemokine receptors in human endothelial cells. Functional expression of CXCR4 and its transcriptional regulation by inflammatory cytokines. J Biol Chem 273: 4282–4287.
9. Nagasawa T, Kikutani H, Kishimoto T (1994) Molecular cloning and structure of a pre-B-cell growth-stimulating factor. Proc Natl Acad Sci U S A 91: 2305–2309.
10. Janowski M (2009) Functional diversity of SDF-1 splicing variants. Cell Adh Migr 3: 243–249.
11. Tachibana K, Hirota S, Iizasa H, Yoshida H, Kawabata K, et al. (1998) The chemokine receptor CXCR4 is essential for vascularization of the gastrointestinal tract. Nature 393: 591–594.
12. Yuen DA, Stead BE, Zhang Y, White KE, Kabir MG, et al. (2012) eNOS deficiency predisposes podocytes to injury in diabetes. J Am Soc Nephrol 23: 1810–1823.
13. Stokman G, Stroo I, Claessen N, Teske GJ, Florquin S, et al. (2010) SDF-1 provides morphological and functional protection against renal ischaemia/reperfusion injury. Nephrol Dial Transplant 25: 3852–3859.
14. Ding M, Cui S, Li C, Jothy S, Haase V, et al. (2006) Loss of the tumor suppressor Vhlh leads to upregulation of Cxcr4 and rapidly progressive glomerulonephritis in mice. Nat Med 12: 1081–1087.
15. Floege J, Smeets B, Moeller MJ (2009) The SDF-1/CXCR4 axis is a novel driver of vascular development of the glomerulus. J Am Soc Nephrol 20: 1659–1661.
16. Advani A, Gilbert RE, Thai K, Gow RM, Langham RG, et al. (2009) Expression, localization, and function of the thioredoxin system in diabetic nephropathy. J Am Soc Nephrol 20: 730–741.
17. Yuen DA, Connelly KA, Advani A, Liao C, Kuliszewski MA, et al. (2010) Culture-modified bone marrow cells attenuate cardiac and renal injury in a chronic kidney disease rat model via a novel antifibrotic mechanism. PLoS One 5: e9543.
18. Advani A, Connelly KA, Yuen DA, Zhang Y, Advani SL, et al. (2011) Fluorescent microangiography is a novel and widely applicable technique for delineating the renal microvasculature. PLoS ONE 6: e24695.
19. Kanki S, Segers VF, Wu W, Kakkar R, Gannon J, et al. (2011) Stromal-cell derived factor-1 retention and cardioprotection for ischemic myocardium. Circ Heart Fail 4: 509–518.
20. Burlington H, Cronkite EP (1973) Characteristics of cell cultures derived from renal glomeruli. Proc Soc Exp Biol Med 142: 143–149.
21. Kelly DJ, Hepper C, Wu LL, Cox AJ, Gilbert RE (2003) Vascular endothelial growth factor expression and glomerular endothelial cell loss in the remnant kidney model. Nephrol Dial Transplant 18: 1286–1292.
22. Advani A, Kelly DJ, Cox AJ, White KE, Advani SL, et al. (2009) The (Pro)renin receptor: site-specific and functional linkage to the vacuolar H+-ATPase in the kidney. Hypertension 54: 261–269.
23. Advani A, Huang Q, Thai K, Advani SL, White KE, et al. (2011) Long-Term Administration of the Histone Deacetylase Inhibitor Vorinostat Attenuates Renal Injury in Experimental Diabetes through an Endothelial Nitric Oxide Synthase-Dependent Mechanism. Am J Pathol 178: 2205–2214.
24. Yuan H, Reddy MA, Sun G, Lanting L, Wang M, et al. (2013) Involvement of p300/CBP and epigenetic histone acetylation in TGF-beta1-mediated gene transcription in mesangial cells. Am J Physiol Renal Physiol 304: F601–613.
25. Fricker SP, Anastassov V, Cox J, Darkes MC, Grujic O, et al. (2006) Characterization of the molecular pharmacology of AMD3100: a specific antagonist of the G-protein coupled chemokine receptor, CXCR4. Biochem Pharmacol 72: 588–596.
26. Rosenkilde MM, Gerlach LO, Jakobsen JS, Skerlj RT, Bridger GJ, et al. (2004) Molecular mechanism of AMD3100 antagonism in the CXCR4 receptor: transfer of binding site to the CXCR3 receptor. J Biol Chem 279: 3033–3041.
27. Kim YG, Suga SI, Kang DH, Jefferson JA, Mazzali M, et al. (2000) Vascular endothelial growth factor accelerates renal recovery in experimental thrombotic microangiopathy. Kidney Int 58: 2390–2399.
28. Sameermahmood Z, Balasubramanyam M, Saravanan T, Rema M (2008) Curcumin modulates SDF-1alpha/CXCR4-induced migration of human retinal endothelial cells (HRECs). Invest Ophthalmol Vis Sci 49: 3305–3311.
29. Johnson RJ (1997) What mediates progressive glomerulosclerosis? The glomerular infiltration comes of age. Am J Pathol 151: 1179–1181.
30. Yano T, Liu Z, Donovan J, Thomas MK, Habener JF (2007) Stromal cell derived factor-1 (SDF-1)/CXCL12 attenuates diabetes in mice and promotes pancreatic beta-cell survival by activation of the prosurvival kinase Akt. Diabetes 56: 2946–2957.
31. De Falco V, Guarino V, Avilla E, Castellone MD, Salerno P, et al. (2007) Biological role and potential therapeutic targeting of the chemokine receptor CXCR4 in undifferentiated thyroid cancer. Cancer Res 67: 11821–11829.
32. Kanda S, Mochizuki Y, Kanetake H (2003) Stromal cell-derived factor-1alpha induces tube-like structure formation of endothelial cells through phosphoinositide 3-kinase. J Biol Chem 278: 257–262.
33. Grunewald M, Avraham I, Dor Y, Bachar-Lustig E, Itin A, et al. (2006) VEGF-induced adult neovascularization: recruitment, retention, and role of accessory cells. Cell 124: 175–189.
34. Dai S, Yuan F, Mu J, Li C, Chen N, et al. (2010) Chronic AMD3100 antagonism of SDF-1alpha-CXCR4 exacerbates cardiac dysfunction and remodeling after myocardial infarction. J Mol Cell Cardiol 49: 587–597.
35. Neusser MA, Lindenmeyer MT, Moll AG, Segerer S, Edenhofer I, et al. (2010) Human nephrosclerosis triggers a hypoxia-related glomerulopathy. Am J Pathol 176: 594–607.
36. Ceradini DJ, Kulkarni AR, Callaghan MJ, Tepper OM, Bastidas N, et al. (2004) Progenitor cell trafficking is regulated by hypoxic gradients through HIF-1 induction of SDF-1. Nat Med 10: 858–864.
37. Daly AJ, McIlreavey L, Irwin CR (2008) Regulation of HGF and SDF-1 expression by oral fibroblasts—implications for invasion of oral cancer. Oral Oncol 44: 646–651.
38. Kouzarides T (2000) Acetylation: a regulatory modification to rival phosphorylation? EMBO J 19: 1176–1179.

39. Simonsson M, Kanduri M, Gronroos E, Heldin CH, Ericsson J (2006) The DNA binding activities of Smad2 and Smad3 are regulated by coactivator-mediated acetylation. J Biol Chem 281: 39870–39880.

40. Chabane N, Li X, Fahmi H (2009) HDAC4 contributes to IL-1-induced mPGES-1 expression in human synovial fibroblasts through up-regulation of Egr-1 transcriptional activity. J Cell Biochem 106: 453–463.

41. Gilbert RE, Wu LL, Kelly DJ, Cox A, Wilkinson-Berka JL, et al. (1999) Pathological expression of renin and angiotensin II in the renal tubule after subtotal nephrectomy. Implications for the pathogenesis of tubulointerstitial fibrosis. Am J Pathol 155: 429–440.

42. Remuzzi A, Gagliardini E, Sangalli F, Bonomelli M, Piccinelli M, et al. (2006) ACE inhibition reduces glomerulosclerosis and regenerates glomerular tissue in a model of progressive renal disease. Kidney Int 69: 1124–1130.

43. Feng Y, Broder CC, Kennedy PE, Berger EA (1996) HIV-1 entry cofactor: functional cDNA cloning of a seven-transmembrane, G protein-coupled receptor. Science 272: 872–877.

44. Saini V, Marchese A, Majetschak M (2010) CXC chemokine receptor 4 is a cell surface receptor for extracellular ubiquitin. J Biol Chem 285: 15566–15576.

45. Mazzinghi B, Ronconi E, Lazzeri E, Sagrinati C, Ballerini L, et al. (2008) Essential but differential role for CXCR4 and CXCR7 in the therapeutic homing of human renal progenitor cells. J Exp Med 205: 479–490.

46. Naumann U, Cameroni E, Pruenster M, Mahabaleshwar H, Raz E, et al. (2010) CXCR7 functions as a scavenger for CXCL12 and CXCL11. PLoS One 5: e9175.

47. Chu PY, Zatta A, Kiriazis H, Chin-Dusting J, Du XJ, et al. (2011) CXCR4 antagonism attenuates the cardiorenal consequences of mineralocorticoid excess. Circ Heart Fail 4: 651–658.

48. Petruzziello-Pellegrini TN, Yuen DA, Page AV, Patel S, Soltyk AM, et al. (2012) The CXCR4/CXCR7/SDF-1 pathway contributes to the pathogenesis of Shiga toxin-associated hemolytic uremic syndrome in humans and mice. J Clin Invest 122: 759–776.

7

Does Erythropoietin Cause Hemoglobin Variability- Is It 'Normal'?

Ashwani K Gupta*, Waseem David

Department of Nephrology, University of Florida-Jacksonville, Jacksonville, Florida, United States of America

Abstract

Hemoglobin variability (Hb-var) in patients with chronic kidney disease has been stipulated to be a result of exogenous treatment with erythropoiesis stimulating agents (ESA) and has been related to mortality in dialysis patients. We hypothesized the existence of Hb-var independent of ESA administration and compared it to that in healthy adults using data from the Scripps-Kaiser and NHANES III databases. We studied the Hb-var in 1571 peritoneal dialysis patients which included 116 patients not requiring treatment with erythropoietin. We systematically studied the differences between the groups that needed ESA therapy and those who did not. White race and male sex were significant predictors of need for erythropoietin therapy. We found peritoneal dialysis patients to exhibit significantly increased Hb-var independent of treatment with exogenous erythropoietin (0.99 gm/dL vs. 1.17 gm/dL, p-value<0.001). We found age to be a significant determinant of Hb-var in the ESA treated group. Hb-var in younger patients (<30 years) was increased by 50% compared to young healthy adults. The Hb-var in elderly (>60 years) peritoneal dialysis patients was similar to that seen in healthy elders, suggesting similarity with anemia of aging. We conclude that exogenous ESA administration does not explain Hb-var entirely but may enhance it. Intrinsic factors affecting erythropoiesis including age may be the major determinants of Hb-var.

Editor: Zoran Ivanovic, French Blood Institute, France

Funding: The authors have no support or funding to report.

Competing Interests: The authors have declared that no competing interests exist.

* E-mail: akgupta@ufl.edu

Introduction

The basal rate of Red Blood Cell (RBC) production is diminished in patients with chronic kidney disease (CKD). Usually, the anemia is proportional to the severity of renal dysfunction, caused due to a deficiency of erythropoietin (EPO) [1]. Supplementation with exogenous Erythropoiesis Stimulating Agents (ESA) partially corrects the EPO deficiency and is used for its treatment [2]. Treatment of anemia in this population has several benefits including improvement in exercise tolerance, functional and sexual capacity [3], along with reduction in left ventricular hypertrophy [4], and improved cardiovascular functioning. A large variability has been observed in the hemoglobin level of dialysis patients treated with ESAs [5]. The physiologic basis underlying hemoglobin variability (Hb-var) is poorly understood. It is thought that patient demographics, comorbidities, concurrent events (infections and hospitalizations) as well practice patterns of ESA and iron administration are related to Hb-var. Several investigations [6–11] have focused exclusively on the effects of ESA on Hb-var in hemodialysis patients. This phenomenon has been called Hb cycling [5,12] by clinical epidemiologists and has been related to mortality [13–16] and cardiovascular outcomes.

Data on Hb-var in peritoneal dialysis (PD) patients are limited to small reports from the Netherlands [17], the United Kingdom [18] and China [19]. Walker et al. [20] have reported the largest group of 558 PD patients receiving Erythropoietin and 528 PD patients receiving Darbepoetin from the Australian continent. They observed an Hb standard deviation of 1.5 gm/dL in the Darbepoetin group, as compared to 1.1 gm/dL in the erythropoietin treated group. No data have been reported from the United States or Canada. A large cohort of European dialysis patients [21] included data on 967 patients not receiving ESA, but the authors did not analyze this data separately. We hypothesize the existence of Hb-var in PD patients not receiving any ESA and that the Hb-var in PD patients would be comparable to or greater than healthy adults. This has not been reported in the literature previously. In this study, we examined Hb-var data on 1571 PD patients who received dialysis at various Dialysis Clinics Inc. (a large non-profit dialysis provider) facilities throughout the United States between January 2007 and December 2009. The study attempts to define "normal" Hb-var in CKD by comparing our results with population normal in healthy adults obtained from the Scripps-Kaiser and NHANESIII databases [22]. In order to determine the relationship of Hb variability to ESA administration, we compared the subset of PD patients not receiving any ESA to the group receiving ESAs. The study of the subset of CKD patients not receiving ESA is a natural first step in understanding the red blood cell dynamics in renal failure. We will attempt to describe how this subset of patients differs in characteristics from those who require ESA therapy. We will further attempt to investigate the factors that determine Hb variability in both subsets of patients.

Methods

Study Design

This was a retrospective observational study. The study protocol was approved by the University of Florida Institutional Review Board and adhered to the declaration of Helsinki. A limited data set consisting of de-identified data was provided by Dialysis Clinics Inc. through a data use agreement. It was not possible to identify individual patients directly or through identifiers linked to the patients. Therefore, it was exempted from requiring informed consent by the IRB. Prevalent peritoneal dialysis patients receiving services for 6 months or longer at any of the centers operated by Dialysis Clinic Inc., a large nonprofit dialysis provider in the United States between January 2007 and December 2009 were included in this study. Children less than 18 years of age were excluded from the study population. Demographic data including - age, sex, race, dialysis vintage were included in the data provided. Date of clinic visit, Hb measured per clinic protocol (monthly); ESA dose administered, types of ESA used were also recorded. Laboratory values obtained during routine clinical care including serum iron, ferritin, TIBC, percent saturation (usually every 3 months), serum Albumin, PTH, and Kt/V measured per clinic protocol were recorded.

Data Analysis

All data analysis was carried out using STATA v.9.0. Patients were stratified into those requiring any ESA therapy (n = 1455) and those not requiring ESA therapy (n = 116). Patients who were administered even a single dose of an ESA during the study period were stratified in the ESA group. ESA naïve patients did not receive any doses of an ESA during the entire follow-up period. Hb-var was calculated using a 1 month standard deviation (SD-Hb) and the coefficient of hemoglobin variation. The coefficient of hemoglobin variation is defined as the ratio of the SD-Hb to the mean Hb. Results are reported as mean ± standard deviation. Comparisons between groups were based on a two sided student's t-test of means. The patients were divided into deciles of age to compare Hb-var with the population means reported in the Scripps-Kaiser and NHANESIII databases [22]. A regression model was fit to SD-Hb in the ESA treated group to study the effect of various parameters on SD-Hb.

Results

Data was available for a total of 1571 patients followed over a mean 19 months (range 7–156 weeks). The data revealed that 7.4% (n = 116) of our sample did not require any ESA therapy over the entire follow-up period. The two groups did not differ with regards to mean patient age, dialysis vintage and follow up period in the study. The proportion of diabetics in either group was also similar. Table 1 shows the differences between the no-ESA vs. ESA group. As expected, the mean Hb in the no-ESA group was 13.0 explaining the lack of need for ESA therapy. The ESA group was treated to a mean Hb of 11.7. The standard deviation of hemoglobin in the ESA group was 1.17 gm/dL compared to 0.99 gm/dL in the no-ESA group (p-value<0.001).

The group not requiring ESA had a greater proportion of males (69%). The proportion of sexes was equally distributed in the ESA group (53% males vs. 47% females). Since females may have menstrual blood losses which can partly account for variability in their hemoglobin, males were analyzed separately as well. By limiting the analysis to males only, the results did not change. The male no-ESA group still had a standard deviation of 1.0 gm/dL compared to 1.15 gm/dL in males who received ESA.

Patients in the no-ESA group had significantly more residual renal function, perhaps explaining the lack of EPO requirement in this group. The no-ESA group had slightly higher serum albumin and lower ferritins and PTH. Other iron indices (TIBC, Transferrin and total iron) were lower in the ESA treated group. A racial difference was noted in EPO requirement. A greater proportion of whites than blacks (9.1% vs. 4.2%) did not need ESA therapy to maintain similar levels of Hb. Separate subgroup analysis of the no-ESA group by race did not find any significant differences in Hb levels, iron indices, ratio of sexes, dialysis vintage or Kt/V. The black patients had significantly higher PTH overall-an effect that was consistent across the ESA and no-ESA groups.

Figure 1a and 1b compare the SD-Hb seen in Peritoneal Dialysis not requiring any ESA therapy patients with population normals obtained from the Scripps-Kaiser database (Fig. 1a), and NHANESIII(Fig. 1b). Figure 2a and 2b compare the SD-Hb seen in ESA treated Peritoneal Dialysis patients with population normals obtained from the Scripps-Kaiser database (Fig. 2a), and NHANESIII (Fig. 2b). Hb-var in the ESA naïve group was similar in magnitude and trend as observed in the NHANESIII and Scripps-Kaiser populations (Fig. 3). In contrast the ESA treated group was distinctively different and the Hb-var was highest in younger patients. In older patients the Hb-var approached the population means and tended to decline in the patients with age more than 60 years. This was observed in both males and females as well as in Caucasians and African American patients.

Table 2 shows the results of a regression model with the p-values of significant predictors of SD-Hb in the ESA treated group. Age was again found to be a significant predictor of SD-Hb. SD-Hb declined by 0.05 gm/dL with each decile of age. Iron saturation and dialysis clearance (KT/V) were also found to be significant predictors of SD-Hb. Patient sex, race, vintage on dialysis, serum albumin, serum iron, transferrin and ferritin were not found to be significant predictors of SD-Hb. Using a stepwise regression model, in the ESA naïve group none of the factors studied were predictive of Hb-var.

Discussion

Hemoglobin Variability - Normal or Abnormal

In the absence of a disease condition RBC production is controlled by a negative feedback system. The rate of change of RBC concentration is the difference between their rates of production and destruction. Within the bone marrow there exists a population of committed lineage specific pluripotent stem cells, also called colony forming units (CFU). CFUs are capable of differentiating into mature RBC under the influence of hormone erythropoietin produced by the kidneys. Low density of circulating RBC signals EPO production, whereas an increase in the numbers of circulating RBCs provides negative feedback to EPO. The pluripotent cells in the bone marrow exist in either a resting state (G_0) or a proliferative state. In dialysis patients the effects of peripheral factors such as varying iron stores and circulating inflammatory mediators such as hepcidin [23] affecting bone marrow responsiveness to EPO have been studied extensively. It is not known, if these factors can also influence cell replication times within the marrow or change the rates of entry and exit of cells between the resting and proliferative states. Theoretically, hemoglobin variability in patients with CKD may originate from an altered rate of apoptosis of precursor cells within the proliferating compartment of the marrow(due to EPO deficiency), or it may occur due to an increased delay in cell maturation times within the marrow. Exogenous ESA administration may enhance

Table 1. Differences between ESA treated and ESA Naïve PD Patients.

Variable	No-ESA			ESA			P-value
	Obs(n)	Mean	Std. Dev.	Obs(n)	Mean	Std. Dev.	
Mean-Hb(gm/dL)	116	13.0	1.7	1455	11.7	0.9	<0.0001
SD-Hb*(gm/dL)	116	0.99	0.45	1455	1.17	0.43	<0.0001
CV-Hb#	116	7.70	3.60	1455	10.00	3.80	<0.0001
Age(years)	116	59.9	13.37	1455	59.9	14.25	0.9
Sex							
Male	80	69%		773	53%		0.004
Female	36	31%		682	47%		
Vintage(years)	114	6.3	2.8	1454	6.9	3.4	0.08
Race							
White	88	75%		883	60%		0.004
Black	20	17.20%		460	31.60%		
Other	8	7.80%		111	8.40%		
Follow-up	116	17.7	10.0	1455	19.5	10.0	0.06
Diabetes	29	25.0%		1455	32.3%		0.12
Albumin(gm/dL)	116	3.6	0.4	1455	3.4	0.4	<0.0001
Serum Ferritin(ng/dL)	116	442.3	87.8	1455	594.4	13.5	0.005
Serum Iron(μg/dL)	115	82.4	25.5	1442	73.9	23.7	0.0003
TSAT(%)	98	28.5	14.2	1279	27.3	9.6	0.29
TIBC(μg/dL)	98	312.7	61.1	1287	274.7	56.1	<0.0001
Transferrin(mg/dL)	113	218.4	40.6	1441	192.1	38.3	<0.0001
K/tV	113	2.47	0.74	1425	2.25	0.57	0.0002
Renal	113	0.99	0.86	1425	0.55	0.68	<0.0001
Peritoneal	114	1.43	0.48	1447	1.68	0.52	<0.0001
PTH	116	284.9	146.9	1453	322.6	192.1	0.0395

*Standard Deviation of Hemoglobin.
#Coefficient of Hemoglobin Variability.

(as is evident by a significantly greater Hb-var in the ESA treated group) or ameliorate this hemoglobin variability, but does not account for it entirely.

The existence of hemoglobin variability in the patients on dialysis not requiring ESA therapy provides useful insights into understanding RBC dynamics in CKD patients. Previous investigations have focused on the relationship between ESAs and Hb-var [6–11]; we think the Hb-var is inherent to the normal hematopoietic processes. In a review, Arneson et al. [24] have compared four different methodologies used to characterize hemoglobin variability. Using the mean, standard deviation or the absolute hemoglobin change [25], provides us with a summary measure that is easy to understand conceptually. A residual standard deviation methodology has been proposed by Feldman et al. It measures the deviation from a regression line and therefore controls for linear trends only in the data. Gilbertson et al. [8] have also used fluctuation across thresholds to characterize hemoglobin variability. These methods attempt to describe Hb-var but can be difficult to comprehend. They do not address the reasons for the hemoglobin variability and have not found clinical applications.

Peritoneal dialysis patients lack large volume shifts and do not have ongoing blood losses into dialysis tubings and dialyzers, which characterize hemodialysis which can affect Hb-var. Access related blood loss and use of hemodialysis catheters are also known

to effect Hb-var [21] in hemodialysis patients but are not relevant to peritoneal dialysis patients. To test our hypothesis that Hb-var is present in chronic kidney disease independent of these factors, we chose to study patients on peritoneal dialysis. To exclude the effects of exogenous ESA on Hb-var, we studied patients who were not treated with any ESA. We found that patients on peritoneal dialysis with significantly preserved residual renal function still exhibited fluctuations in their Hb level. Hemoglobin variability (~1 gm/dL) was present in ESA naïve patients and was significantly increased to 1.17 gm/dL by ESA therapy. This indicates that variability in Hb is inherent to disturbed RBC dynamics in CKD, independent of exogenous ESA administration.

Determinants of Hemoglobin Variability

The inverse relationship between age and Hb-var in ESA treated hemodialysis patients has been observed previously [6,21], but no teleological argument has been made to explain it. In our study of peritoneal dialysis patients, we found that the youngest patients had the maximum degree of variation in their Hb and also the maximum deviation from the population means. It can be hypothesized that the inflammatory cytokines and uremic milieu characteristic of chronic kidney disease disrupts the hemostatic processes that maintain Hb in a narrow range in healthy adults. Aging has been associated with a pro-inflammatory state and higher levels of IL-6, a key regulator of hepcidin [26,27]. These

A

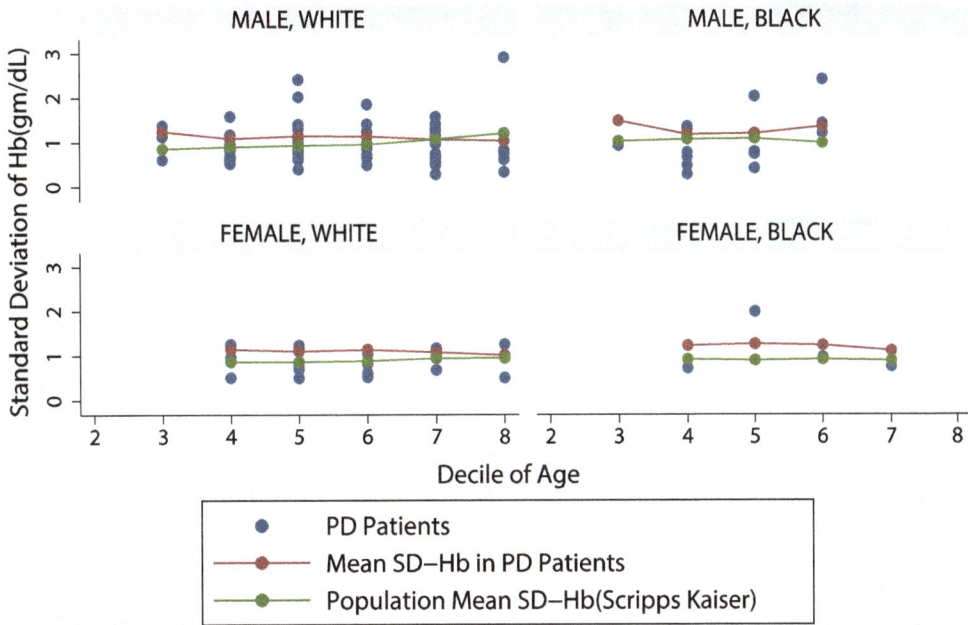

B

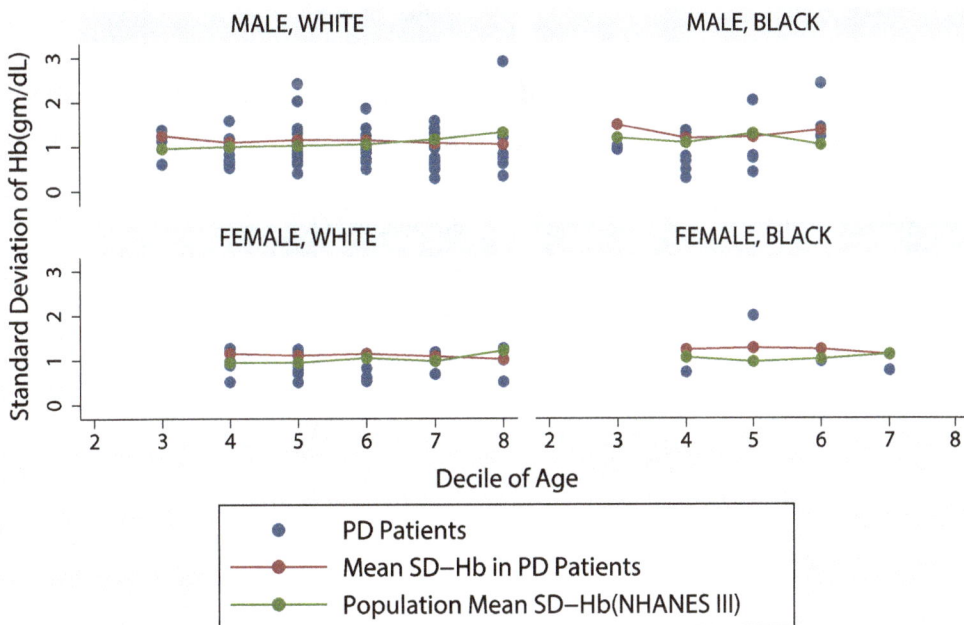

Figure 1. Hemoglobin Variability in ESA naïve Peritoneal Dialysis Patients.

Figure 2. Hemoglobin Variability in ESA treated Peritoneal Dialysis Patients.

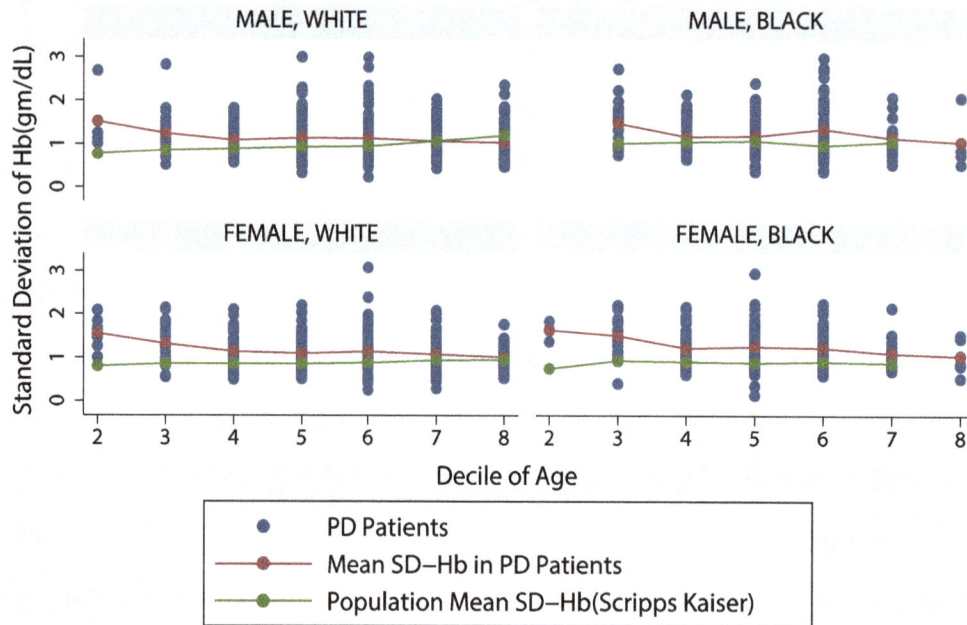

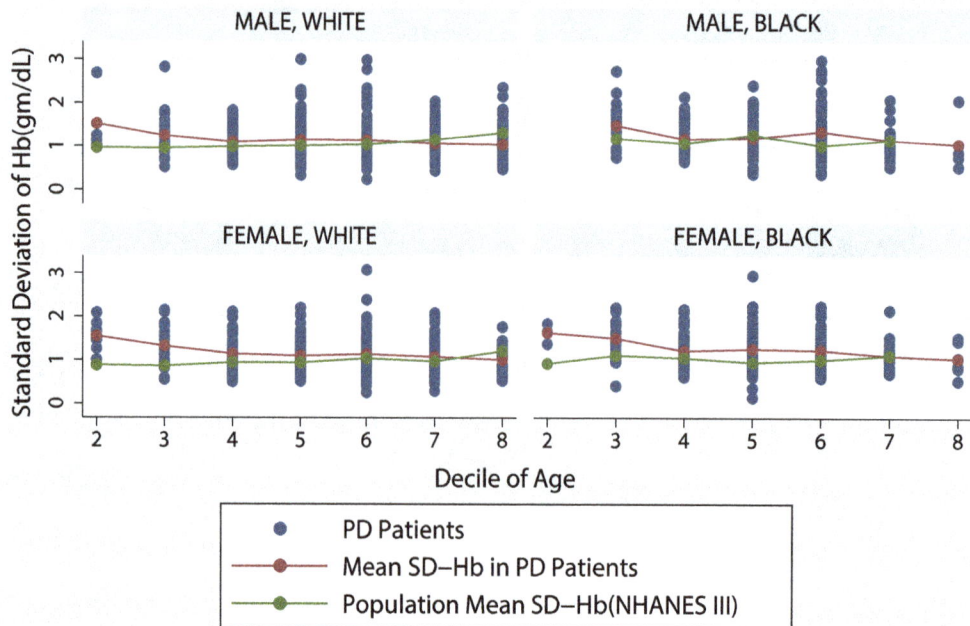

SD–Hb in different Population Groups

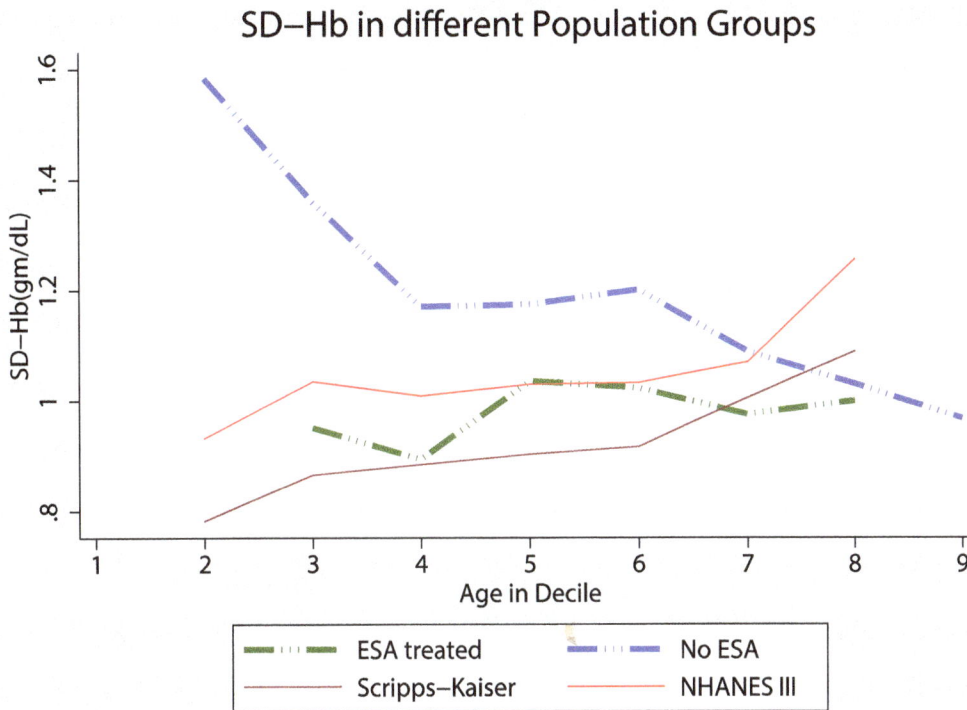

Figure 3. Hemoglobin Variability in different Population groups.

similarities with CKD may explain the closer degree of resemblance between elderly ESA treated peritoneal dialysis patients and the apparently healthy elders in the general population. Studying the factors that affect cell replication and control movement of cells between the resting and actively proliferating marrow pools may help us devise new treatments for anemia in CKD patients. Mathematical models of RBC dynamics can help us travel the path from normal physiology to disease pathophysiology and ultimately, allow us to devise more rational therapies. The factors affecting Hb-var in patients not treated with ESA have not been investigated before. In our regression models none of the clinical parameters being studied were significant predictors of Hb-var in this subgroup of patients. This may be a result of relatively small number of patients, to have enough power to detect a difference. Indeed however, this is the first time a

systematic study of patients not needing ESA has been undertaken. Larger analysis will be needed to confirm this finding.

Determinants of Need for ESA therapy

Higher EPO requirements have been observed in African American patients on dialysis in previous observational studies [28,29]. A race related genetic influence on hematopoiesis has been postulated earlier by Kauffman et al. [30]. Our finding that significantly more white patients did not need any ESA points to a stronger link to genetic factors effecting hematopoiesis. Similarly, greater proportion of males did not need ESA therapy. We did not have data related to hospitalizations, blood loss and infections which can also explain this apparent EPO hypo-responsiveness. The greater degree of residual renal function and total delivered dialysis dose (Kt/V) in the no-ESA group is not unexpected. The no-ESA group also had lower levels of various inflammatory markers including lower PTH, lower ferritin, and higher albumin level, once again pointing towards a role of inflammation in modulating erythropoiesis. Albumin levels have been found to be inversely correlated with inflammation in end stage renal disease patients [31–36]. Increased levels of cytokines INF-γ, TNF-α, IL-1 and IL-6 [37–39] have been implicated in producing ESA resistance and low hemoglobin levels. The low levels or absence of activation of these in patients not requiring ESA can be hypothesized but needs to be investigated. On the other hand ESA administration downregulates hepcidin [40,41] and may also suppress cytokine levels [42,43]. Lower levels hepcidin and proinflammatory cytokines may exert competing influence on erythropoiesis and can help explain the increased level of Hb-var in these patients. HFE gene mutations have been linked to lower ESA requirement [44], but their role in patients not needing ESA needs to be investigated. The prevalence of polymorphisms in

Table 2. Stepwise regression model of SD-Hb.

SD-Hb	Coef.	Std. Err.	t	P>t	[95% Conf.	Interval]
Kt/V	−0.05859	0.031955	−1.83	0.067	−0.12139	0.004215
T-Sat	0.011898	0.001898	6.27	0	0.008168	0.015629
Age	−0.0048	0.001315	−3.65	0	−0.00738	−0.00221
Followup	−0.00454	0.00177	−2.56	0.011	−0.00802	−0.00106
Regression Constant	1.322492	0.132143	10.01	0	1.062788	1.582196

Patient Sex, Race, Vintage on Diaysis, Serum Albumin, Iron, Transferrin and Ferretin were removed at a threshold level of p = 0.1.

genes for cytokine production can also provide useful insights. Compared to the study in hemodialysis patients [21] where inflammatory markers were significant predictors of Hb-var, serum albumin, PTH and ferritins were not found to be predictive of Hb-var in peritoneal dialysis patients. This is likely because peritoneal dialysis patients overall have lesser degree of inflammatory response compared to hemodialysis patients.

Conclusions

We conclude that Hb-var cannot be attributed to exogenous ESA administration alone. The physiologic bases of Hb-var are not completely understood. Deregulated homeostatic mechanisms in chronic kidney disease may enhance Hb-var. Hb-var in peritoneal dialysis patients younger than 50 years of age may be 50% greater than in healthy adults. The normal biology of aging may determine Hb-var. Effects of aging such as increased levels of inflammatory mediators and diminished capacity to secrete erythropoietin may mimic chronic kidney disease. The interaction

and effects of exogenous ESA administration on these factors remains poorly understood and should be investigated. Identification of these mechanisms may help us identify unique targets for novel therapies. By choosing appropriate physiologic targets for therapy we may be able to improve patient outcomes and enhance our understanding of disease processes.

Acknowledgments

The authors would like to acknowledge James Leighton, MD and Charles W. Heilig, MD at the University of Florida-Jacksonville, for their support and help with reading the manuscript proofs and suggesting improvements. The authors would also like to thank Karen Majchrzak at Dialysis Clinics Inc. for administrative help with obtaining the database for analysis.

Author Contributions

Conceived and designed the experiments: AKG. Analyzed the data: AKG WD. Wrote the paper: AKG WD.

References

1. Eschbach JW, Adamson JW (1988) Modern aspects of the pathophysiology of renal anemia. Contrib Nephrol 66: 63–70.
2. Ahmad R, Hand M (1987) Recombinant erythropoietin for the anemia of chronic renal failure. N Engl J Med 317: 169–170.
3. Johansen KL, Finkelstein FO, Revicki DA, Gitlin M, Evans C, et al. (2011) Systematic review and meta-analysis of exercise tolerance and physical functioning in dialysis patients treated with erythropoiesis-stimulating agents. Am J Kidney Dis 55: 535–548.
4. Massimetti C, Pontillo D, Feriozzi S, Costantini S, Capezzuto A, et al. (1998) Impact of recombinant human erythropoietin treatment on left ventricular hypertrophy and cardiac function in dialysis patients. Blood Purif 16: 317–324.
5. Fishbane S, Berns JS (2005) Hemoglobin cycling in hemodialysis patients treated with recombinant human erythropoietin. Kidney Int 68: 1337–1343.
6. Berns JS, Elzein H, Lynn RI, Fishbane S, Meisels IS, et al. (2003) Hemoglobin variability in epoetin-treated hemodialysis patients. Kidney Int 64: 1514–1521.
7. Ebben JP, Gilbertson DT, Foley RN, Collins AJ (2006) Hemoglobin level variability: associations with comorbidity, intercurrent events, and hospitalizations. Clin J Am Soc Nephrol 1: 1205–1210.
8. Gilbertson DT, Ebben JP, Foley RN, Weinhandl ED, Bradbury BD, et al. (2008) Hemoglobin level variability: associations with mortality. Clin J Am Soc Nephrol 3: 133–138.
9. Gilbertson DT, Peng Y, Bradbury B, Ebben JP, Collins AJ (2009) Hemoglobin level variability: anemia management among variability groups. Am J Nephrol 30: 491–498.
10. Kainz A, Mayer B, Kramar R, Oberbauer R (2010) Association of ESA hypo-responsiveness and haemoglobin variability with mortality in haemodialysis patients. Nephrol Dial Transplant 25: 3701–3706.
11. Lau JH, Gangji AS, Rabbat CG, Brimble KS (2010) Impact of haemoglobin and erythropoietin dose changes on mortality: a secondary analysis of results from a randomized anaemia management trial. Nephrol Dial Transplant 25: 4002–4009.
12. Singh AK, Milford E, Fishbane S, Keithi-Reddy SR (2008) Managing anemia in dialysis patients: hemoglobin cycling and overshoot. Kidney Int 74: 679–683.
13. Brunelli SM, Lynch KE, Ankers ED, Joffe MM, Yang W, et al. (2008) Association of hemoglobin variability and mortality among contemporary incident hemodialysis patients. Clin J Am Soc Nephrol 3: 1733–1740.
14. Ishani A, Solid CA, Weinhandl ED, Gilbertson DT, Foley RN, et al. (2008) Association between number of months below K/DOQI haemoglobin target and risk of hospitalization and death. Nephrol Dial Transplant 23: 1682–1689.
15. Kainz A, Wilflingseder J, Fugger R, Kramar R, Oberbauer R (2012) Hemoglobin variability after renal transplantation is associated with mortality. Transpl Int 25: 323–327.
16. Weinhandl ED, Peng Y, Gilbertson DT, Bradbury BD, Collins AJ (2011) Hemoglobin variability and mortality: confounding by disease severity. Am J Kidney Dis 57: 255–265.
17. van der Putten K, van der Baan FH, Schellekens H, Gaillard CA (2009) Hemoglobin variability in patients with chronic kidney disease in the Netherlands. Int J Artif Organs 32: 787–793.
18. Selby NM, Fonseca SA, Fluck RJ, Taal MW (2012) Hemoglobin variability with epoetin beta and continuous erythropoietin receptor activator in patients on peritoneal dialysis. Perit Dial Int 32: 177–182.
19. Chen HC, Chen KH, Lin YJ, Chang CJ, Tian YC, et al. (2012) Hemoglobin variability does not predict mortality in peritoneal dialysis patients. Chang Gung Med J 35: 79–87.
20. Walker R, Pussell BA (2009) Fluctuations in haemoglobin levels in haemodialysis, pre-dialysis and peritoneal dialysis patients receiving epoetin alpha or darbepoetin alpha. Nephrology (Carlton) 14: 689–695.
21. Eckardt KU, Kim J, Kronenberg F, Aljama P, Anker SD, et al. (2010) Hemoglobin variability does not predict mortality in European hemodialysis patients. J Am Soc Nephrol 21: 1765–1775.
22. Beutler E, Waalen J (2006) The definition of anemia: what is the lower limit of normal of the blood hemoglobin concentration? Blood 107: 1747–1750.
23. Canavesi E, Alfieri C, Pelusi S, Valenti L (2012) Hepcidin and HFE protein: Iron metabolism as a target for the anemia of chronic kidney disease. World J Nephrol 1: 166–176.
24. Arneson TJ, Zaun D, Peng Y, Solid CA, Dunning S, et al. (2009) Comparison of methodologies to characterize haemoglobin variability in the US Medicare haemodialysis population. Nephrol Dial Transplant 24: 1378–1383.
25. Yang W, Israni RK, Brunelli SM, Joffe MM, Fishbane S, et al. (2007) Hemoglobin variability and mortality in ESRD. J Am Soc Nephrol 18: 3164–3170.
26. Ferrucci L, Balducci L (2008) Anemia of aging: the role of chronic inflammation and cancer. Semin Hematol 45: 242–249.
27. McCranor BJ, Langdon JM, Prince OD, Femnou LK, Berger AE, et al. (2013) Investigation of the role of interleukin-6 and hepcidin antimicrobial peptide in the development of anemia with age. Haematologica.
28. Kausz AT, Solid C, Pereira BJ, Collins AJ, St Peter W (2005) Intractable anemia among hemodialysis patients: a sign of suboptimal management or a marker of disease? Am J Kidney Dis 45: 136–147.
29. Lacson E, Jr., Rogus J, Teng M, Lazarus JM, Hakim RM (2008) The association of race with erythropoietin dose in patients on long-term hemodialysis. Am J Kidney Dis 52: 1104–1114.
30. Kaufman JS (2008) Racial differences in erythropoietin responsiveness. Am J Kidney Dis 52: 1035–1038.
31. Yeun JY, Kaysen GA (1997) Acute phase proteins and peritoneal dialysate albumin loss are the main determinants of serum albumin in peritoneal dialysis patients. Am J Kidney Dis 30: 923–927.
32. Yeun JY, Kaysen GA (1998) Factors influencing serum albumin in dialysis patients. Am J Kidney Dis 32: S118–125.
33. Kaysen GA, Dubin JA, Muller HG, Rosales LM, Levin NW (2000) The acute-phase response varies with time and predicts serum albumin levels in hemodialysis patients. The HEMO Study Group. Kidney Int 58: 346–352.
34. Kaysen GA, Chertow GM, Adhikarla R, Young B, Ronco C, et al. (2001) Inflammation and dietary protein intake exert competing effects on serum albumin and creatinine in hemodialysis patients. Kidney Int 60: 333–340.
35. Kaysen GA, Dubin JA, Muller HG, Mitch WE, Rosales LM, et al. (2002) Relationships among inflammation nutrition and physiologic mechanisms establishing albumin levels in hemodialysis patients. Kidney Int 61: 2240–2249.
36. Kaysen GA, Dubin JA, Muller HG, Rosales L, Levin NW, et al. (2004) Inflammation and reduced albumin synthesis associated with stable decline in serum albumin in hemodialysis patients. Kidney Int 65: 1408–1415.
37. Cooper AC, Mikhail A, Lethbridge MW, Kemeny DM, Macdougall IC (2003) Increased expression of erythropoiesis inhibiting cytokines (IFN-gamma, TNF-alpha, IL-10, and IL-13) by T cells in patients exhibiting a poor response to erythropoietin therapy. J Am Soc Nephrol 14: 1776–1784.
38. Faquin WC, Schneider TJ, Goldberg MA (1992) Effect of inflammatory cytokines on hypoxia-induced erythropoietin production. Blood 79: 1987–1994.
39. Yilmaz MI, Solak Y, Covic A, Goldsmith D, Kanbay M (2011) Renal anemia of inflammation: the name is self-explanatory. Blood Purif 32: 220–225.

40. Ashby DR, Gale DP, Busbridge M, Murphy KG, Duncan ND, et al. (2010) Erythropoietin administration in humans causes a marked and prolonged reduction in circulating hepcidin. Haematologica 95: 505–508.

41. Ashby DR, Gale DP, Busbridge M, Murphy KG, Duncan ND, et al. (2009) Plasma hepcidin levels are elevated but responsive to erythropoietin therapy in renal disease. Kidney Int 75: 976–981.

42. Bian XX, Yuan XS, Qj CP (2010) Effect of recombinant human erythropoietin on serum S100B protein and interleukin-6 levels after traumatic brain injury in the rat. Neurol Med Chir (Tokyo) 50: 361–366.

43. Shen Y, Wang Y, Li D, Wang C, Xu B, et al. (2010) Recombinant human erythropoietin pretreatment attenuates heart ischemia-reperfusion injury in rats by suppressing the systemic inflammatory response. Transplant Proc 42: 1595–1597.

44. Canavese C, Bergamo D, Barbieri S, Timbaldi M, Thea A, et al. (2002) Clinical relevance of hemochromatosis-related HFE C282Y/H63D gene mutations in patients on chronic dialysis. Clin Nephrol 58: 438–444.

8

Impact of Vitamin D Supplementation on Arterial Vasomotion, Stiffness and Endothelial Biomarkers in Chronic Kidney Disease Patients

Nihil Chitalia[1,2], Tuan Ismail[2], Laura Tooth[3], Frances Boa[3], Geeta Hampson[4], David Goldsmith[4], Juan Carlos Kaski[2¶], Debasish Banerjee[1,2*¶]

1 Renal and Transplantation Unit, St George's Healthcare NHS Trust, London, United Kingdom, 2 Cardiovascular Research Centre, St George's, University of London, London, United Kingdom, 3 Chemical Pathology, St George's Healthcare NHS Trust, London, United Kingdom, 4 Renal and Clinical Chemistry Departments, Guy's and St Thomas, NHS Foundation Trust, London, United Kingdom

Abstract

Background: Cardiovascular events are frequent and vascular endothelial function is abnormal in patients with chronic kidney disease (CKD). We demonstrated endothelial dysfunction with vitamin D deficiency in CKD patients; however the impact of cholecalciferol supplementation on vascular stiffness and vasomotor function, endothelial and bone biomarkers in CKD patients with low 25-hydroxy vitamin D [25(OH)D] is unknown, which this study investigated.

Methods: We assessed non-diabetic patients with CKD stage 3/4, age 17–80 years and serum 25(OH)D <75 nmol/L. Brachial artery Flow Mediated Dilation (FMD), Pulse Wave Velocity (PWV), Augmentation Index (AI) and circulating blood biomarkers were evaluated at baseline and at 16 weeks. Oral 300,000 units cholecalciferol was administered at baseline and 8-weeks.

Results: Clinical characteristics of 26 patients were: age 50 ± 14 (mean $\pm$ 1SD) years, eGFR 41 ± 11 ml/min/1.73 m^2, males 73%, dyslipidaemia 36%, smokers 23% and hypertensives 87%. At 16-week serum 25(OH)D and calcium increased (43 ± 16 to 84 ± 29 nmol/L, $p < 0.001$ and 2.37 ± 0.09 to 2.42 ± 0.09 mmol/L; $p = 0.004$, respectively) and parathyroid hormone decreased (10.8 ± 8.6 to 7.4 ± 4.4; $p = 0.001$). FMD improved from $3.1 \pm 3.3\%$ to $6.1 \pm 3.7\%$, $p = 0.001$. Endothelial biomarker concentrations decreased: E-Selectin from 5666 ± 2123 to 5256 ± 2058 pg/mL; $p = 0.032$, ICAM-1, 3.45 ± 0.01 to 3.10 ± 1.04 ng/mL; $p = 0.038$ and VCAM-1, 54 ± 33 to 42 ± 33 ng/mL; $p = 0.006$. eGFR, BP, PWV, AI, hsCRP, von Willebrand factor and Fibroblast Growth Factor-23, remained unchanged.

Conclusion: This study demonstrates for the first time improvement of endothelial vasomotor and secretory functions with vitamin D in CKD patients without significant adverse effects on arterial stiffness, serum calcium or FGF-23.

Editor: Yiqing Song, Indiana University Richard M. Fairbanks School of Public Health, United States of America

Funding: This study was partially funded by the St Georges Hospital Charity (http://www.givingtogeorges.org.uk/). The funders had no role in study design, data collection and analysis, decision to publish, or preparation of the manuscript. No additional funding received for this study.

Competing Interests: The authors have declared that no competing interests exist.

* E-mail: Debasish.Banerjee@stgeorges.nhs.uk

¶ These authors are joint last authors on this work.

Introduction

Patients with chronic kidney disease (CKD) have up to 3.5 fold increased risk of cardiovascular (CV) events and cardiovascular disease (CVD) is the most common cause of mortality and morbidity [1]. Evidence from general population surveys has shown that CKD is an independent risk factor for CVD [2].

Vascular atherosclerosis is a predominant cause of CV events in CKD, with endothelial cell activation as its primary inciting event [3,4]. Endothelial dysfunction is the final common pathway of vascular injury mediated by both traditional and non-traditional risk factors of CVD [5]. Circulating biomarkers of endothelial cell activation such as Intracellular Adhesion Molecule (ICAM), Vascular Adhesion Molecule (VCAM), Endothelial leucocyte adhesion molecule (E-Selectin) and platelet adhesion molecule, such as von willebrand factor (vWF), have been validated for assessment of endothelial function [6]. Flow mediated dilatation (FMD) of the brachial artery in response to distal ischaemia, has been validated for assessment of endothelial function in-vivo [6]. Brachial artery FMD is a surrogate for CV disease, as it correlates with coronary atherosclerosis [7]. FMD has been shown to predict future CV events and mortality in the general population and in patients with mild to moderate CKD [8,9]. Additionally, it has been used extensively to study the effects of pharmacological therapies on vascular function in-vivo [10–12]. More importantly, an improvement in endothelial function, as measured by brachial artery FMD, may relate to better prognosis in patients with atherosclerotic disease [13].

Low vitamin D is associated with endothelial dysfunction and high CV mortality in patients with CKD [14,15]. Native vitamin D treatment has been shown to improve endothelium mediated vascular responses in experimental studies. Studies on spontaneously hypertensive rats show an improvement in vascular response to acetylcholine following a 6 week treatment with vitamin D [16,17]. In type II diabetic patients and 25-hydroxy vitamin D [25(OH)D] deficiency, vitamin D2 treatment over 8 weeks significantly improved brachial artery FMD [18]. We have previously reported an association between reduced vitamin D levels and impaired brachial artery FMD in CKD patients [14]. However, it is unknown if vitamin D supplementation is associated with an improvement in endothelial function in patients with CKD.

Serum Fibroblast Growth Factor-23 (FGF-23) a phosphaturic hormone secreted by osteoblasts, inhibits 1 alpha hydroxylase enzyme, preventing conversion of 25 (OH)D to 1,25 dihydroxy vitamin D [1,25 $(OH)_2D$] is elevated in CKD, and associated with mortality, coronary artery atherosclerosis and left ventricular hypertrophy [19–21]. However, it is not known if nutritional vitamin D treatment in vitamin D insufficient/deficient CKD patients, changes serum FGF-23 levels.

As the impact of Vitamin D supplementation on arterial vasomotor and stiffness function, endothelial and bone biomarkers has not been investigated systematically, this study tested the effect of treatment with oral cholecalciferol on endothelial function, arterial stiffness, biomarkers of endothelial cell activation and serum FGF-23, in relatively healthy non-diabetic CKD stage 3 and 4 patients with low levels of vitamin D.

Methods

The protocol for this trial and supporting CONSORT checklist are available as supporting information; see Checklist S1 and Protocol S1. The brief methods are as follows.

1. Patients

Stable (past 6 months) stage 3–4 CKD patients, with low vitamin D (25(OH)D<75 nmol/L), were recruited. Baseline serum 25 (OH)D were measured during routine clinic visits for patients. Patients were excluded from the study if they were known to have diabetes mellitus, malignancy, heart failure (Ejection fraction on ECHO<40% or N-terminal pro Brain natriuretic peptide (NT-proBNP)>500 pg/ml), active inflammation, active autoimmune conditions, recent acute coronary syndrome (within last 3 months), rapidly deteriorating renal function, corrected serum calcium>2.55 mmol/L and if already on Vitamin D supplementation. Patients were considered to have diabetes mellitus if they were on insulin, oral hypoglycaemic agents, diagnosed as diet controlled diabetes, had a fasting blood sugar ≥7 mmol/L or random glucose ≥11.1 mmol/L. The study was approved by NRES Surrey Research Ethics committee (REC reference 10/H1109/14) and all patients provided written informed consent. Patient recruitment and follow up is represented in figure 1. Patients were recruited between June 2010 and May 2012 follow up completed in September 2012. The trial was registered after study completion to ensure proper conduct and we confirm that all on-going and related trials with Vitamin D are registered.

2. Brachial artery FMD

Brachial artery FMD was estimated at baseline and on follow up at 16 weeks. All study subjects were assessed in our vascular laboratory, in a quiet purpose-built room maintained at constant temperature of 22–24°C, after 10 min of rest in the supine position, and after 12 hour overnight fasting. Patients were asked to withhold their regular medications for the day, until after the scan. Caffeine and tobacco were disallowed in the 6 hours prior to the scan. A standard HDI (High Definition Imaging) 3000 ultrasound system (ATL, Bothell, WA, USA) equipped with a 12–5 MHz linear array transducer was used for endothelial function measurements. The same trained physician performed all scans. The overall mean (SD) intra patient variability of this technique within our department is 0.9 (0.48) % (range 0.21–2%) [22].

The right arm brachial artery was scanned in a longitudinal section 2–10 cm above the elbow and its diameter measured continuously with on-line, wall-tracking software for 1 min at baseline, during 4.5 min of induced distal ischaemia (induced by inflation to 300 mmHg of a pneumatic cuff placed at a site distal to the segment of the artery being analysed), and for another 5 min during reactive hyperaemia after cuff release. After return to baseline, vessel diameter was again measured continuously up to 3 min for baseline measurements and for 5 min after administration of 50 μg sublingual glyceryl trinitrate, a direct nitric oxide donor. FMD was defined as the maximum percentage increase in vessel diameter during reactive hyperaemia; endothelium independent FMD was defined as the maximum percentage increase in vessel diameter after sublingual glyceryl trinitrate.

3. Pulse wave velocity and Augmentation index

The pulse wave velocity (PWV) was measured at baseline and at week 16. This was done at the same time as the brachial artery FMD. Arterial stiffness was assessed non-invasively using a pressure tonometer coupled to a SphygmoCor PWV system. A simultaneously recorded ECG signal (continuous recording of 3 chest leads) provided an R-wave timing reference. Pulsation from two contra lateral recording sites, the common carotid artery and the femoral artery were identified and marked. The distance between the suprasternal notch and common carotid pulsation was subtracted from the distance between the suprasternal notch and the femoral artery pulse to obtain the PWV distance. A pressure tonometer was then placed at the two recording sites to obtain 10 homogenous continuous waveforms. The software processed each set of pulse waveforms and ECG waveform data to calculate the mean time difference between the arrivals of the pulse at the two peripheral recording sites on a beat to beat basis. The PWV was then calculated using the mean time difference and the arterial path length between the two recording sites. At the same time blood pressure was recorded over the right arm and a mean of three readings was considered. Height (without footwear) and weight (in street clothes) was measured and recorded in the SphygmoCor PWV system. Using the same equipment, the radial pulse waveform was analysed and the corresponding central aortic waveform generated using a transfer function. The augmentation index (AI) was calculated as the ratio of the difference between early and peak systolic pressure versus the early systolic pressure from the derived aortic wave form.

4. Measurement of circulating biomarkers

Whole blood samples were obtained in SST tubes during baseline and follow-up scans. The samples were centrifuged immediately at 4000 rpm for 15 minutes and the serum separated. Serum was analysed for baseline 25(OH)D levels using a

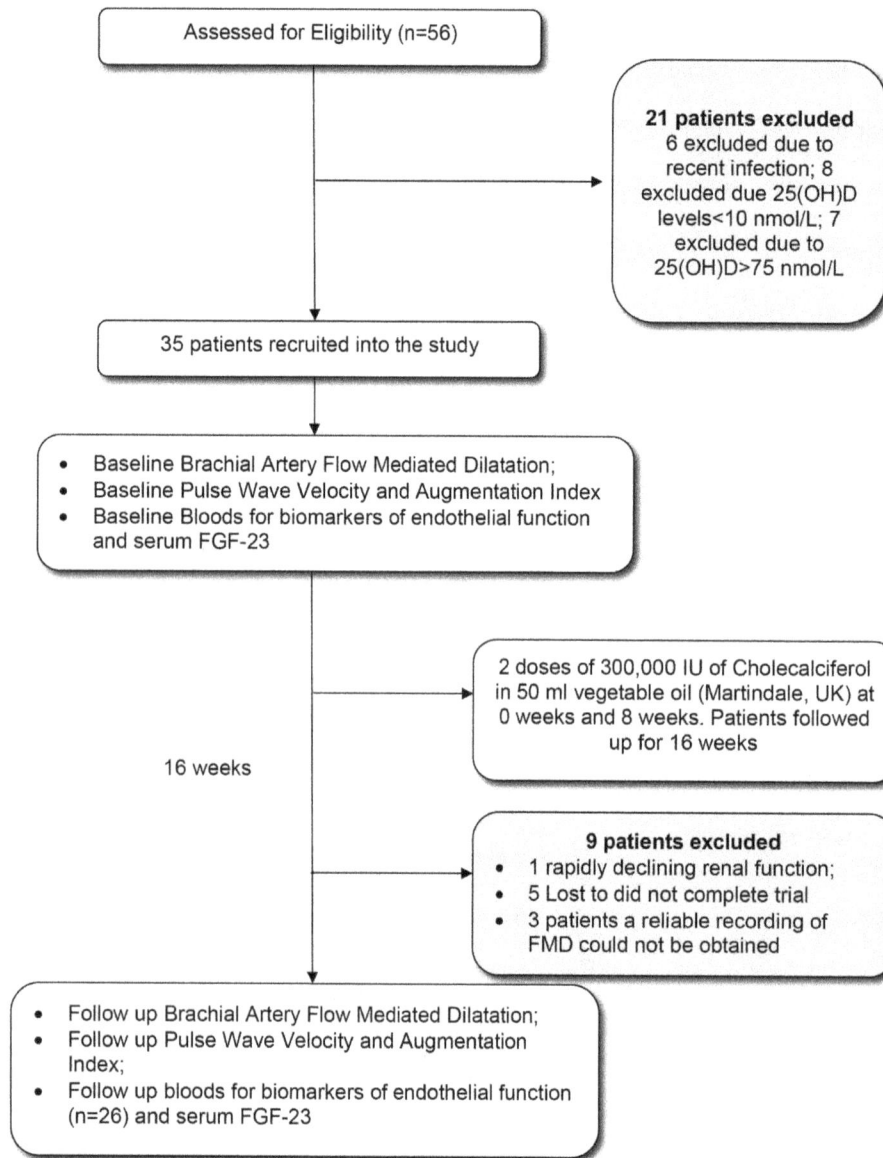

Figure 1. Number of patients recruited into the study and completed the follow-up. Legend: Flow Diagram of the patient pathway recruited into the effects of oral vitamin D on endothelial function intervention study. Thirty five patients were recruited into the study after excluding twenty one patients. Twenty six patients completed the study.

chemiluminescent immunoassay on an automated IDS-iSYS analyser. The analytical range was 12.5–350 nmol/L and inter-batch co-efficient of variation (CV) <12%. High sensitivity C-reactive protein (hsCRP) was measured using the hsCRP latex-enhanced immunoturbidimetric assay (Siemens Healthcare Diagnostics) on an ADVIA 2400 analyser. The analytical range was 0.16–10 mg/L and the inter batch CV<10%. The remaining serum was stored at −70°C.

Baseline and follow-up serum samples for each patient were measured simultaneously in duplicates for endothelial function biomarkers, with mean value of the two concentrations taken as the representative concentration of the biomarker in the sample.

Serum E-Selectin was measured using ELISA (Abcam). The samples and the standards were diluted 1:100. The assay range for this ELISA is 1600–50,000 pg/ml and the intra-assay and inter-assay CV% is 5.4 and 6.0%, respectively.

Serum ICAM was measured using ELISA (Thermo Scientific). The samples were diluted in the ratio of 1:100. The assay range for this ELISA is 0.3–10 ng/ml and the intra-assay CV% is <10%.

Serum vWF was measured using ELISA (Abcam). The samples were diluted in the ratio of 1:100. The assay range for this ELISA is 3–30 mU/ml and the intra-assay and inter-assay CV% is 5.1 and 7.2%, respectively (note 1 IU/ml = 9.8 µg/ml).

Soluble VCAM-1 (sVCAM-1) was measured using ELISA (Invitrogen). The samples were diluted in the ratio of 1:50. The assay range for this ELISA is 0–75 ng/ml and the intra-assay and inter-assay CV% is <4.6 and <8.2%.

Serum FGF-23 was measured by second-generation ELISA (Immutopics, Inc, San Clemente, California) detecting both intact FGF-23 and C-terminal fragments. The interassay CV for this assay was 8.6% and 7.8% at plasma concentrations of 34.6 and 280.8 RU/mL, respectively.

5. Vitamin D therapy

All patients recruited received 2 doses of oral 300,000 units of Cholecalciferol in vegetable oil (Martindale Pharma) at the beginning of the study and at week 8. This dose of cholecalciferol has been found to be safe and effective in lowering serum parathyroid hormone (PTH) levels in CKD 3/4 patients, without hypercalcemia [23]. A study from our hospital in patients with 25 (OH)D<40 nmol/L, using 300,000 IU of the same preparation showed a significant decline of 25 (OH)D levels at 12 weeks post administration [24], hence we chose to readminister 300,000 units at 8 weeks to maintain a biological effect of vitamin D3.

6. Statistical analysis

Data were analysed using Statistical Package for Social Sciences (SPSSv.16, Chicago, IL). Continuous and normally distributed variables are expressed as mean±1SD. Continuous and non-normally distributed variables are expressed as median±Inter-quartile range (IQR). Categorical variables are expressed as percentages (%). Comparison of means for continuous, parametric variables was performed using dependent sample T-test and for non-parametric variables using Wilcoxon signed rank test. Comparison of categorical variables was performed using Chi-squared testing. A twosided p-value of <0.05 was considered to indicate statistical significance.

7. Sample Size Calculation

The sample size was calculated to show a 10% improvement in mean FMD with vitamin D treatment. The mean FMD of patients recruited into our previous study was 3.8%. The standard deviation of the intra-patient variability in FMD measurements, is 0.48% (range: 0.21–2%) [22]. Taking $\alpha = 0.05$ and a $\beta = 20$, twenty-seven patients were required to show a 10% change in FMD measurements. Assuming a dropout rate of 30% due to failure of study follow-up, progression to ESRD, transfer to other renal units or death, 35 patients were recruited into the study.

Results

Thirty five patients were recruited. Twenty six patients completed the 16 week follow-up (figure 1). The baseline clinical characteristics of these 26 patients are represented in table 1. Thirteen patients were Caucasians with 6 South-East Asians, 6 Afro-Caribbeans and 1 of Chinese origin. Six patients had a family history of ischaemic heart disease. Three patients had a history of ischaemic heart disease, but none had suffered a myocardial infarction (MI) or stroke in the preceding 3 months.

There was no significant change in the number of patients on angiotensin converting enzyme inhibitors or angiotensin receptor blockers or their dosages during the study.

All patients had a low baseline 25(OH)D level with a mean level of 43±16 nmol/L; range 13–74 nmol/L (normal reference range 75–200 nmol/L). The calcium levels were within normal limits 2.37±0.09 mmol/L (normal reference range 2.2–2.6 mmol/L). The parathyroid hormone levels were high with a mean of 10.8 pmol/L, range 3–41 pmol/L (normal reference range 1.1–6.9 pmol/L).

At the end of 16 weeks vitamin D concentrations improved from 43±16 to 84±29 nmol/L, p<0.001. The calcium increased (2.37±0.09 to 2.42±0.09 mmol/L; p=0.004); and the parathyroid hormone decreased (10.8±8.6 to 7.4±4.4; p=0.001). The estimated GFR (eGFR) and systolic and diastolic blood pressure remained very stable.

Table 1. Characteristics of the study population at baseline (n = 26).

Variables	Mean± 1SD or n(%)
Age (years)	50±14
Males (%)	19 (73%)
Ethnicity (%)	
Caucasian	13 (50%)
South-east Asian	6 (23%)
Afro Caribbean	6 (23%)
Chinese	1 (4%)
Hypertension (%)	22 (87%)
Current Smokers (%)	6 (23%)
Hyperlipidaemia (%)	9 (36%)
Family history of CVD (%)	6 (23%)
History of CVD (%)	3 (11%)
MDRD estimated GFR (ml/min/1.73 m²)	41±11
Treatment	
ACEi or AT II RA	20 (77%)
Statins	11 (42%)
Aspirin	4 (15%)
Betablockers	4 (15%)
Nitrates	0 (0%)

Legend: Baseline demographics and characteristics of study population that completed the study: MDRD eGFR: Abbreviated four variable Modified Diet of Renal Disease estimated Glomerular Filtration Rate[48]. Mean automated sitting clinic blood pressure taken thrice using appropriate size cuff was measured. Hypertension was defined as clinic blood pressure of ≥140/80 mmHg or on antihypertensives medications. Diabetes Mellitus was defined by WHO guidelines 2006 for definition of diabetes. Hyperlipidemia was defined as Total cholesterol >5 mmol/L and/or LDL>2.5 and or HDL<1.55 or on lipid lowering therapy (National cholesterol Education Program ATP III guidelines 2001). ACEi-Angiotensin converting enzyme inhibitor, AT II RA- Angiotensin II receptor antagonist.

Impact on Vascular function

The brachial artery FMD improved from 3.1±3.3% to 6.1±3.7%, p<0.001 (figure 2). The PWV and AI tended to improve but did not reach statistical significance, as shown in table 2. There was no significant change in haemoglobin or haematocrit values during the study.

Impact on blood biomarkers

The circulating biomarkers for endothelial function also showed an improvement. The E-Selectin decreased from 5666±2123 to 5256±2058 pg/mL, p=0.032. The ICAM-1 levels decreased from 3.45±1.01 to 3.10±1.04 ng/mL, p=0.038. The VCAM-1 level decreased from 54±33 to 42±33 ng/mL, p=0.006. The vWF levels improved, but the change was not statistically significant 23.7±12.2 to 21.6±12.2 mU/mL, p=0.076. There was no change in hsCRP concentrations or urine protein creatinine ratio. There was no change in FGF-23 levels before and after vitamin D therapy (131±81 vs. 132±67 RU/ml; p=0.862).

Discussion

The present study demonstrate that supplementation with cholecalciferol in stable, moderate CKD was associated with

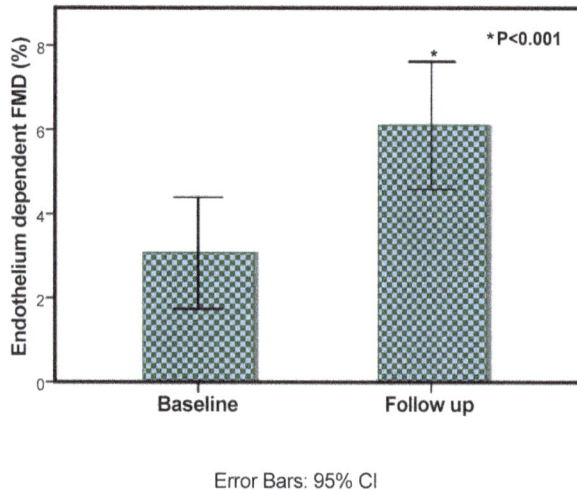

Error Bars: 95% CI

Figure 2. Measure of endothelial function before and after Vitamin D Therapy. Legend: The endothelial function as measured by brachial artery flow mediated dilatation improves from 3.1±3.3% to 6.1±3.7%. Error bars show 95% CI, p<0.001.

improvement of vascular endothelial function. Vitamin D3 administration over 16 weeks almost doubled the vitamin D levels, and this was associated with an appropriate decrease in parathyroid hormone levels. The calcium levels, increased slightly, but none of the patients developed hypercalcaemia (serum calcium >2.60 mmol/L). There were reductions in concentrations of circulating biomarkers of endothelial dysfunction, E-selectin, ICAM-1 and VCAM-1. There were no changes in hsCRP, FGF-23 levels and arterial stiffness over the 16 weeks.

In the present study we have measured 25(OH)D, and not 1,25 di-hydroxy vitamin D [1,25(OH)$_2$D], because studies have shown that the deficiency is reliably related to low 25(OH)D levels and measurement of 1,25(OH)$_2$D levels is challenging, unreliable and expensive and therefore not available to most clinicians [25]. Furthermore, 25(OH)D is inexpensive, easy to administer and has few side effects, even when administered in large doses. Moreover, studies have shown that 25(OH)D levels do stimulate Vitamin D receptors, with less affinity but with higher availability for binding due to its 1000-fold higher concentration in serum [26,27]. There have been no reports of hypercalcaemia with high dose vitamin D supplementation in this population, and this was also true in our study [28].

Vitamin D is an excellent target for treatment in the context of CKD because of its association with CV disease and endothelial function. In the general population, vitamin D deficiency is associated with increased all-cause mortality, as well as CV event rates [28,29]. In patients with CKD, relationship of low vitamin D with mortality and CV event rate have been demonstrated in both dialysis and pre-dialysis patients [15,30]. We and others have previously demonstrated an association of 25(OH)D deficiency with endothelial function [14]. However the present study was the first to investigate the impact of cholecalciferol therapy on endothelial dysfunction in vitamin D deficient/insufficient pre-dialysis CKD patients.

Endothelial dysfunction is a harbinger of atherosclerosis. It is often the first abnormality demonstrated which can predict the initiation and progression of atherosclerotic artery disease [4]. We and others have demonstrated highly abnormal endothelial function in CKD, associated with increased carotid intima-media thickness, hence it is a possible mechanism of initiation and

progression of atherosclerosis in CKD [5]. In the general population, endothelial dysfunction within coronary arteries, predicts future CV events [3]. In large general population studies, endothelial dysfunction measured by brachial artery FMD predicts both CV events and mortality [9]. In CKD patients, endothelial dysfunction is an independent predictor of adverse CV outcomes [31].

Endothelial function measured in the peripheral arteries has been used in different patient groups to study the effect of vitamin D supplementation on vascular function. Amongst several such studies which we could identify, three studies demonstrated an improvement of endothelial function with cholecalciferol therapy but the rest did not. In overweight African-Americans the flow mediated dilatation improved by 1.8%; in post stroke patients with FMD improved by 6.9%, and in diabetic patients the FMD improved by 2.3% [18,32,33]. The studies where vitamin D therapy was unable to show improvement often used low dose vitamin D supplementation; such as 1,000 units per day for two weeks in a randomised control trial of diabetic patients; and 2,500 IU units per day for four months in post menopausal women [34,35]. It is conceivable that these studies were unable to show a benefit as the dose of vitamin D used was physiologically inadequate. In other negative studies, vitamin D was supplemented even when the baseline levels were within normal limits, for example, in the studies involving post MI and type 2 diabetic patients, serum 25(OH) D concentrations up to 100 nmol/L at baseline. Supplementing 25(OH)D3 may not be as effective in these patients, as supplementing in patients with low 25(OH)D concentrations [36,37]. Our study included patients with low 25(OH)D and the treatment dose was high.

Impact of Vitamin D on circulating biomarkers of endothelial function has been variable. In post-MI patients or with coronary artery disease, E-selectin did not improve with vitamin D, whereas, in diabetic patients it did [35,37,38]. Our study showed improvement in E-selectin, VCAM-1, ICAM-1 together with the improvement in FMD, hence confirming our findings on in-vivo vascular endothelial function analysis.

CKD patients have immune dysregulation [39,40]. This results in an increased predisposition to infections as well as chronic systemic inflammation adversely affecting the CV system. Vitamin D has pleiotropic effects on the immune system with evidence that it modulates the adaptive immune system. We know from experimental studies, that vitamin D down regulates Th1 activity, dendritic cell maturation and up regulates Th17 regulator activity, thereby possibly suppressing the low grade inflammation in the blood vessel and the heart [41–43]. The present study demonstrated improvement in circulating biomarkers of endothelial function but did not investigate the mechanism any further.

This study did not demonstrate any change of FGF-23 concentrations with Vitamin D therapy. FGF-23 concentrations increase with kidney failure and elevated FGF-23 has been associated with abnormal endothelial function, adverse cardiovascular outcomes, and has recently shown to cause left ventricular hypertrophy [44]. Vitamin D therapy has usually been shown to lead to increases in FGF-23 concentrations in CKD and dialysis, though this effect is not consistent; in our repletion study, we did not see any effect on FGF-23 concentration [45–47].

This study has demonstrated that abnormal vasomotor and secretory endothelial function can be rapidly improved with 600,000 IU of Cholecalciferol. There were no adverse changes in arterial stiffness. However, 16 weeks is too short a time period to exclude the possibility of later with vitamin D therapy. The rise in serum calcium concentration was very modest, but was statistically significant.

Table 2. Analysis of baseline and follow up parameters after Cholecalciferol therapy.

Variables (n = 26)	Baseline (week 0)	Follow up (16 weeks)	p value
Haemoglobin (g/dl)	14.1±1.8	13.8±6.7	0.379
Haematocrit (%)	44±6	43±5	0.486
Serum Albumin (mmol/L)	36±6	38±4	0.283
Urine Protein Creatinine Ratio (mg/mmol)[†]	35.7±124.2	30.15±221.3	0.866
Serum 25 (OH)D (nmol/L)	43±16	84±29	<0.001*
Serum Calcium (mmol/L)	2.37±0.09	2.42±0.09	0.004*
Serum Phosphate (mmol/L)	1.07±0.20	1.10±0.19	0.459
Serum Parathyroid hormone (pmol/L)	10.8±8.6	7.4±4.4	0.001*
MDRD eGFR (ml/min/1.73 m^2)	41±11	40±12	0.559
Systolic Blood Pressure (mmHg)	133±12	133±17	0.991
Diastolic Blood pressure (mmHg)	87±9	85±10	0.309
Central pulse pressure (mmHg)	33±12	35±14	0.349
Baseline brachial artery diameter (mm)	4.6±0.9	4.6±0.7	0.945
Endothelium dependent FMD (%)	3.1±3.3	6.1±3.7	0.001*
Endothelium independent FMD (%)	7.34±4.5	10.38±6.7	0.121
PWV (m/s)	7.9±1.9	7.7±2.2	0.059
AI (%)	22±16	18±20	0.055
On ACE I or AT II RA [n(%)]	20(77%)	20(77%)	NC
On Statin	11(42%)	11(42%)	NC
On Nitrate	0%	0%	NC
HsCRP (mg/L)[†]	3.35±4.75	4.00±4.42	0.272
E selectin (pg/ml)	5666±2123	5256±2058	0.032*
ICAM (ng/ml)	3.45±1.01	3.10±1.04	0.038*
sVCAM 1 (ng/ml)	54±33	42±33	0.006*
vWF (mU/ml)	23.7±12.2	21.6±12.2	0.076
FGF-23 (RU/ml)	131±81	132±67	0.862

Legend: MDRD eGFR: Abbreviated four variable Modified Diet of Renal Disease estimated Glomerular Filtration Rate (REF). Mean automated, sitting, clinic, blood pressure taken thrice using appropriate size cuff was recorded.
* denotes p<0.05.
[†]Distribution non-parametric variable represented as median±IQR, Wilcoxon Signed Rank Test used to analyse the difference in distribution of baseline and follow up values.
ACE I- Angiotensin converting enzyme inhibitor, AT II RA- Angiotensin II receptor antagonist. NC: No Change.

A limitation of this study is that it was conducted over a short period; so long term effect of vitamin D therapy cannot be assessed. Logistic reasons precluded randomisation; and potential bias cannot be excluded. However the study demonstrates improvement of both endothelial vasomotor and secretory function with cholecalciferol i.e there were improvements of flow mediated dilatation as well as the levels of VCAM-1, ICAM-1 and E-Selectin without adverse effects on arterial stiffness and FGF-23. These findings strongly suggest an effect of Vitamin D on the endothelial cells and potentially will lead to further studies investigating the mechanisms of such benefits of cholecalciferol on vascular function. The study excluded patients with CKD due to diabetes; so in this particular patient cohort, which forms a large proportion of the patients we see in our clinics, these results cannot be extrapolated. The study was restricted to pre-dialysis stage 3/4 CKD; so in patients with early CKD (stages 1 and 2), post kidney transplant and dialysis patients the impact of vitamin D supplementation on endothelial function remains unknown. A randomised control trial with a longer duration of follow up is required to confirm the present findings and plan future clinical outcome driven trials.

In conclusion, this study for the first time demonstrates that Cholecalciferol improves endothelial vasomotor and secretory function, in stable non-diabetes stage 3/4 CKD patients without any significant effect on arterial stiffness, calcium and FGF-23 levels.

Acknowledgments

Part of this work was presented at the ASN Kidney Week 2012.

Author Contributions

Conceived and designed the experiments: The authors have contributed towards the design and planning (DB, NC, DG, JCK), patient recruitment (DB, NC, TI), patient study (DB, NC, TI) biomarker analysis (LT, FB, GH, DB, NC, TI) and writing (DB, NC, JCK, DG, GH, LT, FB) of the study.

References

1. Go AS, Chertow GM, Fan D, McCulloch CE, Hsu CY (2004) Chronic kidney disease and the risks of death, cardiovascular events, and hospitalization. N Engl J Med 351: 1296–1305

2. Tonelli M, Muntner P, Lloyd A, Manns BJ, Klarenbach S, et al. (2012) Risk of coronary events in people with chronic kidney disease compared with those with diabetes: a population-level cohort study. Lancet 380: 807–814

3. Halcox JP, Schenke WH, Zalos G, Mincemoyer R, Prasad A, et al. (2002) Prognostic value of coronary vascular endothelial dysfunction. Circulation 106: 653–658

4. Suwaidi JA, Hamasaki S, Higano ST, Nishimura RA, Holmes DR Jr, et al (2000) Long-term follow-up of patients with mild coronary artery disease and endothelial dysfunction. Circulation 101: 948–954

5. Recio-Mayoral A, Banerjee D, Streather C, Kaski JC (2011) Endothelial dysfunction, inflammation and atherosclerosis in chronic kidney disease–a cross-sectional study of predialysis, dialysis and kidney-transplantation patients. Atherosclerosis 216: 446–451

6. Deanfield J, Donald A, Ferri C, Giannattasio C, Halcox J, et al. (2005) Endothelial function and dysfunction. Part I: Methodological issues for assessment in the different vascular beds: a statement by the Working Group on Endothelin and Endothelial Factors of the European Society of Hypertension. J Hypertens 23: 7–17

7. Anderson TJ, Uehata A, Gerhard MD, Meredith IT, Knab S, et al. (1995) Close relation of endothelial function in the human coronary and peripheral circulations. J Am Coll Cardiol 26: 1235–1241

8. Stam F, van GC, Becker A, Dekker JM, Heine RJ, et al. (2006) Endothelial dysfunction contributes to renal function-associated cardiovascular mortality in a population with mild renal insufficiency: the Hoorn study. J Am Soc Nephrol 17: 537–545

9. Yeboah J, Folsom AR, Burke GL, Johnson C, Polak JF, et al. (2009) Predictive value of brachial flow-mediated dilation for incident cardiovascular events in a population-based study: the multi-ethnic study of atherosclerosis. Circulation 120: 502–509

10. Bae JH, Bassenge E, Lee HJ, Park KR, Park CG, et al (2001) Impact of postprandial hypertriglyceridemia on vascular responses in patients with coronary artery disease: effects of ACE inhibitors and fibrates. Atherosclerosis 158: 165–171

11. Sidhu JS, Cowan D, Kaski JC (2004) Effects of rosiglitazone on endothelial function in men with coronary artery disease without diabetes mellitus. Am J Cardiol 94: 151–156

12. Timimi FK, Ting HH, Haley EA, Roddy MA, Ganz P, et al. (1998) Vitamin C improves endothelium-dependent vasodilation in patients with insulin-dependent diabetes mellitus. J Am Coll Cardiol 31: 552–557

13. Suessenbacher A, Frick M, Alber HF, Barbieri V, Pachinger O, et al. (2006) Association of improvement of brachial artery flow-mediated vasodilation with cardiovascular events. Vasc Med 11: 239–244

14. Chitalia N, Recio-Mayoral A, Kaski JC, Banerjee D (2012) Vitamin D deficiency and endothelial dysfunction in non-dialysis chronic kidney disease patients. Atherosclerosis 220: 265–268

15. Pilz S, Tomaschitz A, Friedl C, Amrein K, Drechsler C, et al (2011) Vitamin D status and mortality in chronic kidney disease. Nephrol Dial Transplant 26: 3603–3609

16. Borges AC, Feres T, Vianna LM, Paiva TB (1999) Effect of cholecalciferol treatment on the relaxant responses of spontaneously hypertensive rat arteries to acetylcholine. Hypertension 34: 897–901

17. Wong MS, Delansorne R, Man RY, Svenningsen P, Vanhoutte PM (2010) Chronic treatment with vitamin D lowers arterial blood pressure and reduces endothelium-dependent contractions in the aorta of the spontaneously hypertensive rat. Am J Physiol Heart Circ Physiol 299: H1226–H1234

18. Sugden JA, Davies JI, Witham MD, Morris AD, Struthers AD (2008) Vitamin D improves endothelial function in patients with Type 2 diabetes mellitus and low vitamin D levels. Diabet Med 25: 320–325

19. Gutierrez OM, Mannstadt M, Isakova T, Rauh-Hain JA, Tamez H,et al (2008) Fibroblast growth factor 23 and mortality among patients undergoing hemodialysis. N Engl J Med 359: 584–592

20. Kanbay M, Huddam B, Azak A, Solak Y, Kadioglu GK, et al (2011) A randomized study of allopurinol on endothelial function and estimated glomular filtration rate in asymptomatic hyperuricemic subjects with normal renal function. Clin J Am Soc Nephrol 6: 1887–1894

21. Wolf M, Molnar MZ, Amaral AP, Czira ME, Rudas A, et al. (2011) Elevated fibroblast growth factor 23 is a risk factor for kidney transplant loss and mortality. J Am Soc Nephrol 22: 956–966

22. Sidhu JS, Newey VR, Nassiri DK, Kaski JC (2002) A rapid and reproducible on line automated technique to determine endothelial function. Heart 88: 289–292

23. Chandra P, Binongo JN, Ziegler TR, Schlanger LE, Wang W,et al (2008) Cholecalciferol (vitamin D3) therapy and vitamin D insufficiency in patients with

chronic kidney disease: a randomized controlled pilot study. Endocr Pract 14: 10–17

24. Leventis P, Kiely PD (2009) The tolerability and biochemical effects of high-dose bolus vitamin D2 and D3 supplementation in patients with vitamin D insufficiency. Scand J Rheumatol 38: 149–153

25. Fraser WD, Milan AM (2013) Vitamin D assays: past and present debates, difficulties, and developments. Calcif Tissue Int 92: 118–127

26. Procsal DA, Okamura WH, Norman AW (1975) Structural requirements for the interaction of 1 alpha, 25-(OH) 2- vitiamin D3 with its chick interestinal receptor system. J Biol Chem 250: 8382–8388

27. Lou YR, Molnar F, Perakyla M, Qiao S, Kalueff AV, et al (2010) 25-Hydroxyvitamin D(3) is an agonistic vitamin D receptor ligand. J Steroid Biochem Mol Biol 118: 162–170

28. Dobnig H, Pilz S, Scharnagl H, Renner W, Seelhorst U, et al. (2008) Independent association of low serum 25-hydroxyvitamin d and 1,25-dihydroxyvitamin D levels with all-cause and cardiovascular mortality. Arch Intern Med 168: 1340–1349

29. Kestenbaum B, Katz R, de Boer I, Hoofnagle A, Sarnak MJ, et al S (2011) Vitamin D, parathyroid hormone, and cardiovascular events among older adults. J Am Coll Cardiol 58: 1433–1441

30. Drechsler C, Verduijn M, Pilz S, Dekker FW, Krediet RT, et al (2011) Vitamin D status and clinical outcomes in incident dialysis patients: results from the NECOSAD study. Nephrol Dial Transplant 26: 1024–1032

31. Yilmaz MI, Stenvinkel P, Sonmez A, Saglam M, Yaman H, et al. (2011) Vascular health, systemic inflammation and progressive reduction in kidney function; clinical determinants and impact on cardiovascular outcomes. Nephrol Dial Transplant 26: 3537–3543

32. Harris RA, Pedersen-White J, Guo DH, Stallmann-Jorgensen IS, Keeton D, et al. (2011) Vitamin D3 supplementation for 16 weeks improves flow-mediated dilation in overweight African-American adults. Am J Hypertens 24: 557–562

33. Witham MD, Dove FJ, Sugden JA, Doney AS, Struthers AD (2012) The effect of vitamin D replacement on markers of vascular health in stroke patients - a randomised controlled trial. Nutr Metab Cardiovasc Dis 22: 864–870

34. Gepner AD, Ramamurthy R, Krueger DC, Korcarz CE, Binkley N, et al. (2012) A prospective randomized controlled trial of the effects of vitamin D supplementation on cardiovascular disease risk. PLoS One 7: e36617

35. Shab-Bidar S, Neyestani TR, Djazayery A, Eshraghian MR, Houshiarrad A, et al (2011) Regular consumption of vitamin D-fortified yogurt drink (Doogh) improved endothelial biomarkers in subjects with type 2 diabetes: a randomized double-blind clinical trial. BMC Med 9: 125

36. Witham MD, Dove FJ, Dryburgh M, Sugden JA, Morris AD, et al. (2010) The effect of different doses of vitamin D(3) on markers of vascular health in patients with type 2 diabetes: a randomised controlled trial. Diabetologia 53: 2112–2119

37. Witham MD, Dove FJ, Khan F, Lang CC, Belch JJ, et al. (2012) Effects of Vitamin D supplementation on markers of vascular function after myocardial infarction-A randomised controlled trial. Int J Cardiol

38. Sokol SI, Srinivas V, Crandall JP, Kim M, Tellides G, et al. (2012) The effects of vitamin D repletion on endothelial function and inflammation in patients with coronary artery disease. Vasc Med 17: 394–404

39. Herbelin A, Urena P, Nguyen AT, Zingraff J, scamps-Latscha B (1991) Elevated circulating levels of interleukin-6 in patients with chronic renal failure. Kidney Int 39: 954–960

40. scamps-Latscha B, Herbelin A, Nguyen AT, Zingraff J, Jungers P, et al 1994) Immune system dysregulation in uremia. Semin Nephrol 14: 253–260

41. Barrat FJ, Cua DJ, Boonstra A, Richards DF, Crain C, et al. (2002) In vitro generation of interleukin 10-producing regulatory CD4(+) T cells is induced by immunosuppressive drugs and inhibited by T helper type 1 (Th1)- and Th2-inducing cytokines. J Exp Med 195: 603–616

42. Froicu M, Weaver V, Wynn TA, McDowell MA, Welsh JE, et al. (2003) A crucial role for the vitamin D receptor in experimental inflammatory bowel diseases. Mol Endocrinol 17: 2386–2392

43. Muller K, Bendtzen K (1996) 1,25-Dihydroxyvitamin D3 as a natural regulator of human immune functions. J Investig Dermatol Symp Proc 1: 68–71

44. Faul C, Amaral AP, Oskouei B, Hu MC, Sloan A, et al. (2011) FGF23 induces left ventricular hypertrophy. J Clin Invest 121: 4393–4408

45. Gutierrez OM (2010) Fibroblast growth factor 23 and disordered vitamin D metabolism in chronic kidney disease: updating the "trade-off" hypothesis. Clin J Am Soc Nephrol 5: 1710–1716

46. Turner C, Dalton N, Inaoui R, Fogelman I, Fraser WD, et al. (2013) Effect of a 300 000-IU Loading Dose of Ergocalciferol (Vitamin D2) on Circulating 1,25(OH)2-Vitamin D and Fibroblast Growth Factor-23 (FGF-23) in Vitamin D Insufficiency. J Clin Endocrinol Metab

47. Uzum AK, Salman S, Telci A, Boztepe H, Tanakol R, et al (2010) Effects of vitamin D replacement therapy on serum FGF23 concentrations in vitamin D-deficient women in short term. Eur J Endocrinol 163: 825–831

9

Comparison of the Impact of High-Flux Dialysis on Mortality in Hemodialysis Patients with and without Residual Renal Function

Hyung Wook Kim[1,7], Su-Hyun Kim[2], Young Ok Kim[1], Dong Chan Jin[1], Ho Chul Song[1], Euy Jin Choi[1], Yong-Lim Kim[3], Yon-Su Kim[4], Shin-Wook Kang[5], Nam-Ho Kim[6], Chul Woo Yang[1], Yong Kyun Kim[1,8]*

1 Department of Internal Medicine, College of Medicine, The Catholic University of Korea, Seoul, Korea, 2 Department of Internal Medicine, College of Medicine, Chung-Ang University, Seoul, Korea, 3 Department of Internal Medicine, Kyungpook National University School of Medicine, Daegu, Korea, 4 Department of Internal Medicine, College of Medicine, Seoul National University, Seoul, Korea, 5 Department of Internal Medicine, College of Medicine, Yonsei University, Seoul, Korea, 6 Department of Internal Medicine, Chonnam National University Medical School, Gwangju, Korea, 7 St. Vincent's Hospital, Suwon, Korea, 8 MRC for Cell Death Disease Research Center, The Catholic University of Korea, Seoul, Korea

Abstract

Background: The effect of flux membranes on mortality in hemodialysis (HD) patients is controversial. Residual renal function (RRF) has shown to not only be as a predictor of mortality but also a contributor to β2-microglobulin clearance in HD patients. Our study aimed to determine the interaction of residual renal function with dialyzer membrane flux on mortality in HD patients.

Methods: HD Patients were included from the Clinical Research Center registry for End Stage Renal Disease, a prospective observational cohort study in Korea. Cox proportional hazards regression models were used to study the association between use of high-flux dialysis membranes and all-cause mortality with RRF and without RRF. The primary outcome was all-cause mortality.

Results: This study included 893 patients with 24 h-residual urine volume $\geq$100 ml (569 and 324 dialyzed using low-flux and high-flux dialysis membranes, respectively) and 913 patients with 24 h-residual urine volume <100 ml (570 and 343 dialyzed using low-flux and high-flux dialysis membranes, respectively). After a median follow-up period of 31 months, mortality was not significantly different between the high and low-flux groups in patients with 24 h-residual urine volume $\geq$100 ml (HR 0.86, 95% CI, 0.38–1.95, P = 0.723). In patients with 24 h-residual urine volume <100 ml, HD using high-flux dialysis membrane was associated with decreased mortality compared to HD using low-flux dialysis membrane in multivariate analysis (HR 0.40, 95% CI, 0.21–0.78, P = 0.007).

Conclusions: Our data showed that HD using high-flux dialysis membranes had a survival benefit in patients with 24 h-residual urine volume <100 ml, but not in patients with 24 h-residual urine volume $\geq$100 ml. These findings suggest that high-flux dialysis rather than low-flux dialysis might be considered in HD patients without RRF.

Editor: Martin H. de Borst, University Medical Center Groningen and University of Groningen, Netherlands

Funding: This work was supported by a grant of the Korea Healthcare Technology R & D Project, Ministry of Health and Welfare, Republic of Korea (HI10C2020). The funders had no role in study design, data collection and analysis, decision to publish, or preparation of the manuscript.

Competing Interests: The authors have declared that no competing interests exist.

* E-mail: drkimyk@catholic.ac.kr

Introduction

Patients with End-stage renal disease (ESRD) undergoing maintenance hemodialysis (HD) have a high risk of morbidity and mortality [1]. Therefore, the most effective and best-tolerated HD treatment may improve clinical outcomes in this patient population [2]. In particular, the dialyzer used in HD treatment is one of the important determinants of the effectiveness of dialysis. HD using high-flux dialysis membrane can clear more middle molecular weight uremic toxins such as β2-microglobulin than HD using low-flux dialysis membrane because of its higher porosity [3].

Despite the beneficial effects of middle-molecule removal by high-flux dialysis, the effects of dialyzer membrane flux on mortality are controversial. A number of observational studies have suggested that HD using high-flux dialysis membrane results in improved outcomes compared with low-flux dialysis [4–7]. However, two large randomized clinical trials, the HEMO study and the European Membrane Permeability Outcome (MPO) study, showed no significant survival difference between HD using high-flux dialysis membrane and HD using low-flux dialysis membrane [8,9]. This discrepancy may be due to differences in the populations studied or study design.

Residual renal function is known to be an important determinant of serum β2-microglobulin level and a contributor of β2-microglobulin clearance in patients with HD [10,11]. In patients with greater residual renal function, the beneficial effects of β2-microglobulin removal by high-flux dialysis may not be apparent. Therefore, it may be postulated that the beneficial effect of high-flux dialysis on mortality may be different between patients with different degrees of residual renal function.

This study aimed to determine the interaction of residual renal function with dialyzer membrane flux on mortality in patients enrolled in the Clinical Research Center (CRC) registry for ESRD cohort which is an observational prospective cohort study conducted in Korea.

Materials and Methods

Study Population

All patients included in this study were enrolled in the CRC registry for ESRD. This is an ongoing observational prospective cohort study patients with ESRD from 31 medical centers in Korea. The cohort started in April 2009 and included adult (>18 years of age) dialysis patients. A total 3,067 patients undergoing HD were enrolled in this cohort. For the present study, we excluded patients for whom information about the dialysis membrane used or 24 h-urine volume was not available (n = 1,261). So, 1,806 patients were included in the final analysis.

Demographic and clinical data were collected at the time of enrollment. Assessment of dialysis characteristics and measurements of health were done every 6 months until follow-up was complete. Dates and causes of mortality were reported throughout the follow-up period.

Ethics

The study was approved by the institutional review board at each center [The Catholic University of Korea, Bucheon St. Mary's Hospital; The Catholic University of Korea, Incheon St. Mary's Hospital; The Catholic University of Korea, Seoul St. Mary's Hospital; The Catholic University of Korea, St. Mary's Hospital; The Catholic University of Korea, St. Vincent's Hospital; The Catholic University of Korea, Uijeongbu St. Mary's Hospital; Cheju Halla General Hospital; Chonbuk National University Hospital; Chonnam National University Hospital; Chung-Ang University Medical Center; Chungbuk National University Hospital; Chungnam National University Hospital; Dong-A University Medical Center; Ehwa Womens University Medical Center; Fatima Hospital, Daegu; Gachon University Gil Medical Center; Inje University Pusan Paik Hospital; Kyungpook National University Hospital; Kwandong University College of Medicine, Myongji Hospital; National Health Insurance Corporation Ilsan Hospital; National Medical Center; Pusan National University Hospital; Samsung Medical Center, Seoul; Seoul Metropolitan Government, Seoul National University, Boramae Medical Center; Seoul National University Hospital; Seoul National University, Bundang Hospital; Yeungnam University Medical Center; Yonsei University, Severance Hospital; Yonsei University, Gangnam Severance Hospital; Ulsan University Hospital; Wonju Christian Hospital (in alphabetical order)] and performed in accordance to the Declaration of Helsinki. Written informed consent was obtained from all patients.

Clinical and Dialysis Parameters

In the CRC registry for ESRD study, baseline demographic and clinical data including age, sex, body mass index (BMI), type of dialysis membrane, primary causes of ESRD, comorbidities (cardiovascular disease and DM), laboratory values, and therapeutic characteristics were recorded. Cardiovascular disease was defined as the presence of coronary artery disease, congestive heart failure, peripheral vascular disease, cerebrovascular disease, or atrial fibrillation. Serum hemoglobin, serum albumin, serum creatinine, blood urea nitrogen, serum potassium and serum total cholesterol (TC) were measured. The single-pool Kt/V (spKt/V) was determined by two-point urea modeling based on the intradialytic reduction in blood urea and intradialytic weight loss. Timed 24 h urine collection was performed during the interdialytic intervals at the time of enrollment and 24 h-urine volume was recorded. Zero- residual renal function was operationally defined as having 24 h-urine volume <100 ml. Patients were grouped as having zero- residual renal function or non-zero residual renal function. To estimate the residual glomerular filtration rate, residual renal clearance (ml/min) was calculated as the mean of the creatinine clearance and urea clearance in patients with 24 h-urine volume ≥100 ml [12].

In order to analyze the effects of the dialysis membrane type on mortality in patients with zero- and non-zero residual renal function, the patients were further divided into high-flux and low-flux dialysis groups according to the type of dialysis membrane used. High-flux dialysis was defined as an ultrafiltration coefficient of ≥20 ml/mm Hg per hour and a sieving coefficient for β2-microglobulin >0.6. Low-flux dialysis was defined as an ultrafiltration coefficient of ≤10 ml/mm Hg per hour and a sieving coefficient for β2-microglobulin = 0 [9].

A total of 21 types of low-flux dialyzer and 26 types of high-flux dialyzers were used in this study. The most common low-flux dialyzer was the Gambro polyflux 14L (used in 34.2% of cases) and the most common high-flux dialyzer was the Gambro polyflux 170H (used in 18.9% of cases). All of the dialysis membrane materials were synthetic membranes in the high-flux dialyzer group, whereas 99.0% contained synthetic membranes and 1.0% contained substituted cellulose membranes in low-flux dialyzer group. All dialysis sessions were performed without reuse of the dialyzers. All dialysate solutions were bicarbonate-based. Dialysate complied with the criteria adopted by the European Best Practice Guidelines [13] and the ultrapure dialysates were used in all patients using high-flux dialyzer.

Outcomes

The clinical outcome of this study was all-cause mortality. For each death, the principal investigator at that given institution completed a form that included cause of death according to the CRC registry for ESRD study classification.

Statistical Analyses

Data with continuous variables and normal distribution are presented as means ± SD, and those without normal distribution are presented as the median with ranges as appropriate for the type of variable. Student's t-tests, Mann–Whitney U tests, one-way ANOVA tests and Kruskal-Wallis tests were used to determine the differences in continuous variables. Categorical variables are presented as percentages. Pearson's chi-square test or Fisher's exact test were used to determine the differences in categorical variables.

Absolute mortality rates were calculated per 100 person-years of follow-up. The survival curves were estimated using the Kaplan–Meier method and compared by the log-rank tests between the high- and low-flux dialysis groups. The Cox proportional hazard regression model was used to calculate hazard ratio (HR) with 95% confidence interval (CI) for all-cause mortality. Analyses were adjusted for potential confounders including age, gender, use of high-flux membrane, BMI, diabetes mellitus, cardiovascular disease, primary cause of ESRD, duration of dialysis therapy, systolic blood pressure (BP), diastolic BP, hemoglobin, serum albumin, serum β2-microglobulin, serum TC, type of vascular access, residual renal clearance, and spKt/V. A value of P<0.05 was considered to be statistically significant. All statistical analyses were performed using SPSS 11.5 software (Chicago, IL, USA).

Results

Patients Characteristics

A total of 893 patients with 24 h-residual urine volume ≥ 100 ml and 913 patients with 24 h-residual urine volume < 100 ml were included in this study. Table 1 shows the baseline characteristics of participants.

In the patients with 24 h-residual urine volume ≥100 ml, 64% (569 of 893) patients were dialyzed using low-flux dialysis membranes and 36% (324 of 893) were dialyzed using high-flux dialysis membranes. The high-flux group had a higher prevalence of cardiovascular diseases and lower serum β2-microglobulin levels than the low-flux group. Arteriovenous fistula as the vascular

access was more used in high-flux group and catheter was more used in low-flux group. There was no significant difference in rate of arteriovenous graft use between the high- and the low-flux groups. There were no significant differences in age, gender, BMI, prevalence of diabetes mellitus, primary cause of ESRD, duration of dialysis therapy, systolic BP, diastolic BP, serum hemoglobin levels, serum albumin levels, serum TC levels, 24-h urine volume, residual renal clearance and spKt/V between the high- and the low-flux groups.

In the patients with 24 h-residual urine volume <100 ml, 62% (570 of 913) were dialyzed using low-flux dialysis membranes and 38% (343 of 913) were dialyzed using high-flux dialysis membranes. The high-flux group was younger and had a lower prevalence of diabetes mellitus. Diabetes mellitus as a primary cause of ESRD was more prevalent in lower flux group. The high-flux group had a longer duration of dialysis therapy, higher serum albumin levels and lower spKt/V than the low-flux group. Arteriovenous fistula as the vascular access was more used in high-flux group and catheter was more used in low-flux group. There was no significant difference in rate of arteriovenous graft use between the high- and the low-flux groups. There were no

Table 1. Baseline characteristics of the study populations.

Characteristics	24 h-residual urine volume ≥100 ml (n = 893)			24 h-residual urine volume <100 ml (n = 913)		
	Low-Flux (n = 569)	High-Flux (n = 324)	p	Low-Flux (n = 570)	High-Flux (n = 343)	p
Age (years)	59±14	58±13	0.504	59±13	57±13	0.027
Male, n (%)	338 (9.4)	205 (63.3)	0.255	331 (58.1)	184 (53.6)	0.192
Body mass index (kg/m²)	23.0±3.7	22.6±3.1	0.082	22.6±3.3	22.2±3.5	0.137
Comorbidities						
Diabetes mellitus, n (%)	303 (53.3)	192 (59.3)	0.108	339 (59.5)	165 (48.1)	0.001
Cardiovascular diseases, n (%)	207 (36.4)	144 (44.4)	0.029	253 (44.4)	146 (42.6)	0.865
Causes of ESRD, n (%)			0.059			0.001
Diabetes mellitus	302 (53.1)	189 (58.3)		300 (52.6)	150 (43.7)	
Glomerulonephritis	89 (15.6)	40 (12.3)		83 (14.6)	49 (14.3)	
Renal vascular disease	99 (17.4)	44 (13.6)		74 (13.0)	48 (22.7)	
Others/unknown	79 (13.9)	51 (15.7)		113 (19.8)	66 (19.2)	
Duration of dialysis therapy (months)	0 (0–3)	0 (0–7)	0.114	17 (0–53)	46 (17–84)	<0.001
Measurement before dialysis						
Systolic BP (mmHg)	141±24	143±25	0.233	142±21	143±20	0.438
Diastolic BP (mmHg)	77±14	76±14	0.278	79±13	80±12	0.073
Hemoglobin (g/dl)	9.0±1.7	9.2±1.7	0.060	10.1±1.5	10.3±1.4	0.071
Serum albumin (g/dl)	3.5±0.6	3.4±0.6	0.067	3.7±0.6	3.9±0.5	<0.001
Serum TC (mg/dl)	154±43	154±47	0.988	158±44	155±37	0.275
Serum β2-microglobulin (mg/L)	22.2 (17.2–29.3)	20.3 (15.4–26.2)	0.011	34.4 (23.0–44.9)	30.0 (24.0–44.3)	0.788
Vascular access			<0.001			<0.001
Arteriovenous fistula, n (%)	174 (30.9)	139 (43.6)		330 (58.8)	247 (74.2)	
Arteriovenous graft, n (%)	49 (8.7)	35 (11.0)		98 (17.5)	47 (14.1)	
Catheter, n (%)	340 (60.4)	145 (45.5)		133 (23.7)	39 (11.7)	
24 h-urine volume (ml)	900 (518–1300)	810 (465–1300)	0.285	0 (0–0)	0 (0–0)	0.829
Residual renal clearance (ml/min)	2.9 (1.4–5.2)	2.7 (1.4–4.2)	0.062	-	-	
spKt/V	1.43±0.66	1.46±0.44	0.539	1.52±0.39	1.35±0.78	0.001

Data are expressed as mean ± SD or medians (interquartile percentile) or numbers (percentages).
Abbreviations: ESRD, end-stage renal disease; BP, blood pressure; TC, total cholesterol; Kt/V: K, dialyzer clearance; t, time; V, volume of water a patient's body contains.

significant differences in gender, BMI, prevalence of cardiovascular diseases, systolic BP, diastolic BP, serum hemoglobin levels, serum TC levels, serum β2-microglobulin level and 24-h urine volume between the high- and the low-flux groups.

Effect of Membrane Flux on All-cause Mortality

The median follow-up period was 31 months (interquartile range, 13–40 months). Total of 170 deaths occurred during the follow-up period. Cardiovascular diseases were the leading cause of death (32.9% of all deaths). Table 2 shows the causes of death in each group. The distribution of causes of death was not significantly different between high- and low-flux groups in patients with 24 h-residual urine volume ≥100 ml or in patients with 24 h-residual urine volume <100 ml (p = 0.239 and p = 0.938, respectively).

In patients with 24 h-residual urine volume ≥100 ml, 197 patients left the study during the follow-up period for reasons other than death, including 38 patients who received kidney transplantation, 81 patients who transferred to a nonparticipating hospital, 44 patients who refused further participation and 34 for unspecified reasons. There were 69 deaths in this group during the follow-up period. The leading cause of death was cardiovascular diseases (36.2% of all deaths) (Table 2). The absolute mortality rate during the follow-up period was 4.2 deaths per 100 person-years. In univariate Cox regression analysis, use of high-flux membrane was not associated with mortality (HR 1.08, 95% CI, 0.66–1.76, P = 0.765). Figure 1A shows the Kaplan-Meier plot for all-cause mortality in the high- and the low-flux groups for the patients with 24 h-residual urine volume ≥100 ml. As shown, there was no significant difference in survival between the high-flux group and the low-flux group (P = 0.764 by log-rank test). After adjustment for demographics, comorbid conditions, and laboratory data, the adjusted HR for mortality in the high-flux group was 0.86 (95% CI, 0.38–1.95, P = 0.723), implying the mortality was not significantly different between the high- and the low-flux groups in the patients with 24 h-residual urine volume ≥ 100 ml (Table 3).

In patients with 24 h-residual urine volume <100 ml, 174 patients left the study during the follow-up period for reasons other than death, including 51 patients who received kidney transplantation, 78 patients who transferred to a nonparticipating hospital, 21 patients who refused further participation and 24 for unspecified reasons. There were a total of 101 deaths in this group during the follow-up period. The leading causes of death were cardiovascular diseases (30.7% of all deaths) and infectious diseases (30.7% of all deaths) (Table 2). The absolute mortality rate during the follow-up period was 4.2 deaths per 100 person-years. In univariate Cox regression analysis, the high-flux group was

significantly associated with reduced mortality (HR 0.53, 95% CI, 0.34–0.83, P = 0.005). Figure 1B shows the Kaplan-Meier plot for all-cause mortality in the high- and the low-flux groups in patients with 24 h-residual urine volume <100 ml. Survival was increased in the high-flux group compared to the low-flux group (P = 0.005 by log-rank test). Even after adjustment for demographics, comorbid conditions, and laboratory data, the adjusted HR for mortality in the high-flux group was 0.40 (95% CI, 0.21–0.78, P = 0.007), implying that the high-flux group had a risk of death that was 60% lower than the low-flux group in patients with 24 h-residual urine volume <100 ml (Table 3).

Discussion

The major findings of this study were that HD using high-flux dialysis membrane was associated with decreased mortality compared to HD using low-flux dialysis membrane in patients with 24 h-residual urine volume <100 ml, whereas there was no significant difference in mortality between the high- and the low-flux dialysis group in patients with 24 h-residual urine volume ≥ 100 ml. These data suggest that high-flux dialysis impacts survival differently according to residual renal function and that high-flux dialysis is superior to low-flux dialysis in patients without residual renal function.

Residual renal function is associated with improved survival and clinical outcomes such as hospitalization, nutrition, anemia, and serum phosphorous control in HD patients [14–16]. Furthermore, residual renal function is a strong predictor of serum β2-microglobulin levels, since the kidney is the primary organ for the clearance of β2-microglobulin [11]. In this study, serum β2-microglobulin levels were significantly higher in patients with 24 h-residual urine volume <100 ml (31 mg/L, interquartile range, 23–45 mg/L) than in those with 24 h-residual urine volume ≥100 ml (21 mg/L, interquartile range, 16–28 mg/L) (p<0.001) (data not shown). A previous study also reported that increment of residual renal function was associated with a decrease in serum β2-microglobulin levels in dependent of years on dialysis [11]. Therefore, the beneficial effects of high-flux dialysis by clearance of middle molecules such as β2-microglobulin on clinical outcomes may be overshadowed by residual renal function in HD patients. Thus, it could be postulated that the beneficial effect of high-flux dialysis may be more apparent in patients with lesser residual renal function.

The HEMO study showed that there was no statistically significant interaction between baseline residual renal function and the type of flux intervention with respect to all-cause mortality although there was a trend towards decreased mortality in patients with lesser residual renal function [17]. They reported that all-

Table 2. Causes of deaths in each group.

	24 h-residual urine volume ≥100 ml		24 h-residual urine volume <100 ml	
	Low-Flux (44 deaths)	High-Flux (25 deaths)	Low-Flux (75 deaths)	High-Flux (26 deaths)
Cardiovascular diseases including cerebrovascular diseases, n (%)	13 (29.5)	12 (48.0)	23 (30.7)	8 (30.8)
Infectious diseases, n (%)	14 (31.8)	2 (8.0)	24 (32.0)	7 (26.9)
Malignancy, n (%)	2 (4.5)	1 (4.0)	7 (9.3)	2 (7.7)
Others, n	15 (34.1)	10 (40.0)	21 (28.0)	9 (34.6)

(A)   Residual urine volume ≥ 100 ml

(B)   Residual urine volume < 100 ml

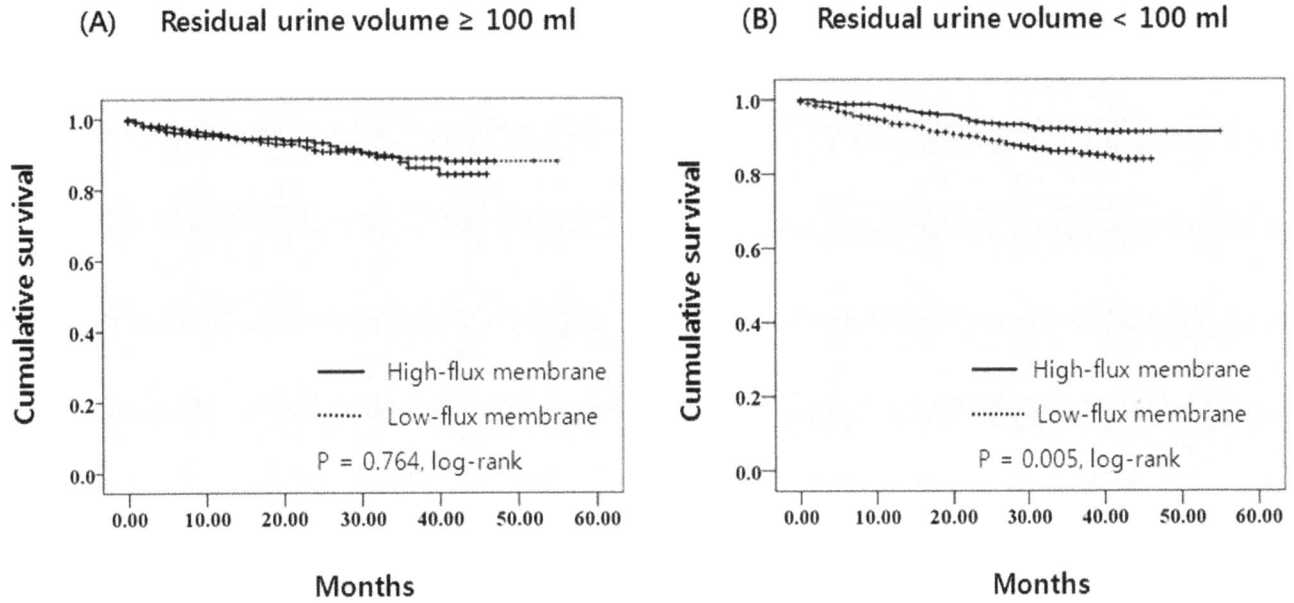

Figure 1. Kaplan-Meier survival curve for mortality in (A) patients with 24 h-residual urine volume ≥100 ml (P = 0.764 by log-rank test) and in (B) patients with 24 h-residual urine volume <100 ml (P = 0.005 by log-rank test).

cause mortality rates were not significantly different between patients with residual urea clearance ≤0.24 ml/min and those with residual urea clearance >0.24 ml/min (P = 0.24) [17], which is not consistent with our results. There are a number of possible explanations for this discrepancy.

First, it should be noted that the HEMO study only included patients with residual urea clearance <1.5 ml/min/35L of urea. Because the impact of high-flux dialysis on mortality may be less apparent in patients with greater residual renal function, the exclusion of patients with greater residual renal function may be a

Table 3. Multivariate Cox regression analysis of mortality in study populations.

	24 h-residual urine volume ≥100 ml			24 h-residual urine volume <100 ml		
	HR	95% CI	P	HR	95% CI	P
High-flux membrane (versus low-flux)	0.86	0.38–1.95	0.723	0.40	0.21–0.78	0.007
Age (1-yearincrement)	1.09	1.05–1.14	<0.001	1.04	1.01–1.07	0.005
Male (versus female)	0.72	0.32–1.64	0.431	0.86	0.45–1.62	0.633
BMI (per increment of 1 kg/m²)	0.98	0.87–1.10	0.743	0.95	0.86–1.05	0.325
Comorbidities						
Diabetes mellitus (versus none)	0.85	0.12–5.88	0.869	2.19	0.73–6.57	0.162
Cardiovascular diseases (versus none)	1.54	0.74–3.22	0.250	1.28	0.69–2.36	0.437
Causes of ESRD						
Diabetes mellitus (versus non diabetes mellitus)	1.32	0.19–9.23	0.78	2.01	0.71–5.89	0.183
Systolic BP (per increment of 10 mmHg)	1.00	0.98–1.02	0.998	1.01	0.99–1.03	0.276
Diastolic BP (per increment of 10 mmHg)	1.02	0.98–1.06	0.385	1.00	0.97–1.04	0.858
Hemoglobin (per increment of 1 g/dl)	0.86	0.67–1.11	0.256	1.05	0.85–1.30	0.645
Serum albumin (per increment of 1 g/dl)	0.41	0.20–0.82	0.012	0.81	0.41–1.61	0.552
Serum β2-microglobulin ((per increment of 1 mg/L)	1.00	1.00–1.00	0.801	1.00	0.99–1.01	0.769
Serum TC (per increment of 10 mg/dl)	1.00	0.99–1.01	0.993	1.00	0.99–1.01	0.686
Residual renal clearance (per increment of 1 ml/min)	1.10	0.97–1.25	0.131			
spKt/V	1.15	0.51–2.62	0.735	0.57	0.31–1.04	0.067

Multivariate model includes age, gender, use of high-flux membrane, BMI, diabetes mellitus, cardiovascular disease, causes of ESRD, duration of dialysis therapy, systolic BP, diastolic BP, hemoglobin, serum albumin, serum β2-microglobulin, serum TC, type of vascular access, residual renal clearance and spKt/V.
Abbreviations: BMI, body mass index; HR, hazard ratio; TC, total cholesterol.

confounding factor in comparing the impact of high-flux dialysis on mortality according to residual renal function.

Additionally, the HEMO study included HD patients in which dialyzers were reused. Although the relationship between reuse of the dialyzer and effectiveness of removal of middle molecules has been controversial, reuse of dialyzers may be associated with structural damage of the membrane and a reduced permeability to middle molecules [18,19]. Therefore, reuse of dialyzer also may be a confounder to determine the impact of dialyzer membrane flux on mortality.

Another large randomized controlled trial, the MPO study, showed that there was no significant difference in mortality between high- and low-flux dialysis in the whole cohort [9]. In subgroup analysis, the MPO study showed a survival benefit with high-flux dialysis in patients with serum albumin level ≤4 mg/dl, while there was no significant difference in mortality between high- and low-flux dialysis in patients with serum albumin level > 4 mg/dl. Data on interaction between residual renal function and the type of flux intervention with respect to all-cause mortality were not shown in the MPO study. However, the MPO study provides some interesting clues on the impact of residual renal function on the relationship between high flux dialysis and mortality. First, patients with serum albumin level ≤4 mg/dl in the MPO study had longer duration of follow-up than the patients with serum albumin level >4 mg/dl because the study protocol was amended during the course of the study [9]. The longer duration of follow-up in patients with serum albumin level ≤ 4 mg/dl may explain the relationship between survival benefit with high-flux dialysis and residual renal function. Long duration of dialysis may cause accumulation of toxic middle molecules and decrease residual renal function to remove them. Therefore, in the MPO study, the patients with serum albumin level ≤ mg/dl could have benefited more from the removal of toxic middle molecules with high-flux dialysis than the patients with serum albumin level >4 mg/dl because of the longer follow up. Second, the survival benefit of high-flux dialysis in the patients with serum albumin level ≤4 mg/dl was evident only after about 12 months of follow-up period, possibly when the residual renal function was lost. These findings of the MPO study therefore support the results of our study.

Our findings have a number of clinical implications. The European Best Practice Guideline (EBPG) relating to dialyzer membrane permeability recommends that the use of synthetic high-flux membranes should be considered to delay long-term complications of HD therapy [20]. The EBPG suggests the specific indication for high-flux dialysis to reduce dialysis-related amyloidosis, to improve control of hyperphosphatemia, to reduce the increased cardiovascular risk, and to improve control of anemia [20]. Our findings support the evidence for use of high-flux dialysis membrane and further contribute to the indications established for high-flux dialysis therapy in HD patients without residual renal function.

Our study has several limitations. First, the design of our study was not a randomized, controlled study but rather was a prospective observational study. The prescription of the dialyzer might be influenced by the results of previous study for the membrane flux on mortality such as MPO study. Accordingly, some baseline characteristics between the high-flux dialysis group and low-flux dialysis group differed in our study, indicating potential selection bias. In addition, the median follow-up period of 31 months was relatively short. Finally, despite the multicenter nature of the study, our cohort consisted of solely Korean patients. Therefore, it is uncertain whether our results can be generalized to other ethnic groups with HD treatment.

In conclusion, we found that HD using high-flux dialysis membranes had survival benefit in patients with 24 h-residual urine volume <100 ml, but not in patients with 24 h-residual urine volume ≥100 ml. These findings suggest that dialyzer membrane flux impacts survival differently according to residual renal function. Thus, high-flux dialysis rather than low-flux dialysis might be considered in HD patients without residual renal function.

Acknowledgments

We thank the study coordinators Hye Young Lim, Nam Hee Kim, Mi Joung Moon, Hwa Young Lee, Mi Joung Kwon, Su Yeon An, Su Joung Oh and Hye Young Kwak for contribution to this study.

Author Contributions

Conceived and designed the experiments: YKK CWY. Performed the experiments: HWK SHK YKK YOK DCJ HCS EJC. Analyzed the data: HWK YKK CWY. Contributed reagents/materials/analysis tools: SHK YKK YOK DCJ YLK YSK SWK NHK CWY. Wrote the paper: HWK YKK.

References

1. Yoshino M, Kuhlmann MK, Kotanko P, Greenwood RN, et al. (2006) International differences in dialysis mortality reflect background general population atherosclerotic cardiovascular mortality. J Am Soc Nephrol 17: 3510–3519.

2. Ward RA (2011) Do clinical outcomes in chronic hemodialysis depend on the choice of a dialyzer? Semin Dial 24: 65–71.

3. DiRaimondo CR, Pollak VE (1989) Beta 2-microglobulin kinetics in maintenance hemodialysis: a comparison of conventional and high-flux dialyzers and the effects of dialyzer reuse. Am J Kidney Dis 13: 390–395.

4. Hornberger JC, Chernew M, Petersen J, Garber AM (1992) A multivariate analysis of mortality and hospital admissions with high-flux dialysis. J Am Soc Nephrol 3: 1227–1237.

5. Port FK, Wolfe RA, Hulbert-Shearon TE, Daugirdas JT, Agodoa LY, et al. (2001) Mortality risk by hemodialyzer reuse practice and dialyzer membrane characteristics: results from the usrds dialysis morbidity and mortality study. Am J Kidney Dis 37: 276–286.

6. Chauveau P, Nguyen H, Combe C, Chêne G, Azar R, et al. (2005) Dialyzer membrane permeability and survival in hemodialysis patients. Am J Kidney Dis 45: 565–571.

7. Krane V, Krieter DH, Olschewski M, März W, Mann JF, et al. (2007) Dialyzer membrane characteristics and outcome of patients with type 2 diabetes on maintenance hemodialysis. Am J Kidney Dis 49: 267–275.

8. Eknoyan G, Beck GJ, Cheung AK, Daugirdas JT, Greene T, et al. (2002) Effect of dialysis dose and membrane flux in maintenance hemodialysis. N Engl J Med 347: 2010–2019.

9. Locatelli F, Martin-Malo A, Hannedouche T, Loureiro A, Papadimitriou M, et al. (2009) Effect of membrane permeability on survival of hemodialysis patients. J Am Soc Nephrol 20: 645–654.

10. McCarthy JT, Williams AW, Johnson WJ (1994) Serum beta 2-microglobulin concentration in dialysis patients: importance of intrinsic renal function. J Lab Clin Med 123: 495–505.

11. Cheung AK, Rocco MV, Yan G, Leypoldt JK, Levin NW, et al. (2006) Serum beta-2 microglobulin levels predict mortality in dialysis patients: results of the HEMO study. J Am Soc Nephrol 17: 546–555.

12. Peritoneal Dialysis Adequacy 2006 Work Group. (2006) Clinical practice guidelines for peritoneal adequacy, update 2006. Am J Kidney Dis 48 Suppl 1: S91–97.

13. Ward RA (2004) Ultrapure dialysate. Semin Dial. 17: 489–497.

14. Shemin D, Bostom AG, Laliberty P, Dworkin LD (2001) Residual renal function and mortality risk in hemodialysis patients. Am J Kidney Dis 38: 85–90.

15. Vilar E, Wellsted D, Chandna SM, Greenwood RN, Farrington K (2009) Residual renal function improves outcome in incremental haemodialysis despite reduced dialysis dose. Nephrol Dial Transplant 24: 2502–2510.

16. van der Wal WM, Noordzij M, Dekker FW, Boeschoten EW, Krediet RT, et al. (2011) Full loss of residual renal function causes higher mortality in dialysis

patients; findings from a marginal structural model. Nephrol Dial Transplant 2011: 2978–2983.

17. Cheung AK, Levin NW, Greene T, Agodoa L, Bailey J, et al. (2003) Effects of high-flux hemodialysis on clinical outcomes: results of the HEMO study. J Am Soc Nephrol 14: 3251–3263.

18. Matos JP, André MB, Rembold SM, Caldeira FE, Lugon JR (2000) Effects of dialyzer reuse on the permeability of low-flux membranes. Am J Kidney Dis 35: 839–844.

19. Cheung AK, Agodoa LY, Daugirdas JT, Depner TA, Gotch FA, et al. (1999) Effects of hemodialyzer reuse on clearances of urea and beta2-microglobulin. The Hemodialysis (HEMO) Study Group. J Am Soc Nephrol 10: 117–127.

20. Tattersall J, Canaud B, Heimburger O, Pedrini L, Schneditz D, et al. (2010) High-flux or low-flux dialysis: a position statement following publication of the Membrane Permeability Outcome study. Nephrol Dial Transplant 25: 1230–1232.

10

Urine Osmolarity and Risk of Dialysis Initiation in a Chronic Kidney Disease Cohort – a Possible Titration Target?

Max Plischke[1], Maria Kohl[2], Lise Bankir[3], Sascha Shayganfar[4], Ammon Handisurya[1], Georg Heinze[2], Martin Haas[1]*

1 Division of Nephrology and Dialysis, Department of Internal Medicine III, Medical University Vienna, Vienna, Austria, 2 Section for Clinical Biometrics, Center of Medical Statistics, Informatics and Intelligent Systems, Medical University of Vienna, Vienna, Austria, 3 INSERM UMRS 1138, Equipe 2, Centre de Recherche des Cordeliers, Paris, France, 4 Division of Cardiology, Pulmonology, and Vascular Medicine, Medical Faculty, University Hospital Düsseldorf, Düsseldorf, Germany

Abstract

Background: Increasing evidence is linking fluid intake, vasopressin suppression and osmotic control with chronic kidney disease progression. Interestingly, the association between urine volume, urine osmolarity and risk of dialysis initiation has not been studied in chronic kidney disease patients before.

Objective: To study the relationship between urine volume, urine osmolarity and the risk of initiating dialysis in chronic kidney disease.

Design: In a retrospective cohort analysis of 273 patients with chronic kidney disease stage 1–4 we assessed the association between urine volume, urine osmolarity and the risk of dialysis by a multivariate proportional sub-distribution hazards model for competing risk data according to Fine and Gray. Co-variables were selected via the purposeful selection algorithm.

Results: Dialysis was reached in 105 patients over a median follow-up period of 92 months. After adjustment for age, baseline creatinine clearance, other risk factors and diuretics, a higher risk for initiation of dialysis was found in patients with higher urine osmolarity. The adjusted sub-distribution hazard ratio for initiation of dialysis was 2.04 (95% confidence interval, 1.06 to 3.92) for each doubling of urine osmolarity. After 72 months, the estimated adjusted cumulative incidence probabilities of dialysis were 15%, 24%, and 34% in patients with a baseline urine osmolarity of 315, 510, and 775 mosm/L, respectively.

Conclusions: We conclude that higher urine osmolarity is associated with a higher risk of initiating dialysis. As urine osmolarity is a potentially modifiable risk factor, it thus deserves further, prospective research as a potential target in chronic kidney disease progression.

Editor: Kathrin Eller, Medical University of Graz, Austria

Funding: Maria Kohl (statistician) was supported by the European Community's Seventh Framework Programme, grant number 241544. The funders had no role in study design, data collection and analysis, decision to publish, or preparation of the manuscript. Maria Kohl was involved in study design, analysis, and preparation of the manuscript. Mortality data, obtained via Statistics Austria, was payed for using the authors' departments (Department of Internal Med. III, Division of Nephrology and Dialysis, Medical University Vienna) research budget, which is not tied to any external funding institution. As this was a retrospective study, other expenses (laboratory, etc) were fully covered by routine patient care at the authors' outpatient department.

Competing Interests: The authors have declared that no competing interests exist.

* E-mail: martin.haas@meduniwien.ac.at

Introduction

Medicinal use of water in chronic kidney disease (CKD) has gained research interest lately [1], as established efforts to retard CKD progression remain far from satisfactory [2]. Epidemiological data associating fluid intake or urine volume with GFR decline in humans have not been fully conclusive [3–7]. Nonetheless, there is increasing evidence linking fluid intake, vasopressin suppression and osmotic control with CKD and ADPKD progression [8–12]. Kidney excretion is adjusted according to water and dietary solute intake, as well as water and solute losses by lungs, skin, and the gastrointestinal tract. The required urine volume can be determined by dividing the daily osmolar excretion, to maintain the body's solute content at steady state, by the maximal urine osmolality, with failing kidneys losing capacity to concentrate urine maximally. As such, water intake required to achieve comparable urinary solute dilution varies considerably between individuals. [1]

Interestingly, median 24-hour urine osmolality is greater than that of plasma in humans, suggesting continuous antidiuretic action [13], which has been associated with renal function decline [10]. Consequentially, Wang et al. recently devised a quantitative method to determine the amount of water needed on a case-by-case basis to achieve a mean urine osmolality equivalent to that of plasma [13]. Relationships between urine osmolarity (given as mosm/L compared to mosm/kg H_2O for osmolality) and GFR decline have been described in two studies [3,7] with contrasting results. We were interested in studying urine volume and urine osmolarity in terms of harder endpoints in chronic kidney disease. Thus we set out to study these variables in terms of risk of initiating dialysis, with death as a competing event.

Subjects and Methods

Patients

All patients attending our nephrology outpatient department between 1 January 2000 and 31 December 2002 were included in a single-centre cohort study. The study baseline was defined as one year after the first visit, while the time period between the first visit and baseline was defined as the run-in phase. Baseline demographic data for each patient were collected from outpatient files including medication, co-morbidities, and the nature of renal disease. A minimum of two visits, with 24-hour urine samples taken before and after baseline, were defined as inclusion criteria. Exclusion criteria were a reported urine volume less than 500 ml/d or a creatinine clearance below 15 ml/min (CKD 5). The mean of all measurements taken during the run-in phase (median: 5 [25th–75th percentiles: 3–8]) was used as the baseline value for each parameter.

The primary endpoint of the study was time to dialysis, with death as the competing event. Mortality data and data on the initiation of dialysis until 31 December 2008 were obtained from Statistics Austria (the national statistics institution) and the Austrian Dialysis and Transplantation Registry (ÖDTR), respectively. Patients starting dialysis had no loss of follow-up according to ÖDTR. Because of a possible relocation of a patient to a country other than Austria, a minor loss of follow-up for mortality data from Statistics Austria cannot be excluded.

Ethics Statement

This was a retrospective study making use of data already collected during routine patient care at our outpatient department. The processing and analysis of data was done after anonymization. Therefore no informed consent was requested from patients. This approach was reviewed and approved by the local ethics committee (Ethikkommission Medizinische Universität Wien).

Laboratory data

Standard 24-hour urine samples of the patients were analysed in regard of proteinuria, creatinine, sodium, urea nitrogen, and potassium levels, in accordance with routinely used methods at our central laboratory (Clinical Institute of Medical and Chemical Laboratory Diagnostics, Medical University of Vienna). On the day of each visit, serum samples were analysed for creatinine, sodium, potassium, glucose and urea nitrogen levels in accordance with routine methods.

After conversion of glucose and urea nitrogen from mg/dl in mmol/L the estimated urine osmolarity (U_{osm}) (mosm/L) was calculated as follows:

$$Uosm = 2 \times (UNa + UK) + Uurea$$

Estimated plasma osmolarity (P_{osm}) (mosm/L) was calculated as follows:

$$Posm = 2 \times (PNa + PK) + Purea + Pglucose$$

U_{Na}, U_K, and U_{urea} are the concentrations of sodium, potassium and urea in the urine (all in mmol/L), and P_{Na}, P_K, P_{urea}, and $P_{glucose}$ are the concentrations of sodium, potassium, urea and glucose in plasma (in mmol/L).

Statistical analysis

Continuous variables were described by medians (25th to 75th percentiles), and compared between groups using Wilcoxon's rank sum tests. Correlations between continuous variables were assessed by Spearman's rank correlation coefficient. For further analysis, osmolarity, proteinuria and creatinine clearance were log-base-2 transformed because of the skewed distributions of these variables. To describe intra- versus inter-individual variance of urine osmolarity, we conducted a variance component analysis including all run-in urine osmolarity values that were available for each patient using a mixed model with patients as levels of a random factor. The outcome variable was time to dialysis, with death as the competing event. Patients who were alive without dialysis at the time of their last visit were censored. Absolute event rates were computed as the number of events divided by the total follow-up time for all patients. Observations with missing values were not used in the calculated models. We described the distribution of time to dialysis using cumulative incidence functions, and compared groups using Gray's test [14].

Due to the established relationship between baseline creatinine clearance and risk of initiating dialysis/ESRD, and the known progressive loss in urine concentration ability with decreasing renal function [1], it seemed important to introduce creatinine clearance as an adjustment factor in all further analyses.

We fitted two multivariate proportional sub-distribution hazards models for competing risk data according to Fine and Gray [15] in order to assess the effect of urine osmolarity or volume on the risk for initiating dialysis. In these models, we considered osmolarity or urine volume and included those variables that either proved significant in a multivariate model (P<0.10) or changed the log hazard ratio of osmolarity or urine volume by more than 15% when those variables were excluded from the analyses (purposeful selection algorithm) [16]. We assumed that any variable not selected would have no relevant impact on our conclusions. All variables listed in Table 1 (except 24-hour proteinuria, 24-hour osmolar excretion and 24-hour sodium excretion) were considered as potential confounders. Results from multivariate competing risk regression were described by means of sub-distribution hazard ratios (SHR) and 95% confidence intervals (95% CI), and by computing and visualising estimated cumulative incidence curves at specific covariate values. As urine osmolarity and creatinine clearance were log-base-2 transformed, their SHR correspond to each doubling of these variables. We checked for significant pairwise interactions of variables and for time-dependent effects by including interactions with follow-up time. Non-linear effects were assessed by the method of fractional polynomials [17]. For sensitivity analysis, we also estimated a cause-specific (death-censored) Cox regression model. The R-software, version 2.12 (www.r-project.org), was used for statistical analysis.

Results

Baseline data

Three hundred and seventy-two patients were examined for eligibility. After applying all inclusion and exclusion criteria, a total of 273 patients (56% male) with CKD class 1-4 and a median age of 56 years (42 to 67 years) were confirmed eligible and included in the study (**Table 1**). Median creatinine clearance was 48 (30 to 79) ml/min. Kidney disease was unknown in 46% of the patients; the

Table 1. Demographic and clinical characteristics of all patients at baseline, and in the subgroups of CKD patients stages 1-3a (creatinine clearance $\geq$45 ml/min) and stage 3b-4 (creatinine clearance $\geq$15 and <45 ml/min).

	Total	CKD 1-3a	CKD 3b-4
	(n = 273)	(n = 141)	(n = 132)
Age (years)	56 (42–67)	50 (37–61)	59 (46–71)
Male	153 (56%)	87 (62%)	66 (50%)
BMI	26 (23–30)	26 (23–30)	26 (23–30)
CCl (ml/min)	48 (30–79)	78 (60–105)	30 (25–35)
MAP (mmHg)	97 (93–102)	97 (93–103)	98 (94–102)
P_{osm} (mosm/L)	308 (302–315)	303 (300–308)	313 (308–318)
Urine analysis			
Proteinuria (g/L)	0.87 (0.24–2.34)	0.76 (0.21–2.34)	1.01 (0.26–2.31)
Proteinuria 24 h (g/24 h)	2.05 (0.53–5.63)	1.72 (0.53–5.2)	2.21 (0.57–6.12)
Volume (ml/24 h)	2220 (1935–2871)	2157 (1839–2700)	2325 (2000–3000)
U_{osm} (mosm/L)	510 (414–622)	607 (477–740)	445 (370–519)
Osmolar excretion (mosm/24 h)	1200 (930–1412)	1309 (1091–1636)	1018 (810–1254)
Sodium (mmol/L)	84 (68–104)	96 (75–116)	75 (61–93)
Sodium excretion (mmol/24 h)	201 (141–251)	215 (167–265)	181 (134–234)
Underlying kidney disease			
Polycystic kidney disease	18 (7%)	6 (4%)	12 (9%)
Diabetic nephropathy	20 (7%)	7 (5%)	13 (10%)
Glomerular disease	98 (36%)	73 (52%)	25 (19%)
Other	11 (4%)	4 (3%)	7 (5%)
Unknown	126 (46%)	51 (36%)	75 (57%)
Comorbidities			
Chronic heart failure	8 (3%)	3 (2%)	5 (4%)
Diabetes mellitus	59 (23%)	23 (18%)	36 (27%)
Liver cirrhosis (child C)	0 (0%)	0 (0%)	0 (0%)
Medication			
ACEI/AT-II Blocker	216 (85%)	111 (85%)	105 (84%)
Diuretics	120 (47%)	45 (35%)	75 (60%)
Beta-blocker	119 (47%)	47 (36%)	72 (58%)
Non-dihydropyridine CCB	39 (15%)	21 (16%)	18 (14%)

Abbreviations: BMI, body mass index; CCl, creatinine clearance; MAP, mean arterial pressure; P_{osm}, plasma osmolarity; U_{osm}, urine osmolarity; ACEI/AT-II, angiotensin converting enzyme/angiotensin II receptor antagonist; CCB, calcium channel blocker. Values are given as median (Q1-Q3), if not stated otherwise.

remaining patients had mainly polycystic kidney disease, different forms of glomerulonephritis, or diabetic nephropathy (Table 1). Nearly all patients received antihypertensive drugs with an effect on protein excretion, such as inhibitors of the renin angiotensin aldosterone system, non-dihydropyridine calcium channel blockers, or beta-blockers.

There was a significant inverse correlation between average run-in 24-hour urine volume and average run-in urine osmolarity (R = -0.45; P<0.001). Urine osmolarity was significantly higher in men than in women (522 [446 to 629] vs. 458 [385 to 596] mosm/L; P<0.01), in patients without diuretics (520 [422 to 679] vs. 490 [408 to 577] mosm/L; P<0.05), and in patients without beta-blocker therapy (526 [429 to 673] vs. 463 [392 to 557] mosm/L;

P<0.01). Urine osmolarity and creatinine clearance were positively correlated (R = 0.6, p<0.01). The total variance for run-in urine osmolarity was 45253; the intra-individual variance was about one fourth ($\sigma2 = 11349$), i.e., random fluctuation within a patient explained 25% of the total variance, while the inter-individual variance component explained about 75% of the total variance. One patient was missing data for proteinuria, and 20 patients each were missing data for diuretics and beta-blocker therapy.

Follow-up

Median follow-up until death or censoring was 92 (76 to 95) months. End-stage renal disease developed in 105 patients (39%).

Thirty-eight patients (14%) died on dialysis and 35 patients (13%) died with functioning kidneys.

The absolute event rate for ESRD was 0.07/year. Event rates were 0.05/year for patients with mild to moderate chronic kidney disease (CKD stage 1–3, creatinine clearance ≥30 ml/min), and 0.22/year for those with severe CKD (stage 4, creatinine clearance 15–29 ml/min).

Urine osmolarity and risk of initiating dialysis

Univariate analysis, without adjustment for baseline creatinine clearance (see correlation above), suggested a higher cumulative incidence of dialysis in patients with lower-than-median urine osmolarities (p<0.01). Multivariate competing risk regression analysis, with death as the competing risk, adjusted for age, creatinine clearance, proteinuria, type of underlying renal disease, beta-blocker and diuretic therapies, showed that a higher urine osmolarity was associated with a higher risk of initiating dialysis (**Table 2**).

Based on this model, we estimated the adjusted cumulative incidence probabilities of dialysis for patients with three different urine osmolalities (10th, 50th and 90th percentile), assuming average values for all other covariates. A constant and stepwise significant increase was seen in patients with low (315 mosm/L), intermediate (510 mosm/L), and high (775 mosm/L) baseline urine osmolarity (**Figure 1**; p<0.05). At 72 months, the estimated cumulative incidence probabilities of dialysis in these patients were 15%, 24% and 34%, respectively. Lower baseline creatinine clearance, higher baseline protein excretion, the type of underlying renal disease, and treatment with diuretics were also independently associated with a higher risk of dialysis (Table 2). No significant interactions of urine osmolarity with other variables in the model were found. There was no evidence of time-dependent effects or a non-linear effect of urine osmolarity or any other metric covariate. The cause-specific Cox model yielded a similar result for the adjusted effect of urine osmolarity (cause-specific hazard ratio 2.19, 95% CI 1.21 to 3.95).

Urine volume and risk of initiating dialysis

There was a significant inverse association between average 24-hour urine volume and average urine osmolarity (R = −0.46; P<0.01). Therefore, we did not adjust for urine osmolarity in the multivariate regression analysis for urine volume. In this model, higher protein excretion, lower creatinine clearance, and the underlying renal disease but not urine volume were associated with a higher risk of dialysis (**Table 3**).

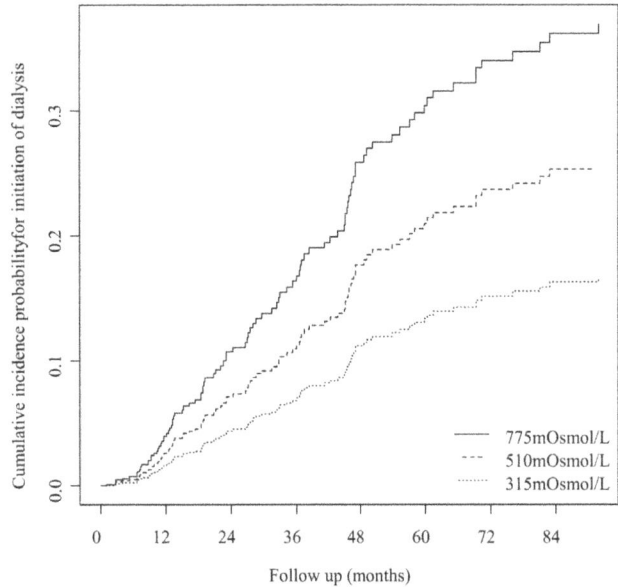

Figure 1. Cumulative incidence probabilities of dialysis initiation for different baseline urine osmolarities. Cumulative incidence probabilities of dialysis initiation for a baseline urine osmolarity of 315, 510 or 775 mosm/L (10th, 50th, and 90th percentile), estimated from the proportional sub-distribution hazards model. Given the estimated adjusted subdistribution hazard ratio (SHR) of 2.04 (p = 0.033) per doubling of urine osmolarity, the SHRs comparing patients with 775 mosm/L or 315 mosm/L to patients with 510 mosm/L were 1.54 (95%CI:1.03 to 2.28) or 0.61 (95%CI: 0.39 to 0.96), respectively.

Discussion

The present study demonstrates an independent, positive relationship between urine osmolarity and risk of initiating dialysis in a cohort of CKD patients stage 1 through 4. Competing risk models were adjusted for age, creatinine clearance, proteinuria, type of underlying renal disease, beta-blocker and diuretic therapies.

Two published studies have described relationships between 24-h urine osmolarity and GFR change over time. Hebert et al. reported a significant inverse relationship between baseline urine osmolarity and GFR decline in non-polycystic kidney disease patients (subgroup of full cohort), adjusted for diet, blood pressure and body surface area. Adjusting for additional covariates such as baseline GFR or diuretics use failed to result in statistically

Table 2. The independent effect of urine osmolarity, age, protein excretion, kidney function, renal disease and different drugs, on the risk of initiating dialysis in the competing risk regression analysis.

	SH Ratio	95% confidence interval		p-value
Urine osmolarity (per doubling)	2.04	1.06	3.92	0.03
Age (per decade)	0.87	0.74	1.02	0.08
Proteinuria (per doubling)	1.85	1.60	2.13	<0.001
Creatinine clearance (per doubling)	0.15	0.09	0.23	<0.001
Renal disease (PKD vs. other renal diseases)	3.44	1.73	6.81	<0.001
Beta-blocker therapy (yes vs. no)	1.54	0.97	2.43	0.07
Diuretic therapy (yes vs. no)	1.62	1.03	2.55	0.04

Abbreviations: SH Ratio, subdistribution hazard ratio; PKD, polycystic kidney disease

Table 3. The independent effect of urine volume, age, protein excretion, kidney function, renal disease and different drugs, on the risk of of initiating dialysis in the competing risk regression analysis.

	SH Ratio	95% confidence interval		p-value
Urine volume (per 0.5 L/d)	1.05	0.92	1.20	0.49
Age (per decade)	0.90	0.77	1.05	0.18
Proteinuria (per doubling)	1.79	1.54	2.07	<0.001
Creatinine clearance (per doubling)	0.20	0.13	0.30	<0.001
Renal disease (PKD vs. other renal diseases)	3.76	1.92	7.34	<0.001
Beta-blocker therapy (yes vs. no)	1.58	0.98	2.54	0.06
Diuretic therapy (yes vs. no)	1.59	0.99	2.54	0.05

Abbreviations: SH Ratio, subdistribution hazard ratio; PKD, polycystic kidney disease

significant models. Other models were calculated for follow-up urine osmolarities (collected after the study baseline; thus, not fully comparable) and did stay significant after further adjustments. [3] Torres et al. in turn suggested that higher baseline 24-h Uosm was associated with higher GFR decline across time in a cohort of ADPKD patients. [7]

The association between urine osmolarity and the risk of initiating dialysis, a stronger marker for end stage renal disease, has not been previously investigated. Our data thus adds to the existing evidence. The data is in line with Torres et al. suggesting a faster renal function decline in patients with higher urine osmolarity. Our cohort appeared to have the highest urine osmolarity with a median of 510 (IQR: 414–622) mosm/L versus a mean of 368 ± 159 mosm/L (Torres et al.), and a mean of 270 to 334 mosm/L (depending on protein diet group and polycystic kidney disease status) (Hebert et al.). It is therefore conceivable that lowering urine osmolarity below a specific threshold might be harmful to the kidney as well. A recent study addressing the association between sodium excretion, an important part of total urine osmolarity, and end-stage renal disease in patients with type 1 diabetes mellitus showed an inverse association with end stage renal disease [18]. Furthermore, a U-shaped curve was described for sodium excretion and mortality, such that subjects with the highest and the lowest sodium excretion had the highest mortality, partly supporting the hypothesis of low urine osmolarity being associated with harmful effects. Interestingly, in the univariate versus the multivariable analysis the strong effect of impaired renal function seems to obscure the positive correlation of osmolarity with the incidence of ESRD. Adjusting for creatinine clearance reveals this relationship. We conclude that among patients with equal renal function those with higher osmolarity values are more likely to progress to ESRD than those with lower osmolarity values in our cohort.

As described in the methods, estimated urine osmolarity was calculated from urine sodium, potassium and urea concentrations in 24 hour urine samples. These are the dominant solutes in the urine (plus the anions associated with sodium and potassium). Other solutes represent less than 10% of total urinary solutes (in the absence of glucosuria). Thus, estimated urine osmolarity is often used as an approximation of true osmolarity. Regarding the difference between osmolality (in mosm/kg H_2O) and osmolarity (in mosm/L), it is negligible in our study because the density of urine is very close to that of pure water in the range of values considered here. Other authors have used estimated urine osmolarity in several studies. [3,19]

Several authors have studied urine volume and GFR decline. Opposed to the prevailing view that water is beneficial in CKD,

Hebert et al. reported higher GFR decline in higher urine volume quartiles. However, multivariable adjustment seemed to diminish the association.[1,3] In support of Hebert et al., Wang et al. found a weak, but significant association between higher urine volume and GFR decline.[4] A large study by Clark et al. showed a relationship between higher urine volume and lower rate of eGFR decline, which stayed significant after multivariable adjustment. [5] Another large study reported worse kidney function in individuals with a lower self-reported fluid intake [6]; however, neither urine volume nor urine osmolarity were evaluated. It has been suggested that lower mean baseline GFR in cohorts of Hebert et al. and Wang et al., which is associated with alterations in water metabolism, might explain these paradoxical findings. With falling GFR, the ability to concentrate urine to osmolalities greater than that of plasma is progressively lost. [1] As such, in contrast to the general population, solute excretion and urine volume are closely interrelated in severe chronic kidney disease [20,21]. In our study we did not find a significant relationship between urine volume and a higher risk of dialysis. The rather weak association between urine volume and 24-hour urine osmolarity in the present study suggests that, in contrast to patients with severe kidney failure, urine concentration by vasopressin was still effective in the vast majority of the patients.

Stimulation of vasopressin secretion is supposed to be the cause of the more rapid decline of kidney function in patients with a high urine osmolarity. Vasopressin exerts a range of different effects and interacts through the three receptors V1a, V2 and V1b [22]. The antidiuretic effect is mainly mediated by the V2 receptor and includes increased tubular permeability for water and urea, and stimulation of ENaC-mediated sodium reabsorption [22]. Chronic administration of vasopressin in rats was shown to increase renal blood flow, glomerular filtration rate, and renal mass [23–25]. Vice versa, prevention of hyperfiltration in 5/6 nephrectomised rats by chronic inhibition of vasopressin secretion led to less glomerular sclerosis, less interstitial fibrosis and slower progression of renal failure [8,9,26]. However, precise plasma levels of vasopressin are difficult to obtain. Furthermore, non-detectable changes of vasopressin lead to a broad range of different urine osmolalities [22].

The optimal range of urine osmolality is difficult to define. Studies in normal rats and healthy humans have shown that urine concentration above an osmolarity of about 300 mosm/L induces a significant hyperfiltration [22,27]. In accordance with these findings we registered the lowest risk of initiation dialysis in patients with a urine osmolarity of a similar range. On the other hand we cannot rule out that urine osmolarity values below those in our cohort range might worsen the risk of renal function decline as suggested by the cohort of Hebert et al. (see above).

Either increasing fluid intake or decreasing the intake of osmolytes could achieve a reduction of urine osmolality. A recently published formula could be used to estimate the quantity of fluid needed to achieve a urine osmolality equivalent to that of plasma [13]. An alternative approach might be the use of vaptans, which suppress vasopressin activity by antagonistic binding to the VP receptors. Recently a protective effect of dual V1a/V2 blockade on the progression of CKD has been reported in rats [28]. A similar effect has been shown in diabetic rats, where the rise in albuminuria was prevented by a V2 antagonist [29].

Our study is limited by its design. As an observational cohort study can only prove associations and not causality, it remains to be proven in a prospective trial that changing urine osmolarity indeed has a positive effect on rate of renal function decline in CKD, before any therapeutic recommendation can be made. Furthermore, our study cohort showed a high event rate for ESRD, which might be explained by the cohort's relatively high baseline proteinuria. Thus, it is not clear if the study results are applicable to CKD populations with different demographics. Nonetheless, our study further strengthens the link between urine osmolarity and renal function decline by establishing a relationship with risk of dialysis initiation. In addition to the hard end-point of ESRD, a long follow-up period, the use of baseline variables issued from several measurements over a 1 year run-in phase reducing the impact of possible occasional sampling errors, and the application of competing risk analysis techniques strengthen the conclusions of this study.

While it is indisputable that, in the presence of a competing risk such as death, cumulative incidence curves are the method of choice rather than conventional Kaplan-Meier estimates, there is some controversy as to whether the standard cause-specific (death-censored) Cox regression analysis or the proportional sub-distribution hazards (Fine-Gray) model should be used to obtain adjusted hazard ratios. We decided to use the latter because it directly models differences in cumulative incidences and permits the investigator to predict the cumulative incidence of ESRD based on the covariate values of a patient. This would not have been possible when using the cause-specific Cox model. Our competing risk analysis using the Fine-Gray model mirrors more precisely the association between a covariate and the cumulative incidence of ESRD in patients at high risk of death during the observation period. Our observation that urine osmolarity might be positively associated with the risk for ESRD is robust as regards the type of analysis used, as results of the cause-specific Cox model were very similar.

In conclusion, we demonstrate that higher urine osmolarity is independently associated with a higher risk of initiating dialysis in a cohort of patients with CKD stage 1 to 4. Modifying urine osmolarity by dietary counselling or pharmaceutical interventions might evolve into a further treatment option in ESRD.

Author Contributions

Conceived and designed the experiments: MP MK LB GH MH. Performed the experiments: SS AH. Analyzed the data: MP MK LB GH MH. Contributed reagents/materials/analysis tools: MP MK GH MH. Wrote the paper: MP MK LB GH MH.

References

1. Wang CJ, Grantham JJ, Wetmore JB (2013) The medicinal use of water in renal disease. Kidney Int 84: 45–53.
2. Bankir L, Bouby N, Ritz E (2013) Vasopressin: a novel target for the prevention and retardation of kidney disease? Nat Rev Nephrol 9: 223–239.
3. Hebert LA, Greene T, Levey A, Falkenhain ME, Klahr S (2003) High urine volume and low urine osmolality are risk factors for faster progression of renal disease. Am J Kidney Dis 41: 962–971.
4. Wang X, Lewis J, Appel L, Cheek D, Contreras G, et al. (2006) Validation of creatinine-based estimates of GFR when evaluating risk factors in longitudinal studies of kidney disease. J Am Soc Nephrol 17: 2900–2909.
5. Clark WF, Sontrop JM, Macnab JJ, Suri RS, Moist L, et al. (2011) Urine volume and change in estimated GFR in a community-based cohort study. Clin J Am Soc Nephrol 6: 2634–2641.
6. Strippoli GF, Craig JC, Rochtchina E, Flood VM, Wang JJ, et al. (2011) Fluid and nutrient intake and risk of chronic kidney disease. Nephrology (Carlton) 16: 326–334.
7. Torres VE, Grantham JJ, Chapman AB, Mrug M, Bae KT, et al. (2011) Potentially modifiable factors affecting the progression of autosomal dominant polycystic kidney disease. Clin J Am Soc Nephrol 6: 640–647.
8. Bouby N, Bachmann S, Bichet D, Bankir L (1990) Effect of water intake on the progression of chronic renal failure in the 5/6 nephrectomized rat. Am J Physiol 258: F973–979.
9. Sugiura T, Yamauchi A, Kitamura H, Matsuoka Y, Horio M, et al. (1999) High water intake ameliorates tubulointerstitial injury in rats with subtotal nephrectomy: possible role of TGF-beta. Kidney Int 55: 1800–1810.
10. Meijer E, Bakker SJ, de Jong PE, Homan van der Heide JJ, van Son WJ, et al. (2009) Copeptin, a surrogate marker of vasopressin, is associated with accelerated renal function decline in renal transplant recipients. Transplantation 88: 561–567.
11. Meijer E, Bakker SJ, Halbesma N, de Jong PE, Struck J, et al. (2010) Copeptin, a surrogate marker of vasopressin, is associated with microalbuminuria in a large population cohort. Kidney Int 77: 29–36.
12. Nagao S, Nishii K, Katsuyama M, Kurahashi H, Marunouchi T, et al. (2006) Increased water intake decreases progression of polycystic kidney disease in the PCK rat. J Am Soc Nephrol 17: 2220–2227.
13. Wang CJ, Creed C, Winklhofer FT, Grantham JJ (2011) Water prescription in autosomal dominant polycystic kidney disease: a pilot study. Clin J Am Soc Nephrol 6: 192–197.
14. Gray RJ (1988) A class of K-sample tests for comparing the cumulative incidence of a competing risk. The annals of statistics: 1141–1154.
15. Fine JP, Gray RJ (1999) A proportional hazards model for the subdistribution of a competing risk. Journal of the American statistical association: 496–509.
16. Hosmer DW, Lemeshow S, May S (2008) Applied Survival Analysis: Regression Modeling of Time to Event Data. Chickester, UK: Wiley.
17. Royston P, Altman DG (1994) Regression using fractional polynomials of continuous covariates: parsimonious parametric modelling. Applied Statistics: 429–467.
18. Thomas MC, Moran J, Forsblom C, Harjutsalo V, Thorn L, et al. (2011) The association between dietary sodium intake, ESRD, and all-cause mortality in patients with type 1 diabetes. Diabetes Care 34: 861–866.
19. Perucca J, Bouby N, Valeix P, Bankir L (2007) Sex difference in urine concentration across differing ages, sodium intake, and level of kidney disease. Am J Physiol Regul Integr Comp Physiol 292: R700–705.
20. Feinfeld DA, Danovitch GM (1987) Factors affecting urine volume in chronic renal failure. Am J Kidney Dis 10: 231–235.
21. Luft FC, Fineberg NS, Sloan RS, Hunt JN (1983) The effect of dietary sodium and protein on urine volume and water intake. J Lab Clin Med 101: 605–610.
22. Bankir L (2001) Antidiuretic action of vasopressin: quantitative aspects and interaction between V1a and V2 receptor-mediated effects. Cardiovasc Res 51: 372–390.
23. Bouby N, Ahloulay M, Nsegbe E, Dechaux M, Schmitt F, et al. (1996) Vasopressin increases glomerular filtration rate in conscious rats through its antidiuretic action. J Am Soc Nephrol 7: 842–851.
24. Gellai M, Silverstein JH, Hwang JC, LaRochelle FT Jr., Valtin H (1984) Influence of vasopressin on renal hemodynamics in conscious Brattleboro rats. Am J Physiol 246: F819–827.
25. Bankir L, Bouby N, Trinh-Trang-Tan MM (1991) Vasopressin-dependent kidney hypertrophy: role of urinary concentration in protein-induced hypertrophy and in the progression of chronic renal failure. Am J Kidney Dis 17: 661–665.
26. Bouby N, Fernandes S (2003) Mild dehydration, vasopressin and the kidney: animal and human studies. Eur J Clin Nutr 57 Suppl 2: S39–46.
27. Anastasio P, Cirillo M, Spitali L, Frangiosa A, Pollastro RM, et al. (2001) Level of hydration and renal function in healthy humans. Kidney Int 60: 748–756.
28. Perico N, Zoja C, Corna D, Rottoli D, Gaspari F, et al. (2009) V1/V2 Vasopressin receptor antagonism potentiates the renoprotection of renin-angiotensin system inhibition in rats with renal mass reduction. Kidney Int 76: 960–967.
29. Bardoux P, Bruneval P, Heudes D, Bouby N, Bankir L (2003) Diabetes-induced albuminuria: role of antidiuretic hormone as revealed by chronic V2 receptor antagonism in rats. Nephrol Dial Transplant 18: 1755–1763.

11

Indoxyl Sulfate Downregulates Expression of Mas Receptor via OAT3/AhR/Stat3 Pathway in Proximal Tubular Cells

Hwee-Yeong Ng[1,2], Maimaiti Yisireyili[1], Shinichi Saito[1], Chien-Te Lee[2], Yelixiati Adelibieke[1], Fuyuhiko Nishijima[3], Toshimitsu Niwa[1]*

1 Department of Advanced Medicine for Uremia, Nagoya University Graduate School of Medicine, Nagoya, Japan, 2 Division of Nephrology, Department of Internal Medicine, Kaohsiung Chang Gung Memorial Hospital and Chang Gung University College of Medicine, Kaohsiung, Taiwan, 3 Biomedical Research Laboratories, Kureha Co., Tokyo, Japan

Abstract

Renin-angiotensin system (RAS) plays a pivotal role in chronic kidney disease (CKD). Angiotensin converting enzyme-related carboxypeptidase 2 (ACE2)/angiotensin (Ang)-(1–7)/Mas receptor axis counteracts the deleterious actions of Ang II. ACE2 exerts its actions by cleaving Ang II into Ang-(1–7) which activates Mas receptor. This study aimed to determine if the expression of Mas receptor is altered in the kidneys of CKD rats, and if indoxyl sulfate (IS), a uremic toxin, affects the expression of Mas receptor in rat kidneys and cultured human proximal tubular cells (HK-2 cells). The expression of Mas receptor was examined in the kidneys of CKD and AST-120-treated CKD rats using immunohistochemistry. Further, the effects of IS on Mas receptor expression in the kidneys of normotensive and hypertensive rats were examined. The effects of IS on the expression of Mas receptor and phosphorylation of endothelial nitric oxide synthase (eNOS) in HK-2 cells were examined using immunoblotting. CKD rats showed reduced renal expression of Mas receptor, while AST-120 restored its expression. Administration of IS downregulated Mas receptor expression in the kidneys of normotensive and hypertensive rats. IS downregulated Mas receptor expression in HK-2 cells in a time- and dose-dependent manner. Knockdown of organic anion transporter 3 (OAT3), aryl hydrocarbon receptor (AhR), and signal transducer and activator of transcription 3 (Stat3) inhibited IS-induced downregulation of Mas receptor and phosphorylated eNOS. N-acetylcysteine, an antioxidant, also inhibited IS-induced downregulation of Mas receptor and phosphorylated eNOS. Ang-(1–7) attenuated IS-induced transforming growth factor-β1 (TGF-β1) expression.

Conclusion: Mas receptor expression is reduced in the kidneys of CKD rats. IS downregulates renal expression of Mas receptor via OAT3/AhR/Stat3 pathway in proximal tubular cells. IS-induced downregulation of Mas receptor might be involved in upregulation of TGF-β1 in proximal tubular cells.

Editor: Shree Ram Singh, National Cancer Institute, United States of America

Funding: This work was supported by the research grant from Aichi Kidney Foundation, and a grant from Kureha Corporation, Japan. The funder provided support in the form of salaries for FN, but did not have additional role in the study design, data collection and analysis, decision to publish, or preparation of the manuscript. The specific role of these authors are articulated in the 'author contributions' section.

Competing Interests: FN is employed by Kureha. The other authors declare no competing interests.

* E-mail: tniwa@med.nagoya-u.ac.jp

Introduction

Renin-angiotensin system (RAS) plays a pivotal role in chronic kidney disease (CKD). RAS is regulated and modulated by two axes. The first axis primarily consists of angiotensin converting enzyme (ACE), angiotensin (Ang) II and Ang II type 1 receptor. This axis induces vasoconstriction, proliferation and oxidative stress [1]. The second axis, which consists of angiotensin converting enzyme-related carboxypeptidase 2 (ACE2), Ang-(1–7), and Mas receptor, counteracts the deleterious actions of Ang II as an endogenous regulator of RAS. ACE2 degrades Ang II into Ang-(1–7), which binds to Mas receptor [2], and then induces vasodilatation, and attenuates inflammation and fibrosis [3]. Mas receptor deficiency mice demonstrated a variety of complications including metabolic syndrome-like state, impaired heart function,

increased blood pressure, and endothelial dysfunction [4]. The ACE2/Ang-(1–7)/Mas axis is protective in renal disease [5,6], proven by the transgenic and knockout mouse models. However, the expression of ACE2 in diseased kidneys in previous studies is divergent [7]. In addition, there are controversial data on the renoprotective effect of Ang-(1–7), including stimulation of inflammation by Ang-(1–7) [8]. Little is known about Mas receptor expression in CKD. Indoxyl sulfate (IS), one of protein-bound uremic toxins, elicits a variety of cytotoxic effects, and exacerbates CKD [9,10]. The role of IS on the Mas receptor has not been elucidated. This study aimed to determine if the expression of Mas receptor is altered in the kidneys of CKD rats, and if IS affects the expression of Mas receptor in rat kidneys and cultured human proximal tubular cells.

(A)

(B)

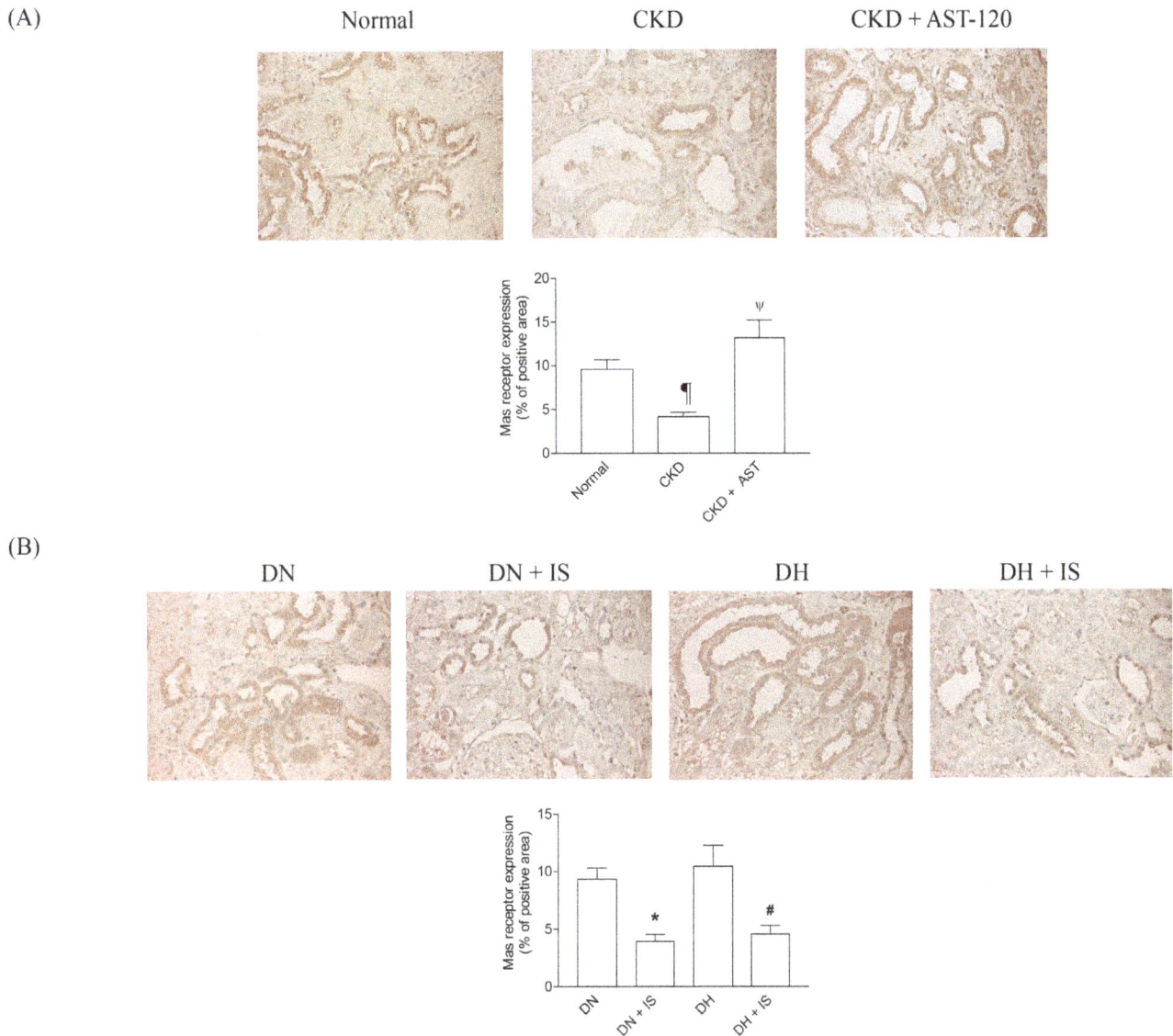

Figure 1. Immunohistochemical staining of Mas receptor in kidneys of CKD and Dahl rats. CKD rats showed significantly lower level of Mas receptor expression than normal. By administrating AST-120, Mas receptor expression was restored (A). The expression of Mas receptor was downregulated by IS in normotensive and hypertensive Dahl rats with normal renal function (B). The pictures were taken under ×400 magnification (n = 8 for each group). Data are expressed as mean±SE. ¶$p < 0.05$ *vs.* normal; ψ$p < 0.05$ *vs.* CKD; *$p < 0.05$ *vs.* DN; #$p < 0.05$ *vs.* DH.

Materials and Methods

Reagents

Antibodies were obtained from the following suppliers: anti-Mas receptor (AAR-013) (Alomone Laboratories, Ltd., Jerusalem, Israel); anti-endothelial nitric oxide synthase (eNOS) (BD Biosciences, Mississauga, ON, Canada); anti-aryl hydrocarbon receptor (AhR) (Santa Cruz Biotechnology, Santa Cruz, CA, USA); anti-α-tubulin (Calbiochem, La Jolla, CA, USA); anti-signal transducer and activator of transcription 3 (Stat3), anti-phosphorylated eNOS (Ser1177) (peNOS), anti-transforming growth factor-β1 (TGF-β1), anti-rabbit IgG horseradish peroxidase-linked antibody and anti-mouse IgG horseradish peroxidase-linked antibody (Cell Signaling Technology, Beverly, MA, USA). IS was obtained from Alfa Aesar (Morecambe, Lancs., UK). Ang-(1–7) was purchased from Bachem California (Torrance, CA, USA). N-acetylcysteine (NAC), an antioxidant, was from Calbiochem (La Jolla, CA,

USA). Dulbecco's modified Eagle's medium/F12 was purchased from Wako (Osaka, Japan). Trypsin-EDTA, fetal bovine serum, and insulin transferrin-selenium were purchased from Gibco (Grand Island, NY, USA). Penicillin and streptomycin were purchased from Nacalai Tesque Inc. (Kyoto, Japan).

Cell Culture

HK-2 cells derived from human proximal tubular cells were purchased from ATCC (Manassas, VA, USA). The cells were incubated at 37°C under 5% CO_2 humidified atmosphere, and were maintained in Dulbecco's modified Eagle's medium/F12 supplemented with 10% FBS, insulin-transferrin-selenium, 100 U/mL penicillin, and 100 μg/mL streptomycin.

HK-2 cells were starved in Dulbecco's modified Eagle's medium/F12 for 24 h before stimulation. In the time course-experiment, HK-2 cells were incubated with IS (250 μM) for 1, 3, 6, 12, 24, or 48 h. In the dose-experiment, the cells were incubated

Table 1. Biochemical data of the animals at the end of the study.

Animal study 1	Normal	CKD	CKD+AST-120	
	(n = 9)	(n = 8)	(n = 8)	
Serum creatinine (mg/dL)	0.40±0.01	1.41±0.23¶	1.17±0.06	
Creatinine clearance (mL/min)	3.68±0.13	1.14±0.16¶	1.20±0.09	
Serum indoxyl sulfate (mg/dL)	0.08±0.007	0.52±0.16¶	0.12±0.02ψ	
Animal study 2	**DN**	**DN+IS**	**DH**	**DH+IS**
	(n = 8)	(n = 8)	(n = 8)	(n = 8)
Systolic blood pressure (mmHg)	143±3	141±3	158±5	158±9
Serum creatinine (mg/dL)	0.56±0.01	0.58±0.01	0.55±0.01	0.58±0.01
Creatinine clearance (mL/min)	1.91±0.09	1.81±0.07	1.90±0.09	1.79±0.05
Serum indoxyl sulfate (mg/dL)	0.10±0.01	0.94±0.13*	0.06±0.01	1.89±0.26#

Data were cited from reference [11] for animal study 1 and [12] for animal study 2.
Data are expressed as mean±SE.
Abbreviation: CKD, chronic kidney disease; DN, Dahl normotensive rats; DH, Dahl hypertensive rats; IS, indoxyl sulfate.
¶$p < 0.05$ vs. normal, ψ$p < 0.05$ vs. CKD.
*$p < 0.05$ vs. DN, #$p < 0.05$ vs. DH.

with IS at a concentration of 0, 50, 100, 200, or 250 μM. In the experiments with NAC and Ang-(1–7), the cells were incubated with or without NAC (5 mM) or Ang-(1–7) ($10^{-8} \sim 10^{-6}$ M) for 30 min followed by indoxyl sulfate (250 μM) for 48 h (for Mas receptor) or 72 h (for TGF-β1).

Preparation of Small Interfering RNAs Specific to OAT3, AhR, and Stat3

Small interfering RNAs (siRNAs) specific to Stat3 were obtained from Nippon Gene Material (Tokyo, Japan). The sense sequences of the Stat3 siRNAs were 5-GGAGCAGCACCUUCAG-GAUdTdT-3. OAT3 and AhR siRNA were purchased from Santa Cruz Biotechnology (Santa Cruz, CA, USA). Lipofectamin RNAiMAX (Invitrogen, Life Technologies, Carlsbad, CA, USA) was used to transfect siRNAs into HK-2 cells according to the manufacturer's protocol. HK-2 cells were treated with or without OAT3 (10 nM), AhR siRNA (30 nM) or Stat3 siRNA (10 nM) for 24 h. Then, the cells were washed twice with PBS, and lysed in the lysis buffer.

Animal Experiments

The following animal studies were approved by Animal Care Committee of Biomedical Research Laboratories of Kureha, and were performed according to the Guiding Principles for the Care and Use of Laboratory Animals of the Japanese Pharmacological Society.

Animal study 1. Experimental rats were produced as reported previously [11]. Briefly, 7-week-old male Sprague-Dawley rats (Clea, Tokyo, Japan) were used to produce CKD by 5/6-nephrectomy. In the first session, while the renal artery and vein of the left kidney were ligated, two-thirds of the left kidney was removed with a razor, and thrombin was applied onto the cut surface for hemostasis. Then, the artery and vein of the left kidney were unligated. One week after the first operation, the right kidney was removed after ligation of the renal artery and vein. These operations were performed under anesthesia with sodium pento-barbital (Schering-Plough, Corp., NJ, USA). Eleven weeks after 5/6-nephrectomy, the rats were randomized into two groups CKD

(n = 8), and AST-120-treated CKD rats (n = 8). AST-120 was administered to the rats at a dose of 4 g/kg with powder chow (CE-2, Clea) for 16 weeks, whereas powder chow alone was administered to control and CKD rats. Normal rats (n = 9) were used as a control group.

Animal study 2. To test the direct effect of IS on Mas receptor, animals with normal renal function were fed with or without IS (200 mg/kg of IS in drinking water). Experimental rats were produced as reported previously [12]. Briefly, 5-week-old male Dahl salt-sensitive rats (Dahl-Iwai S, n = 32) were purchased from Japan SLC (Hamamatsu, Shizuoka, Japan), and were fed with powder rat chow (CE-2; Clea, Tokyo, Japan) and water. At 16th week of age, the rats were divided into four groups: 1) Dahl normotensive rats (DN), and 2) Dahl normotensive indoxyl sulfate-administered rats (DN+IS; 200 mg/kg/day of indoxyl sulfate in drinking water), 3) Dahl hypertensive rats (DH), and 4) Dahl hypertensive indoxyl sulfate-administered rats (DH+IS). After 32 weeks, blood pressure was measured using the tails of the rats with a pneumatic cuff and a sphygmomanometer for small animals (UR-5000, Ueda Avancer Co., Tokyo, Japan), then the rats were anesthetized, and renal cortices were isolated.

Immunohistochemistry

Immunohistochemistry was performed using the streptavidin-biotin complex method. Paraffin-embedded fixed tissue sections (4 μm) were deparaffinized with xylene, and rehydrated with ethanol. Antigen retrieval was carried out with 10 mM citrate buffer (pH 6.0) twice for 5 min microwave treatment. The sections were incubated with 3% H_2O_2 methanol for 10 min, and then incubated with 10% serum (Nichirei Co., Tokyo, Japan) for 30 min at room temperature. After that, anti-Mas receptor antibody (1:100) was added, and incubated at 4°C overnight. The next day, the sections were incubated with the secondary antibody at room temperature for 30 min, and then with peroxidase-conjugated streptavidin (Nichirei Co.) at 37°C for 30 min. The localization of Mas receptor was visualized using 3,3'-diaminobenzidine tetrahydrochloride (Merck KGaA, Darm-stadt, Germany) at a concentration of 30 mg/mL, containing

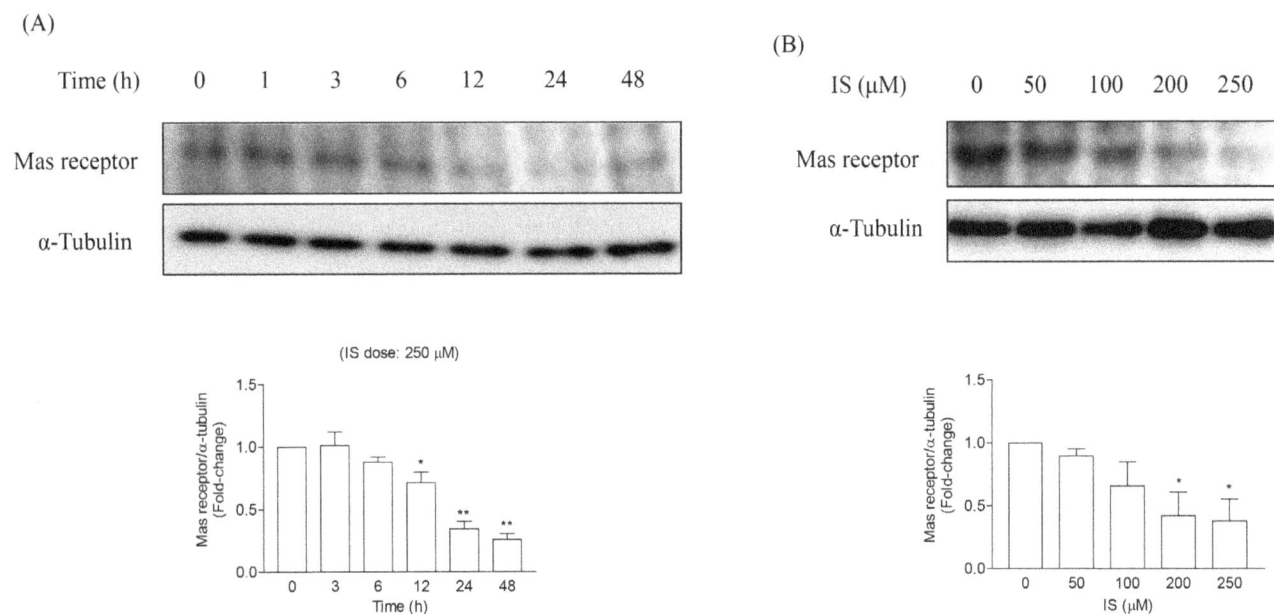

Figure 2. Time- and dose-dependent effects of IS on Mas receptor protein expression in HK-2 cells. Mas receptor in the HK-2 was reduced by IS in a time- (A) and dose- (B) dependent manner. Bars represent means±SE, expressed as relative change in comparison with the basal value (n≥3 for every experiment).*p<0.05 vs. basal value; **p<0.001 vs. basal value.

0.03% H_2O_2. The sections were photographed (DN100, E600; Nikon, Tokyo, Japan). The immunostaining-positive areas were then quantified in 20 random renal cortex sections using NIH Image 1.62.

Immunoblotting

Immunoblotting was performed as described previously [13,14]. In brief, cell lysates were fractionated by sodium dodecyl sulfate-polyacylamide gel electrophoresis (SDS-PAGE) on polyacrylamide gels (8~12%), and proteins were transferred to polyvinylidene fluoride membranes (Immobilon-P, Millipore, Bedford, MA, USA). Mas receptor, peNOS, AhR, OAT3, Stat3, and TGF-β1 were detected using their specific antibodies. To normalize the blots for protein levels, after being immunoblotted with the specific antibodies, the blots were stripped and reprobed with either anti-α-tubulin or anti-eNOS antibodies (for peNOS). The protein bands were visualized using the enhanced Chemi-Lumi One system (Nacalai Tesque).

Statistical Analysis

Data analysis was performed with SPSS Statistics version 17 (IBM, Armonk, NY, USA). Results are expressed as mean±SE. Student t-test was used to analyze the difference of mean values between two groups. Comparison among different groups was performed by using one-way analysis of variance (ANOVA), and then examined by least significance difference (LSD) test. A p value <0.05 is considered to be statistically significant.

Results

Mas Receptor Expression is Reduced in Kidneys of CKD Rats

We first examined whether the expression of Mas receptor is altered in the kidneys of CKD rats, and whether AST-120, an oral sorbent, affects its expression. AST-120 reduces the serum level of

indoxyl sulfate by adsorbing its precursor, indole, in the intestine [10,15,16]. Laboratory parameters of these rats, which have been reported previously [11], are cited in Table 1. Immunohistochemisty revealed that Mas receptor was mainly localized in renal proximal tubular cells (Fig. 1). CKD rats showed significantly decreased Mas receptor-positive area in the kidney as compared with normal (Fig. 1A). However, AST-120 treatment significantly alleviated the decrease of Mas receptor-positive area in the kidney (Fig. 1A). Thus, the expression of Mas receptor was decreased in the kidneys of CKD rats, and AST-120 restored its expression.

Administration of Indoxyl Sulfate Reduces Mas Receptor Expression in Rat Kidneys

We next determined whether administration of indoxyl sulfate reduces the expression of Mas receptor in rat kidneys. Laboratory parameters as reported previously [12] are cited in Table 1. Both DN+IS and DH+IS rats showed significantly decreased Mas receptor-positive areas as compared with DN and DH rats, respectively (Fig. 1B). However, there was no significant difference in Mas receptor-positive area between DN and DH groups (Fig. 1B). Thus, administration of indoxyl sulfate reduced Mas receptor expression in the kidneys of normotensive and hypertensive rats.

Indoxyl Sulfate Downregulates Mas Receptor Expression in Proximal Tubular Cells

We examined the effects of IS on Mas receptor expression in HK-2 cells at different time durations and doses. IS reduced the expression of Mas receptor in a time- and dose-dependent manner (Fig. 2). IS at a concentration of 250 µM, which is comparable to its average serum level observed in uremic patients [10], decreased Mas receptor expression.

(A)

OAT3

α-Tubulin

siOAT3   -   +

(B)

Mas receptor

α-Tubulin

IS (250 μM)   -   +   -   +
siOAT3 (10 nM)   -   -   +   +

(C)

peNOS

eNOS

IS (250 μM)   -   +   -   +
siOAT- (10 nM)   -   -   +   +

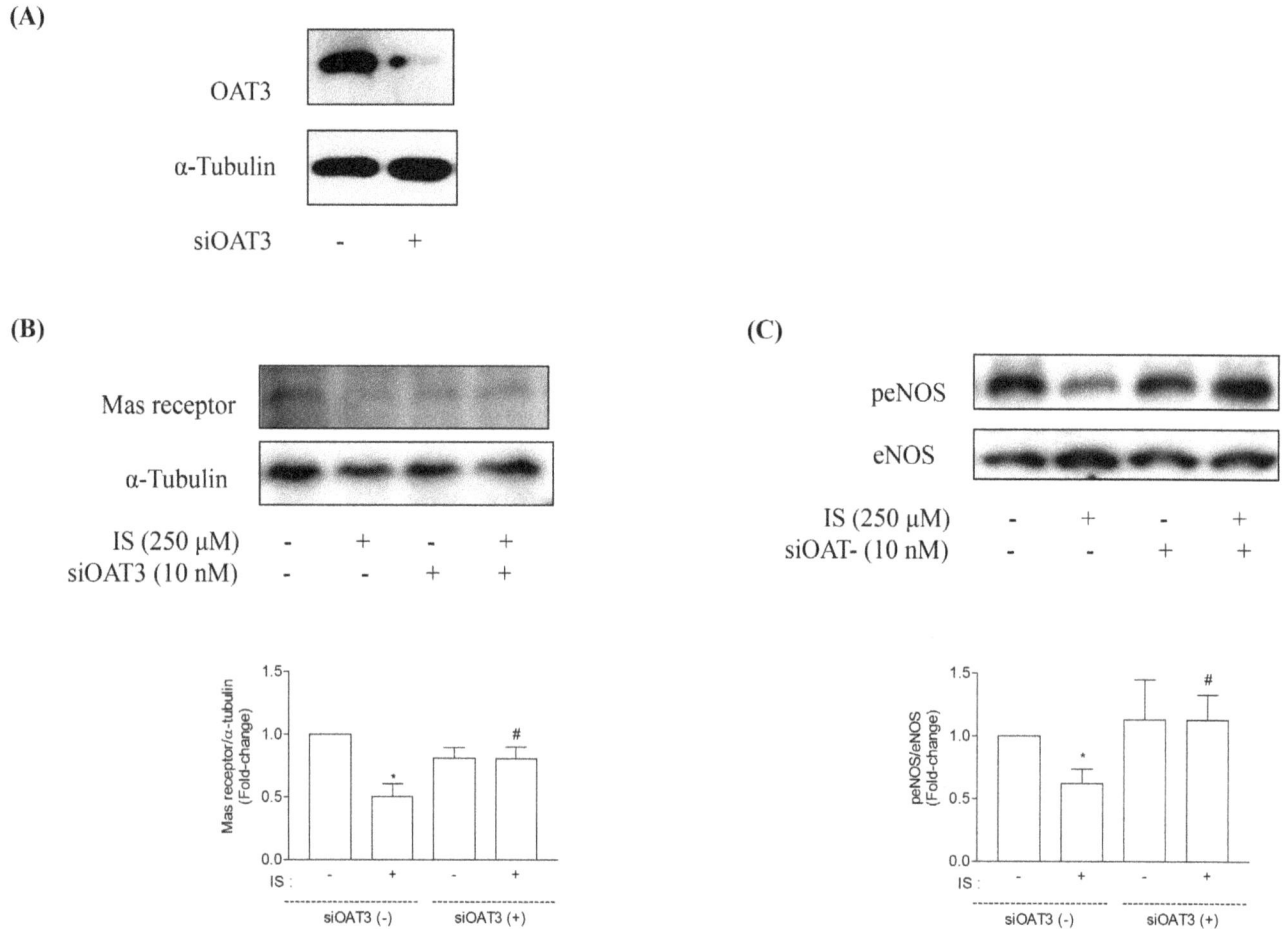

Figure 3. Effects of OAT3 siRNA on Mas receptor and peNOS expression in HK-2 cells. HK-2 cells were treated with or without OAT3 siRNA (siOAT3, 10 nM) (A). Mas receptor (B) and peNOS (C) protein expression was abolished by knocking down OAT3. Data are means±SE, expressed as relative change in comparison with the basal value (n≥3 for every experiment). *p<0.05 *vs.* control; #p<0.05 *vs.* IS.

Accumulation of IS via OAT3 in Proximal Tubular Cells Downregulates Mas Receptor Expression

We investigated the mechanism how IS induced downregulation of Mas receptor. OAT3 is the major transporter for transcellular transport of IS into proximal tubular cells [17]. To confirm the effect of IS on Mas receptor, we also investigated the alteration of peNOS, because Mas receptor activates Akt/eNOS pathway [18] by phosphorylation of eNOS. Under physiological conditions, renal nitric oxide (NO) is derived mainly from constitutive NOS, including eNOS and neuronal NOS [19]. HK-2 cells were treated with or without 10 nM OAT3 siRNA for 24 h (Fig. 3A). IS reduced the expression of Mas receptor and peNOS (Fig. 3B, C). Knockdown of OAT3 blocked the inhibitory effects of IS on Mas receptor and peNOS (Fig. 3B, C).

AhR and Stat3 are Involved in IS-induced Downregulation of Mas Receptor in Proximal Tubular Cells

AhR has been demonstrated to form a complex with IS in cytoplasm [20]. HK-2 cells were treated with or without 30 nM AhR siRNA for 24 h (Fig. 4A). Knockdown of AhR blocked the inhibitory effects of IS on Mas receptor and peNOS (Fig. 4B, C).

Furthermore, AhR interacts with the other transcription factors such as Stat3 [21] in the cytoplasm after binding with its ligand. Previously, we have demonstrated that Stat3 is involved in IS-induced fibrogenesis and inflammation [22]. We then investigated the role of Stat3 in the downregulation of Mas receptor. HK-2 cells were treated with or without 10 nM Stat3 siRNA (Fig. 5A). Knockdown of Stat3 blocked the inhibitory effects of IS on Mas receptor and peNOS (Fig. 5B, C).

Reactive Oxygen Species are Involved in IS-induced Downregulation of Mas Receptor in Proximal Tubular Cells

To study the influence of reactive oxygen species on IS-induced downregulation of Mas receptor, NAC, an antioxidant, was used. NAC blocked the inhibitory effects of IS on Mas receptor and peNOS (Fig. 6A, B). Thus, reactive oxygen species are also involved in IS-induced downregulation of Mas receptor.

Activation of Mas Receptor by Ang-(1–7) Inhibits IS-induced Production of TGF-β1 in Proximal Tubular Cells

It is unclear whether activation of Mas receptor could provide beneficial effects on lowering renal toxicity of IS. We examined the

(A)

(B)

(C)

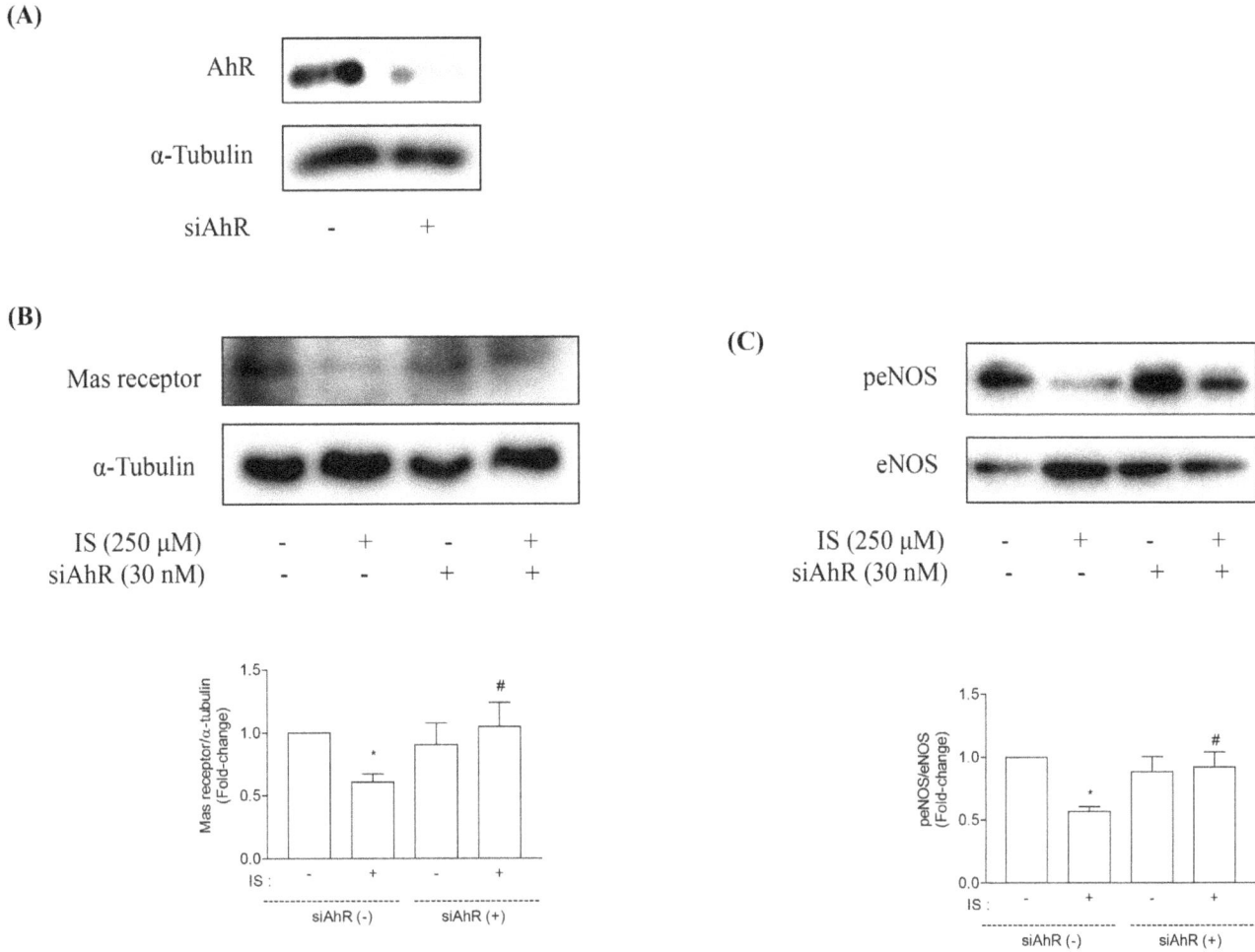

Figure 4. Effects of AhR siRNA on Mas receptor and peNOS expression in HK-2 cells. HK-2 cells were treated with or without AhR siRNA (siAhR, 30 nM) (A). Knockdown of AhR inhibited IS-induced downregulation of Mas receptor (B) and peNOS (C) expression. Data are means±SE, expressed as relative change in comparison with the basal value (n≥3 for every experiment). *$p<0.05$ vs. control; #$p<0.05$ vs. IS.

effects of Ang-(1–7) on TGF-β1 expression in HK-2 cells treated with IS for 72 h. IS significantly upregulated expression of TGF-β1 (Fig. 7). Pretreatment of Ang-(1–7) at a concentration of 10^{-8} and 10^{-7} M significantly inhibited IS-induced upregulation of TGF-β1 (Fig. 7). Thus, activation of Mas receptor by Ang-(1–7) inhibits IS-induced upregulation of TGF-β1.

Discussion

The main pathophysiological mechanism associated with CKD results from the activation of RAS. IS upregulates most of the ACE/Ang II/Ang II type 1 receptor axis components, including renin, angiotensinogen and Ang II type 1 receptor, but downregulates Ang II type 2 receptor [23,24]. Our study provides new evidence that IS has a negative effect on ACE2/Ang-(1–7)/Mas receptor axis. IS accumulates in renal tubular cells via OAT3-mediated uptake (Fig. 8), and serves as a ligand of AhR in the cytoplasm [20]. The complex of IS-AhR might interact with Stat3, and translocate into the nucleus to recognize and regulate Mas

receptor gene other than classical dioxin response elements motifs [25]. However, AhR itself is also a transcription factor, and influences the immune response [26]. It is also possible that AhR alters Mas receptor expression directly without interacting with Stat3. In the present study, we could not discriminate the two pathways. Apart from IS and reactive oxygen species, the increased Ang II in CKD might also act as a negative regulator of ACE2/Ang-(1–7)/Mas receptor axis [27]. Taken together, the effects of IS on RAS and CKD progression are extensive and deleterious.

To confirm the alteration of Mas receptor and its signaling, peNOS was selected to represent the activation of Mas receptor. Our results clearly demonstrated that the change of activated eNOS was completely in parallel with that of Mas receptor. The importance of eNOS in tubular epithelium is rarely discussed. NO produced by eNOS is a paracrine factor to regulate NaCl absorption in the proximal tubules [28], suggesting its involvement in the glomerulotubular feedback and glomerular filtration rate

(A)

Stat3

α-Tubulin

siStat3   -   +

(B)

Mas receptor

α-Tubulin

| IS (250 µM) | - | + | - | + |
| siStat3 (10 nM) | - | - | + | + |

(C)

peNOS

eNOS

| IS (250 µM) | - | + | - | + |
| siStat3 (10 nM) | - | - | + | + |

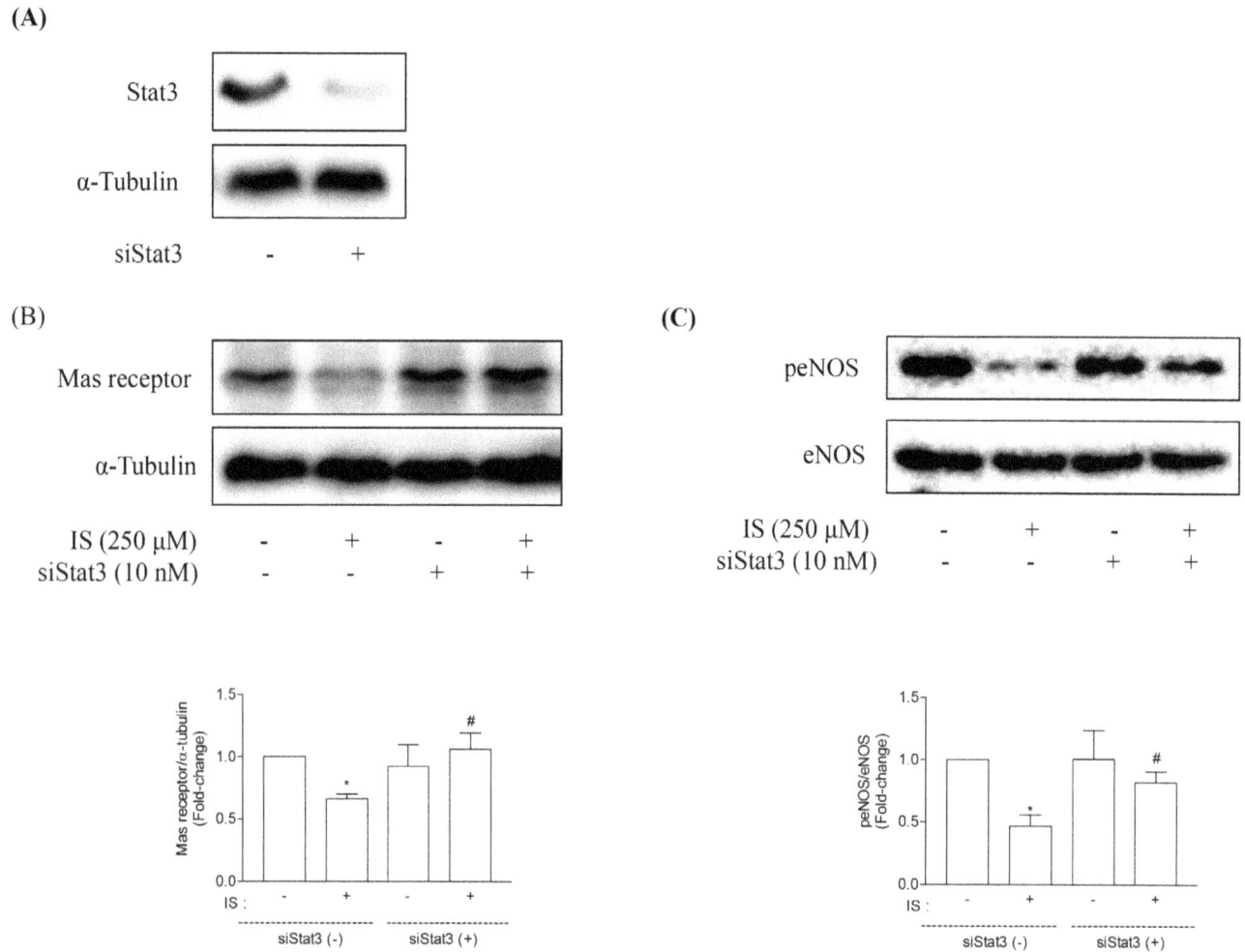

Figure 5. Effects of Stat3 siRNA on Mas receptor and peNOS expression in HK-2 cells. HK-2 cells were treated with or without Stat3 siRNA (siStat3, 10 nM) (A). Knockdown of Stat3 inhibited IS-induced downregulation of Mas receptor (B) and peNOS (C) expression. Data are means±SE, expressed as relative change in comparison with the basal value (n≥3 for every experiment). *p<0.05 *vs.* control; #p<0.05 *vs.* IS.

[29]. Reduction of activated eNOS in renal tubules might alter renal microcirculatory dynamic, which then exacerbates renal microenvironmental ischemia [30]. In human study, elevated eNOS expression in the renal vessels and tubules is associated with recovery from ischemia [31]. Furthermore, eNOS inhibits cellular senescence [32], and reduces oxidative stress. Downregulation of Mas receptor/peNOS by IS might be responsible for the renal toxicity of IS, such as oxidative stress, cellular senescence, and abnormal oxygen consumption [14,33].

In the present study, Ang-(1–7) inhibited IS-induced production of TGF-β1. This finding highlightens the importance of Ang-(1–7)/Mas receptor in the IS-induced renal injury. Administration of Ang-(1–7) has been reported to be beneficial in adriamycin-related kidney failure, 5/6-nephrectomized mice, and experimental diabetes [34]. Ang-(1–7)/Mas receptor axis contributes to their renoprotective effects, at least in part, by counteracting Ang II [35]. Like most of the ACE inhibitors and Ang II type 1 receptor

blockers, Ang-(1–7) might provide protective effects independent of blood pressure lowering [36]. The possible mechanism includes modulation of oxidative stress, inflammation, and fibrosis [34]. Ang-(1–7) is also effective in inhibiting IS-related renal toxicity. However, Ang-(1–7) has been shown to exacerbate renal disease with increased ACE activity [8,37]. This might be due to divergent roles of Ang-(1–7)/Mas receptor in renal cell types such as mesangial cells vs. tubular cells. In addition, treatment dose may be another factor affecting the outcome. Because Ang-(1–7) is metabolized by ACE, overdose of Ang-(1–7) activates ACE [37] and subsequently Ang II pathway. The present study also showed that higher doses of Ang-(1–7) did not provide a better effect in inhibiting TGF-β1 production. The abundance of Mas receptor in the kidney might determine the effect of Ang-(1–7). Thus, reduction of Mas receptor is speculated to accelerate nephron loss in CKD. Novel drugs which stimulate expression and

(A)

(B)

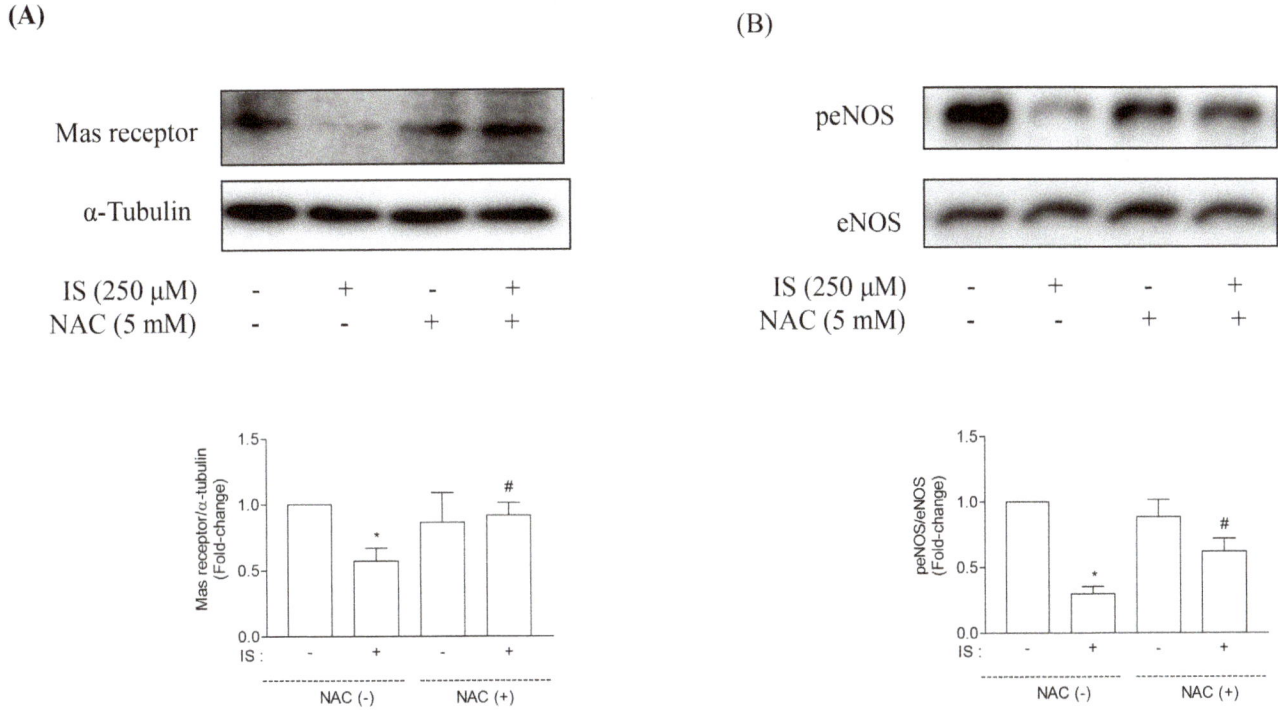

Figure 6. Effects of NAC on Mas receptor and peNOS expression in HK-2 cells. NAC (5 mM) inhibited IS-induced downregulation of Mas receptor (A) and peNOS (B) expression. Data are means±SE, expressed as relative change in comparison with the basal value (n≥3 for every experiment). *$p < 0.05$ vs. control; #$p < 0.05$ vs. IS.

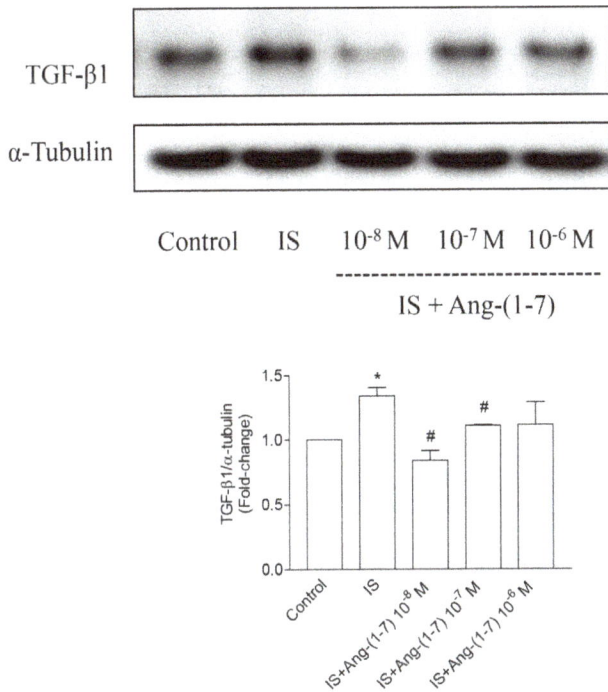

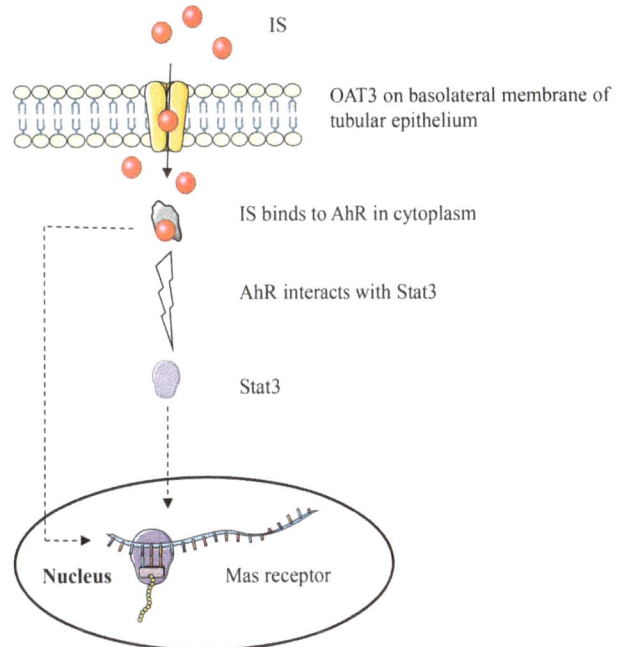

Figure 7. Effect of Ang-(1–7) on TGF-β1 expression in IS-treated HK2 cells. IS enhanced the expression of TGF-β1, whereas Ang-(1–7) inhibited it. Data are means±SE, expressed as relative change in comparison with the basal value (n≥3 for every experiment). *$p < 0.05$ vs. control; #$p < 0.05$ vs. IS.

Figure 8. Schema of mechanism of IS-induced Mas receptor downregulation. IS accumulates in HK-2 cells via OAT3. In the cells, IS acts as a ligand of AhR. The IS-AhR complex then interacts with Stat3. In turn, Mas receptor is downregulated by IS-AhR-Stat3 or IS-AhR complex. This figure was created using Servier Medical Art (www.servier.com).

activation of Mas receptor should be developed for the treatment of CKD patients.

In conclusion, Mas receptor expression is reduced in the kidney of CKD rats. IS downregulates renal expression of Mas receptor via OAT3/AhR/Stat3 pathway in proximal tubular cells. IS-induced downregulation of Mas receptor might be involved in upregulation of TGF-β1 in proximal tubular cells.

References

1. Ruster C, Wolf G. (2006) Renin-angiotensin-aldosterone system and progression of renal disease. J Am Soc Nephrol 17: 2985–2991.
2. Fressatto de Godoy MA, Pernomian L, de Oliveira AM, Rattan S. (2012) Biosynthetic pathways and the role of the MAS receptor in the effects of Angiotensin-(1–7) in smooth muscles. Int J Hypertens 2012: 121740.
3. Pinheiro SV, Simoes E Silva AC. (2012) Angiotensin converting enzyme 2, Angiotensin-(1–7), and receptor MAS axis in the kidney. Int J Hypertens 2012: 414128.
4. Santos RA, Ferreira AJ, Verano-Braga T, Bader M. (2013) Angiotensin-converting enzyme 2, angiotensin-(1–7) and Mas: new players of the renin-angiotensin system. J Endocrinol 216: R1–R17.
5. Nadarajah R, Milagres R, Dilauro M, Gutsol A, Xiao F, et al. (2012) Podocyte-specific overexpression of human angiotensin-converting enzyme 2 attenuates diabetic nephropathy in mice. Kidney Int 82: 292–303.
6. Pinheiro SV, Ferreira AJ, Kitten GT, da Silveira KD, da Silva DA, et al. (2009) Genetic deletion of the angiotensin-(1–7) receptor Mas leads to glomerular hyperfiltration and microalbuminuria. Kidney Int 75: 1184–1193.
7. Soler MJ, Wysocki J, Battle D. (2013) ACE2 alterations in kidney disease. Nephrol Dial Transplant 28: 2687–2697.
8. Esteban V, Heringer-Walther S, Sterner-Kock A, de Bruin R, van den Engel S, et al. (2009) Angiotensin-(1–7) and the g protein-coupled receptor MAS are key players in renal inflammation. PLoS One 4: e5406.
9. Niwa T. (2010) Indoxyl sulfate is a nephro-vascular toxin. J Ren Nutr 20(5 Suppl): S2–6.
10. Niwa T, Ise M. (1994) Indoxyl sulfate, a circulating uremic toxin, stimulates the progression of glomerular sclerosis. J Lab Clin Med 124: 96–104.
11. Bolati D, Shimizu H, Niwa T. (2012) AST-120 ameliorates epithelial-to-mesenchymal transition and interstitial fibrosis in the kidneys of chronic kidney disease rats. J Ren Nutr 22: 176–180.
12. Adijiang A, Shimizu H, Higuchi Y, Nishijima F, Niwa T. (2011) Indoxyl sulfate reduces klotho expression and promotes senescence in the kidneys of hypertensive rats. J Ren Nutr 21: 105–109.
13. Ng HY, Chen HC, Tsai YC, Yang YK, Lee CT. (2011) Activation of intrarenal renin-angiotensin system during metabolic acidosis. Am J Nephrol 34: 55–63.
14. Shimizu H, Bolati D, Adijiang A, Enomoto A, Nishijima F, et al. (2010) Senescence and dysfunction of proximal tubular cells are associated with activated p53 expression by indoxyl sulfate. Am J Physiol Cell Physiol 299: C1110–C1117.
15. Niwa T, Nomura T, Sugiyama S, Miyazaki T, Tsukushi S, et al. (1997) The protein metabolite hypothesis, a model for the progression of renal failure: An oral adsorbent lowers indoxyl sulfate levels in undialyzed uremic patients. Kidney Int Suppl 62: S23–28.
16. Miyazaki T, Aoyama I, Ise M, Seo H, Niwa T. (2000) An oral sorbent reduces overload of indoxyl sulfate and gene expression of TGF-β1 in uremic rat kidneys. Nephrol Dial Transplant 15: 1773–1781.
17. Enomoto A, Takeda M, Tojo A, Sekine T, Cha SH, et al. (2002) Role of organic anion transporters in the tubular transport of indoxyl sulfate and the induction of its nephrotoxicity. J Am Soc Nephrol 13: 1711–1720.
18. Tassone EJ, Sciacqua A, Andreozzi F, Presta I, Perticone M, et al. (2013) Angiotensin-(1–7) counteracts the negative effect of angiotensin II on insulin signalling in HUVECs. Cardiovasc Res 99: 129–136.
19. Raij L, Baylis C. (1995) Glomerular actions of nitric oxide. Kidney Int 48: 20–32.
20. Gondouin B, Cerini C, Dou L, Sallée M, Duval-Sabatier A, et al. (2013) Indolic uremic solutes increase tissue factor production in endothelial cells by the aryl hydrocarbon receptor pathway. Kidney Int 84: 733–744.
21. Hankinson O. (2005) Role of coactivators in transcriptional activation by the aryl hydrocarbon receptor. Arch Biochem Biophys 433: 379–386.
22. Shimizu H, Yisireyili M, Nishijima F, Niwa T. (2012) Stat3 contributes to indoxyl sulfate-induced inflammatory and fibrotic gene expression and cellular senescence. Am J Nephrol 36: 184–189.
23. Sun CY, Chang SC, Wu MS. (2012) Uremic toxins induce kidney fibrosis by activating intrarenal renin-angiotensin-aldosterone system associated epithelial-to-mesenchymal transition. PLoS One 7: e34026.
24. Shimizu H, Saito S, Higashiyama Y, Nishijima F, Niwa T. (2013) CREB, NF-κB, and NADPH oxidase coordinately upregulate indoxyl sulfate-induced angiotensinogen expression in proximal tubular cells. Am J Physiol Cell Physiol 304: C685–692.
25. Patel RD, Murray IA, Flaveny CA, Kusnadi A, Perdew GH. (2009) Ah receptor represses acute-phase response gene expression without binding to its cognate response element. Lab Invest 89: 695–707.
26. Quintana FJ. (2013) The aryl hydrocarbon receptor: a molecular pathway for the environmental control of the immune response. Immunology 138: 183–189.
27. Koka V, Huang XR, Chung AC, Wang W, Truong LD, et al. (2008) Angiotensin II up-regulates angiotensin I-converting enzyme (ACE), but down-regulates ACE2 via the AT1-ERK/p38 MAP kinase pathway. Am J Pathol 172: 1174–1183.
28. Plato CF, Shesely EG, Garvin JL. (2000) eNOS mediates L-arginine-induced inhibition of thick ascending limb chloride flux. Hypertension 35: 319–323.
29. Wang H, Carretero OA, Garvin JL. (2002) Nitric oxide produced by THAL nitric oxide synthase inhibits TGF. Hypertension 39: 662–666.
30. Manucha W, Oliveros L, Carrizo L, Seltzer A, Vallés P. (2004) Losartan modulation on NOS isoforms and COX-2 expression in early renal fibrogenesis in unilateral obstruction. Kidney Int 65: 2091–2107.
31. Ishimura T, Fujisawa M, Isotani S, Iijima K, Yoshikawa N, et al. (2002) Endothelial nitric oxide synthase expression in ischemia-reperfusion injury after living related-donor renal transplantation. Transpl Int 15: 635–640.
32. Hayashi T, Matsui-Hirai H, Miyazaki-Akita A, Fukatsu A, Funami J, et al. (2006) Endothelial cellular senescence is inhibited by nitric oxide: implications in atherosclerosis associated with menopause and diabetes. Proc Natl Acad Sci USA 103: 17018–17023.
33. Palm F, Nangaku M, Fasching A, Tanaka T, Nordquist L, et al. (2010) Uremia induces abnormal oxygen consumption in tubules and aggravates chronic hypoxia of the kidney via oxidative stress. Am J Physiol Renal Physiol 299: F380–F386.
34. Simões e Silva AC, Silveira KD, Ferreira AJ, Teixeira MM. (2013) ACE2, angiotensin-(1–7) and Mas receptor axis in inflammation and fibrosis. Br J Pharmacol 169: 477–492.
35. Katovich MJ, Grobe JL, Raizada MK. (2008) Angiotensin-(1–7) as an antihypertensive, antifibrotic target. Curr Hypertens Rep 10: 227–232.
36. Li Y, Wu J, He Q, Shou Z, Zhang P, et al. (2009) Angiotensin (1–7) prevent heart dysfunction and left ventricular remodeling caused by renal dysfunction in 5/6 nephrectomy mice. Hypertens Res 32: 369–374.
37. Velkoska E, Dean RG, Griggs K, Burchill L, Burrell LM. (2011) Angiotensin-(1–7) infusion is associated with increased blood pressure and adverse cardiac remodelling in rats with subtotal nephrectomy. Clin Sci 120: 335–345.

Author Contributions

Conceived and designed the experiments: HN TN. Performed the experiments: HN MY SS YA FN. Analyzed the data: HN TN. Contributed reagents/materials/analysis tools: CL TN. Wrote the paper: HN TN.

12

Structural and Functional Brain Alterations in End Stage Renal Disease Patients on Routine Hemodialysis: A Voxel-Based Morphometry and Resting State Functional Connectivity Study

Yingwei Qiu[1,2][*][9], Xiaofei Lv[3][9], Huanhuan Su[1][9], Guihua Jiang[1], Cheng Li[4], Junzhang Tian[1]

1 Department of Medical Imaging, Guangdong No. 2 Provincial People's Hospital, Guangzhou, PR China, 2 Department of Medical Imaging, The First Affiliated Hospital of Gannan Medical University, Ganzhou, PR China, 3 Departments of Medical Imaging and Interventional Radiology, Cancer Center, Sun Yat-Sen University, Guangzhou, PR China, 4 Department of Renal Transplantation, Guangdong No. 2 Provincial People's Hospital, Guangzhou, PR China

Abstract

Background and Purpose: Cognitive impairment is a well-described phenomenon in end-stage renal disease (ESRD) patients. However, its pathogenesis remains poorly understood. The primary focus of this study was to examine structural and functional brain deficits in ESRD patients.

Materials and Methods: Thirty ESRD patients on hemodialysis (without clinical neurological disease) and 30 age- and gender-matched control individuals (without renal or neurological problems) were recruited in a prospective, single-center study. High-resolution structural magnetic resonance imaging (MRI) and resting state functional MRI were performed on both groups to detect the subtle cerebral deficits in ESRD patients. Voxel-based morphometry was used to characterize gray matter deficits in ESRD patients. The impact of abnormal morphometry on the cerebral functional integrity was investigated by evaluating the alterations in resting state functional connectivity when brain regions with gray matter volume reduction were used as seed areas.

Results: A significant decrease in gray matter volume was observed in ESRD patients in the bilateral medial orbito-prefrontal cortices, bilateral dorsal lateral prefrontal cortices, and the left middle temporal cortex. When brain regions with gray matter volume reduction were used as seed areas, the integration was found to be significantly decreased in ESRD patients in the fronto-cerebellum circuits and within prefrontal circuits. In addition, significantly enhanced functional connectivity was found between the prefrontal cortex and the left temporal cortex and within the prefrontal circuits.

Conclusions: Our study revealed that both the structural and functional cerebral cortices were impaired in ESRD patients on routine hemodialysis.

Editor: Satoru Hayasaka, Wake Forest School of Medicine, United States of America

Funding: This work was supported by the grants from the Natural Scientific Foundation of China [Grant No. 81201084 for YQ], and the Planned Science and Technology Project of Guangdong Province, China [Grant No. 2011B031800044 for GJ]. The funders had no role in study design, data collection and analysis, decision to publish, or preparation of the manuscript.

Competing Interests: The authors have declared that no competing interests exist.

* E-mail: qiuyw1201@gmail.com

[9] These authors contributed equally to this work.

Introduction

End stage renal disease (ESRD) is the last stage (stage 5) of chronic kidney disease (CKD), and corresponds to complete or almost complete loss of kidney function. Cognitive impairment is highly prevalent in ESRD patients [1,2]. Deficits involve a range of cognitive domains, including concentration, memory and planning, which may be associated with increased staff time in caring for the patients, greater utilization of healthcare resources, more frequent hospitalizations and an increased number of days spent in the hospital [3,4]. Recognizing the cerebral deficits of ESRD could help us understand the underlying neuronal mechanisms and lead to earlier interventions that might reduce morbidity.

Imaging plays an important role in detecting structural and functional abnormalities of the brain in ESRD patients. Conventional MR and computed tomography (CT) imaging studies with visual assessment and manual measurements of structures of interest have demonstrated that patients with ESRD have reduced brain volumes, reduced deep white matter volumes, a high prevalence of subcortical white matter lesions, and a high incidence rate for stroke [5–8]. MR spectroscopy (MRS) studies have demonstrated that CKD patients (stage 4–5) without clinical signs of uremic encephalopathy showed metabolic disturbances in multiple brain regions, including the parieto-occipital white matter, the occipital grey matter, the basal ganglia and the pons [8–10]. Positron emission tomography (PET) studies have displayed that hemispheric oxygen [11] and glucose metabolism [12], especially for bilateral pre-frontal cortices (PFC), are depressed in patients with ESRD. However, due to the methodological limitations, insensitivity to the early and small lesions (conventional MRI and CT with visual assessment and manual measurements of structures of interest) [13], need for a predetermined region of interest, time-consuming manual measurements or subjective visual assessments (conventional MRI and CT with visual assessment and manual measurements of structures of interest and single-voxel MRS) [13,14], and radiation exposure and low spatial resolution (PET) [15], their applications are restricted in a large cohort.

Resting state functional MRI (rs-fMRI) has the ability to record spontaneous brain activity fluctuations when subjects lie still in the scanner. Low-frequency (0.01–0.8 Hz) fluctuations of the blood-oxygen-level-dependent (BOLD) signal in the resting state are considered to be physiologically meaningful and related to spontaneous neural activity [16]. Recently, using rs-fMRI and the regional homogeneity analysis method, Liang et al. found that patients with ESRD showed decreased regional homogeneity in multiple areas of the bilateral frontal, parietal and temporal lobes. Moreover, they found the progressively decreased regional homogeneity in the default mode network (DMN), indicating that frontal and parietal lobes might be trait-related in ESRD patients with minimal nephro-encephalopathy [17]. Voxel-based morphometry (VBM) is a spatially specific and unbiased method of analyzing MR images reflecting the regional gray matter volume at a voxel scale [18]. This technique has already been successfully applied to normal aging [18], schizophrenia [19], dementia [20], mild cognitive impairment (MCI) [21], drug addicts [22] and hepatic encephalopathy [23]. In ESRD patients, Zhang and colleagues found diffusely decreased gray matter volume that was further decreased in the presence of encephalopathy [24]; while Prohovnik and coworkers found significant cerebral atrophy, most notably bilaterally in the caudate nuclei in ESRD patients [25]. These morphometric deficits may also relate to the functional integrity alterations in the ESRD patients. However, no studies have investigated the effects of the observed gray matter impairment on functional integrity. Studies combining VBM with rs-fMRI can explore the structural and functional cerebral deficits simultaneously [26,27]. This method can be an ideal way to explore the neurobiological mechanisms of ESRD patients.

The purposes of the present study were to 1) identify brain regions with gray matter volume deficits, using voxel-based morphometry, and 2) investigate the brain network effect of these anatomic deficits in ESRD patients using the observed structural deficits as seed regions in functional connectivity analysis.

Materials and Methods

Participants

This prospective study was approved by the Research Ethics Review Board of the Institute of Mental Health at the Guangdong No. 2 Provincial People's Hospital. Written informed consent was obtained from all subjects. Sixty subjects, including 30 control subjects and 30 ESRD patients participated in this study. The ESRD patients were recruited from the Renal and Hemodialysis Clinics and Department of Renal Transplantation at Guangdong No. 2 Provincial People's Hospital. Demographic characteristics and chronic health conditions of each ESRD patient were obtained from the patient's electronic medical records. Laboratory values from ESRD patients included serum calcium, serum

phosphorus, serum uric acid and creatinine. As part of the routine clinical care, these laboratory tests were drawn monthly on dialysis days prior to the treatment. Values for serum calcium, serum phosphorus, serum uric acid and serum urea were calculated by averaging the monthly laboratory tests for 3 consecutive months prior to MR imaging. All tests were performed at a single central laboratory using standard methods. Measured blood pressure was determined by averaging the 3 office blood pressure readings prior to MR imaging. The control group was recruited from the local community.

Exclusion criteria for both groups were as follows: a history of stroke or dementia either reported or documented in the medical chart, a history of Parkinson's or neurodegenerative disease, diabetes, alcoholism, drug abuse, psychiatric disorder, or major neurologic disorders (severe head injury, stroke, epilepsy, or visible lesions), liver function enzymes (AST and ALT) more than twice the upper limit of normal, or a hemoglobin level <10 g. In all of the ESRD patients MRI was performed on non-dialysis days to limit the effect of the potential temporal relationship between brain changes and time since last dialysis.

MR imaging

MR data were obtained on a Philips Achieva 1.5 T Nova dual MR scanner using a 16-channel Neuro-Vascular (NV) coil. None of the subjects were taking any medications at the time of the scans. Tight but comfortable foam padding was used to minimize head motion, and earplugs were used to reduce scanner noise. Sagittal structural images (160 sagittal slices, TR = 25 ms, TE = 4.1 ms, thickness = 1.0 mm, no gap, in-plane resolution = 231×232, FOV = 230×230 mm^2, flip angle = 30°) were acquired using a fast field echo (FFE) three-dimensional T1 weighted sequence. Resting-state functional MRI (fMRI) scans were performed by an echo planar imaging (EPI) sequence with scan parameters of TR = 3000 ms, TE = 50 ms, flip angle = 90°, matrix = 64×64, FOV = 230×230 mm^2, slice thickness = 4.5 mm and slice gap = 0 mm. Each brain volume comprised 33 axial slices and each functional run contained 160 volumes (8 minutes). During resting state fMRI scanning, subjects were instructed to close their eyes and keep as still as possible, and not to think of anything systematically or fall asleep.

After the scan, all the participants were asked the following questions to verify the degree of their cooperation: "what were you thinking during the scan?", "did you fall asleep just now?", "were your eyes closed during the scan?" and "did you feel uncomfortable during the scan?" Only when the participant answered "nothing", "no, I did not", "yes, I kept my eyes closed" and "no, I did not feel any uncomfortable", were their data used in the present study.

Voxel-Based Morphometry Analysis

Structural image processing was conducted using the Voxel-based morphometry toolbox (VBM8) (http://dbm.neuro.uni-jena.de/vbm/) implemented in Statistical Parametric Mapping-8 (SPM8) (http://www.fil.ion.ucl.ac.uk/spm, Welcome Department of Imaging Neuroscience, London). VBM8 in SPM8 combines tissue segmentation, bias correction, and spatial normalization into a unified model [27]. Hidden Markov Random Fields were applied to improve accuracy of tissue segmentation (medium HMRF 0.3). Otherwise, default parameters were used. Individual brains were normalized to tissue probability maps provided by International Consortium for Brain Mapping (ICBM). The optimally processed images were smoothed with an isotropic Gaussian kernel (full-width half maximum = 12 mm). At the second level, whole brain data were modeled across the groups using analysis of covariance (ANCOVA) with total gray matter volume and age as covariates. The effects of total gray matter volume were removed to allow inferences between regional differences in gray matter volume. An absolute threshold mask of .1 was used. The significance of group differences in each region was estimated by distributional approximations from the theory of random Gaussian fields, and significance levels were set at p<0.05 (corrected for multiple comparisons). To identify the association between structural abnormalities and clinical severity of kidney disease and times of hemodialysis, the average gray matter volume values for all voxels in the abnormal areas, revealed by voxel-based morphometry, were extracted and correlated with the duration of chronic kidney disease, duration of hemodialysis and the laboratory values (serum calcium level, serum phosphorus level, serum uric acid level and serum urea values) in individual ESRD patient.

Functional Connectivity Analysis

Preprocessing and statistical analysis of functional images were conducted using SPM8. For each subject, the first ten time points were discarded to avoid transient signal changes before magnetization reached steady-state and to allow subjects to get used to the fMRI scanning noise. Then echo-planar images were slice-time corrected and realigned to the first image in the first series and were subsequently unwarped to correct for susceptibility-by-movement interaction, subjects with head motion exceeding 1.0 mm of maximal translation (in any direction of x, y or z) or 1.0° of maximal rotation through the resting-state run were excluded from further analysis. All realigned images were spatially normalized to the Montreal Neurological Institute (MNI) echo-planar imaging template in SPM8, and each voxel was resampled to $3 \times 3 \times 3$ mm^3. Functional connectivity was examined using a method based on a seed voxel correlation approach [27,28]. Since voxel-based morphometry analysis showed anatomic deficits in the bilateral medial PFC, the bilateral dorsal lateral PFC (dlPFC) and the left middle temporal gyrus, areas with gray matter volume reduction were defined as seeds for functional connectivity analysis. A reference time series for each seed was obtained by averaging the fMRI time series for all voxels within the region with anatomic deficits. Next, each time series was temporally bandpass filtered (0.01–0.08 Hz). Correlation analysis was conducted between the seed reference and the rest of the whole brain in a voxel-wise manner using the realigned images. To combine results across subjects and compute statistical significance, correlation coefficients were converted to a normal distribution by Fisher's z transform [29,30].

For each group, individual z value maps were analyzed with a random effect one-sample t test to identify voxels showing a significant positive or negative correlation to the seed time series, with correlations thresholded using a family-wise error correction at p<0.05. For between-group comparison, two-sample t tests were used to compare z value maps between ESRD patients and matched controls, with the significance threshold of group differences set at p<0.05 using AlphaSim correction in the REST software (http://www. restfmri.net), which applied Monte Carlo simulation to calculated the probability of false positive detection by taking both the individual voxel probability thresholding and cluster size into consideration [31]. To identify the association between functional connectivity and clinical severity of kidney disease in ESRD patients, the z value of the regions that showed aberrant functional connectivity with the anatomic abnormalities (revealed by group comparison) were extracted and correlated with the duration of chronic kidney disease, duration of hemodialysis and the laboratory values (serum calcium, serum

phosphorus, serum uric acid and serum urea values) in individual ESRD patient.

A complementary analysis was carried out to investigate the link between the structural and functional results, i.e., we wanted to address whether the effects observed on functional connectivity in ESRD patients could be explained by the reduced gray matter volume observed in the seed areas. Therefor, we replicated the four between-groups comparisons of the functional connectivity maps in using the gray matter volume of the respective seed areas as covariates.

Results

Demographic Results

Table 1 demonstrates the basic characteristics of ESRD patients and controls. There were no significant differences in age (p = 0.737), education (p = 0.506), sex composition (p = 0.559) between the ESRD and control groups. Table 2 demonstrates systolic blood pressure, diastolic blood pressure and hematocrit at the start and end of hemodialysis treatment session. In these patients, ESRD was secondary to glomerulonephritis.

Morphometry Analysis

Relative to controls, ESRD patients showed significantly decreased gray matter volume in bilateral medial orbito-prefrontal cortex (OFC, Brodmann's area 10, 11, 32, Talairach coordinates: 1.5, 43.5, −13.5; voxel size = 328 mm^3), left middle temporal gyrus (Brodmann's area 10, 11, 32, Talairach coordinates: −55.5, −9, −12; voxel size = 533 mm^3), left dorsal lateral prefrontal cortex (dlPFC, Brodmann's area 10, Talairach coordinates: −30, 51, 0; voxel size = 340 mm^3) and right dlPFC (Brodmann's area 11, Talairach coordinates: 27, 54, −9; voxel size = 182 mm^3) (Figure 1). No significant increases in gray matter volume were found in ESRD patients compared to controls. No significant negative/positive correlations were found between the abnormal gray matter volume and the duration of chronic kidney disease, duration of hemodialysis and laboratory values for serum calcium level, phosphorus, uric acid and urea levels in ESRD patients.

Functional Connectivity Analysis

The four seed areas, where reduced gray matter volume was detected among ESRD patients, were selected for functional connectivity analysis. When the seed was located in the bilateral medial OFC, the ESRD patients showed reduced functional connectivity in the bilateral posterior cerebellar lobes, right dlPFC, bilateral ACC, and enhanced FC in bilateral OFC, bilateral superior parietal lobe than controls (Table 3, Figure 2). When the seed was located in the left dlPFC, the ESRD patients demonstrated enhanced functional connectivity in the superior temporal gyrus compared to controls (Table 3, Figure 2). When the seed was located in the right dlPFC, the ESRD patients demonstrated reduced FC in bilateral posterior cerebellar lobes, the left inferior temporal gyrus, the right dlPFC, and enhanced FC in bilateral OFC, and the left posterior gyrus (Table 3, Figure 2). When the seed was located in the left middle temporal gyrus, enhanced FC was found in the right medial PFC in ESRD patients when compared to controls (Table 3, Figure 2).

The replication of the group comparisons for the four functional connectivity maps with the corresponding gray matter volume of the seeds as covariates resulted in similar results, except for the network corresponding to the seed of left dorsal lateral prefrontal cortex, which showed no significant differences between the two groups.

Table 1. Demographic and Clinical Characteristics for End Stage Renal Disease (ESRD) Patients and Controls.

Characteristic	Group				
	ESRD Patients (N = 30)		Controls (N = 30)		
	Mean	SD	Mean	SD	P
Age (years)	38.8	9.6	38.1	7.0	0.737
Education (years)	9.8	5.1	10.6	4.5	0.506
Laboratory tests					
S. uric acid (mg/dl)	5.98	1.20	N/A	N/A	-
S. urea (mmol/l)	19.2	5.4	N/A	N/A	-
S. calcium (mmol/l)	2.32	0.25	N/A	N/A	-
S. Phosphorus (mmol/l)	1.30	0.24	N/A	N/A	-
Illness duration (years)	12.5	4.8	N/A	N/A	-
Dialysis duration (mouths)	17.2	6.8	N/A	N/A	-
Mean hemodialysis duration (h/w)	14.5	3.5	N/A	N/A	-
	N	%	N	%	P
Gender					
Female	7	23.3	9	30	0.559
Male	23	76.7	21	70	0.559

There were no significant differences in age (p = 0.737), education (p = 0.506), sex composition (p = 0.559) between ESRD patients and controls.
Note. N/A = not applicable.

No significant positive or negative correlation was found between any of the Z values and the duration of chronic kidney disease, duration of hemodialysis and laboratory values for serum calcium, serum phosphorus, serum uric acid and serum serum urea values in ESRD patients.

Discussion

Our study revealed the following important findings. First, ESRD patients have several areas of decreased gray matter volume (including the bilateral medial OFC, the bilateral dlPFC and the left middle temporal gyrus) compared with healthy controls. Second, the decrease in gray matter volume in these regions was related to the functional network integrity deficits in ESRD patients. To the best of our knowledge, this is the first systemic investigation of anatomic and functional deficits in ESRD patients on routine hemodialysis with VBM and functional connectivity methods.

The loss of gray matter volumes includes the bilateral dlPFC, the bilateral medial OFC, and the left middle temporal gyrus. The reduced gray matter volume of the prefrontal cortex in ESRD patients observed in the present study is supported by a recent histological study by Migliori and coworkers [32]. These Authors compared normal rats, nephrectomized rats and nephrectomized rats treated with Fluoxetin, and found a significant decrease in brain derived neurotrophic factor (BDNF) at the level of the prefrontal cortex in the nephrectomized rats compared to normal rats. Moreover, they showed a partial recovery in the Nx-F rats [32]. The reduced BDNF had been widely related to atrophy and cellular death of glia and neurons in neurodegenerative disorder [32]. Previous PET studies also revealed abnormalities in these areas. In an F-18-fluorodeoxyglucose (FDG) PET study, Song et al. found several voxel clusters of significantly decreased cerebral glucose metabolism in pre-dialysis CKD patients, including the left prefrontal cortex (Brodmann's area 9), the right prefrontal cortex (Brodmann's area 10) and the right basolateral prefrontal cortex (Brodmann's area 46), the left anterior cingulate gyrus (Brodmann's area 32), the left premotor cortex (Brodmann's area 6), the left transverse temporal gyrus (Brodmann's area 41), the left superior temporal gyrus (Brodmann's area 42), the right basolateral prefrontal cortex (Brodmann's area 44), the right inferior parietal lobule (Brodmann's area 39), the left middle temporal gyrus (Brodmann's area 19), and the left angular gyrus (Brodmann's area 39). Moreover, they found a negative correlation between the cerebral glucose metabolism of the right orbitofrontal cortex and the Hamilton Depression Rating Scale (HDRS) in pre-dialysis CKD patients (Brodmann's area 11) [12]. Through measuring brain oxygen metabolism, Kanai et al.

Table 2. Blood pressure systolic, Blood pressure diastolic and Hematocrit of the ESRD patients at the start and end of hemodialysis treatment session.

variable	Pre	Post	p
Blood pressure systolic (mm Hg)	143±21	138±19	0.67
Blood pressure diastolic (mm Hg)	81±8	83±7	0.52
Hematocrit (vol%)	36.1±3.12	36.7±3.75	0.46

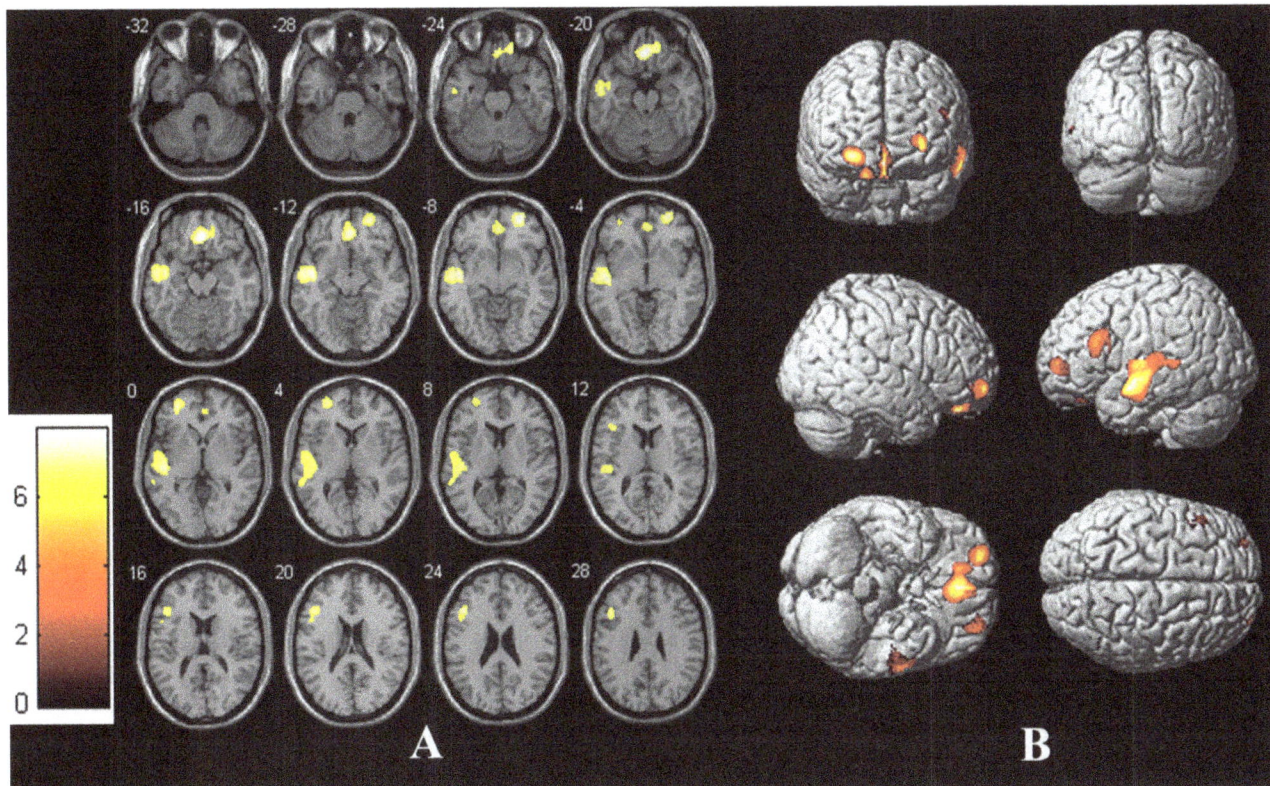

Figure 1. Statistical Parametric Images of Voxel-Based Morphometry Analysis for ESRD Patients and controls (Panels A: slices view, Panels B: whole brain rendering). Relative to controls, ERSD patients had significantly reduced gray matter volume in the bilateral medial orbitofrontal cortex, bilateral dorsal lateral prefrontal cortex and right middle temporal gyrus.

demonstrated significantly lower values of hemispheric and cerebral cortex oxygen metabolism in both hemodialysis and CKD patients compared with controls, and the frontal cortices tended to show the lowest values in patients with renal failure [11].

However, our VBM findings were somewhat different from previous VBM studies. Through comparing minimal nephro-encephalopathy (MNE) and Non-MNE, with controls, Zhang et al. reported diffusely decreased gray matter volumes in ESRD patients. In addition, they found that serum urea was negatively associated with changes in gray matter volume in many regions (bilateral occipital lobes, bilateral lingual lobes, bilateral calcarine, bilateral superior temporal gyri, bilateral temporal poles, bilateral uncus, posterior cingulate cortex/precuneus/cuneus, right fusiform, right parahippocampus, right amygdala, left hippocampus/parahippocampus) [24]. Thus, the differences in the laboratory tests (especially for the serum urea) might be one of the potential reasons. Another possible mechanism might be the hemodialysis differences in the ESRD patients between the two studies. In contrast to our present study, in which all the ESRD patients were undergoing hemodialysis, only 33 of 57 ESRD patients were on hemodialysis in their study [24]. Studies based on transcranial Doppler have indicated a decrease in the mean flow velocity (mfv) at the level of the middle cerebral artery (MCA) during hemodialysis, MCAmfv has been proposed as a reliable proxy for cerebral blood flow [33–35]. In addiction, lower cerebral blood flow has always been associated with lower brain gray matter volume and lower cortical thickness [36–38]. In a study by Prohovnik et al., 10 ESRD patients on hemodialysis and 6 controls were compared, and they found decreased gray volume only in bilateral caudate nuclei but not in other regions [25]. The most

likely cause for the difference from our study may be the sample size.

The dorsal lateral prefrontal cortex serves as the highest cortical area responsible for motor planning, organization, and regulation [39]. OFC is involved in cognitive processing of decision-making [40]. Damage to either of these regions can result in the dysexecutive syndrome [41], which leads to problems with emotion, social judgment, executive memory, abstract thinking and intentionality. The decreased gray matter volume in these regions observed in the present study may imply executive function deficits in ESRD patients, which is supported by previous neuropsychological studies indicating that executive function deficits were the prominent feature of cognitive impairment among ESRD patients [42].

How the gray matter structural abnormalities in ESRD patients relate to cerebral functional integrity deficits is an interesting question. In the present study, regions with abnormal gray matter volume were used as seeds for functional connectivity analysis. We found a disconnect between the prefrontal cortex and the bilateral cerebellum (consist fronto-cerebellar circuits), and within the prefrontal cortex. We also found enhanced functional connectivity between the prefrontal cortex and left middle temporal gyrus as well as within the prefrontal cortex in ESRD patients when compared to the healthy controls (Figure 2, Table 3). Moreover, supplementary analysis showed that most of the results remained significant when local gray matter volumes (except the left dorsal lateral prefrontal cortex) were statistically controlled for. This suggests that local gray matter volumes partially influenced the functional results, but that the abnormalities we found regarding

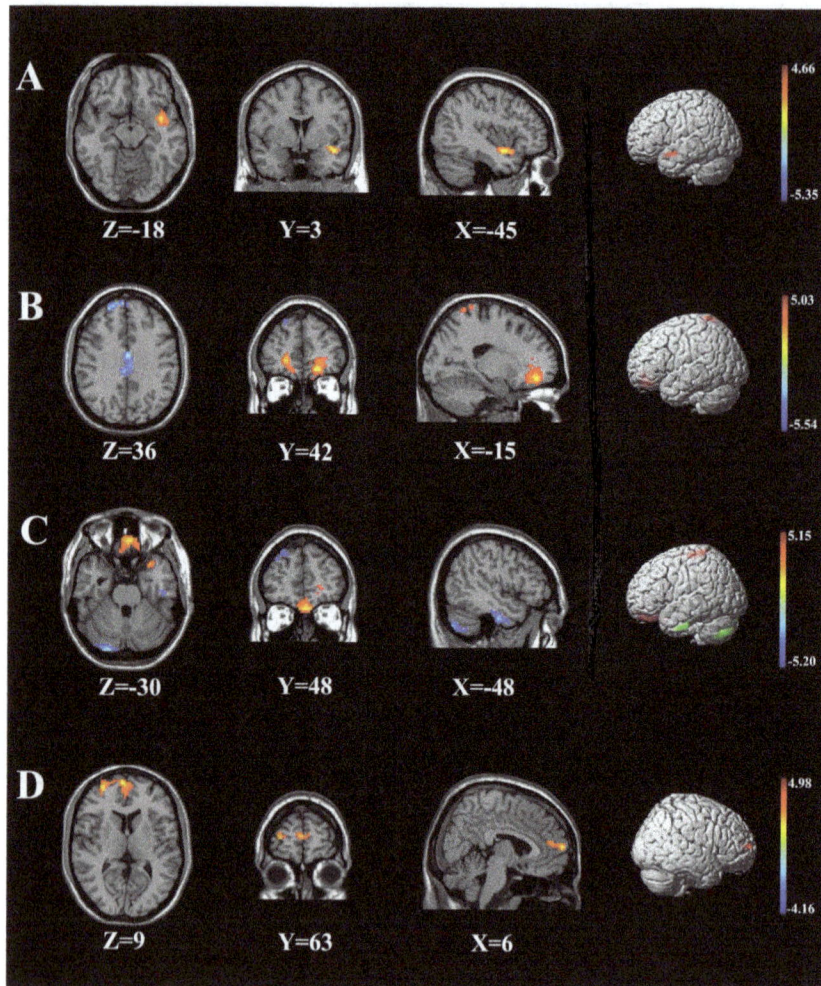

Figure 2. Statistical Parametric Images of Between-Group Functional Connectivity Analysis for ESRD Patients and Controls. Panels A demonstrated enhanced functional connectivity in superior temporal gyrus (Red) in ESRD patients when the seed areas were located in the left dorsal lateral prefrontal cortex ([Brodmann's area 10], panels B demonstrated reduced functional connectivity in bilateral cerebellum posterior lobe, left inferior temporal gyrus, right dlPFC (Blue), and enhanced functional connectivity in bilateral OFC, left posterior gyrus (Red) in ESRD patients when the seed areas were located in the right dorsal lateral prefrontal cortex ([Brodmann's area 11], panels C demonstrated reduced functional connectivity in bilateral cerebellum posterior lobe, right dlPFC, bilateral ACC (Blue), enhanced FC in bilateral OFC, bilateral superior parietal lobe (Red) when the seed areas were located in the medial orbito-frontal cortex ([Brodmann's area 10, 11, 32], and panels D demonstrated enhanced functional connectivity in right medial PFC (Red) in ESRD patients when the seed areas were located in the left middle temporal gyrus [Brodmann's area 10, 11, 32].

resting state functional connectivity in the ESRD group cannot entirely be explained by their lower gray matter volume.

Fronta-frontal circuits including the dorsolateral circuit, orbito-frontal circuit and anterior cingulate cortex circuit are thought to be involved in attention, cognition, action and emotion [43]. The separation performances of functional connectivity (enhance and reduce) within fronta-frontal circuits may represent different neural mechanisms, while reduced functional connectivity within the fronta-frontal circuits implies that the ESRD-related functional impairment, and enhanced functional connectivity may indicate compensatory mechanisms. Ideally, task-fMRI studies combined quantitative MRI imaging with neuropsychological testing should be planned to prove this hypothesis.

Fronto-cerebellar circuits include three distinct circuits that associate with the prefrontal cortex. These fronto-cerebellar circuits are thought to be involved in higher-order cognitive functioning. Studies have consistently demonstrated that the fronto-cerebellar circuits are associated with cognitive function

[44,45]. Disconnection of the fronto-cerebellar connectivity observed in the present study may contribute to cognitive deficits in ESRD patients. This hypothesis can be partly supported by previous studies on alcoholism, which indicated that the disconnection between the fronto-cerebeller circuits related to the cognitive deficits in alcoholics and alcohol-naïve youth with a family history of alcoholism [44,45]. Further support to this hypothesis is also provided by a recent study performed in children with attention-deficit/hyperactivity disorder (ADHD), which found that the frontal and cerebellar circuits neural activity was enhanced in ADHD patients after cognitive training [46]. If this hypothesis holds, cognitive training can be used to enhance fronto-cerebellar connectivity of ESRD patients, which may improve the cognitive function in ESRD patients.

We also observed an enhanced FC between the left middle temporal gyrus and the medial PFC (Brodmann's area 10), while the fronto-temporal circuits function in language processing. The

Table 3. Significant differences between ESRD Patients and Controls in resting state functional connectivity for the four seed areas (showed different in group comparison) and the rest of the brain.

Seed area	Cluster anatomical locations (Brodmann Area)	Cluster size (voxel)	Primary peak location	t-score	ESRD n = 30 Mean (zFC)	Controls n = 30 Mean (zFC)
ESRD<Controls						
Bilateral medial OFC	Right cerebellum posterior lobe	388	36, −84, −33	−5.5361	−0.28	−0.04
	Left cerebellum posterior lobe	258	−36, −78, −45	−4.059	−0.28	−0.03
	right dlPFC (8,9,10)	139	24,51,36	−4.371	−0.13	0.08
	bilateral ACC(23,24,31)	234	18, −39,36	−4.6875	−0.10	0.08
Right DLPFC	Left Cerebellum Posterior Lobe	92	−48, −72, −48	−4.1573	−0.15	0.05
	Right Cerebellum Posterior Lobe	89	24, −93, −30	−5.196	−0.19	0.01
	Left Inferior Temporal Gyrus (20)	120	−48, −15, −36	−4.625	−0.14	0.07
	right dlPFC	110	42,33,42	−3.749	−0.11	0.10
ESRD>Controls						
Bilateral medial OFC	Left OFC (10, 11, 32)	276	−21,42, −15	5.0312	0.49	0.21
	Right OFC (10, 11)	153	21,45, −3	4.8567	0.56	0.25
	Left superior parietal lobe (4,5,7)	127	−12, −45,75	4.0437	0.14	−0.08
	Right superior parietal lobe (7)	108	24, −81,51	4.7056	0.11	−0.12
Left DLPFC	Left Superior Temporal Gyrus (38)	100	−45,3, −18	4.6605	0.09	−0.15
Right DLPFC	Bilateral OFC (10,11,25,38,47)	366	0,48, −30	4.5486	0.23	0.01
	Bilateral postcentral gyrus (1,2,3,4,5,6)	110	−36, −39,66	4.8554	0.13	−0.07
Left middle temporal gyurs	Right medial PFC (10,32)	129	6 63 9	4.2882	0.12	−0.09

All the coordinates are donated by Montreal Neurological Institute (MNI) space coordinates. t-score donates the statistic value of two sample t-test by contrasting ESRD patients to controls at p<0.05 AlphaSim corrected.

enhanced FC in this circuit may be compensatory for the GM volume reduction in the left temporal gyrus.

We did not find any correlation between the brain deficits (structural and functional) and clinical parameters in ESRD patients. Several factors might explain these findings. First, depression is the most common psychological disorder in ESRD patients with a prevalence as high as 20–25% by some contemporary estimates [47]. The reduced gray matter volume in the bilateral OFC, the left middle temporal gyrus and the bilateral dlPFC observed in present study is also found in patients with depression [48]. Thus, the brain deficits observed in the present study may result from the complication (depression) and not from the ESRD itself. A more rigorous experiment to exclude the effects of depression is needed in the future. Second, a relatively small sample size may lead to insufficient power. Although we did not find any significant correlation between the brain deficits and clinical parameters in ESRD patients, we found negative trends between the serum urea levels and the bilateral OFC, the left middle temporal gyrus and the right dlPFC gray matter volume. A larger sample size is needed in future studies.

Limitations

We acknowledge that our study has some limitations. The main limitation of the study is that all of the ESRD patients received regular hemodialysis at the time of the fMRI study. Whether and how hemodialysis itself can affect the brain is unknown; however, it can affect the patient's cognitive function [49,50]. Although we did not find any significant correlation between the abnormal gray matter volume, FC and times of hemodialysis, a more detailed experiment with chronic kidney disease (stage 4–5) without hemodialysis is required in the future study. Second, although we temporally bandpass filtered all fMRI data (0.01–0.08 Hz), and

removed components with high correlation to cerebrospinal fluid or white matter or with low correlation to gray matter, we cannot completely rule out the influence of physiological noise on our findings due to its variation over time and across subjects. Simultaneous recording of heart rate and respiratory rate and depth during fMRI scanning might help further reduce physiological noise artifacts. Another limitation is that the current study did not include cognitive testing to allow the examination of any correlation with the structural brain abnormalities and functional connectivity. Such an investigation might potentially improve our understanding of the pathophysiological mechanisms of ESRD. In addition, this study is preliminary and our results are limited to a small sample size, which may affect the statistical analysis. Further studies with large-cohort are needed.

Conclusions

In conclusion, the present study applied morphometry analysis and resting-state functional connectivity to examine the structural and functional integrity changes in ESRD patients. Our findings document that patients with ESRD undergoing routine hemodialysis display clear-cut structural alterations in selected gray matter areas, Moreover, regions with gray matter volume reduction have significantly altered resting state functional connectivity with other brain regions. Our results provide support for future efforts to combine anatomical and functional data to explore the cognitive deficits of ESRD patients.

Acknowledgments

The authors express their appreciation to Zheng Guo at the University of Kentucky for her help on preparing this manuscript. Also, the authors are highly grateful to the anonymous reviewers for their significant and constructive comments and suggestions, which greatly improve the article.

Author Contributions

Conceived and designed the experiments: YQ HS XL. Performed the experiments: YQ GJ CL. Analyzed the data: YQ HS. Contributed reagents/materials/analysis tools: YQ JT. Wrote the paper: YQ.

References

1. Etgen T, Chonchol M, Förstl H, Sander D (2012) Chronic kidney disease and cognitive impairment: a systematic review and meta-analysis. Am J Nephrol 35(5):474–82.
2. Kurella M, Chertow GM, Luan J, Yaffe K (2004) Cognitive impairment in chronic kidney disease. J Am Geriatr Soc 52(11):1863–9.
3. Sehgal AR, Grey SF, DeOreo PB, Whitehouse PJ (1997) Prevalence, recognition and implications of mental impairment among hemodialysis patients. Am J Kidney Dis 30:41–49.
4. Bremer BA, Wert KM, Durica AL (1997) Neuropsychological, physical, and psychosocial functioning of individuals with end-stage renal disease. Ann Behav Med 19:348–352.
5. Fazekas G, Fazekas F, Schmidt R, Kapeller P, Offenbacher H, et al. (1995) Brain MRI findings and cognitive impairment in patients undergoing chronic hemodialysis treatment. J Neurol Sci 134:83–88.
6. Ikram MA, Vernooij MW, Hofman A, Niessen WJ, van der Lugt A, et al. (2008) Kidney function is related to cerebral small vessel disease. Stroke 39(1):55–61.
7. Kamata T, Hishida A, Takita T, Sawada K, Ikegaya N, et al. (2000) Morphologic abnormalities in the brain of chronically hemodialyzed patients without cerebrovascular disease. Am J Nephrol 20(1):27–31.
8. Savazzi GM, Cusmano F, Musini S (2001) Cerebral imaging changes in patients with chronic renal failure treated conservatively or in hemodialysis. Nephron 89(1):31–6.
9. Chiu ML, Li CW, Chang JM, Chiang IC, Ko CH, et al. (2010) Cerebral metabolic changes in neurologically presymptomatic patients undergoing haemodialysis: in vivo proton MR spectroscopic findings. Eur Radiol 20(6):1502–7.
10. Tryc AB, Alwan G, Bokemeyer M, Goldbecker A, Hecker H, et al. (2011) Cerebral metabolic alterations and cognitive dysfunction in chronic kidney disease. Nephrol Dial Transplant 26(8):2635–41.
11. Kanai H, Hirakata H, Nakane H, Fujii K, Hirakata E, et al. (2001) Depressed cerebral oxygen metabolism in patients with chronic renal failure: a positron emission tomography study. Am J Kidney Dis 38(4 Suppl 1):S129–33.
12. Song SH, Kim IJ, Kim SJ, Kwak IS, Kim YK (2008) Cerebral glucose metabolism abnormalities in patients with major depressive symptoms in pre-dialytic chronic kidney disease: statistical parametric mapping analysis of F-18-FDG PET, a preliminary study. Psychiatry Clin Neurosci 62(5):554–61.
13. Whitwell JL (2009) Voxel-based morphometry: an automated technique for assessing structural changes in the brain. J Neurosci 29(31):9661–4.
14. Maudsley AA, Domenig C, Ramsay RE, Bowen BC (2010) Application of volumetric MR spectroscopic imaging for localization of neocortical epilepsy. Epilepsy Res 88(2–3):127–38.
15. Kuperman S, Gaffney GR, Hamdan-Allen G, Preston DF, Venkatesh L (1990) Neuroimaging in child and adolescent psychiatry. J Am Acad Child Adolesc Psychiatry 29(2):159–72.
16. Rauch A, Rainer G, Logothetis NK (2008) The effect of a serotonin-induced dissociation between spiking and perisynaptic activity on BOLD functional MRI. Proc Natl Acad Sci U S A 105(18):6759–64.
17. Liang X, Wen J, Ni L, Zhong J, Qi R, et al. (2013) Altered Pattern of Spontaneous Brain Activity in the Patients with End-Stage Renal Disease: A Resting State Functional MRI Study with Regional Homogeneity Analysis. PLoS ONE 8(8): e71507.
18. Good CD, Johnsrude IS, Ashburner J, Henson RN, Friston KJ, et al. (2001) A voxel-based morphometric study of ageing in 465 normal adult human brains. Neuroimage 14:21–36.
19. Pomarol-Clotet E, Canales-Rodríguez EJ, Salvador R, Sarró S, Gomar JJ, et al. (2010) Medial prefrontal cortex pathology in schizophrenia as revealed by convergent findings from multimodal imaging. Mol Psychiatry 15(8):823–30.
20. Chételat G, Desgranges B, Landeau B, Mézenge F, Poline JB, et al. (2008) Direct voxel-based comparison between grey matter hypometabolism and atrophy in Alzheimer's disease. Brain 131(Pt 1):60–71.
21. Gili T, Cercignani M, Serra L, Perri R, Giove F, et al. (2011) Regional brain atrophy and functional disconnection across Alzheimer's disease evolution. J Neurol Neurosurg Psychiatry 82(1):58–66.
22. Qiu YW, Jiang GH, Su HH, Lv XF, Tian JZ, et al. (2013) The impulsivity behavior is correlated with prefrontal cortex gray matter volume reduction in heroin-dependent individuals. Neurosci Lett 538: 43–48.
23. Zhang LJ, Qi R, Zhong J, Xu Q, Zheng G, et al. (2012) The Effect of Hepatic Encephalopathy, Hepatic Failure, and Portosystemic Shunt on Brain Volume of Cirrhotic Patients: A Voxel-Based Morphometry Study. PLoS ONE 7(8): e42824.
24. Zhang LJ, Wen J, Ni L, Zhong J, Liang X, et al. (2013) Predominant gray matter volume loss in patients with end-stage renal disease: a voxel-based morphometry study. Metab Brain Dis 28(4):647–54.
25. Prohovnik I, Post J, Uribarri J, Lee H, Sandu O, et al. (2007) Cerebrovascular effects of hemodialysis in chronic kidney disease. J Cereb Blood Flow Metab 27(11):1861–1869.
26. Qiu YW, Lv XF, Jiang GH, Su HH, Yu T, et al. (2014) Reduced ventral medial prefrontal cortex (vmPFC) volume and impaired vmPFC-default mode network integration in codeine-containing cough syrups users. Drug Alcohol Depend 134:314–21.
27. Lui S, Deng W, Huang X, Jiang L, Ma X, et al. (2009) Association of cerebral deficits with clinical symptoms in antipsychotic-naive first-episode schizophrenia: an optimized voxel-based morphometry and resting state functional connectivity study. Am J Psychiatry 166: 196–205.
28. Horwitz B, Rumsey JM, Donohue BC (1998) Functional connectivity of the angular gyrus in normal reading and dyslexia. Proc Natl Acad Sci U S A 95:8939–8944.
29. Fox MD, Snyder AZ, Vincent JL, Corbetta M, Van Essen DC, et al. (2005) The human brain is intrinsically organized into dynamic, anticorrelated functional networks. Proc Natl Acad Sci U S A 102:9673–9678.
30. Jenkins GM, Watts DG (1968) Spectral Analysis and Its Applications. San Francisco
31. Yan CG, Zang YF (2010) DPARSF: A MATLAB Toolbox for "Pipeline" Data Analysis of Resting-State fMRI. Front Syst Neurosci 4:13.
32. Miglior M, Mannari C (2009) Role of brain derived neurotrophic factor (BDNF) in the development of neuropsychiatric disorders in chronic renal failure. Metabolic and other complications of ESRD – 1. abstract.
33. Regolisti G, Maggiore U, Cademartiri C, Cabassi A, Caiazza A, et al. (2013) Cerebral blood flow decreases during intermittent hemodialysis in patients with acute kidney injury, but not in patients with end-stage renal disease. Nephrol Dial Transplant 28(1):79–85.
34. Skinner H, Mackaness C, Bedforth N, Mahajan R (2005) Cerebral haemodynamics in patients with chronic renal failure: effects of haemodialysis. Br J Anaesth 94(2):203–5.
35. Stefanidis I, Bach R, Mertens PR, Liakopoulos V, Liapi G, et al. (2005) Influence of hemodialysis on the mean blood flow velocity in the middle cerebral artery. Clin Nephrol 64(2):129–37.
36. Denier N, Schmidt A, Gerber H, Schmid O, Riecher-Rössler A, et al. (2013) Association of frontal gray matter volume and cerebral perfusion in heroin addiction: a multimodal neuroimaging study. Front Psychiatry 4:135.
37. Alosco ML, Gunstad J, Jerskey BA, Xu X, Clark US, et al. (2013) The adverse effects of reduced cerebral perfusion on cognition and brain structure in older adults with cardiovascular disease. Brain Behav 3(6):626–36.
38. Drew DA, Bhadelia R, Tighiouart H, Novak V, Scott TM, et al. (2013) Anatomic brain changes in hemodialysis patients: a cross-sectional study. Am J Kidney Dis 61(2):271–8.
39. Zelazo PD, Müller U (2010) Executive Function in Typical and Atypical Development, in The Wiley-Blackwell Handbook of Childhood Cognitive Development, Second edition (ed U. Goswami), Wiley-Blackwell, Oxford, UK. doi: 10.1002/9781444325485.ch22.
40. Kringelbach ML (2005) The orbitofrontal cortex: linking reward to hedonic experience. Nature Reviews Neuroscience 6: 691–702.
41. John JP (2009) Fronto-temporal dysfunction in schizophrenia: A selective review. Indian J Psychiatry 51:180–90.
42. Kurella Tamura M, Yaffe K (2011) Dementia and cognitive impairment in ESRD: diagnostic and therapeutic strategies. Kidney Int 79(1):14–22.
43. Burruss JW, Hurley RA, Taber KH, Rauch RA, Norton RE, et al. (2000) Functional neuroanatomy of the frontal lobe circuits. Radiology 214(1):227–30.
44. Herting MM, Fair D, Nagel BJ (2011) Altered fronto-cerebellar connectivity in alcohol-naïve youth with a family history of alcoholism. Neuroimage 54(4):2582–9.
45. Rogers BP, Parks MH, Nickel MK, Katwal SB, Martin PR (2012) Reduced fronto-cerebellar functional connectivity in chronic alcoholic patients. Alcohol Clin Exp Res 36(2):294–301.
46. Hoekzema E, Carmona S, Tremols V, Gispert JD, Guitart M, et al. (2010) Enhanced neural activity in frontal and cerebellar circuits after cognitive training in children with attention-deficit/hyperactivity disorder. Hum Brain Mapp 31(12):1942–50.
47. Kimmel PL, Cukor D, Cohen SD, Peterson RA (2007) Depression in end-stage renal disease patients: a critical review. Adv Chronic Kidney Dis 14(4):328–34.
48. Grieve SM, Korgaonkar MS, Koslow SH, Gordon E, Williams LM (2013) Widespread reductions in gray matter volume in depression. Neuroimage Clin 3:332–9.
49. Nasser Mel T, Shawki S, El Shahawy Y, Sany D (2012) Assessment of cognitive dysfunction in kidney disease. Saudi J Kidney Dis Transpl 23(6):1208–14.
50. Kurella Tamura M, Unruh ML, Nissenson AR, Larive B, Eggers PW, et al. (2012) Effect of More Frequent Hemodialysis on Cognitive Function in the Frequent Hemodialysis Network Trials. Am J Kidney Dis 61(2):228–37.

13

Variation in Genes that Regulate Blood Pressure Are Associated with Glomerular Filtration Rate

May E. Montasser[1*¤], **Lawrence C. Shimmin**[1], **Dongfeng Gu**[2], **Jing Chen**[3], **Charles Gu**[4], **Tanika N. Kelly**[5], **Cashell E. Jaquish**[6], **Treva K. Rice**[4], **Dabeeru C. Rao**[4], **Jie Cao**[2], **Jichun Chen**[2], **De-Pei Liu**[7], **Paul K. Whelton**[5], **Lotuce Lee Hamm**[3], **Jiang He**[5], **James E. Hixson**[1]

1 Human Genetics Center, School of Public Health, University of Texas Health Science Center at Houston, Houston, Texas, United States of America, 2 Cardiovascular Institute and Fu Wai Hospital, Chinese Academy of Medical Sciences, Beijing, China, 3 Tulane University School of Medicine, New Orleans, Louisiana, United States of America, 4 Washington University in School of Medicine, St. Louis, Missouri, United States of America, 5 Tulane University School of Public Health and Tropical Medicine, New Orleans, Louisiana, United States of America, 6 National Heart, Lung and Blood Institute, National Institute of Health, Bethesda, Maryland, United States of America, 7 National Laboratory of Medical Molecular Biology, Institute of Basic Medical Sciences, Chinese Academy of Medical Sciences, Beijing, China

Abstract

Chronic kidney disease (CKD) can be a consequence of diabetes, hypertension, immunologic disorders, and other exposures, as well as genetic factors that are still largely unknown. Glomerular filtration rate (GFR), which is widely used to measure kidney function, has a heritability ranging from 25% to 75%, but only 1.5% of this heritability is explained by genetic loci that have been identified to date. In this study we tested for associations between GFR and 234 SNPs in 26 genes from pathways of blood pressure regulation in 3,025 rural Chinese participants of the "Genetic Epidemiology Network of Salt Sensitivity" (GenSalt) study. We estimated GFR (eGFR) using baseline serum creatinine measurements obtained prior to dietary intervention. We identified significant associations between eGFR and 12 SNPs in 6 genes (ACE, ADD1, AGT, GRK4, HSD11B1, and SCNN1G). The cumulative effect of the protective alleles was an increase in mean eGFR of 4 mL/min per 1.73 m^2, while the cumulative effect of the risk alleles was a decrease in mean eGFR of 3 mL/min per 1.73 m^2. In addition, we identified a significant interaction between SNPs in CYP11B1 and ADRB2. We have identified common variants in genes from pathways that regulate blood pressure and influence kidney function as measured by eGFR, providing new insights into the genetic determinants of kidney function. Complex genetic effects on kidney function likely involve interactions among genes as we observed for CYP11B1 and ADRB2.

Editor: Antonio Carlos Seguro, University of São Paulo School of Medicine, Brazil

Funding: The Genetic Epidemiology Network of Salt Sensitivity (GenSalt) is supported by several grants (U01HL072507, R01HL087263, and R01HL090682) from the National Heart, Lung and Blood Institute, National Institutes of Health, Bethesda, Maryland. The funders had no role in study design, data collection and analysis, decision to publish, or preparation of the manuscript.

Competing Interests: The authors have declared that no competing interests exist.

* E-mail: mmontass@medicine.umaryland.edu

¤ Current address: Division of Endocrinology, Diabetes, and Nutrition, Department of Medicine, University of Maryland School of Medicine, Baltimore, Maryland, United States of America

Introduction

Chronic kidney disease (CKD) is a major risk factor for cardiovascular disease and all-cause mortality, placing a huge burden on the health care system [1,2]. CKD is a complex trait, regulated by interactions of several environmental and genetic factors [3]. CKD can arise as a consequence of diabetes, hypertension, immunologic disorders (such as lupus or primary glomerulonephritis), and a variety of other exposures. While the genetic causes of monogenic forms of renal diseases are well established, those contributing to the common forms of CKD are still largely unknown [4]. Recent meta analyses of genome wide association studies (GWAS) identified several loci for kidney function indices and CKD, collectively explaining a very small fraction of the variability of these traits, leaving most of their genetic components undetermined [5]. Earlier linkage analyses and candidate gene studies also produced inconsistent or unconfirmed results [6–9]. Most study populations were ascertained on the basis of disease status, resulting in enrichment for diabetes, obesity, and hypertension, thus complicating genetic studies of CKD [10,11].

Genetic studies of CKD can benefit from a pathway-based targeted approach that includes testing for genetics and environmental interactions [12] for an intermediate quantitative trait [13] such as glomerular filtration rate (GFR) that is widely used to measure kidney function. GFR is a complex trait with an estimated heritability of 25–75% [14]. However, only about 1.5% of its variability has been explained by the genetic loci that have been identified so far [5].

In the current study, we examined the genetic factors that may influence GFR in rural Chinese participants of the "Genetic Epidemiology Network of Salt Sensitivity" (GenSalt) study, who did not have clinical evidence of overt CKD. Estimated GFR (eGFR) values were calculated from serum creatinine measurements obtained during a three-day observation period preceding dietary intervention, while the participants consumed their usual diet. We tested single nucleotide polymorphisms (SNPs) in 26 genes from pathways of blood pressure regulation for association with eGFR measures. This genetic study of GFR provides insight into the genetic determinants of kidney function in a general population sample of individuals without CKD, and potentially into the initiation and progression of CKD.

Materials and Methods

Ethics statement

Institutional review boards at Tulane University Health Sciences Center, Washington University School of Medicine, University of Texas School of Public Health, Fu Wai Hospital and Chinese National Human Genome Center at Beijing, Chinese Academy of Medical Sciences approved the GenSalt study. Written informed consents for the baseline observation and for the intervention program were obtained from each participant.

Study population

The GenSalt Study was conducted in Han Chinese families living in six rural villages in Northern China. Families were recruited through 18–60 year old probands who were either prehypertensive or had stage-1 hypertension (SBP 130–160 mm Hg and/or DBP 85–100 mm Hg), but had never been treated with antihypertensive medication. Parents, spouses, siblings, and offspring were invited to participate in the study. Family members were excluded if they had stage-2 hypertension, a history of CVD, diabetes, or heavy alcohol consumption, or were pregnant, on a low sodium diet or taking anti-hypertensive medications. A total of 3,025 individuals in 631 families participated in this study. A large number of demographic, anthropomorphic, and medical variables were measured in GenSalt participants. More information regarding participants recruitment and measurements are available elsewhere [15]. Institutional Review Board approval for this study was obtained at all of the participating institutions and all study participants signed an informed consent document.

Phenotype measurements

Serum creatinine was measured during a 3-day baseline observation period while the study participants consumed their usual diet prior to a GenSalt dietary intervention. During this period, an overnight fasting blood sample was obtained from each participant by venipuncture. This was used to measure serum creatinine by the modified kinetic Jaffe reaction method. GFR was estimated using an amended formulation of the Modification of Diet in Renal Disease (MDRD) study equation, specifically designed for use in healthy individuals [16]: eGFR in mL/min per $1.73 \text{ m}^2 = 216 \times$ (serum creatinine in mg/dL)$^{-0.490} \times$ (age in years)$^{-0.192} \times 0.923$ (if female).

Gene and SNP selection and genotyping

The GenSalt genotyping effort focused on 26 blood pressure candidate genes. The genes were selected based on their presumed role in blood pressure homeostasis and being a part of blood pressure regulation pathways such as the renin angiotensinsystem (*REN, RENBP, AGT, AT2R1, AT2R2, ACE*), the aldosterone system (*CYP11B1, CYP11B2, MLR, HSD11B1, HSD11B2, CYP3A5*), the endothelial system (*EDN1, NOS3, SELE*), the sympathetic nervous system (*GRK4, ADRB2*), alternative renin angiotensinsystem pathway (*ACE2, APLN, AGTRL1*), as well as atrial natriuretic peptide genes (*NPR3, NPPA*), sodium channels genes (*SCNN1B, SCNN1G*), and intracellular messengers genes (*GNB3, ADD1*). We selected 234 SNPs within these genes based on linkage disequilibrium (LD) structure in the Chinese population from the International HapMap project [17]. SNP genotyping was performed using the SNPlex platform (Applied Biosystems, Foster City CA) according to the manufacturer's protocol [18]. We excluded 41 SNPs in three genes from the association analysis due to low call rate (<80%), low minor allele frequency (MAF <0.05), or severe deviation from Hardy-Weinberg Equilibrium (HWE) (p<0.001). Detailed information concerning the remaining 193 SNPs within 24 genes is listed in **Table S1**.

Statistical analysis

Plink and PedCheck programs were used to assess the Mendelian consistency of SNP genotype data [19,20]. Programs from the Affected-Sib-Pair Interval Mapping and Exclusion package (ASPEX) and the Graphical Representation of Relationships (GRR) package were used to check for potential misreported relationships within pedigrees [21,22]. Haploview (Broad Institute, Boston MA) was used for SNP descriptive statistics [23]. The Generalized Estimation Equation (GEE) method was used to test for associations between eGFR and the genetic variants, accounting for familial correlation [24]. Values for eGFR were adjusted for significant covariates including age, age^2, age^3, gender, BMI, high density lipoprotein cholesterol (HDL-C), hypertension, and field center. Neither smoking nor alcohol consumption was significantly associated with eGFR and were not included as covariates in statistical analysis. GEE analysis was performed with SAS 9.1 using proc genmod, and exchangeable working correlation matrix. False Discovery Rate (FDR) was used to correct for the multiple testing in GEE analysis [25]. For interactions among genes, we used the Generalized Multifactor Dimensionality Reduction program (GMDR) [26] to determine joint effects of each pair of SNPs. The best model identified by GMDR for eGFR was verified using GEE to account for familial correlation. Several web algorithms and data bases were used for SNP annotation and bioinformatics analysis including UCSC [27], SNPnexus [28,29], PolyPhen-2 [30], SIFT [31], and FastSNP [32].

Results

Table 1 presents the basic characteristics of the 3,025 GenSalt participants who were included in this study. The study sample consisted of healthy free living members of three-generation families with an average age of 50 years, and approximately equal proportions of males and females. Their average values for BMI, HDL-C, serum creatinine, and eGFR were all within normal ranges. **Table S1** shows characteristics of the 193 SNPs within 26 loci involved in blood pressure regulation that were chosen according to LD in the Han Chinese population (International HapMap project).

Table 2 presents results of genetic analysis that identified 12 SNPs in six genes that showed significant associations with eGFR (p<0.05). The four significant SNPs in *ACE* were highly correlated with r^2 ranging from 0.78 to 0.96. The three SNPs in the hydroxysteroid 11-beta dehydrogenase 1 gene (*HSD11B1*) were less correlated (r^2 from 0.35 to 0.43), and the two significant SNPs in the alpha-adducin gene (*ADD1*) were not significantly correlated (r^2 = 0.17). The FDR for all significant p-values was 0.59, which means that seven of these 12 significant SNPs might have been false positives. **Figure 1** shows the average eGFR values for each of the three genotypes for nine of the significant SNPs (excluding three highly correlated *ACE* SNPs). Three of the significant SNPs (AGT_rs4762, GRK4_rs2488815, and SCNN1G_rs4299163) can be considered as risk SNPs where the additive effect of the minor allele was associated with lower values of eGFR. The other

Table 1. Basic characteristics of the study subjects.

	Healthy subjects
N	3025
Age	50.0± 16.6
Male %	51.3
Hypertension %	17
Smokers %	34.5
Alcohol consumers %	27
Body Mass Index	23.1 ± 3.2
HDL (mg/dL)	51.47 ± 11.3
Serum creatinine (mg/dL)	0.93 ± 0.21
eGFR (mL/min per 1.73 m²)	104.91 ± 14.07

HDL: High Density Lipoprotein, eGFR: estimated Glomerular Filtration Rate. Values are mean ± standard deviation for Age, Body Mass Index, HDL, serum creatinine, and eGFR.

significant SNPs can be considered as protective, where the minor allele was associated with higher eGFR values.

Figure 2 shows the cumulative effects on mean adjusted eGFR values for carriers of the minor alleles for all nine significant SNPs (**Panel A**) and separately for the six protective alleles (**Panel B**) and three risk alleles (**Panel C**). Carriers with increasing numbers of the minor protective alleles had up to more than 4 mL/min per 1.73 m² higher mean eGFR values (p = 0.001) (**Figure 2, Panel B**). Carriers with increasing numbers of the minor risk alleles had mean eGFR values that were as much as almost 3 mL/min per 1.73 m² lower (p = 0.006) (**Figure 2, Panel C**).

We also tested the SNPs for effects of gene by gene interactions (GxG) on eGFR. We identified a joint effect on eGFR between a nonsynonymous SNP in the gene for cytochrome P450, family 11, subfamily B, polypeptide 1 (CYP11B1_rs4541, Ala386Val) and a synonymous SNP in the beta-2-adrenergic receptor gene (ADRB2_rs1042718). **Figure 3** shows the joint effects on mean eGFR values of interactions between CYP11B1_rs4541 and ADRB2_rs1042718 genotypes. The mean adjusted eGFR value

in homozygotes for the ADRB2_rs1042718 minor allele (AA) depended on their genotype for CYP11B1_rs4541. Homozygotes for the minor allele of ADRB2_rs1042718 (AA) who are also homozygous for the major allele of CYP11B1_rs4541 (CC) had the lowest mean eGFR values. Homozygotes for the minor allele of ADRB2_rs1042718 (AA) who are heterozygous for CYP11B1_rs4541 (CT) had the highest eGFR. The difference between these two joint genotypes was approximately 5 mL/min per 1.73 m².

Discussion

The overall goal of this study was to conduct a comprehensive examination of the effects of variability in genes from pathways of blood pressure regulation on renal GFR. The GenSalt study cohort was comprised of rural Han Chinese villagers to minimize the genetic heterogeneity that is encountered in most association studies that are conducted in admixed urban populations. None of our study participants were taking antihypertensive medication, so the complexity associated with the antihypertensive drugs is absent from our study. In addition, we employed an amended version of the MDRD eGFR equation that was specifically designed for use in healthy free living individuals and eliminated the underestimation of GFR with the equation that was previously in use [16].

In our analyses of individual SNPs, the Thr207Met polymorphism (rs4762) in the angiotensinogen gene (*AGT*) showed the strongest association with eGFR (**Table 2**). *AGT* plays a role in the renin-angiotensin system (RAS), a primary pathway in blood pressure regulation with strong influences on cardiovascular and renal disease. *AGT* encodes preangiotensinogen in the liver, which is subsequently cleaved by renin to generate angiotensin I. Angiotensin I converting enzyme (*ACE*), converts angiontensin I to angiotensin II [33,34], a potent vasoconstrictor that also affects renal hemodynamics by decreasing renal cortical blood flow, total renal plasma flow, urinary sodium excretion, and GFR [33,34]. Moreover, angiotensin II increases glomerular capillary pressure, potentially contributing to glomerulosclerosis [35,36]. *AGT*_rs4762 (Thr207Met) is a probably damaging SNP [30,31] as it substitutes a non-polar amino acid (methionine) for a polar amino acid (threonine). Furthermore, threonine at this position in *AGT* is highly conserved among divergent species ranging from

Table 2. SNPs that showed significant associations with eGFR in GenSalt participants.

Gene	Chr.	SNP	Region	HWpval	Call Rate	MAF	Maj/Min	P*
ACE	17	rs4316	exon	0.0917	97.2	0.353	T/C	0.0077
ACE	17	rs4343	exon	0.4012	92.7	0.354	A/G	0.0170
ACE	17	rs4353	intron	0.2622	97.6	0.393	G/A	0.0181
ACE	17	rs4331	exon	0.2927	96.2	0.353	G/A	0.0313
ADD1	4	rs3775067	intron	0.934	97.1	0.34	C/T	0.0061
ADD1	4	rs12503220	utr	0.3043	93.1	0.134	G/A	0.0231
AGT	1	rs4762	exon	0.3746	95.6	0.073	C/T	0.0051
GRK4	4	rs2488815	intron	0.0255	96.7	0.206	C/T	0.0279
HSD11B1	1	rs4844880	utr	0.6649	89.5	0.356	T/A	0.0166
HSD11B1	1	rs2235543	utr	0.0703	92.5	0.35	C/T	0.0308
HSD11B1	1	rs846908	intergenic	0.9629	92.5	0.251	G/A	0.0419
SCNN1G	16	rs4299163	intron	0.8433	96.6	0.103	G/C	0.0247

HWpval: Hardy-Weinberg p value, MAF: minor allele frequency, Maj/Min: Major/Minor allele.
*p values adjusted for age, age², age³, gender, BMI, high density lipoprotein cholesterol (HDL-C), hypertension, field center, and family structure.

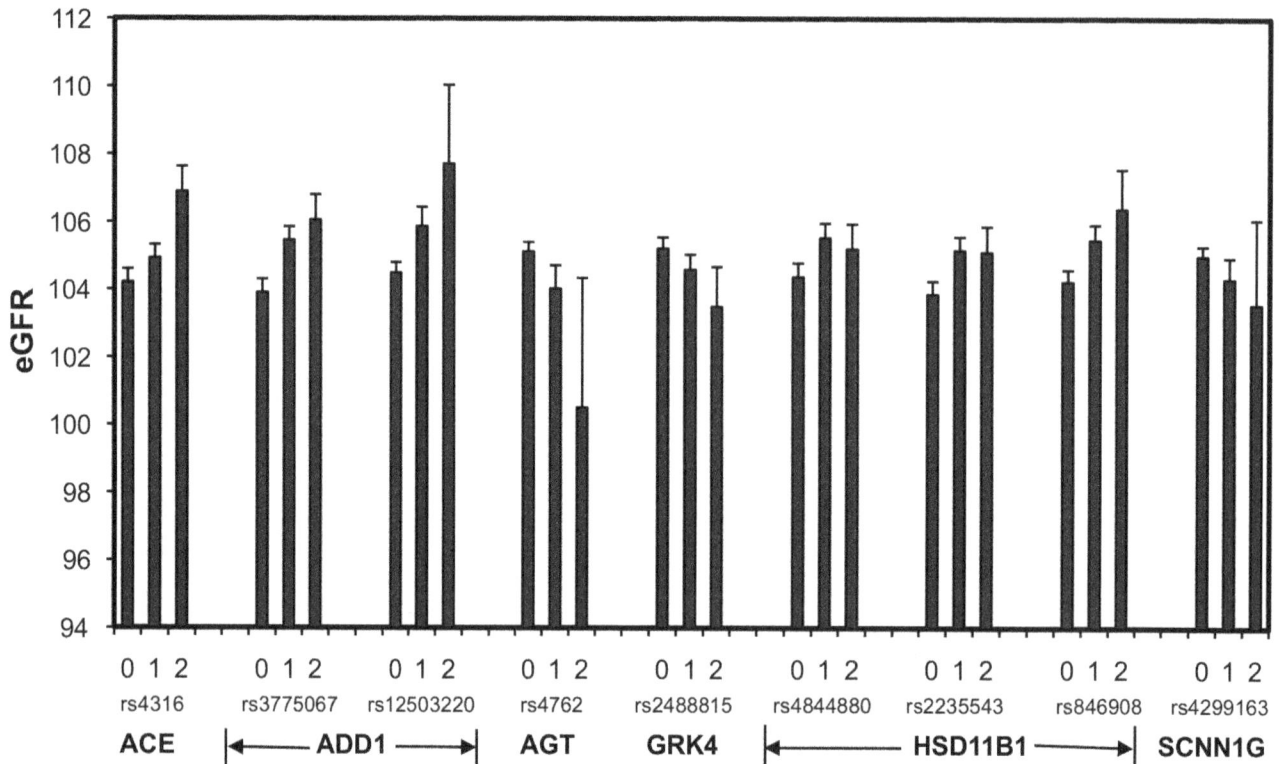

Figure 1. Mean eGFR values and standard errors for genotypes of SNPs that showed significant associations (0, homozygotes for common alleles; 1, heterozygotes; 2, homozygotes for minor alleles).

human to zebrafish [37]. Previous studies in Asians have identified associations of AGT_rs4762 with diabetic nephropathy in Taiwanese patients [38] and hypertension in different Asian populations based on meta-analysis [37].

We also found significant associations with eGFR for four correlated SNPs in the *ACE* gene, another key player in the RAS pathway of blood pressure regulation. Three of these SNPs (ACE_rs4316, ACE_rs4331, ACE_rs4343) are exonic variants, but do not cause amino acid substitutions (synonymous SNPs). ACE_rs4343, was previously reported to be significantly associated with diabetic nephropathy in an Asian Indian population [39].

Our analysis identified a significant association of eGFR with two intronic SNPs (rs3775067 and rs12503220) in the adducin 1 gene (*ADD1*). *ADD1* encodes the alpha subunit of the cytoskeleton protein adducin, which plays an important role in hypertension and renal function via sodium homeostasis [40]. Many previous studies have reported associations of *ADD1* variants with hypertension, renal functions and renal diseases, in different populations including Chinese [40–48].

Another SNP that showed associations in our study was rs2488815, an intronic SNP in the G protein_coupled receptor kinase 4 (*GRK4*) gene, a major player in sodium homeostasis and blood pressure regulation [49]. *GRK4* is expressed in the renal proximal tubule, where about 70% of renal sodium reabsorption takes place. Increased *GRK4* activity leads to decreased dopamine signaling and increased AngII receptor expression and function, both of which increase sodium retention and blood volume which ultimately leads to hypertension [50,51]. *GRK4* variants have been shown to be associated with hypertension and blood pressure traits in different populations including Han Chinese [52].

Three SNPs in the hydroxysteroid 11beta dehydrogenase1 gene (*HSD11B1*) were associated with eGFR in the current study. *HSD11B1* is a NADP dependent enzyme that functions in the proximal tubule and medullary interstitial cells of the human kidney. *HSD11B1* plays a role in the metabolism of the endogenous glucocorticoids, which in turn modulate sodium homeostasis, renal blood flow, and GFR [53]. *HSD11B1* enzymatic activities are thought to be involved in obesity, hypertension, and other components of the metabolic syndrome. *HSD11B1* overexpression in mice has been associated with dose-dependent hypertension and *AGT* expression in liver [54–56].

Our analyses of individual SNPs identified associations of eGFR with an intronic SNP (rs4299163) in the gene encoding the gamma subunit of the epithelial sodium channel gene (*SCNN1G*). Epithelial sodium channels (*ENaC*), are the main regulators for sodium transport in the kidney [57,58], and rare variants in *SCNN1G* cause Liddle Syndrome, a monogenic form of hypertension [59]. Other variants in *SCNN1G* cause pseudohypoaldosteronism type 1, a rare inherited form of renal tubular acidosis [60,61]. Many studies have identified linkage of SBP with the region that contains *SCNN1G* on chromosome 16 [62]. A fine mapping study of this region detected associations of SBP with three *SCNN1G* intronic SNPs, including rs4299163 [62].

In addition to analyses of individual SNPs, we tested for interactions among genes (GxG interactions) that influence eGFR. Our GxG analyses identified a joint effect on eGFR between a conservative nonsynonymous SNP rs4541 (Ala386Val) in *CYP11B1* and a synonymous SNP rs1042718 in *ADRB2*. *CYP11B1* is one of the cytochrome p450 genes encoding 11β hydroxylase, a protein involved in the synthesis of cortisol in the adrenal cortex [63]. Cortisol is associated with Cushing's syndrome, hypertension

A

B

C

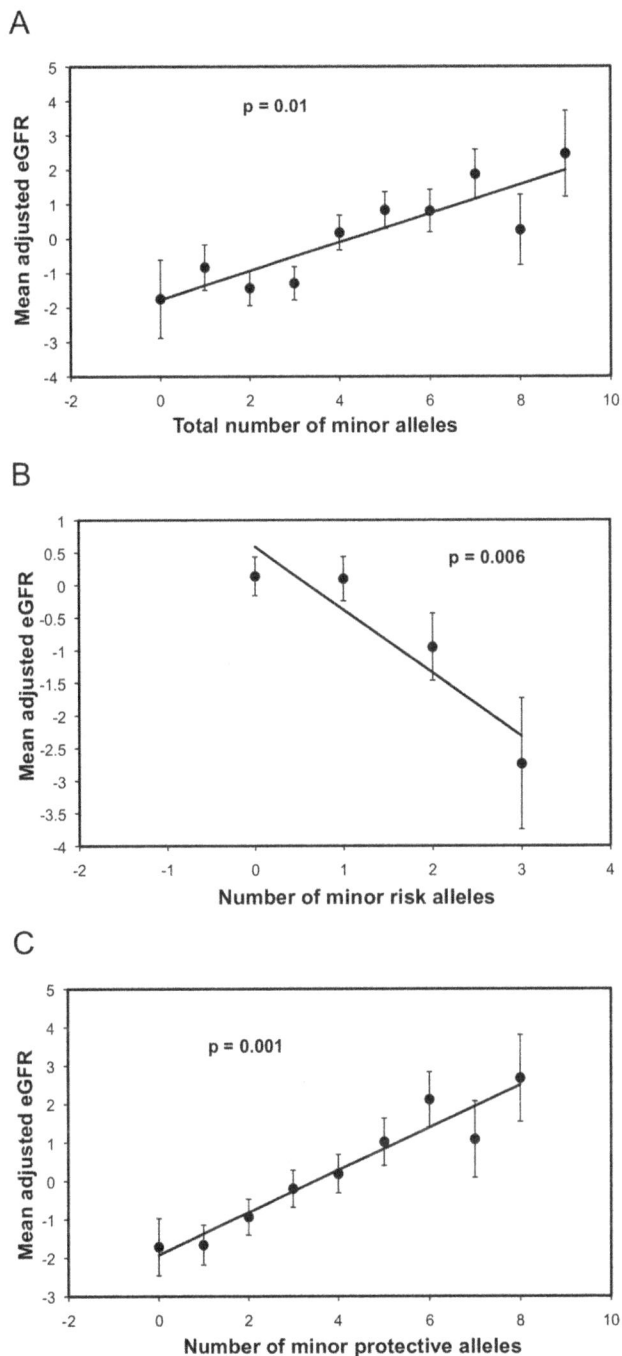

Figure 2. The cumulative effect of the minor alleles in all of the 9 significant SNPs (Panel A), the 6 protective SNPs (Panel B), and the 3 risk SNPs (Panel C) on the value of the mean adjusted eGFR. The best fitting trend line and p value from t-tests between those with no minor allele and those with the largest possible number of minor alleles in each category are shown.

Figure 3. Mean adjusted eGFR as a result of the genotypic interaction between CYP11B1_rs4541 and ADRB2_rs1042718. The data points represent the eGFR for the nine possible combinations of the three *ADRB2* genotypes versus each of the three possible *CYP11B1* genotypes. The number of individuals at each point is provided.

resistance [67,68]. *ADRB2* SNPs were previously found to be associated with hypertension and blood pressure traits in different populations including Han Chinese but many of the results are inconsistent [68–70]. ADRB2_rs1042718, the SNP showing significant GxG interaction, is part of a haplotype recently found to be associated with weight, insulin, and homeostasis model assessment (HOMA) score in Korean adolescents [71]. The exact mechanism of interaction between these two coding region SNPs in relation to eGFR warrants further investigation.

We compared the results of our association study with a recently published meta-analysis of kidney function traits in several East Asian populations, including GenSalt [72]. The SNPs with significant associations in our study (Table 2) were not significantly associated with eGFR in the meta-analysis. This discrepancy could stem from differences in the study populations since we included only Han Chinese from Northern China, while the meta-analysis included Japanese, Malay, Indian, Korean, and Chinese. GenSalt participants were relatively healthy free living individuals from three-generation families, while the meta-analysis included hospital and population based cohorts with no exclusion of diseased individuals. In addition, we employed an equation to calculate eGFR that was specifically designed for use in healthy individuals [16], while the meta-analysis used a different equation specific for Japanese individuals [73].

The genes included in this study were all in pathways known to be involved in regulation of blood pressure which may play an important role in regulating kidney function. However, there are established overlaps, such as the RAS pathway which is involved in renal function decline since treatment of patients with renin-angiotensin inhibitors slows the progression of kidney disease [74–76]. Such protective effect of RAS blocking on kidney function may be through both blood pressure and non-blood pressure dependent mechanisms. Our study was not designed to determine whether these genes impact GFR independent of their effects on blood pressure, or whether their effects on GFR are linked to the same pathophysiologic cascades as their involvement in hyperten-

of chronic renal failure, hypertension related to low birth weight, and essential hypertension [64,65]. Glucocorticoid-Remediable Aldosteronism, a rare form of hypertension, is caused by a gene fusion between *CYP11B1* and *CYP11B2* [66]. *ADRB2* encodes the beta 2 adrenergic receptor, a member of the G-protein superfamily receptors, playing a role in metabolism regulation and also in blood pressure regulation by mediating vasodilation and vascular

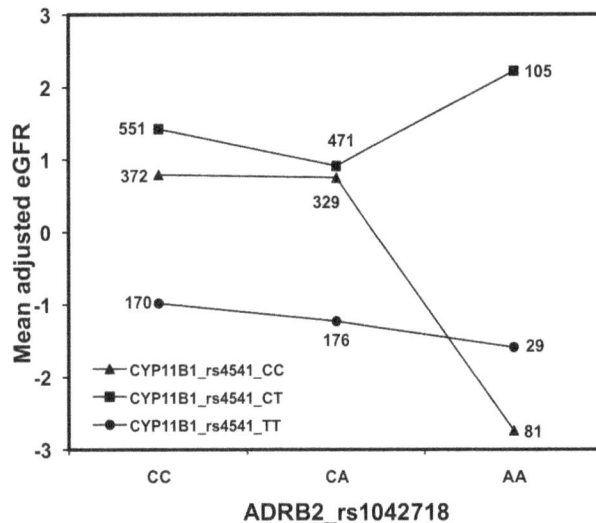

sion. However, their significant association with kidney function remains after adjustment for hypertension.

In conclusion, we have identified common variants in genes from pathways of blood pressure regulation and their interactions that influence kidney function, providing new insights into the genetic determinants of kidney function. A longitudinal association between these common variants and changes in kidney function remains to be investigated.

Acknowledgments

GenSalt Study Steering Committee
Dongfeng Gu, Jiang He (Chair), James E Hixson, Cashell E Jaquish, Depei Liu, Dabeeru C. Rao, Paul K Whelton, and Zhijian Yao.
GenSalt Collaborative Research Group
Tulane University Health Sciences Center, New Orleans, USA: Jiang He (PI), Lydia A Bazzano, Chung-Shiuan Chen, Jing Chen, Mei Hao, Lotuce Lee Hamm, Tanika Kelly, Paul Muntner, Kristi Reynolds, Paul K Whelton, Wenjie Yang, and Qi Zhao.
Washington University School of Medicine, St Louis, USA: Dabeeru C. Rao (PI), Matthew Brown, Charles Gu, Hongyan Huang, Treva Rice, Karen Schwander, and Shiping Wang.
University of Texas Health Sciences Center at Houston: James E Hixson (PI) and Lawrence C Shimmin.
National Heart, Lung, and Blood Institute: Cashell E Jaquish.

Chinese Academy of Medical Sciences, Beijing, China: Dongfeng Gu (PI), Jie Cao, Jichun Chen, Jingping Chen, Zhenhan Du, Jianfeng Huang, Hongwen Jiang, Jianxin Li, Xiaohua Liang, Depei Liu, Xiangfeng Lu, Donghua Liu, Qunxia Mao, Dongling Sun, Hongwei Wang, Qianqian Wang, Xigui Wu, Ying Yang, and Dahai Yu.
Shandong Academy of Medical Sciences, Shandong, China: Fanghong Lu (PI), Zhendong Liu, Shikuan Jin, Yingxin Zhao, Shangwen Sun, Shujian Wang, Qengjie Meng, Baojin Liu, Zhaodong Yang, and Chuanrui Wei.
Shandong Center for Diseases Control and Prevention, Shandong, China: Jixiang Ma (PI), Jiyu Zhang, and Junli Tang.
Zhengzhou University: Dongsheng Hu, Hongwei Wen, Chongjian Wang, Minghui Shen, Jingjing Pan, and Liming Yang.
Xinle Traditional Chinese Medicine Hospital, Hebei, China: Xu Ji (PI), Rongyan Li, Haijun Zu, and Junwei Song.
Ganyu Center for Disease Control and Prevention: Delin Wu (PI), Xushan Wang, and Xiaofeng Zhang.
Xi'an Jiaotong University, Shanxi, China: Jianjun Mu (PI), Enrang Chen,Fuqiang Liu, and Guanji Wu.
Chinese National Human Genome Center at Beijing: Zhi-Jian Yao (PI), Shufeng Chen, Dongfeng Gu, Hongfan Li, Laiyuan Wang, and Penghua Zhang.
The Asian Genetic Epidemiology Network (AGEN): Toshihiro Tanaka.

Author Contributions

Conceived and designed the experiments: DG Jing Chen CG TNK CEJ TR DCR Jie Cao Jichun Chen DPL PW LLH JH JEH. Performed the experiments: LCS DG Jing Chen CG TNK TR DCR Jie Cao Jichun Chen JH JEH. Analyzed the data: MEM. Wrote the paper: MEM LCS TR PW LLH JEH.

References

1. Centers for Disease Control and Prevention (CDC) (2007) Prevalence of chronic kidney disease and associated risk factors-United States, 1999–2004. MMWR Morb Mortal Wkly Rep 56: 161–165.
2. Saran AM, DuBose TD Jr (2008) Cardiovascular disease in chronic kidney disease. Ther Adv Cardiovasc Dis 2: 425–434.
3. Arar NH, Voruganti VS, Nath SD, Thameem F, Bauer R, et al. (2008) A genome-wide search for linkage to chronic kidney disease in a community-based sample: The SAFHS. Nephrol Dial Transplant 23: 3184–3191.
4. Benoit G, Machuca E, Heidet L, Antignac C (2010) Hereditary kidney diseases: Highlighting the importance of classical mendelian phenotypes. Ann N Y Acad Sci 1214: 83–98.
5. Boger CA, Heid IM (2011) Chronic kidney disease: Novel insights from genome-wide association studies. Kidney Blood Press Res 34: 225–234.
6. de Borst MH, Benigni A, Remuzzi G (2008) Primer: Strategies for identifying genes involved in renal disease. Nat Clin Pract Nephrol 4: 265–276.
7. Freedman BI, Bostrom M, Daeihagh P, Bowden DW (2007) Genetic factors in diabetic nephropathy. Clin J Am Soc Nephrol 2: 1306–1316.
8. Maeda S (2008) Genetics of diabetic nephropathy. Ther Adv Cardiovasc Dis 2: 363–371.
9. Adler S (2006) Renal disease: Environment, race, or genes? Ethn Dis 16: S2-35-9.
10. Fox CS, Yang Q, Cupples LA, Guo CY, Larson MG, et al. (2004) Genomewide linkage analysis to serum creatinine, GFR, and creatinine clearance in a community-based population: The framingham heart study. J Am Soc Nephrol 15: 2457–2461.
11. Schelling JR, Abboud HE, Nicholas SB, Pahl MV, Sedor JR, et al. (2008) Genome-wide scan for estimated glomerular filtration rate in multi-ethnic diabetic populations: The family investigation of nephropathy and diabetes (FIND). Diabetes 57: 235–243.
12. Basson J, Simino J, Rao DC (2012) Between candidate genes and whole genomes: Time for alternative approaches in blood pressure genetics. Curr Hypertens Rep 14: 46–61.
13. Carlson CS, Eberle MA, Kruglyak L, Nickerson DA (2004) Mapping complex disease loci in whole-genome association studies. Nature 429: 446–452.
14. Kiryluk K (2008) Quantitative genetics of renal function: Tackling complexities of the eGFR phenotype in gene mapping studies. Kidney Int 74: 1109–1112.
15. GenSalt Collaborative Research Group (2007) GenSalt: Rationale, design, methods and baseline characteristics of study participants. J Hum Hypertens 21: 639–646.
16. Rule AD, Larson TS, Bergstralh EJ, Slezak JM, Jacobsen SJ, et al. (2004) Using serum creatinine to estimate glomerular filtration rate: Accuracy in good health and in chronic kidney disease. Ann Intern Med 141: 929–937.

17. The International HapMap Consortium (2003) The international HapMap project. Nature 426: 789–796.
18. Tobler AR, Short S, Andersen MR, Paner TM, Briggs JC, et al. (2005) The SNPlex genotyping system: A flexible and scalable platform for SNP genotyping. J Biomol Tech 16: 398–406.
19. Purcell S, Neale B, Todd-Brown K, Thomas L, Ferreira MA, et al. (2007) PLINK: A tool set for whole-genome association and population-based linkage analyses. Am J Hum Genet 81: 559–575.
20. O'Connell JR, Weeks DE (1998) PedCheck: A program for identification of genotype incompatibilities in linkage analysis. Am J Hum Genet 63: 259–266.
21. Hinds DR (1999) The ASPEX package:Affected sib-pair exclusion mapping v1.88.
22. Abecasis GR, Cherny SS, Cookson WO, Cardon LR (2001) GRR: Graphical representation of relationship errors. Bioinformatics 17: 742–743.
23. Barrett JC, Fry B, Maller J, Daly MJ (2005) Haploview: Analysis and visualization of LD and haplotype maps. Bioinformatics 21: 263–265.
24. Hanley JA, Negassa A, Edwardes MD, Forrester JE (2003) Statistical analysis of correlated data using generalized estimating equations: An orientation. Am J Epidemiol 157: 364–375.
25. Benjamini Y, Hochberg Y (1995) Controlling the false discovery rate: A practical and powerful approach to multiple testing. Journal of the Royal Statistical Society. Series B (Methodological) 57: 289–300.
26. Lou XY, Chen GB, Yan L, Ma JZ, Zhu J, et al. (2007) A generalized combinatorial approach for detecting gene-by-gene and gene-by-environment interactions with application to nicotine dependence. Am J Hum Genet 80: 1125–1137.
27. University of California Santa Cruz (UCSC) genome browser website. Available: http://genome.ucsc.edu/, 2013.
28. Dayem Ullah AZ, Lemoine NR, Chelala C (2012) SNPnexus: A web server for functional annotation of novel and publicly known genetic variants (2012 update). Nucleic Acids Res 40: W65–70.
29. Chelala C, Khan A, Lemoine NR (2009) SNPnexus: A web database for functional annotation of newly discovered and public domain single nucleotide polymorphisms. Bioinformatics 25: 655–661.
30. Adzhubei IA, Schmidt S, Peshkin L, Ramensky VE, Gerasimova A, et al. (2010) A method and server for predicting damaging missense mutations. Nat Methods 7: 248–249.
31. Kumar P, Henikoff S, Ng PC (2009) Predicting the effects of coding non-synonymous variants on protein function using the SIFT algorithm. Nat Protoc 4: 1073–1081.
32. Yuan HY, Chiou JJ, Tseng WH, Liu CH, Liu CK, et al. (2006) FASTSNP: An always up-to-date and extendable service for SNP function analysis and prioritization. Nucleic Acids Res 34: W635-41.

33. Phillips JK (2005) Pathogenesis of hypertension in renal failure: Role of the sympathetic nervous system and renal afferents. Clin Exp Pharmacol Physiol 32: 415–418.

34. Ritz E, Adamczak M, Zeier M (2003) Kidney and hypertension-causes. update 2003. Herz 28: 663–667.

35. Kim S, Iwao H (2000) Molecular and cellular mechanisms of angiotensin II-mediated cardiovascular and renal diseases. Pharmacol Rev 52: 11–34.

36. Ichihara A, Kobori H, Nishiyama A, Navar LG (2004) Renal renin-angiotensin system. Contrib Nephrol 143: 117–130.

37. Pereira TV, Nunes AC, Rudnicki M, Yamada Y, Pereira AC, et al. (2008) Meta-analysis of the association of 4 angiotensinogen polymorphisms with essential hypertension: A role beyond M235T? Hypertension 51: 778–783.

38. Chang HR, Cheng CH, Shu KH, Chen CH, Lian JD, et al. (2003) Study of the polymorphism of angiotensinogen, anigiotensin-converting enzyme and angiotensin receptor in type II diabetes with end-stage renal disease in Taiwan. J Chin Med Assoc 66: 51–56.

39. Ahluwalia TS, Ahuja M, Rai TS, Kohli HS, Bhansali A, et al. (2009) ACE variants interact with the RAS pathway to confer risk and protection against type 2 diabetic nephropathy. DNA Cell Biol 28: 141–150.

40. Staessen JA, Bianchi G (2005) Adducin and hypertension. Pharmacogenomics 6: 665–669.

41. Shioji K, Kokubo Y, Mannami T, Inamoto N, Morisaki H, et al. (2004) Association between hypertension and the alpha-adducin, beta1-adrenoreceptor, and G-protein beta3 subunit genes in the Japanese population; the suita study. Hypertens Res 27: 31–37.

42. Wang JG, Staessen JA, Barlassina C, Fagard R, Kuznetsova T, et al. (2002) Association between hypertension and variation in the alpha- and beta-adducin genes in a white population. Kidney Int 62: 2152–2159.

43. Ju Z, Zhang H, Sun K, Song Y, Lu H, et al. (2003) Alpha-adducin gene polymorphism is associated with essential hypertension in Chinese: A case-control and family-based study. J Hypertens 21: 1861–1868.

44. Yamagishi K, Iso H, Tanigawa T, Cui R, Kudo M, et al. (2004) Alpha-adducin G460W polymorphism, urinary sodium excretion, and blood pressure in community-based samples. Am J Hypertens 17: 385–390.

45. Bray MS, Li L, Turner ST, Kardia SL, Boerwinkle E (2000) Association and linkage analysis of the alpha-adducin gene and blood pressure. Am J Hypertens 13: 699–703.

46. Bianchi G, Ferrari P, Staessen JA (2005) Adducin polymorphism: Detection and impact on hypertension and related disorders. Hypertension 45: 331–340.

47. Huang XH, Sun K, Song Y, Zhang HY, Yang Y, et al. (2007) Association of alpha-adducin gene and G-protein beta3-subunit gene with essential hypertension in Chinese. Zhonghua Yi Xue Za Zhi 87: 1682–1684.

48. He X, Zhu DL, Chu SL, Jin L, Xiong MM, et al. (2001) Alpha-adducin gene and essential hypertension in china. Clin Exp Hypertens 23: 579–589.

49. Jose PA, Soares-da-Silva P, Eisner GM, Felder RA (2010) Dopamine and G protein-coupled receptor kinase 4 in the kidney: Role in blood pressure regulation. Biochim Biophys Acta 1802: 1259–1267.

50. Morris BJ (2009) GRK4 genetics and response to beta-blocker. Am J Hypertens 22: 235–236.

51. Harris DM, Cohn HI, Pesant S, Eckhart AD (2008) GPCR signalling in hypertension: Role of GRKs. Clin Sci (Lond) 115: 79–89.

52. Zeng C, Villar VA, Eisner GM, Williams SM, Felder RA, et al. (2008) G protein-coupled receptor kinase 4: Role in blood pressure regulation. Hypertension 51: 1449–1455.

53. Gong R, Morris DJ, Brem AS (2008) Human renal 11beta-hydroxysteroid dehydrogenase 1 functions and co-localizes with COX-2. Life Sci 82: 631–637.

54. Paterson JM, Morton NM, Fievet C, Kenyon CJ, Holmes MC, et al. (2004) Metabolic syndrome without obesity: Hepatic overexpression of 11beta-hydroxysteroid dehydrogenase type 1 in transgenic mice. Proc Natl Acad Sci U S A 101: 7088–7093.

55. Stimson RH, Walker BR (2007) Glucocorticoids and 11beta-hydroxysteroid dehydrogenase type 1 in obesity and the metabolic syndrome. Minerva Endocrinol 32: 141–159.

56. Morton NM, Seckl JR (2008) 11beta-hydroxysteroid dehydrogenase type 1 and obesity. Front Horm Res 36: 146-164.

57. Tesson F, Leenen FH (2007) Still building on candidate-gene strategy in hypertension? Hypertension 50: 607–608.

58. Busst CJ, Bloomer LD, Scurrah KJ, Ellis JA, Barnes TA, et al. (2011) The epithelial sodium channel gamma-subunit gene and blood pressure: Family based association, renal gene expression, and physiological analyses. Hypertension 58: 1073–1078.

59. Warnock DG (2001) Liddle syndrome: Genetics and mechanisms of na+ channel defects. Am J Med Sci 322: 302–307.

60. Rodriguez-Soriano J (2000) New insights into the pathogenesis of renal tubular acidosis—from functional to molecular studies. Pediatr Nephrol 14: 1121–1136.

61. Strautnieks SS, Thompson RJ, Gardiner RM, Chung E (1996) A novel splice-site mutation in the gamma subunit of the epithelial sodium channel gene in three pseudohypoaldosteronism type 1 families. Nat Genet 13: 248–250.

62. Busst CJ, Scurrah KJ, Ellis JA, Harrap SB (2007) Selective genotyping reveals association between the epithelial sodium channel gamma-subunit and systolic blood pressure. Hypertension 50: 672–678.

63. Freel EM, Connell JM (2004) Mechanisms of hypertension: The expanding role of aldosterone. Journal of the American Society of Nephrology 15: 1993–2001.

64. Whitworth JA, Brown MA, Kelly JJ, Williamson PM (1995) Mechanisms of cortisol-induced hypertension in humans. Steroids 60: 76–80.

65. Kelly JJ, Mangos G, Williamson PM, Whitworth JA (1998) Cortisol and hypertension. Clin Exp Pharmacol Physiol Suppl 25: S51–6.

66. Dluhy RG, Lifton RP (1999) Glucocorticoid-remediable aldosteronism. J Clin Endocrinol Metab 84: 4341–4344.

67. Gjesing AP, Andersen G, Burgdorf KS, Borch-Johnsen K, Jorgensen T, et al. (2007) Studies of the associations between functional beta2-adrenergic receptor variants and obesity, hypertension and type 2 diabetes in 7,808 white subjects. Diabetologia 50: 563–568.

68. Brodde OE (2008) Beta-1 and beta-2 adrenoceptor polymorphisms: Functional importance, impact on cardiovascular diseases and drug responses. Pharmacol Ther 117: 1–29.

69. Yu SF, Zhou WH, Jiang KY, Gu GZ, Wang S (2008) Job stress, gene polymorphism of beta2-AR, and prevalence of hypertension. Biomed Environ Sci 21: 239–246.

70. Ge D, Huang J, He J, Li B, Duan X, et al. (2005) beta2-adrenergic receptor gene variations associated with stage-2 hypertension in northern Han Chinese. Ann Hum Genet 69: 36–44.

71. Park HS, Shin ES, Lee JE (2008) Genotypes and haplotypes of beta2-adrenergic receptor and parameters of the metabolic syndrome in Korean adolescents. Metabolism 57: 1064–1070.

72. Okada Y, Sim X, Go MJ, Wu JY, Gu D, et al. (2012) Meta-analysis identifies multiple loci associated with kidney function-related traits in east Asian populations. Nat Genet 44: 904–909.

73. Horio M, Imai E, Yasuda Y, Watanabe T, Matsuo S (2010) Modification of the CKD epidemiology collaboration (CKD-EPI) equation for Japanese: Accuracy and use for population estimates. Am J Kidney Dis 56: 32–38.

74. Lu X, Roksnoer LC, Danser AH (2013) The intrarenal renin-angiotensin system: Does it exist? implications from a recent study in renal angiotensin-converting enzyme knockout mice. Nephrol Dial Transplant 28: 2977–2982.

75. Kobori H, Nangaku M, Navar LG, Nishiyama A (2007) The intrarenal renin-angiotensin system: From physiology to the pathobiology of hypertension and kidney disease. Pharmacol Rev 59: 251–287.

76. Zhuo JL, Ferrao FM, Zheng Y, Li XC (2013) New frontiers in the intrarenal renin-angiotensin system: A critical review of classical and new paradigms. Front Endocrinol (Lausanne) 4: 166.

14

Acute Kidney Injury Urinary Biomarker Time-Courses

John W. Pickering[1]*, **Zoltán H. Endre**[2]

1 Department of Medicine, University of Otago Christchurch, Christchurch, New Zealand, **2** Department of Nephrology, Prince of Wales Clinical School, University of New South Wales, Sydney, Australia

Abstract

Factors which modify the excretion profiles of acute kidney injury biomarkers are difficult to measure. To facilitate biomarker choice and interpretation we modelled key modifying factors: extent of hyperfiltration or reduced glomerular filtration rate, structural damage, and reduced nephron number. The time-courses of pre-formed, induced (upregulated), and filtered biomarker concentrations were modelled in single nephrons, then combined to construct three multiple-nephron models: a healthy kidney with normal nephron number, a non-diabetic hyperfiltering kidney with reduced nephron number but maintained total glomerular filtration rate, and a chronic kidney disease kidney with reduced nephron number and reduced glomerular filtration rate. Time-courses for each model were derived for acute kidney injury scenarios of structural damage and/or reduced nephron number. The model predicted that pre-formed biomarkers would respond quickest to injury with a brief period of elevation, which would be easily missed in clinical scenarios. Induced biomarker time-courses would be influenced by biomarker-specific physiology and the balance between insult severity (which increased single nephron excretion), the number of remaining nephrons (reduced total excretion), and the extent of glomerular filtration rate reduction (increased concentration). Filtered biomarkers have the longest time-course because plasma levels increased following glomerular filtration rate decrease. Peak concentration and profile depended on the extent of damage to the reabsorption mechanism and recovery rate. Rapid recovery may be detected through a rapid reduction in urinary concentration. For all biomarkers, impaired hyperfiltration substantially increased concentration, especially with chronic kidney disease. For clinical validation of these model-derived predictions the clinical biomarker of choice will depend on timing in relation to renal insult and interpretation will require the pre-insult nephron number (renal mass) and detection of hyperfiltration.

Editor: Martin H. de Borst, University Medical Center Groningen and University of Groningen, Netherlands

Funding: 1. Marsden Grant UOO1020 administered by the Royal Society of New Zealand. 2. University of Otago Research Grant. The funders had no role in study design, data collection and analysis, decision to publish, or preparation of the manuscript.

Competing Interests: The authors have declared that no competing interests exist.

* Email: john.pickering@otago.ac.nz

Introduction

Proteomics and genomics have identified many candidate urinary biomarkers of acute kidney injury (AKI). The clinical utility of these biomarkers is dependent on the time at which they are sampled following renal injury [1,2]. Some biomarkers have very short time-courses [2] with an early peak followed by rapid decline, for example γ-glutymaltranspeptidase (GGT). Others peak later and have a slower decline, for example Neutrophil Gelatinase Associated Lipocalin (NGAL) [2–4]. Biomarker analysis has concentrated on the association between biomarker concentration and AKI defined by increased plasma creatinine concentration. Little is known about the comparative influence of change in glomerular filtration rate (GFR) and biomarker generation on urinary biomarker concentrations and time-courses. We mathematically modeled the single nephron excretion time-course for a step decrease in GFR for three classes of urinary biomarker, namely those which are: (i) pre-formed in the tubules and released into the urine during injury, (ii) induced or upregulated within the tubules, and (iii) first filtered by the glomerulus and possibly reabsorbed within the tubules. We then describe how urinary concentrations of these biomarkers depend on the pre-insult state of the kidney and the extent of both nephron loss and the GFR reduction in AKI.

Methods

The urinary biomarker concentration depends on the total mass of biomarker released into the urine and the total urine flow. The single nephron biomarker concentration varies as the mass of biomarker excreted into the urine ($E(t)$) divided by the single nephron urine flow rate ($snUFR$).

Single Nephron urine flow rate

The single nephron urine flow rate ($snUFR$) is the single nephron GFR ($snGFR$) minus the rate of water absorption in the proximal tubule (R_1) and in the distal tubule and collection duct (R_2):

$$snUFR = snGFR - (R_1 + R_2). \tag{1}$$

While R_1 may vary along with change in sodium reabsorption and R_2 may increase with increased anti-diuretic hormone activity, we have combined the two and modelled total reabsorption (R) as a percentage of GFR.

Pre-formed biomarkers

Let q_0 be the mass of pre-formed biomarker prior to an insult to the nephron. Let the duration of insult be t_i (from time 0). Under steady state conditions the rate of biomarker excretion into the nephron tubule equals the production rate. Let k_n be the normal rate constant for both excretion and production of the preformed biomarker. At equilibrium,

$$\text{rate of production} = \text{rate of excretion} = k_n q_0. \qquad (2)$$

During an insult $(t \le t_i)$, the rate of excretion depends on the available mass of biomarker, q, and the rate at which the insult results in further biomarker excretion (rate constant k_a). Therefore,

$$\text{rate of excretion} = E(t) = k_n q + k_a q. \qquad (3)$$

Therefore, the net rate of change in biomarker mass is,

$$\frac{dq}{dt} = \text{rate of production} - \text{rate of excretion} \qquad (4)$$

$$= k_n q_0 - (k_n + k_a) q \qquad (5)$$

which has the solution

$$q = q_0 (1 - \frac{k_n}{k_n + k_a}) e^{-(k_n + k_a)t} + \frac{k_n q_0}{k_n + k_a}. \qquad (6)$$

Substituting for q in equation 3 gives,

$$E(t) = q_0(k e^{-(k_n + k_a)t} + k_n) \qquad \text{at} \quad t \le t_i \qquad (7)$$

Following the insult $(t > t_i)$,

$$\text{rate of excretion} = E(t) = k_n q \qquad (8)$$

$$\frac{dq}{dt} = k_n q_0 - k_n q \qquad (9)$$

$$q = (q(t_i) - q_0) e^{-k_n(t - t_i)} + q_0 \qquad (10)$$

$$E(t) = k_n((q(t_i) - q_0) e^{-k_n(t - t_i)} + q_0) \qquad \text{at} \quad t > t_i \qquad (11)$$

Induced biomarkers

Induced biomarker gene expression after renal insult follow approximate log-normal distributions [5,6]. For the purpose of these simulations we assume that protein production follows mRNA expression. Therefore, we modelled the excretion of induced or up-regulated biomarkers, Figure 1c, as log-normal function following the start of insult,

$$E(t) = E_{ss} \left(C \left(\frac{1}{t \sigma \sqrt{2\pi}} e^{-\frac{(\log(t) - \mu)^2}{2\sigma^2}} \right) + 1 \right) \qquad (12)$$

where E_{ss} is the steady state excretion rate in the absence of injury, C is a constant which scales the total excretion, μ and σ are the mean and standard deviation.

The mean and standard deviations in equation 12 may be determined from the time from insult until peak biomarker excretion t_p and the time by which half of the total biomarker is excreted, t_m,

$$\mu = \log(t_m) \qquad (13)$$

$$\sigma = \sqrt{\mu - \log(t_p)} \qquad (14)$$

Filtered biomarkers

Let $F(t)$ be the rate the biomarker filters through the glomerulus, $S(t)$ the secretion rate, T_0 the normal (pre-insult) kidney maximum biomarker reabsorption rate, k_p the rate constant for production of receptors (eg megalin or cubulin), and k_l the rate constant for loss of receptors. Normally $k_p = k_l$ which means that the maximum absorption rate is T_0. If $F > T_0$ then the excretion rate will be,

$$E(t) = F(t) - T_0(e^{-k_l t} + 1 - e^{-k_p t}) + S(t). \qquad (15)$$

The rate of filtration may vary according to either a change in systemic rate of production of the biomarker or a change in GFR. The secretion rate may be zero, a constant, or in proportion to the plasma concentration of the biomarker. If the latter then $S(t)$ is proportional to $F(t)$ because both are proportional to the plasma concentration.

Single nephron scenarios

For each biomarker class three scenarios were constructed: (i) the extreme of no change in rate of single nephron biomarker excretion, but loss of $snGFR$ by 33.3%, 50%, or 66.7% for 48 hours (so called $snGFR$ positive/Biomarker negative), (ii) the extreme of no change in $snGFR$ but increases in biomarker excretion (so called $snGFR$ negative/Biomarker positive), (iii) loss of $snGFR$ and increase in biomarker excretion. For the pre-formed biomarker we compared the single nephron excretion time-courses for three durations of insults, namely 1 hour, 6 hours and 18 hours. For the induced biomarker we modelled peak biomarker excretion at 6 hours an 12 hours following insult, and allowed for half the total excretion to occur over 12, 15 or 24 hours. For the filtered biomarker we assumed a plasma half-life of 2 hours (e.g. as for Cystatin C) and varied the reabsorption factor through varying k_l. All time-courses are shown as fold increases from pre-insult single nephron urinary excretion.

Multiple nephron scenarios

Three kidney models were built,

1. **Healthy**: Two million normally functioning nephrons with pre-insult GFR ($g(0)$) of $100\,ml/min$. Reabsorption (R) was assumed to be 99% of GFR prior to injury, increasing to 99.5%

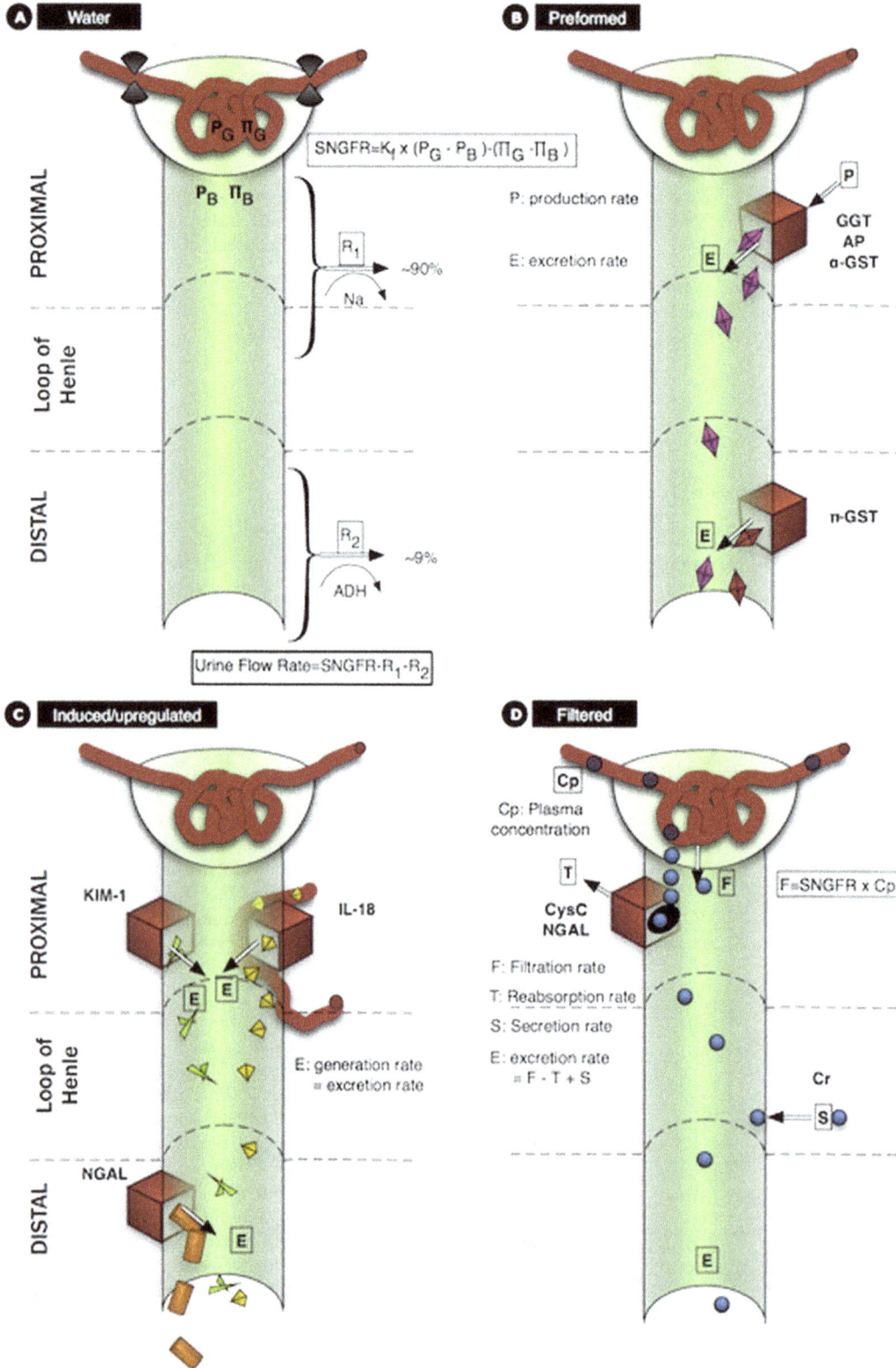

Figure 1. Single Nephron Models. A: Water reabsorption. B: Preformed biomarkers such as α-GST are excreted at a rate (E) dependent on the initial (remaining) mass of biomarker and the production rate (P) of new biomarker. C: Induced biomarkers such as KIM-1 are excreted at a rate approximating a log-normal distribution. D: Filtered biomarkers such as Cystatin C are filtered at a rate (F) dependent on the plasma concentration and single nephron GFR and then reabsorbed at a rate dependent on the number of available transporters (T). Some biomarkers are also secreted (S). The final excretion rate is the sum of the gains minus the losses. The final concentration depends on the excretion rate divided by the urine flow rate. Modified after [34].

with reduction of GFR. This effectively maintains urine output for up to a 50% reduction in GFR.

2. **Non-diabetic hyperfilteration**: Normal pre-insult GFR ($g(0)$) of $100\,ml/min$ with 1.33 million nephrons. To maintain normal GFR these nephrons have increased filtration (hyperfilteration) by an average of 50%. Reabsorption was defined as for the Healthy kidney model.

3. **CKD**: Reduced pre-insult GFR ($g(0)$) of $50\,ml/min$ with 0.67 million nephrons. These nephrons have increased filtration (hyperfilteration) by an average of 50%. Reabsorption was assumed to be 99.5% of GFR prior to injury changing to 99.75% with reaction of GFR. This effectively maintains urine output for up to a 50% reduction in GFR.

In the Healthy kidney N nephrons with $snGFRs$ normally distributed around a mean, $\overline{sn}$. Therefore,

$$GFR = \sum_{i=0}^{i=N} sn_i \qquad (16)$$

$$= N\overline{sn} \qquad (17)$$

where sn_i is the $snGFR$ for the ith nephron. The $snUFR$ is 1% of the $snGFR$. Healthy kidneys are assumed to have the capacity to hyperfilter physiologically, for example following a protein meal or in pregnancy. A similar phenomenon with afferent arteriolar vasodilation occurs in early diabetic kidney disease [7].

In a non-diabetic hyperfiltering kidney there is assumed loss of function of n_l nephrons. The remaining nephrons are hyperfiltering such that the $snGFR$ distribution is no longer normal but skewed towards a distribution of greater single nephron GFRs to compensate for the loss of nehprons [8,9] (see Figure 2). We set the maximum possible snGFR as twice $\overline{sn}$ and modelled the sn_i distribution as a beta-function. In the sub-clinical stages of CKD (the Hyperfilter model) we assume that hyperfiltration compensates for nephron loss (up to 33.3% loss of nephrons compensated for by 50% average increase in $snGFR$, [10]). In the CKD model we assume there has been a further loss of half the remaining nephrons. Although the nephrons are still hyperfiltering, GFR is halved.

The Beta function used in equation 19

$$B(\alpha,\beta) = \int_0^1 t^{\alpha-1}(1-t)^{\beta-1}dt \qquad (18)$$

α and β were chosen so that the maximum single nephron GFR was twice the mean and so as to maintain a total GFR of $100\,ml/min$ given a loss of one-third of nephrons (hyperfilter model) or $50\,ml/min$ given a loss of two-thirds of nephrons (CKD model).

$$GFR = \sum_{i=0}^{i=N-n_l} sn_i \qquad (19)$$

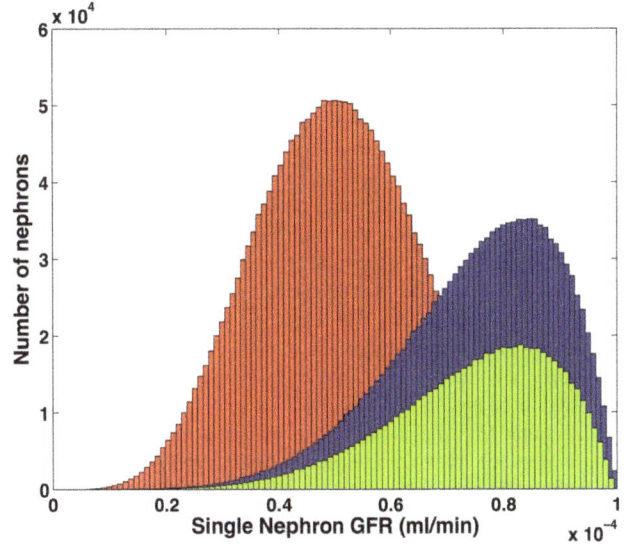

Figure 2. The distribution of single nephron GFRs. Histograms for the Healthy model (dark gray; $\alpha=\beta=5.75$), Hyperfilter model (black; $\alpha=6,\beta=2$) and CKD model (light gray; $\alpha=6,\beta=2$). The Healthy model had 2,000,000 nephrons and GFR of $100\,ml/min$ ($g(0)$), the Hyperfilter model maintained a GFR of $100\,ml/min$ with 33.3% fewer nephrons, and the CKD model had a reduced GFR of $50\,ml/min$ with 66.7% fewer nephrons.

$$= 2\,\overline{sn} \sum_{i=0}^{i=N-n_l} \frac{1}{B(\alpha,\beta)}\left(\frac{i}{N-n_l}\right)^{\alpha-1}\left(1-\frac{i}{N-n_l}\right)^{\beta-1} \qquad (20)$$

For each of the three kidney scenarios sixteen biomarker concentration profiles were constructed based on the combination filtration pressure loss (4 scenarios) and nephron loss (4 scenarios),

1. Filtration pressure loss: The insult caused uniform loss of filtration pressure for all nephrons, causing a reduction in GFR. GFR was assumed to reduce by 0%, 33.3%, 50%, or 66.7% for 48 hours.

2. Nephron loss: The insult caused loss of nephrons with or without hyperfiltration. Nephron loss was assumed to be 0%, 33.3%, 50%, or 66.7%.

The biomarker urinary concentration (Bm) is the sum of each nephron's excretion rate divided by its $snUFR$:

$$Bm = \sum_{i=0}^{i=N-n_l} \frac{E_i(t)}{sn_i(1-R_i)} \qquad (21)$$

where R_i is the proportional reabsorption rate for nephron i ($R_{i1}+R_{i2}$). At time zero prior to insult ($t=0$) we set $R_i = R_i(0) = 0.99$ for all nephrons in the Healthy model, thus maintaining a typical UFR of $1\,ml/min$. Urine output is commonly maintained in CKD patients. Therefore we set $R_i(0) = 0.99$ for all the nephrons in the Hyperfilter model and $R_i(0) = 0.995$ for all the nephrons in the CKD model. We calculated for each of the 16 scenarios the maximum fold increase in biomarker concentration produced contour plots of lines of the same fold increase in biomarker concentration (iso-intensity lines) on a grid of GFR vs nephron number using Matlab function *contourf* to interpolate between points on the grid.

Urinary NGAL: a case study

Urinary NGAL concentrations derive from both induced biomarker production in the distal tubules and loop of Henle, and from filtered NGAL that has not been reabsorbed in the proximal tubules. For this reason and because NGAL is one of the most promising of structural injury biomarkers, we modelled the time-course as a special case. There are few studies in non-diseased adults from which to determine baseline NGAL concentrations. We chose 38 ng/ml for plasma NGAL, which was the mean concentration of a control group of normal adults [11] and 20 ng/ml for urinary NGAL, which was the median concentration in a study of a healthy population [12]. The urinary concentration depends on the plasma concentration which in turn depends on the change in filtration rate and NGAL production rate. The volume of distribution of NGAL has not been measured, but it is known to be distributed over the plasma and its half-life is short, approximately 15 minutes [13]. We therefore, used a plasma volume of 3000 ml as the volume of distribution. We chose the scenario of a two-thirds reduction in GFR with no further loss of nephron number for this case study.

All calculations were performed in Matlab (Matlab 2012b, MathWorks Inc., Natick, MA, USA).

Results

Single nephron scenarios

Pre-formed. AKI results in a rapid loss of the mass of pre-formed biomarker (Figure 3). This is manifest by a many fold increase in excretion rate that exponentially declines during the insult as the pre-formed mass is released into the urine. Should the insult cease before the pre-insult mass is excreted, then the excretion rate drops below the pre-insult excretion rate because the mass available for excretion is smaller than pre-insult. As the mass of biomarker slowly recovers (assuming no permanent

damage to the tubule) the rate of excretion increases until it reaches the pre-AKI equilibrium rate.

Induced. AKI induces some biomarkers to be produced with a portion lost into the tubular filtrate. Pre-AKI excretion rates of induced biomarkers are normally very low and there is a many-fold increase in excretion rate over the space of a few hours (Figure 4). The rate of increase and subsequent decline will vary depending on the biomarker.

Filtered. If there is damage to the reabsorption mechanism of a biomarker that is usually (almost) totally reabsorbed within the proximal tubule, then there will be a many fold increase in urinary excretion of that biomarker assuming that the filtration rate has not changed (Figure 5a). Of the three biomarker classes, only the filtered biomarker excretion rate will change because of a change in GFR (Figure 5b) (not to be confused with change induced by injury which reduces GFR). This has the effect of maintaining a greater fold increase over a longer duration.

Multiple nephron scenarios

For each biomarker class we present contour plots for each kidney type showing the maximum fold increase in biomarkers relative to the pre-insult Healthy kidney model biomarker concentration.

Pre-formed. The maximum concentrations decreased with decreasing number of filtering nephrons and increased with decreasing GFR in each scenario (Figure 6). There is an approximately linear relationship between GFR and nephron number such that a reduction of x% in GFR and x% in nephron number will maintain the same maximal concentrations. The Non-diabetic Hyperfiltering scenario concentrations were lower than in the Healthy scenario at the same GFR's because of fewer nephrons. Conversely concentrations were higher in CKD scenarios despite fewer remaining nephrons because urine output was reduced because of lower GFR.

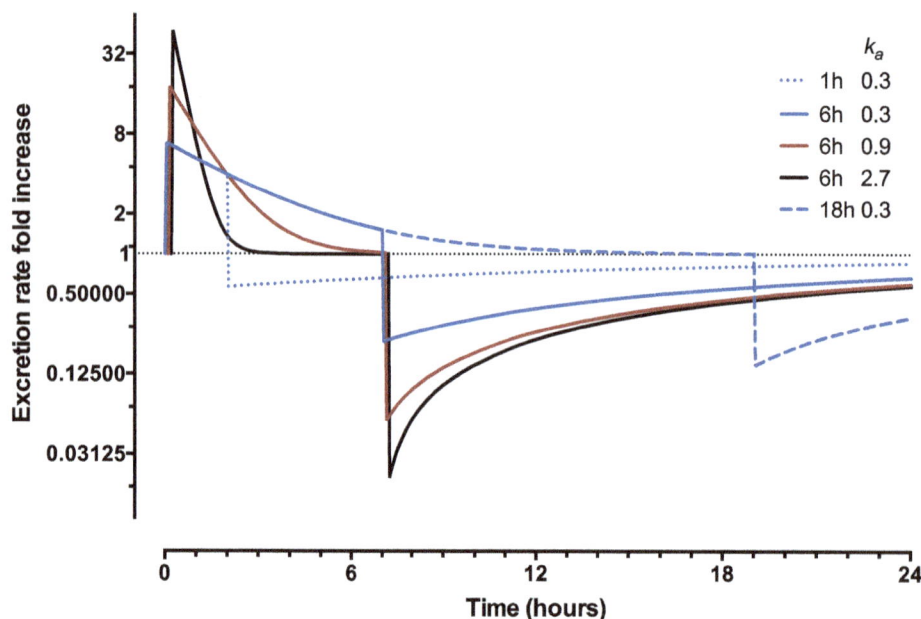

Figure 3. Preformed Biomarkers: single nephron time-course. Fold increase in excretion rate of a pre-formed biomarker for a duration of insult of 1-hour (dotted line), 6-hours (solid lines), 18-hours (dashed line). k_a is the rate constant for additional excretion during insult (h^{-1}). In all cases the excretion rate falls below the pre-AKI excretion rate at the end of the insult because the excretion rate is proportional to the mass of remaining pre-formed biomarker. It is assumed that the biomarker along with the brush border is regenerated at a constant rate, $k_n = 0.05 h^{-1}$.

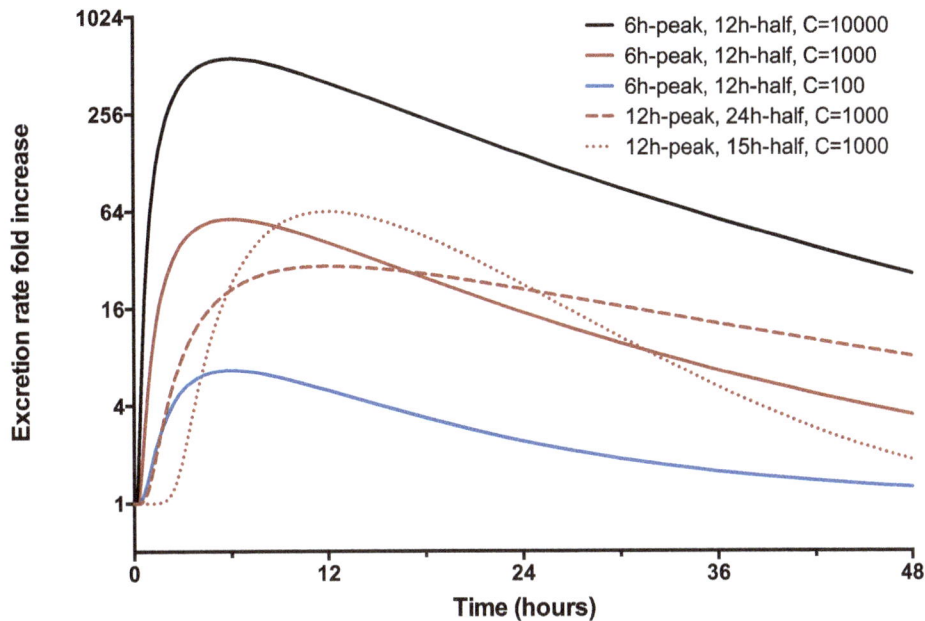

Figure 4. Induced Biomarkers: single nephron time-course. Fold increase in excretion rate of an induced biomarker. Solid lines represent different scaling factors (C) representing greater total damage for a biomarker that peaks at 6 hours and half the total excretion occurs within 12 hours. The dashed line represents the scaling factor of 1000 with a peak at 12 hours and half the total excretion in 24 hours. The dotted line is as for the dashed line but with half the total excretion in 15 hours.

Induced. As with pre-formed biomarkers, the concentration of an induced biomarker depends on the number of nephrons assuming the same rate of induction of biomarker per nephron for each scenario. Hence, the Non-diabetic Hyperfiltering scenario is the same as the Healthy scenario for the same number of functioning nephrons (Figure 7). The CKD scenarios produced greater concentrations despite fewer nephrons contributing less total biomarker mass. This is because reduced urine output resulting from lower GFR increased biomarker concentrations substantially (see equation 21).

Filtered. Unlike pre-formed or induced biomarkers, the concentrations of filtered biomarkers which are normally reabsorbed within the tubules **increase** with decreasing nephron number (Figure 8). In addition, urinary concentrations also depend on plasma concentrations for filtered biomarkers. Because GFR is assumed to fall at time zero and remain low in these scenarios the plasma concentrations increase during the time interval shown. Consequently only in the Healthy Kidney when there is no change in nephron number, but merely a temporary reduction in reabsorption, does the urinary concentration return towards normal levels after 48 hours (Figure 9). In the CKD scenario there was only a small reduction below maximum concentrations by 48 hours.

NGAL. Figure 10 shows the time-courses of urinary and plasma NGAL concentrations for the Healthy, Non-diabetic hyperfiltering, and the CKD scenario after loss of two thirds of GFR without further loss of nephrons. Also shown are the measured plasma and urinary NGAL concentrations in a 90 kg male following cardiac arrest where creatinine changes indicated approximately 70% GFR reduction (more details are given as Case A in [14]). As with plasma creatinine kinetics, a two thirds loss of GFR is expected to result in a three-fold elevation in plasma NGAL [15,16]. However, the typical increase in plasma NGAL exceeded this threshold suggesting that an increased rate of release of NGAL into the plasma. In these models, we set the rate of

NGAL release into the plasma at 50 times that released into the tubules. This resulted in a 10 fold maximal increase in plasma NGAL concentration. The fold increase in urinary NGAL concentration was much greater (over 100 fold) [17].

Discussion

This modeling exercise revealed potentially important differences in the time-course profiles of pre-formed, induced, and filtered urinary biomarkers of AKI which would be difficult to identify empirically and which, if validated experimentally and in human subjects, have clinical consequences. Pre-formed biomarkers respond quickest to injury, but have only very brief periods of elevation even when injury is ongoing. The shape of the induced biomarker time-course is influenced by the specific physiology associated with each induced biomarker while the fold-increase in concentration depends on a balance between the severity of the insult, which increases single nephron excretion, the number of remaining nephrons, to which total excretion is in proportion, and the extent of GFR reduction, which increases total biomarker concentration because of water reabsorption. Filtered biomarkers have the longest time-courses because of the increased plasma levels following GFR decrease. Somewhat surprisingly, peak concentrations are less dependent on the number of remaining nephrons than with induced biomarkers, and there is a small increase in peak-concentration with fewer nephrons. The peak concentration and profile depend on the degree of damage to the reabsorption mechanism and rate of recovery. Rapid recovery may be detectable through a rapid reduction in urinary concentration of a filtered biomarker that is normally reabsorbed. We also demonstrated that for all biomarkers, an inability to hyperfilter substantially increases peak biomarker concentrations, especially where there is substantial loss of nephron number due to chronic illness.

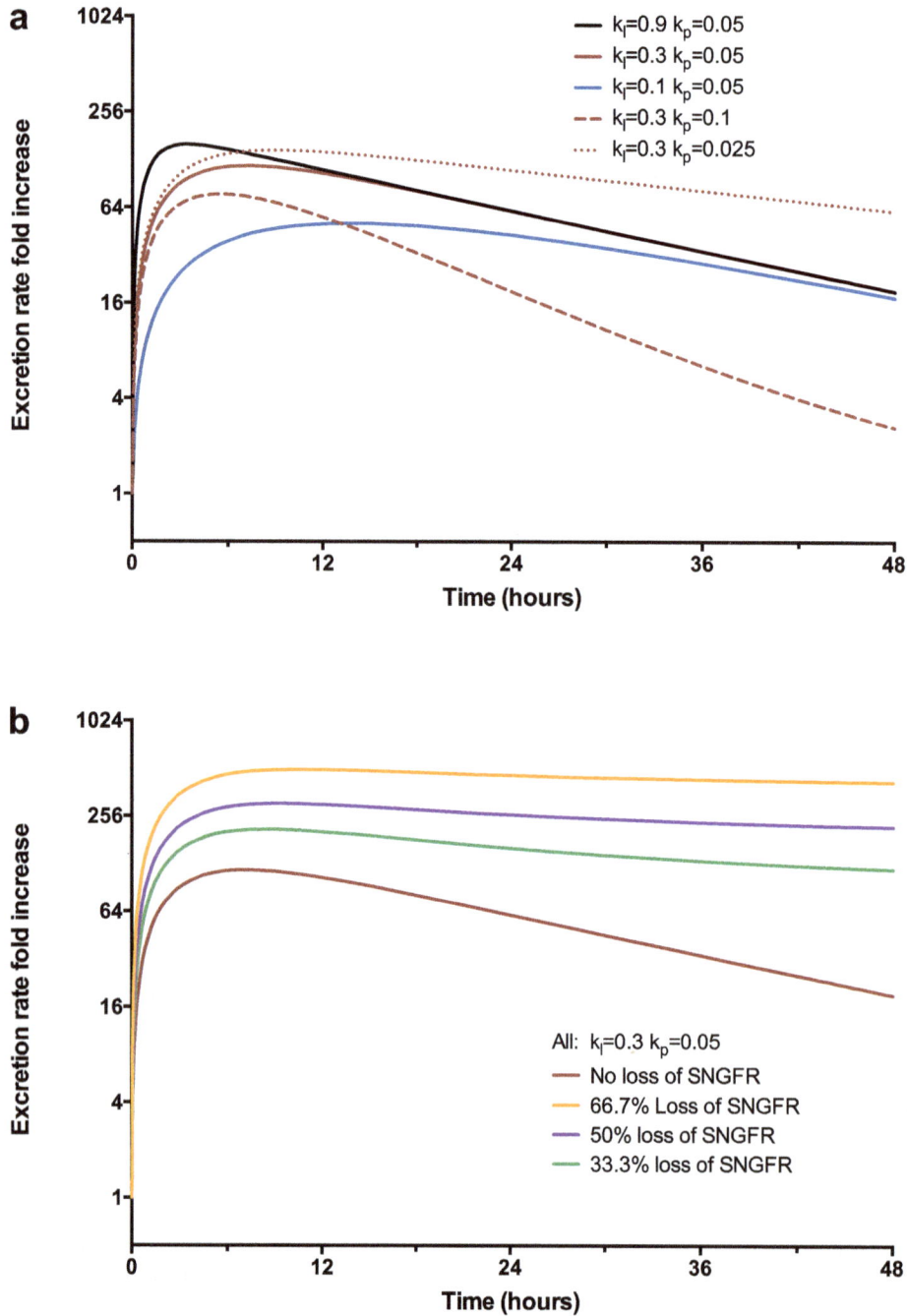

Figure 5. Filtered Biomarkers: single nephron time-course. Fold increase in excretion rate of a filtered biomarker. (a) Solid lines represent different rates of loss of reabsorption receptors. Larger k_l represents greater total damage. Dotted and Dashed lines illustrate the difference the regeneration (production) rate of of the reabsorption receptors makes to the excretion rate. (b) Following a reduction of $snGFR$ and assuming a plasma half-life of 2 hours (e.g. Cystatin C).

A single nephron will release pre-formed biomarkers into the lumen as long as injury continues and biomarker mass remains. The duration of insult is likely a combination of the duration of hypoxia and duration of reperfusion and associated inflammation. As hypoxia is a common cause of brush border damage, we speculate this may contribute to the early release of these pre-formed biomarkers [18,19]. The duration of injury does not necessarily equate to the duration of a decreased GFR. Total biomarker excretion is limited by the pre-formed biomarker mass

and the rate of regeneration. With a large available biomarker mass a very rapid increase in urinary concentration will follow injury. More severe injury will increase the rate of excretion and the peak excretion rate, but also reduce the duration over which excretion occurs (Figure 3). Urinary concentration increases with increasing nephron number because of the greater total available biomarker mass, and also increases with reduced GFR because of increased water reabsorption (Figure 6). The pre-formed biomarker concentrations for the Hyperfiltering and Healthy kidney

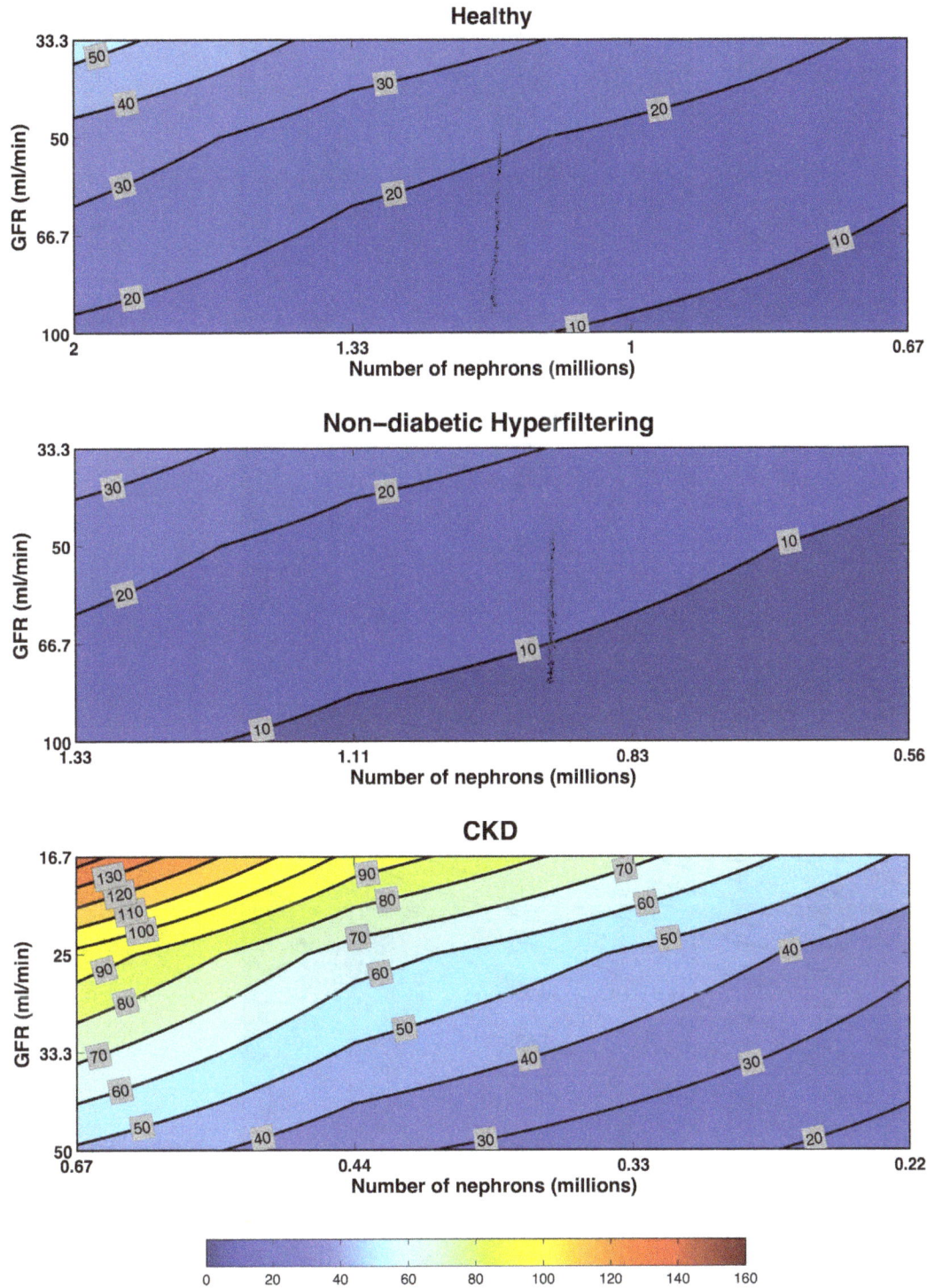

Figure 6. Preformed Biomarkers: multiple-nephron maximum fold concentration increase. Preformed biomarker concentration increases in Healthy, Hyperfiltering and CKD kidneys. Each line of iso-intensity represents the maximal fold increase of a preformed biomarker relative to the pre-injury concentration in a Healthy Kidney with 2 million nephrons and a GFR of $100\,ml/min$. Four GFR scenarios (no change in GFR [$100\,ml/min$ for Healthy and Hyperfiltering kidneys, and $50\,ml/min$ for CKD kidney], one-third, one-half, and two-thirds reduction in GFR) were combined with four nephron number scenarios (no loss [2 M for Healthy, 1.33 M for Hyperfiltering, and 0.67 M for CKD kidneys], one-third, one-half, and two-thirds loss) to produce 16 scenarios. From each of these the maximum fold increase in biomarker concentration was extracted. The iso-intensity lines of fold increase were then interpolated. All scenarios were for a period of AKI of 6 hours, a rate constant of $k_a = 0.9h^{-1}$ for additional excretion of the biomarker, and a brush border generation rate $k_n = 0.05h^{-1}$. Note, the maximum fold-increase in concentration for each scenario occurs at the same time point, namely immediately following insult.

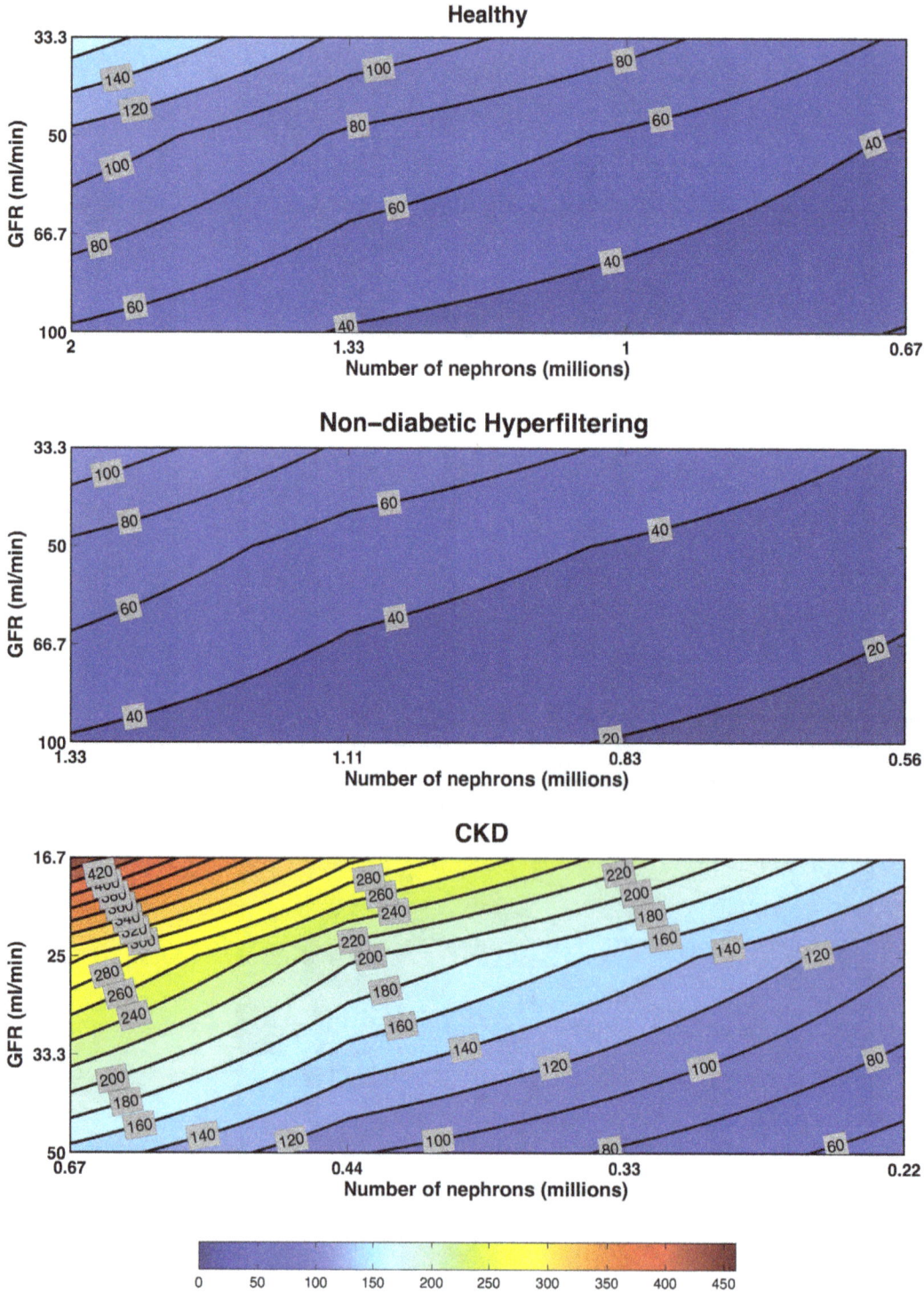

Figure 7. Induced Biomarkers: multiple-nephron maximum fold concentration increase. Induced biomarker concentration increases in Healthy, Hyperfiltering and CKD kidneys. Each line of iso-intensity represents the maximal fold increase of a preformed biomarker relative to the pre-injury concentration in a Healthy Kidney with 2 million nephrons and a GFR of $100\,ml/min$. Four GFR scenarios (no change in GFR [$100\,ml/min$ for Healthy and Hyperfiltering kidneys, and $50\,ml/min$ for CKD kidney], one-third, one-half, and two-thirds reduction in GFR) were combined with four nephron number scenarios (no loss [2 M for Healthy, 1.33 M for Hyperfiltering, and 0.67 M for CKD kidneys], one-third, one-half, and two-thirds loss) to produce 16 scenarios. From each of these the maximum fold increase in biomarker concentration was extracted. The iso-intensity lines of fold increase were then interpolated. All scenarios are for a peak at 6 hours (t_p), half the total excretion occurs within 12 hours (t_m), and a scaling factor (C) of 1000.

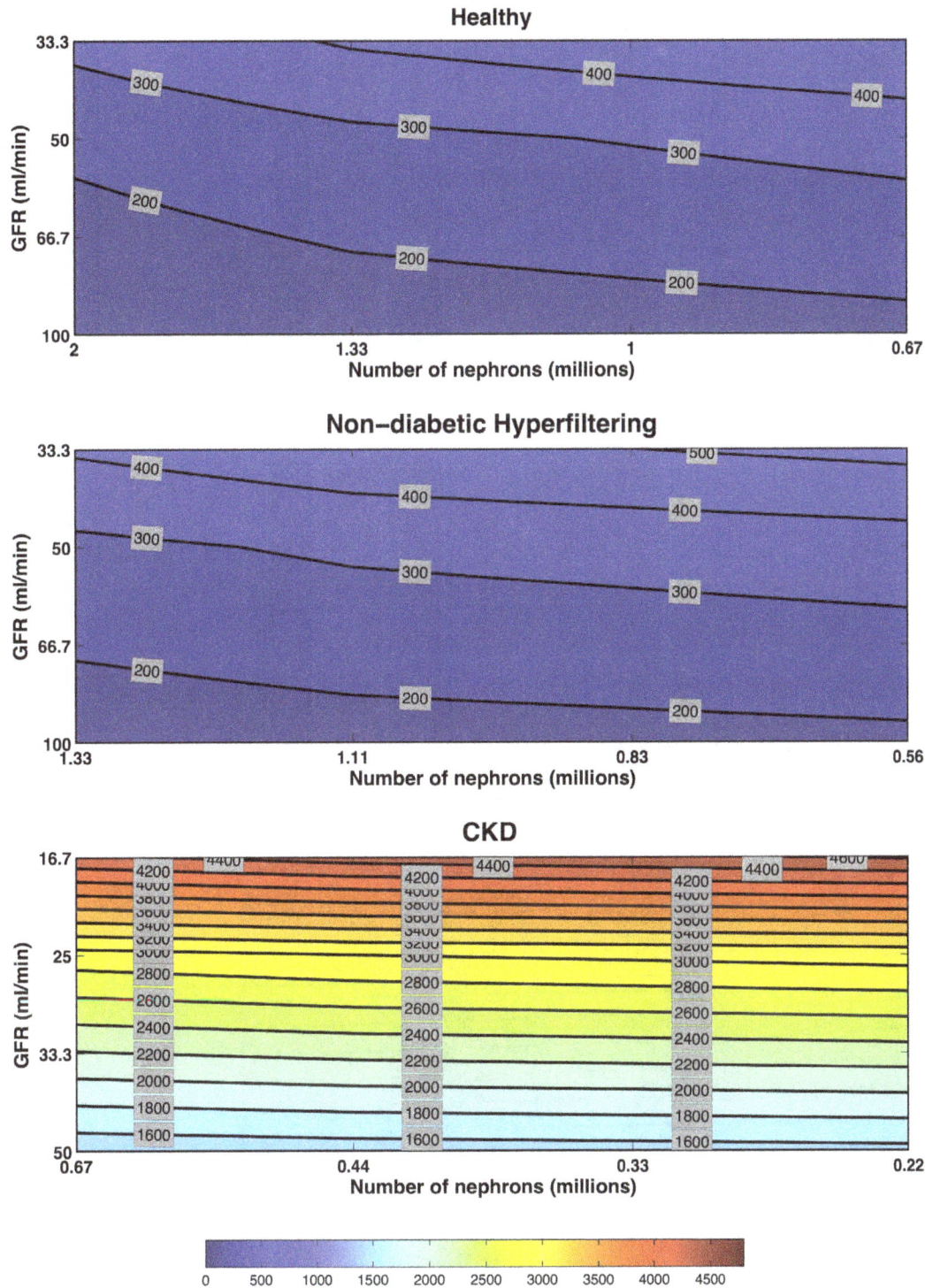

Figure 8. Filtered Biomarkers: multiple-nephron maximum fold concentration increase. Filtered biomarker concentration increases in Healthy, Hyperfiltering and CKD kidneys. Each line of iso-intensity represents the maximal fold increase of a preformed biomarker relative to the pre-injury concentration in a Healthy Kidney with 2 million nephrons and a GFR of $100 ml/min$. Four GFR scenarios (no change in GFR [$100 ml/min$ for Healthy and Hyperfiltering kidneys, and $50 ml/min$ for CKD kidney], one-third, one-half, and two-thirds reduction in GFR) were combined with four nephron number scenarios (no loss [2 M for Healthy, 1.33 M for Hyperfiltering, and 0.67 M for CKD kidneys], one-third, one-half, and two-thirds loss) to produce 16 scenarios. From each of these the maximum fold increase in biomarker concentration was extracted. The iso-intensity lines of fold increase were then interpolated. All scenarios are for a receptor production rate constant $k_p = 0.05$ and loss rate constant $k_l = 0.3$.

models' were similar because hyperfiltration compensated for the loss of nephrons. However, in CKD kidneys, the increased water reabsorption increased biomarker concentrations. The time-courses of urinary biomarker concentrations demonstrates that the most rapid increases in AKI are shown by pre-formed biomarkers γ-GGT, ALP, α-GST and π-GST [2,20]. Shortly

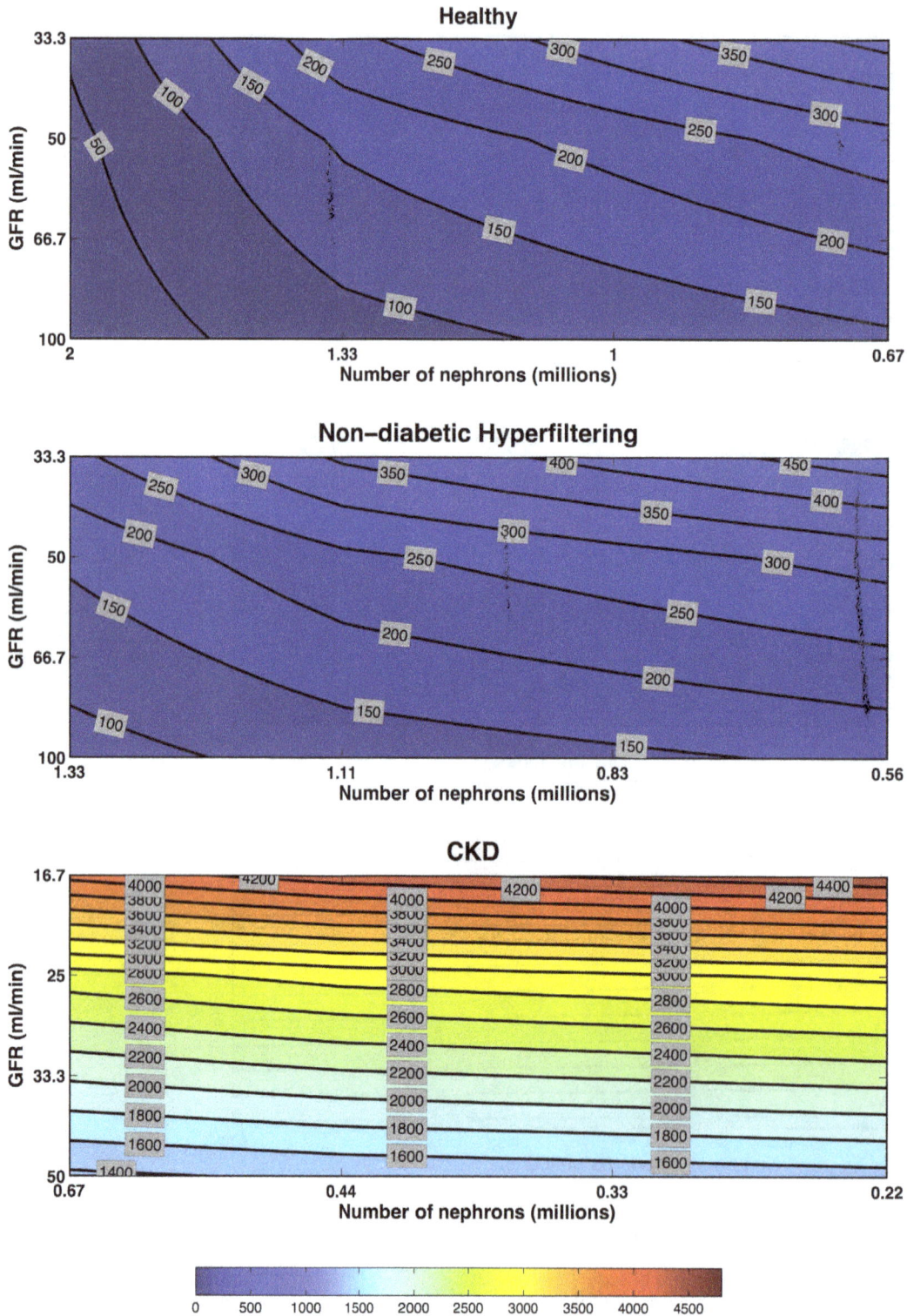

Figure 9. Filtered multiple-nephron fold concentration increase at 48 hours post-insult. Filtered biomarker concentration increases in Healthy, Hyperfiltering and CKD kidneys. Each line of iso-intensity represents the fold increase 48-hours following insult of a preformed biomarker relative to the pre-injury concentration in a Healthy Kidney with 2 million nephrons and a GFR of $100\,ml/min$. Four GFR scenarios (no change in GFR [$100\,ml/min$ for Healthy and Hyperfiltering kidneys, and $50\,ml/min$ for CKD kidney], one-third, one-half, and two-thirds reduction in GFR) were combined with four nephron number scenarios (no loss [2 M for Healthy, 1.33 M for Hyperfiltering, and 0.67 M for CKD kidneys], one-third, one-half, and two-thirds loss) to produce 16 scenarios. From each of these the fold increase in biomarker concentration at 48-hours following insult was extracted. The iso-intensity lines of fold increase were then interpolated. Each scenario from figure 2 is represented for no change in GFR, one-third, one-half, and two-thirds reduction. All scenarios are for a receptor production rate constant $k_p = 0.05$ and loss rate constant $k_l = 0.3$.

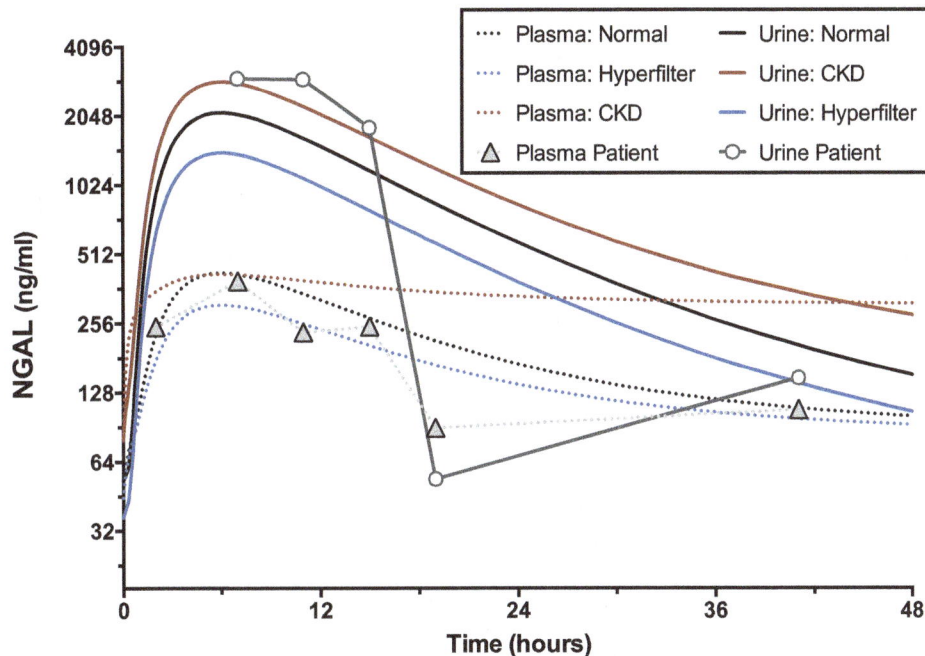

Figure 10. NGAL time-courses. Urinary and plasma NGAL concentration time-courses for the scenario of a 50% loss of GFR with no additional loss of nephrons for the Healthy (black lines), Hyperfiltering (blue lines) and CKD kidneys (red lines). Measured plasma and urinary NGAL values following a cardiac arrest in a 90 kg male with a history of hypertrophic obstructive cardiomyopathy and severely impaired left ventricular function who suffered a cardiac arrest in the emergency department and subsequently lost approximately 70% of GFR (Case A in [14]).

following insult, high concentrations are diagnostic of later increases in plasma creatinine [2]. The "window of detectability" during which pre-formed biomarker excretion can be used to diagnose AKI is short. If the total available biomarker mass is sufficiently reduced, and the rate of regeneration is low, total excretion may fall to levels below that in an uninjured kidney (Figure 3). This may explain why *low* ALP concentrations in the EARLYARF trial at 36 hours post insult were diagnostic of AKI [2].

For induced biomarkers the single nephron excretion may continue indefinitely; mathematically, there is no upper limit to the biomarker mass excreted. In practice, the total mass excreted depends on physiological factors that are not well understood. However, total excretion probably depends on the severity of the insult. We have shown elsewhere that total excretion of several biomarkers is related to AKI severity stage and need for dialysis and death [21]. Nevertheless, the reported time-courses [2,3,22] suggest, that total biomarker and peak biomarker excretion are limited in duration and follow an approximately log-normal curve over time. This also appears true of gene-expression of upregulated biomarkers like NGAL [23]. The peak concentrations in the multiple nephron scenarios, as with pre-formed biomarkers, increase with the available nephrons, increase with lower GFR, and are greatest in CKD patients. Induced biomarkers have differing time-courses, with some reaching a peak much later than others, for example KIM-1 increases more slowly than NGAL or IL18 [24]. This may be modelled by varying the time to maximal biomarker concentrations in the equations for a log-normal distribution of gene expression. In figure 4 the dotted curve illustrates a biomarker with later peak excretion compared to other biomarkers. Over the first few hours the change in concentration is minimal. This mimics the physiological response of KIM-1, which

is involved in the phagocytosis of dead cells in the post-ischemic kidney [25].

The urine concentrations of filtered biomarkers depend on both changes in reabsorption rate, which may be low (e.g. for creatinine), or very high (e.g. for cystatin C), and on the plasma concentration. The temporal profile for a filtered and normally reabsorbed urinary biomarker, like cystatin C, is likely to increase rapidly because of damage to the megalin-cubulin receptors and/or competition for reabsorption [26]. The plasma concentration of such a biomarker increases with time while GFR is reduced which in turn maintains an elevated urinary concentration [2,27]. Unlike pre-formed and induced biomarkers, filtered biomarker concentrations increase with decreasing nephron number because less biomarker mass is reabsorbed. If recovery of GFR is accompanied by recovery of reabsorption then urinary concentrations of a filtered and normally reabsorbed biomarker will reduce more rapidly than their plasma concentrations or plasma creatinine. Thus a filtered and normally reabsorbed urinary marker should be an earlier marker of recovery than a plasma biomarker.

Data in healthy populations of pre-insult normal biomarker concentrations of most of the candidate structural injury biomarkers is sparse. Pennemen and colleagues measured urinary concentrations of KIM-1, NAG, NGAL, and cystatin C in 338 non-smoking healthy volunteers between the ages of 0 and 95 [12]. They noted some sex and age related differences in mean concentrations, but these were diminished when values were normalised to urinary creatinine. Cullen and colleagues measured NGAL in 174 adults and noted age related differences [28]. Other studies have control subjects which provide a pseudo-normal range, for example for IL-18 [29]. This lack of healthy population data needs to be addressed, if only to establish reference ranges. In this study we have deliberated avoided presenting biomarker concentrations, except for the NGAL case study. Instead we presented fold increases from which concentrations may be calculated if a pre-insult concentration is known.

Urinary NGAL is both induced and filtered; it is released into the distal tubule following insult and simultaneously enters the circulation increasing plasma NGAL (which may also increase with systemic bacterial infection) from where it is also filtered where it may be reabsorbed by the megalin-cubulin receptors [17,30,31]. That portion of filtered NGAL not reabsorbed in the proximal tubule (which may be damaged) will reach the final urine. Thus circulating NGAL may increase the duration of increase in the urine beyond that of direct tubular release. We have shown recently that plasma NGAL performs partly as a biomarker of function and partly as a biomarker of structural injury [32]. The plasma concentration typically increases to more than can be explained simply by a loss of GFR and subsequent increase in filtered analyte concentrations. As NGAL is distributed over at least the plasma volume this requires an increase in NGAL production, which may be systemic, from other organs, or from the kidney itself. Our simulation suggests the proportion of induced NGAL released into the circulation must be many times that released into the tubules. This observation begs the question concerning where the NGAL appearing in the plasma is produced and how it enters the plasma? If it is primarily produced in the kidney, then we can be more confident that plasma NGAL relates to kidney injury rather than injury to other organs or a systemic source. One consequence of the kinetics is that whilst urinary NGAL and plasma NGAL may peak at approximately the same time, urinary NGAL concentrations will return to normal more rapidly.

This analysis is subject to the limitations imposed by the model assumptions. For pre-formed biomarkers we assumed that the rate of loss (k_n) was constant for the whole period of the insult. This may be true for well defined insults such as a cardiac arrest or surgery. With other causes of AKI, for example sepsis, this is likely to vary, which may result in a later peak excretion rate and a broadening of the temporal profile. In all the multi-nephron scenarios we could not account for the 'dead' space in the renal pelvis and ureters. From a practical perspective the initial increases in biomarker concentration will be delayed by the time necessary for biomarker to reach the bladder. This will also broaden the temporal profile since not all nephrons are of equal length. We modelled hyperfiltration only for the non-diabetic case where there is loss of nephrons. In diabetic kidney disease, hyperfiltration without loss of nephron number occurs in the early stages of the renal involvement. When GFR is elevated above that of the healthy kidney, the filtered and induced biomarker profiles will only differ from the healthy kidney if the urine flow rate is elevated. In this case, the biomarker concentrations will be lower in proportion to increased urine flow. While the filtered biomarker profiles will be similarly affected by urine flow rate, increased filtration may increase the total filtered biomarker excretion rate.

In all scenarios concentration varies with retention of water. This may be artificially varied in the clinic either through the introduction of a fluid bolus or through loop-diuretics. In both cases the urine is likely to become more diluted and the fold increase reduced. Normalising biomarkers to urinary creatinine has been proposed and discussed in the literature as a way to account for variations in water retention [21,33]. However, we note that urinary creatinine itself is a filtered biomarker with an element of secretion into the tubules, so will be affected by GFR and nephron number differently from other urinary biomarkers. Effectively, this adds noise to a biomarker normalised to creatinine signal meaning that the ratio threshold for diagnosis would need to be greater.

We modelled nephron number as decreased immediately after insult. It seems more likely, that loss of filtration may be slowed progressively, but there is no data to confirm this. The likely effect is broadening of the temporal profiles presented. We also assumed that the water reabsorption rate was constant during AKI and modelled only a step decrease in GFR. As Moran and Myers demonstrated with creatinine kinetics [15], the temporal profiles are likely to change as GFR changes. A change in profile will be greatest for filtered biomarkers.

The ultimate utility of each type of biomarker in each clinical scenario will depend on our understanding of the time-course profiles. Our modeling exercise has highlighted that these will depend on pre-insult GFR, nephron number and renal reserve. As with all modeling exercises, we are limited by the assumptions. What is needed are experimental and clinical studies which measure time-course profiles of multiple biomarkers under known scenarios of GFR, nephron number and renal reserve. Until then, therefore, our conclusions remain speculative. We predict that preformed biomarkers are the earliest indicators of kidney injury, but their brief and early windows of detectability are easily missed in clinical scenarios. Peak urinary concentrations reflect severity of insult, however the temporal profile is reduced by more severe insults. Induced biomarkers have varying durations and times to peak concentration. The window of detectability is extended by the duration and severity of injury. Filtered biomarkers reflect both injury and change of function and have a the broadest time-courses. In a clinical scenario, biomarker choice depends on when measurement is made in relation to the timing of the renal insult, and biomarker interpretation depends on an understanding of the pre-insult kidney size (nephron number) and function (hyperfiltering or not).

Author Contributions

Conceived and designed the experiments: JP. Performed the experiments: JP. Analyzed the data: JP ZH. Wrote the paper: JP ZH. Design of mathematical model: JP.

References

1. Mcilroy DR, Wagener G, Lee HT (2010) Neutrophil gelatinase-associated lipocalin and acute kidney injury after cardiac surgery: the effect of baseline renal function on diagnostic performance. Clin J Am Soc Nephro 5: 211–219.

2. Endre ZH, Pickering JW, Walker RJ, Devarajan P, Edelstein CL, et al. (2011) Improved performance of urinary biomarkers of acute kidney injury in the critically ill by stratification for injury duration and baseline renal function. Kidney Int 79: 1119–1130.

3. Mishra J, Dent CL, Tarabishi R, Mitsnefes MM, Ma Q, et al. (2005) Neutrophil gelatinase-associated lipocalin (NGAL) as a biomarker for acute renal injury after cardiac surgery. Lancet 365: 1231–1238.

4. Han WK, Wagener G, Zhu Y, Wang S, Lee HT (2009) Urinary biomarkers in the early detection of acute kidney injury after cardiac surgery. Clin J Am Soc Nephro 4: 873–882.

5. Mishra J, Ma Q, Prada A, Mitsnefes M, Zahedi K, et al. (2003) Identification of neutrophil gelatinase-associated lipocalin as a novel early urinary biomarker for ischemic renal injury. J Am Soc Nephrol 14: 2534–2543.

6. Ko GJ, Grigoryev DN, Linfert D, Jang HR, Watkins T, et al. (2010) Transcriptional analysis of kidneys during repair from AKI reveals possible roles for NGAL and KIM-1 as biomarkers of AKI-to-CKD transition. Am J Physiol-Renal 298: F1472–83.

7. Brenner BM (1985) Nephron adaptation to renal injury or ablation. Am J Physiol-Renal 249: F324–F337.

8. Kaufman JM, Siegel NJ, Hayslett JP (1975) Functional and hemodynamic adaptation to progressive renal ablation. Circ Res 36: 286–293.

9. Metcalfe W (2007) How does early chronic kidney disease progress? A background paper prepared for the UK Consensus Conference on early chronic kidney disease. Nephrol Dial Transpl 22 Suppl 9: ix26–30.

10. Helal I, Fick-Brosnahan GM, Reed-Gitomer B, Schrier RW (2012) Glomerular hyperfiltration: definitions, mechanisms and clinical implications. Nat Rev Nephrol 8: 293–300.

11. Bolignano D, Basile G, Parisi P, Coppolino G, Nicocia G, et al. (2009) Increased plasma neutrophil gelatinase-associated lipocalin levels predict mortality in elderly patients with chronic heart failure. Rejuvenation Res 12: 7–14.

12. Pennemans V, Rigo JM, Faes C, Reynders C, Penders J, et al. (2013) Establishment of reference values for novel urinary biomarkers for renal damage in the healthy population: are age and gender an issue? Clin Chem Lab Med 51: 1795–1802.

13. Axelsson L, Bergenfeldt M, Ohlsson K (1995) Studies of the release and turnover of a human neutrophil lipocalin. Scand J Clin Lab Inv 55: 577–588.

14. Pickering JW, Ralib AM, Endre ZH (2013) Combining creatinine and volume kinetics identifies missed cases of acute kidney injury following cardiac arrest. Crit Care 17: R7.

15. Moran S, Myers BD (1985) Course of acute renal-failure studied by a model of creatinine kinetics. Kidney Int 27: 928–937.

16. Pickering JW, Endre ZH (2009) GFR shot by RIFLE: errors in staging acute kidney injury. Lancet 373: 1318–1319.

17. Schmidt-Ott KM, Mori K, Li JY, Kalandadze A, Cohen DJ, et al. (2007) Dual action of neutrophil gelatinase-associated lipocalin. J Am Soc Nephrol 18: 407–413.

18. Westhuyzen J, Endre ZH, Reece G, Reith DM, Saltissi D, et al. (2003) Measurement of tubular enzymuria facilitates early detection of acute renal impairment in the intensive care unit. Nephrol Dial Transpl 18: 543–551.

19. Bakońska-Pacoń E, Borkowski J (2003) The effect of the physical effort on the activity of brush border enzymes and lysosomal enzymes of nephron excreted in the urine. Biol Sport 20: 69–78.

20. Koyner JL, Vaidya VS, Bennett MR, Ma Q, Worcester E, et al. (2010) Urinary biomarkers in the clinical prognosis and early detection of acute kidney injury. Clin J Am Soc Nephro 5: 2154–2165.

21. Ralib AM, Pickering JW, Shaw GM, Devarajan P, Edelstein CL, et al. (2012) Test Characteristics of Urinary Biomarkers Depend on Quantitation Method in Acute Kidney Injury. J Am Soc Nephrol 23: 322–333.

22. Krawczeski CD, Goldstein SL,Woo JG,Wang Y, Piyaphanee N, et al. (2011) Temporal relationship and predictive value of urinary acute kidney injury biomarkers after pediatric cardiopulmonary bypass. J Am Coll Cardiol 58: 2301–2309.

23. Han M, Li Y, Liu M, Li Y, Cong B (2012) Renal neutrophil gelatinase associated lipocalin expression in lipopolysaccharide-induced acute kidney injury in the rat. Bmc Nephrol 13: 25.

24. Haase M, Devarajan P, Haase-Fielitz A, Bellomo R, Cruz DN, et al. (2011) The outcome of neutrophil gelatinase-associated lipocalin-positive subclinical acute kidney injury a multicenter pooled analysis of prospective studies. J Am Coll Cardiol 57: 1752–1761.

25. Bonventre JV (2009) Kidney injury molecule-1 (KIM-1): a urinary biomarker and much more. Nephrol Dial Transpl 24: 3265–3268.

26. Nejat M, Hill JV, Pickering JW, Edelstein CL, Devarajan P, et al. (2012) Albuminuria increases cystatin C excretion: implications for urinary biomarkers. Nephrol Dial Transpl 27: iii96–iii103.

27. Molnar AO, Parikh CR, Sint K, Coca SG, Koyner J, et al. (2012) Association of Postoperative Proteinuria with AKI after Cardiac Surgery among Patients at High Risk. Clin J Am Soc Nephro 7: 1749–1760.

28. Cullen MR, Murray PT, Fitzgibbon MC (2012) Establishment of a reference interval for urinary neutrophil gelatinase-associated lipocalin. Ann Clin Biochem 49: 190–193.

29. Blankenberg S, Luc G, Ducimetière P, Arveiler D, Ferrières J, et al. (2003) Interleukin-18 and the risk of coronary heart disease in European men: the Prospective Epidemiological Study of Myocardial Infarction (PRIME). Circulation 108: 2453–2459.

30. Hvidberg V, Jacobsen C, Strong RK, Cowland JB, Moestrup SK, et al. (2005) The endocytic receptor megalin binds the iron transporting neutrophil-gelatinase-associated lipocalin with high affinity and mediates its cellular uptake. FEBS Lett 579: 773–777.

31. Jones RL, Peterson CM, Grady RW, Cerami A (1980) Low molecular weight iron-binding factor from mammalian tissue that potentiates bacterial growth. J Exp Med 151: 418–428.

32. Pickering JW, Endre ZH (2013) The clinical utility of plasma Neutrophil-Gelatinase-Associated-Lipocalin in Acute Kidney Injury. Blood Purif 35: 295–302.

33. Waikar SS, Sabbisetti VS, Bonventre JV (2010) Normalization of urinary biomarkers to creatinine during changes in glomerular filtration rate. Kidney Int 78: 486–494.

34. Endre ZH, Pickering JW, Walker RJ (2011) Clearance and beyond: the complementary roles of GFR measurement and injury biomarkers in acute kidney injury (AKI). Am J Physiol-Renal 301: F697–707.

15

Direct, Acute Effects of Klotho and FGF23 on Vascular Smooth Muscle and Endothelium

Isabelle Six[1,9], Hirokazu Okazaki[1,9], Priscilla Gross[1], Joanna Cagnard[1], Cédric Boudot[1], Julien Maizel[1,2], Tilman B. Drueke[1], Ziad A. Massy[1,2]*

1 INSERM Unit 1088, Jules Verne University of Picardie, Amiens, France, **2** Amiens University Medical Center, Amiens, France

Abstract

Chronic kidney disease (CKD) is regarded as a state of Klotho deficiency and FGF23 excess. In patients with CKD a strong association has been found between increased serum FGF23 and mortality risk, possibly via enhanced atherosclerosis, vascular stiffness, and vascular calcification. The aim of this study was to examine the hypothesis that soluble Klotho and FGF23 exert direct, rapid effects on the vessel wall. We used three in vitro models: mouse aorta rings, human umbilical vein endothelial cells, and human vascular smooth muscle cells (HVSMC). Increasing medium concentrations of soluble Klotho and FGF23 both stimulated aorta contractions and increased ROS production in HVSMC. Klotho partially reverted FGF23 induced vasoconstriction, induced relaxation on phosphate preconstricted aorta and enhanced endothelial NO production in HUVEC. Thus Klotho increased both ROS production in HVSMC and NO production in endothelium. FGF23 induced contraction in phosphate preconstricted vessels and increased ROS production. Phosphate, Klotho and FGF23 together induced no change in vascular tone despite increased ROS production. Moreover, the three compounds combined inhibited relaxation despite increased NO production, probably owing to the concomitant increase in ROS production. In conclusion, although phosphate, soluble Klotho and FGF23 separately stimulate aorta contraction, Klotho mitigates the effects of phosphate and FGF23 on contractility via increased NO production, thereby protecting the vessel to some extent against potentially noxious effects of high phosphate or FGF23 concentrations. This novel observation is in line with the theory that Klotho deficiency is deleterious whereas Klotho sufficiency is protective against the negative effects of phosphate and FGF23 which are additive.

Editor: Michael Bader, Max-Delbrück Center for Molecular Medicine (MDC), Germany

Funding: Hirokazu Okazaki and Priscilla Gross were supported by grants from Conseil Régional de Picardie, Amiens, France (Marno-MPCC for HO and Feder for PG). The funders had no role in study design, data collection and analysis, decision to publish, or preparation of the manuscript.

Competing Interests: The authors have declared that no competing interests exist.

* E-mail: ziad.massy@apr.aphp.fr

9 These authors contributed equally to this work.

Introduction

Cardiovascular disease (CVD) is the leading cause of mortality and morbidity in patients with chronic kidney disease (CKD) [1]. Endothelial dysfunction occurs since the very early stages of CKD [2], and is regarded as an important contributor to increased CVD risk [3]. Endothelial dysfunction is a systemic pathological condition which can be defined as resulting from an imbalance between the actions of vasorelaxing and vasoconstrictor factors. The imbalance is mainly caused by reduced nitric oxide (NO) bioavailability and/or increased generation of reactive oxygen species (ROS) [4].

CKD is considered as a state of Klotho deficiency. α-Klotho (Klotho), originally identified as an anti-aging gene, is predominantly expressed in the kidney but is also detectable in other organs such as parathyroids, choroid plexus and human vascular tissue [5–7]. As a co-factor of fibroblast growth factor 23 (FGF23), Klotho is involved in the control of renal phosphate handling and 1,25 diOH vitamin D synthesis [8–10]. Klotho-deficient and FGF23-deficient mice exhibit similar phenotypes, characterized by accelerated aging, atherosclerosis, ectopic calcifications, bone demineralization, skin atrophy and emphysema [11,12].

Klotho deficiency leads to FGF23 resistance since Klotho acts as an obligatory co-receptor in various tissues probably including the vessel wall [7,13,14]. However, high circulating FGF23 levels can also exert Klotho independent deleterious CV effects [15]. Excessive FGF23 levels were found to be associated with impaired vasodilatation [16], and Klotho gene deficiency to interfere with endothelium-dependent vasodilatation [17]. Klotho gene delivery improves vascular function through increased endothelial-derived NO production and less oxidative stress in VSMCs [18].

Collectively, ample evidence suggests that Klotho and FGF23 play a role in vascular function. However, the interaction between Klotho and FGF23 has recently been found to be more complex than previously thought, requiring further clarification. In the present study, we aimed to determine direct, rapid effects of Klotho and FGF23 on vascular function and to investigate potentially underlying mechanisms. We first examined the vascular reactivity of mouse aorta to exogenous soluble Klotho and FGF23 and observed direct effects. We next asked whether the effects were related to abnormal NO and ROS generation, and then investigated potentially involved signaling pathways using human umbilical vein endothelial cells (HUVEC) and human vascular smooth muscle cells (HVSMC).

Materials and Methods

Ethics Statement

HVSMC were isolated in our laboratory using an explant technique from aortic tissue of healthy donors. Samples were obtained after aortic valve bypass surgery or other types of surgery on the aorta from patients with various cardiovascular diseases (Pr Caus, Pôle Coeur Thorax Vaisseaux, CHU Amiens, France) who gave informed written consent in accordance with French legislation, under PROTOCOL N°2009/19. This protocol was approved by the Ethics Committee, CPP Nord-Ouest II. The investigations were performed according to the principles outlined in the Declaration of Helsinki for use of human tissue or subjects. All of the animal studies were conformed to the principles of European Commission guidelines and all protocols were approved by our Institution's Animal Care and Use Committee (CRE-MEAP, protocol N° 2006/B7).

Products

For the experiments, we used Recombinant Human soluble form of Klotho and Recombinant intact Human FGF23 (R&D Systems, Minneapolis, USA). Endothelial Cell Growth kit-BBE was obtained from ATCC (Manassas, VA, USA). Phosphate (NaH$_2$PO$_4$), Dulbecco's Modified Eagle's Medium (DMEM) and penicillin/streptomycin (P/S) were purchased from Sigma Aldrich (Saint Louis, USA). GlutaMAX^{TM} (Glut) and Fluorescent probe, 2′, 7′dichlorodihydrofluorescein diacetate (DCF) were obtained from Invitrogen, (Saint Aubin, France) and fetal calf serum (FCS) from Dominique Dutcher Laboratories (Brumath, France). FACS Canto II flow cytometer and FACSDiva software were obtained from BD Biosciences (Rungis, France). 4-amino-5-methylamino-2′, 7′-difluorofluorescein diacetate (DAF-FM DA) was obtained from Merck Millipore (St. Quentin-en-Yvelines, France).

All the primary antibodies for western blot analyses were obtained from Cell Signaling, Ozyme (St. Quentin en Yvelines, France).

Animals and diet

All animal studies were performed using C57/BL-6 wild-type female mice at age 8 weeks. The mice were purchased from Charles Rivers Laboratories (Lyon, France). They were housed in polycarbonate cages in temperature- and humidity-controlled rooms with a 12-h light/dark cycle and given free access to water and regular laboratory chow (Diet 2918, Harlan, Oxon, UK).

Mice were anesthetized by intraperitoneal injection of pento-barbital sodium (150 mg/kg) and at the experimental endpoint euthanasia was accomplished by removal of the heart.

Ex vivo models

Vasoreactivity experiments. Wild-type mice were anesthe-tized and a midline incision was made through the sternum to open up the thoracic cavity, and the descending thoracic aorta was carefully isolated. Each aorta was sectioned into 3.5 mm rings devoid of fat and connective tissue. The rings were placed in Kreb's-Henseleit (KH) solution under 5% CO$_2$ and 95% O$_2$ atmosphere at 37 °C. The aorta rings were maintained under a 1.3 g tension (previously determined as the optimal point of their length-tension relationship) and allowed to equilibrate for 60 min. The aorta rings were constricted with KCl (70 mM) and then washed out to reach the resting level.

For the study of potential vasoconstrictor effects of phosphate, Klotho or FGF23, aorta rings were exposed to cumulative treatments with phosphate (1–3 mM), recombinant mouse Klotho (0–2 nM) or recombinant mouse FGF23 (0–400 ng/ml). As the

vessels were not preconstricted, only vasoconstriction was observed. To test the implication of oxygen-derived free radicals or ERK, we incubated vessels in the presence of dimethylthiourea (10 mM), a scavenger of hydroxyl radical or the ERK inhibitor U0126 (10 μM) for 40 min.

The vascular effect of Klotho in association with FGF23 was studied by exposing aorta rings to both Klotho (0.8–1.6 nM) and FGF23 (10–200 ng/ml). Vascular wall tension was supplied by a force-displacement transducer and changes in isometric force recorded continuously. The contractile response was expressed as percentage of KCl contraction, taking into account resting contraction level.

The vascular effect of phosphate in association with Klotho was studied by exposing vessels to phosphate 2.0 mM followed by a range of Klotho concentrations (0.4–2.0 nM). Contraction values were expressed as percentage of contraction obtained with KCl, taking into account resting contraction level. The relaxation obtained with Klotho was calculated taking into account the maximal contraction obtained with phosphate 2.0 mM. A possible involvement of NO was studied by incubating vessels with L-NNA (a competitive inhibitor of nitric oxide synthase, with selectivity for the neuronal and endothelial isoforms of the enzyme) for 30 min before stimulation with phosphate and Klotho. The role of endothelial cells in arterial relaxation was studied by using aortic rings devoid of endothelium. The endothelium was removed by gently rubbing off the intimal surface of the aortic rings with a wooden stick. The effectiveness of this removal was demonstrated by the lack of response to acetylcholine (up to 1.0 μM).

The vascular effect of phosphate in association with FGF23 was studied by stimulating vessels with phosphate 2.0 mM, followed by a range of FGF23 concentrations (10–200 ng/ml). Contraction values were expressed as percentage of contraction obtained with KCl, taking into account resting contraction level.

The vasoconstrictor effects of phosphate and Klotho in association with FGF23 were studied by exposing aortic rings to phosphate (2.0 mM), Klotho (1.6 nM) and FGF23 (10 ng/ml) together.

The effects of these 3 drugs were confirmed by concomitant vessel incubation with phosphate (2 mM), Klotho (1.6 nM) and FGF23 (10 ng/ml) followed by stimulation with phenylephrine (3.10^{-5} M). The contractile response was expressed as percentage of KCl contraction, taking into account resting contraction level.

The relaxation effects of phosphate (2.0 mM), Klotho (1.6 nM) and FGF23 (10 ng/ml) were studied by incubating vessels with these 3 drugs followed by stimulation with acetylcholine (3.10^{-5} M). Relaxation was calculated taking into account the maximal contraction obtained with phenylephrine.

Western blot analysis of mouse aortas

The descending aorta was extracted from mice and placed into DMEM 1%, Glut 1%, P/S, 0% FBS. After stimulation with the respective reagents for 30 min, aortas were lysed. Protein concentration was determined by Bradford assay. Proteins were separated in 10% SDS–polyacrylamide gel electrophoresis and transferred to nitrocellulose membranes. The blots were then incubated overnight at 4°C with the following primary antibodies: anti-ERK1/2 (1:1000) and anti-p-ERK1/2 (1:1000). The blots were then incubated with secondary antibody to detect immuno reactive bands. The membranes were developed with the enhanced chemiluminescence detection system and a specific, peroxidase-conjugated anti-IgG antibody. Band intensity was analyzed using the GeneGenius Bio Imaging System and protein levels were normalized against total ERK1/2 for p-ERK1/2.

A

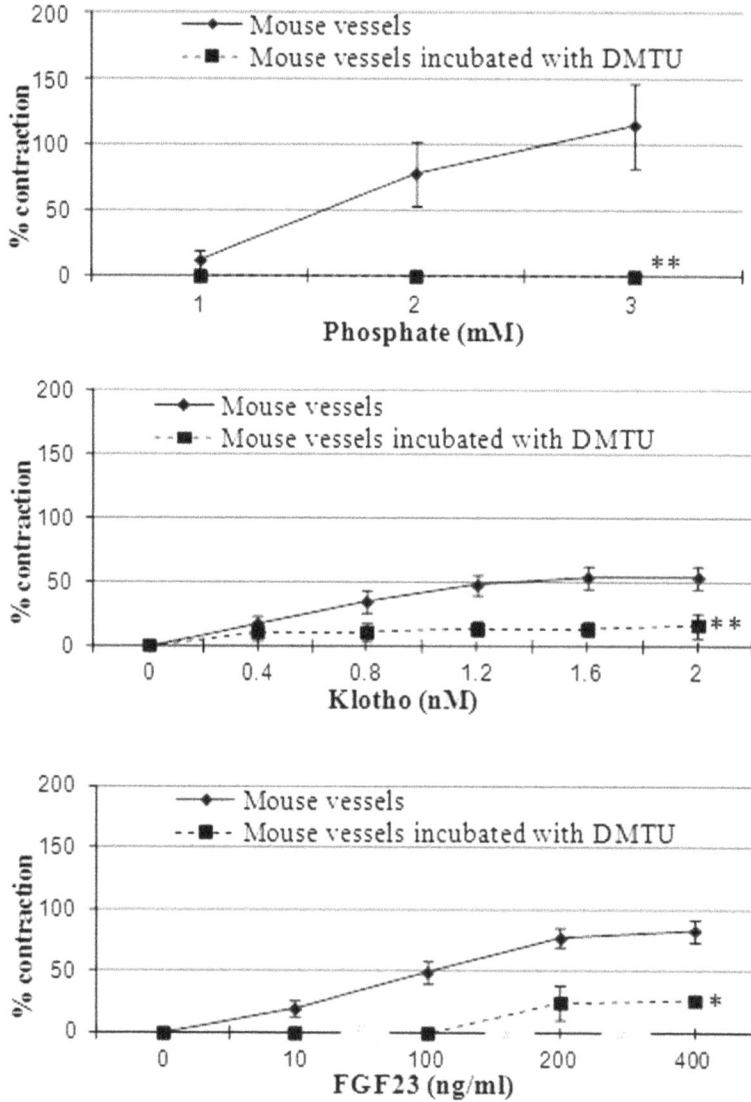

B

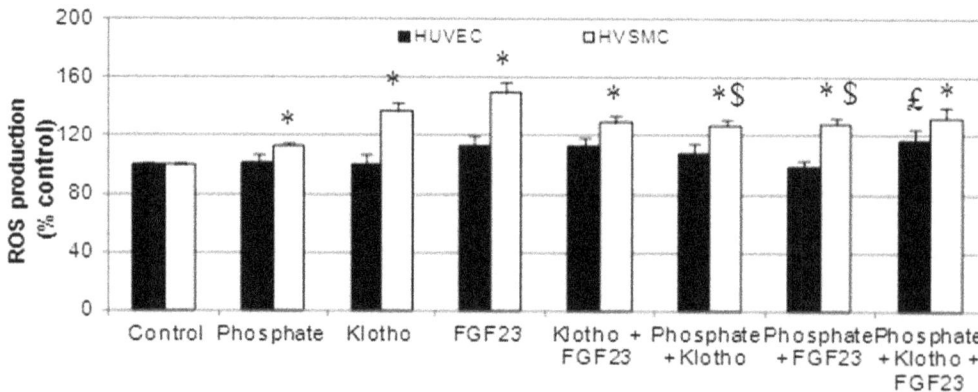

Figure 1. Direct effects of phosphate, Klotho and FGF23 on vascular reactivity and on H$_2$O$_2$ concentration. A.Vascular reactivity on aortic rings *ex vivo*. Direct effects of phosphate (1.0–3.0 mM), Klotho (0–2.0 nM) and FGF23 (0–400 ng/ml) on isolated aortic rings in absence or in the presence of ROS inhibitor, dimethylthiourea (10 mM). Contraction values are expressed as percentage of the contraction obtained with 70 mM KCl. * $p < 0.001$, ** $p < 0.0001$ vs. mouse vessels alone. N, 4 per experiment. B. Direct effects of phosphate (2.0 mM), Klotho (1.6 nM) and FGF23 (10 ng/ml), alone or associated, on H$_2$O$_2$ concentration in human umbilical vein endothelial cells (HUVECs) and human vascular smooth muscle cells (HVSMCs). * $p < 0.0005$ vs. HVSMCs control group, $ $p < 0.005$ vs HVSMCs phosphate group, £ $p < 0.05$ vs. HUVECs control group. N, 7 per experiment.

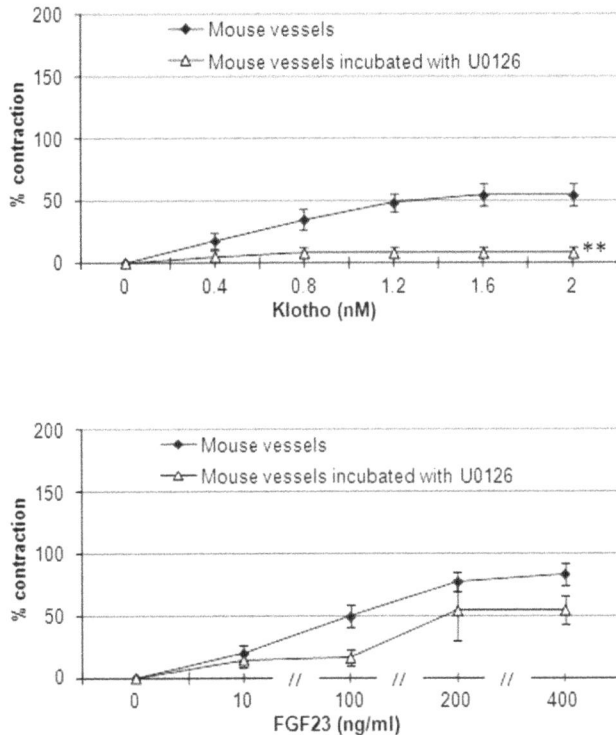

Figure 2. Vascular reactivity on aortic rings *ex vivo*. Direct effects of phosphate (1.0–3.0 mM), Klotho (0–2.0 nM) and FGF23 (0–400 ng/ml) on isolated aortic rings in absence or in the presence of ERK inhibitor, U0126 (10 μM). Contraction values are expressed as percentage of the contraction obtained with 70 mM KCl. ** p<0.0001 vs. mouse vessels alone. N, 4 per experiment.

In vitro models

Human umbilical vein cells (HUVEC). HUVEC, obtained from ATCC, were cultured on 0.1% gelatin-coated flask in a specific culture medium (Vascular Cell Basal Medium) with endothelial Cell Growth kit-BBE.

Human vascular smooth muscle cells (HVSMC). HVSMC were maintained in DMEM with 1% Glut, P/S and supplemented with 15% FCS.

The two cell types were maintained in culture at 37°C (5% CO_2, 90% humidity) and used from passage 3 to passage 8.

Incubation of HUVEC or HVSMC with different drugs

After overnight starvation in DMEM containing P/S, 1% Glut, 0.2% Bovine Serum Albumin (BSA) and 0% FCS, cells were incubated for 10 min at 37°C with DMEM 1% P/S, 1% Glut, containing phosphate (2.0 mM) and/or Recombinant Human Klotho (1.6 nM) and/or Recombinant Human FGF23 (10 ng/mL).

Measurement of intracellular reactive oxygen species (ROS) production by HUVEC or HVSMC using flow cytometry

To evaluate ROS production, hydrogen peroxide (H_2O_2) levels were monitored using fluorescent probe, DCF. After overnight serum starvation, confluent cells were incubated with the different drugs. H_2O_2 production was measured by flow cytometry on detached cells resuspended in PBS and analyzed in a FACS Canto II flow cytometer. The analysis was focused on the whole cell

population. Mean fluorescence intensity was calculated using FACSDiva software and expressed as percentage of control value.

Measurement of intracellular NO production by HUVEC using flow-cytometry

NO production by HUVEC was assessed by measuring the fluorescence of DAF-FM DA, a specific NO probe. After overnight serum starvation, HUVEC were loaded with DAF-FM DA (1.0 μM) for 30 min. Subsequently, cells were stimulated with the different drugs for 10 min. The stimulated cells were then trypsinized and using flow-cytometry (FACSCantoII), a population of 10,000 cells was gated and segregated based on its relative fluorescence intensity. Analyses were done using FACSDiva software.

Western blot analysis

After overnight incubation in starvation medium, HUVECs were stimulated with respective drugs for 10 min. After cell lysis, protein levels were quantified with Bio-Rad Dc Protein Assay kit. Proteins were separated in 10% SDS–polyacrylamide gel electrophoresis and transferred to nitrocellulose membranes. The blots were then incubated overnight at 4°C with the following primary antibodies: anti eNOS (1:1000), anti iNOS (1:1000), and anti phospho-eNOS (serine 1177 or threonine 495, 1:1000). The membranes were developed with the enhanced chemiluminescence detection system and a specific, peroxidase-conjugated anti-IgG antibody. Band intensity was analyzed using the GeneGenius Bio Imaging System and protein levels were normalized against eNOS for phospho-eNOS and β-actin for iNOS.

Statistical analysis

Results were expressed as means ± SEM. Differences between groups were evaluated using analysis of variance (ANOVA) to assess differences between individual mean values. Comparisons between more than two means were performed by using analysis of variance (ANOVA) with or without repeated measurements. If a significant difference was found, Scheffe's test for multiple comparisons was used to identify inter-group differences. For ROS and NO determinations and for western blotting, data were analyzed using a non parametric test (Kruskal-Wallis) to determine significant differences (p<0.05) in mean values between groups followed by Mann-Whitney U test to evaluate the significance of differences between groups. Differences were considered to be significant when p<0.05.

Results

Concentration-dependent vasoconstriction, stimulation of ROS concentration and activation of ERK pathway by phosphate, Klotho, and FGF23 respectively

As demonstrated previously [19], phosphate exhibited a vasoconstrictor effect on aorta rings in a dose-dependent manner and osmolarity kept constant even after addition of phosphate. Exposure of aorta rings to either Klotho or FGF23 induced concentration-dependent contractions within 1 min (**Figure 1A**). This effect was paralleled by an increase of H_2O_2 concentration in HVSMCs by phosphate (2.0 mM), Klotho (1.6 nM) and FGF23 (10 ng/ml) (**Figure 1 B**). The contractions of aortic rings obtained with phosphate, Klotho or FGF23 were abolished by dimethylthiourea (**Figure 1A**). Consistent with the increase in ROS concentration in HVSMCs, ERK phosphorylation of mouse aorta increased in response to phosphate (163±39), Klotho (151±21) or FGF23 (287±119) respectively (p<0.05 vs control).

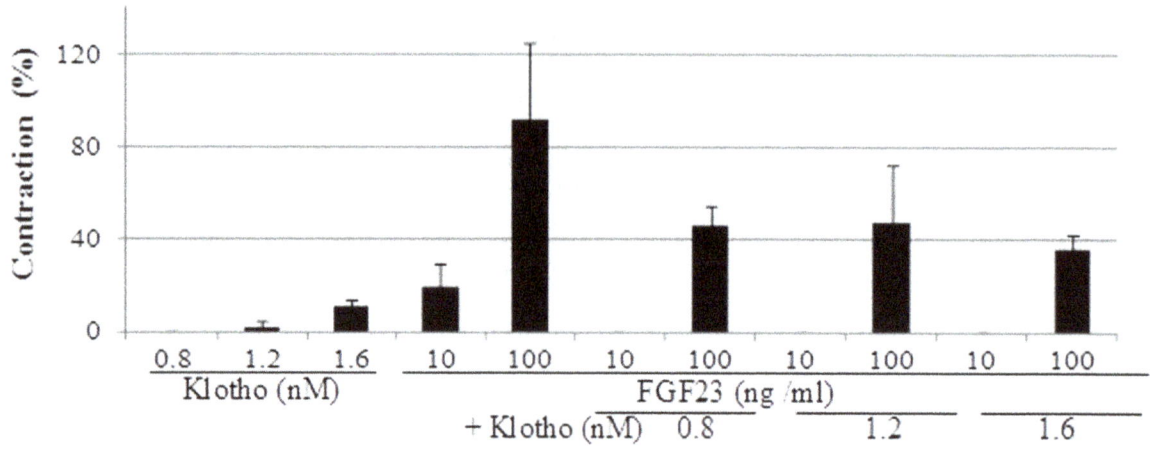

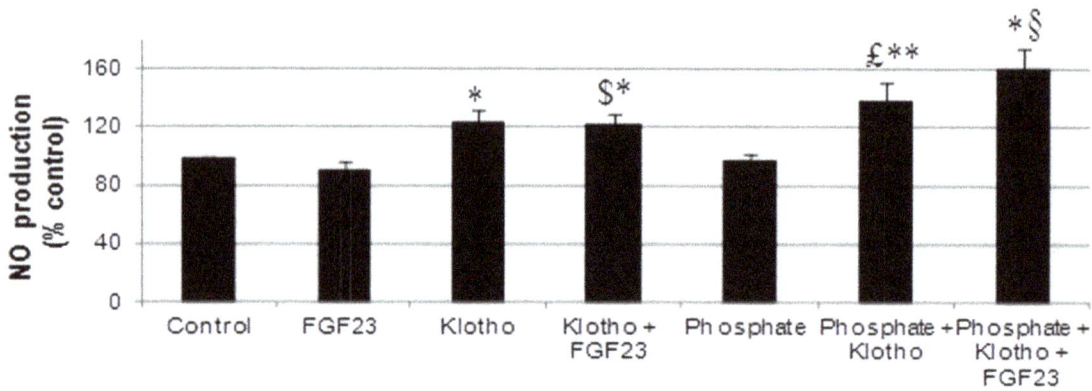

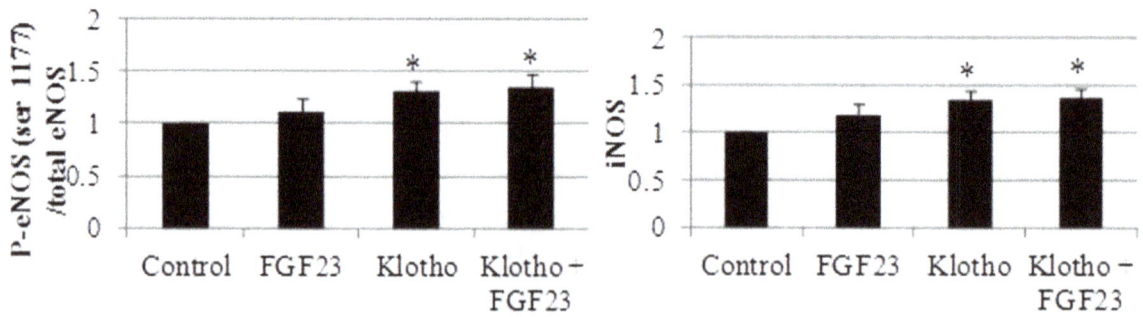

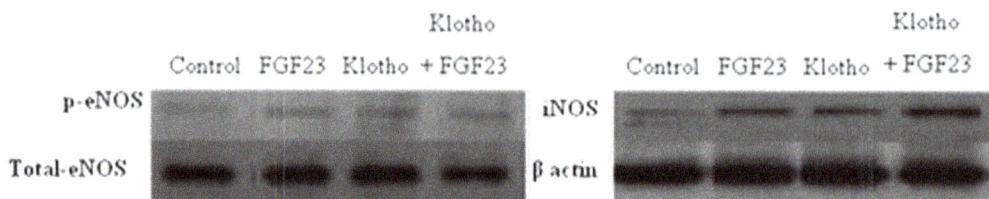

Figure 3. Effects of Klotho associated with FGF23 on vascular reactivity, NO production and eNOS and iNOS expressions. A.Vascular reactivity on aortic rings *ex vivo*. Vascular effects of FGF23 (10, 100 ng/ml) in association with Klotho (0.8, 1.2, 1.6 nM). Contraction values are

expressed as percentage of the contraction obtained with 70 mM KCl. N, 4 per experiment. B. Effects of FGF23 (10 ng/ml), Klotho (1.6 nM) or phosphate (2.0 mM), alone or associated, on NO production, (N, 6 per experiment) in HUVECs. * p<0.05, ** p<0.005 vs. control group, $ p<0.05 vs FGF23 group, £ p<0.005 vs phosphate group, § p<0.05 vs. Klotho group. C. Effects of FGF23 (10 ng/ml), Klotho (1.6 nM), or the two combined on eNOS expression (N, 4–6 per experiment), and iNOS de novo expression (N, 4–6 per experiment) in HUVECs. * p<0.05 vs. control group.

The use of ERK inhibitor U0126 strongly reduced contraction obtained with Klotho. The effect of ERK inhibitor on contraction induced by FGF23 was much less marked (**Figure 2**).

Attenuation of FGF23-induced vasoconstriction by Klotho, probably via enhanced NO generation

In contrast to the vasoconstrictor effects of Klotho or FGF23 alone, the contractile response obtained with FGF23 at 10 ng/ml or 100 ng/ml, was completely abolished or significantly attenuated by pre-treatment with Klotho at 0.8, 1.2 or 1.6 nM (**Figure 3A**).

The increase in H_2O_2 concentration in HVSMCs by exposure to either Klotho or FGF23 remained unchanged by co-exposure to Klotho and FGF23 (**Figure 1B**). Co-exposure to Klotho and FGF23 led to ERK activation in mouse aorta (100±0 for control vs 294±77 for Klotho and FGF23, p<0.05).

Moreover, Klotho increased NO concentration in HUVECs whereas FGF23 did not. Co-exposure maintained Klotho effect (**Figure 3B**).

Exposure of HUVECs to Klotho alone or in association with FGF23 increased eNOS phosphorylation at serine 1177 (the active form of eNOS). Moreover, Klotho induced iNOS de novo expression, and this effect was maintained after co-exposure with FGF23 (**Figure 3C**).

Induction of vascular relaxation by Klotho in phosphate-preconstricted aortic rings, probably via enhanced NO generation

In contrast to the vasoconstrictor effect of Klotho alone, the addition of Klotho induced a concentration-dependent relaxation in phosphate preconstricted vessels (**Figure 4A**) or in phenylephrine preconstricted vessels (data not shown). Maximal Klotho induced vascular relaxation was obtained within 200 sec. This relaxant effect was abolished by endothelium removal (data not shown), indicating the involvement of endothelium-derived factors. Consistent with this hypothesis, the relaxation effect of Klotho on phosphate-preconstricted vessels was blocked by the addition of L-NNA, a competitive inhibitor of NOS with selectivity for the neuronal and endothelial isoforms of the enzyme (**Figure 4A**).

The addition of Klotho significantly augmented the concentration of H_2O_2 induced by phosphate alone only in HVSMCs (**Figure 1B**). Klotho and phosphate alone or in combination induced ERK activation in mouse aortas (100±0 for control vs 261±53 for Klotho and phosphate, p<0.05).

Phosphate induced a significant increase in NO concentration and activated eNOS only in presence of Klotho. Moreover, Klotho alone was able to induce iNOS de novo expression and this effect was maintained even in presence of phosphate (**Figures 3B and 4B**).

Enhancement of vascular contraction by FGF23 in phosphate-preconstricted vessels, possibly by an induction of ROS expression

The addition of FGF23 induced a further, dose-dependent contraction in phosphate preconstricted vessels. Although FGF23 alone was able to induce concentration-dependent contractions this effect was thus enhanced when FGF23 was associated with phosphate (**Figure 5A**). The addition of FGF23 significantly augmented H_2O_2 concentration induced by phosphate alone only in HVSMCs (**Figure 1B**). FGF23 and phosphate alone or in combination induced ERK activation in mouse aortas (100±0 for control vs 290±84 for phosphate and FGF23, p<0.05).

Reduction of endothelium dependent vascular relaxation by Klotho in combination with FGF23 and phosphate

Although phosphate, Klotho, or FGF23 alone exhibited vasoconstrictor effect in mouse aorta rings no contractile response was observed upon co-incubation. The response to phenylephrine was increased by FGF23 and endothelium dependent relaxation decreased by phosphate. Co-incubation with the three compounds decreased endothelium dependent vasorelaxation induced by acetylcholine (**Figure 5B**).

Klotho, phosphate and FGF23 together increased H_2O_2 concentration both in HVSMCs and HUVECs (**Figure 1B**). This combination increased ERK activation in aortas (100±0 for control vs 320±119 for Klotho and phosphate and FGF23, p<0.05).

The three compounds together increased NO concentration in HUVECs via an increase of eNOS expression and induction of de novo iNOS expression (p<0.05 vs control, **Figure 3B**).

Discussion

In the present acute experiments, we demonstrate for the first time that both FGF23 and Klotho directly stimulate arterial vasoconstriction in a concentration-dependent fashion. These actions were found to occur independently of each other. However, their combined effects on the vessel wall are more complex, owing to apparently opposing actions in terms of local oxidant generation and NO production.

In addition to its major expression in kidney, parathyroid, and choroid plexus Klotho is expressed in human vascular tissue [7]. Both Klotho and FGF23 participate in the regulation of vascular tone [16,17]. Moreover, Klotho overexpression improves endothelial function through increased NO production [18].

In the present study we show that Klotho induced a direct dose dependent vasoconstriction. In a previous study using same experimental model, we observed a direct, acute vasoconstrictive effect of phosphate which was associated with enhanced ROS production [19]. According to previous studies done in our *in vitro* HUVEC model Klotho was unable to induce H_2O_2 production [20–22]. In contrast, in the present *in vitro* HVSMC model addition of Klotho induced an excessive H_2O_2 concentration. When using cumulative concentrations of Klotho, the vasoconstriction obtained for each concentration was increased compared to a single concentration (**Figures 1A, 3A**). This led us to suppose that a relaxation factor was stimulated by Klotho as well. This hypothesis was reinforced by the observation of a relaxation effect of Klotho on phosphate preconstricted aorta. Under the same condition, Klotho's relaxant effect was abolished by endothelium removal, indicating the involvement of endothelium-derived factors. Consistent with this hypothesis, the relaxation effect of Klotho was blocked by the addition of L-NNA, a competitive inhibitor of NOS. Moreover, Klotho was able to increase

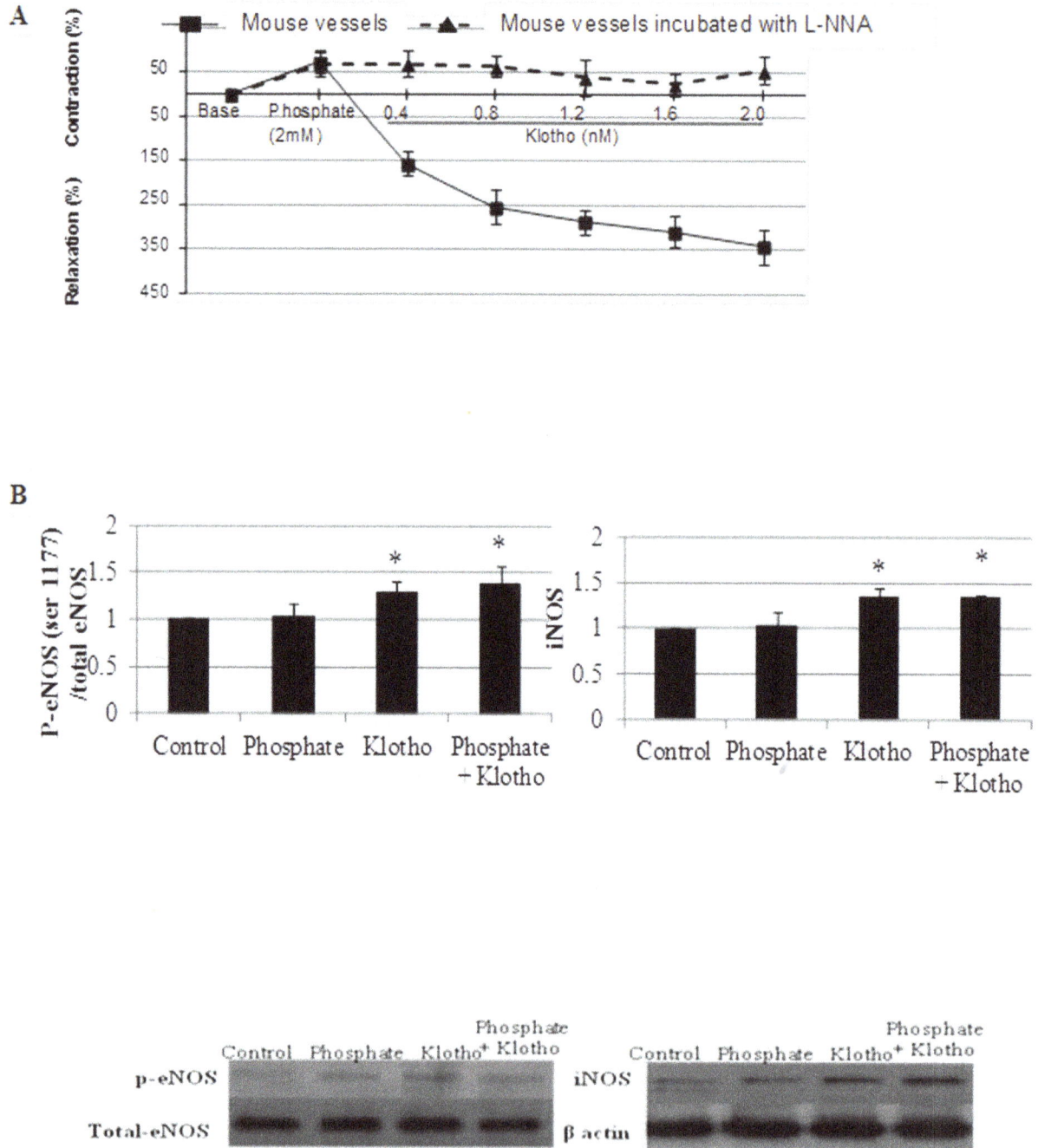

Figure 4. Effects of phosphate associated with Klotho on vascular reactivity and eNOS and iNOS expressions. A. Effects of phosphate (2.0 mM) combined with Klotho (0.4, 0.8, 1.2, 1.6, 2.0 nM) on aortic rings ex vivo. Contraction values are expressed as percentage of the contraction obtained with 70 mM KCl. Relaxation was calculated taking into account the maximal contraction obtained with phosphate 2.0 mM alone. The possible involvement of NO was studied by incubating aortic rings with L-NNA for 30 min before exposure to phosphate and Klotho. N, 4 per experiment. B. Effects of phosphate (2.0 mM), Klotho (1.6 nM) or the two combined on eNOS expression (N, 4–6 per experiment) and iNOS de novo expression (N, 4–6 per experiment). * $p < 0.05$ vs. control group.

endothelial NO concentration. These results are in accordance with previous studies demonstrating a decrease of endothelium-dependent relaxation, NO metabolites such NO_2^- and NO_3^- and NO in aortas of heterozygote Klotho mice, and a total lack of relaxation in aortas of Klotho deficient mice [17,23]. Our study shows that Klotho can directly induce eNOS phosphorylation and iNOS expression, as based on L-NNA experiments which inhibit both enzymes, leading to increased NO concentration and

relaxation of preconstricted aorta. Klotho induced iNOS expression suggesting that it may stimulate inflammatory responses as suggested by other authors [26]. Klotho kept its eNOS phosphorylation capacity even in presence of phosphate and thereby reverted its vasoconstrictor effect. A beneficial vascular role of Klotho has also been demonstrated in the context of hyperphosphatemia. The Klotho concentrations used in the present study were comparable to those used by Hu et al. [24].

A

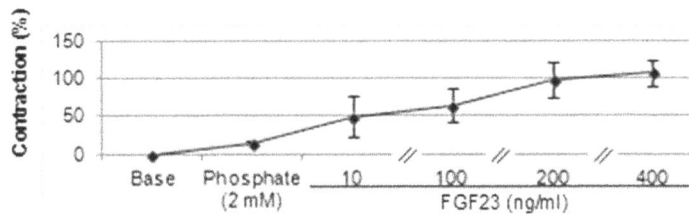

B

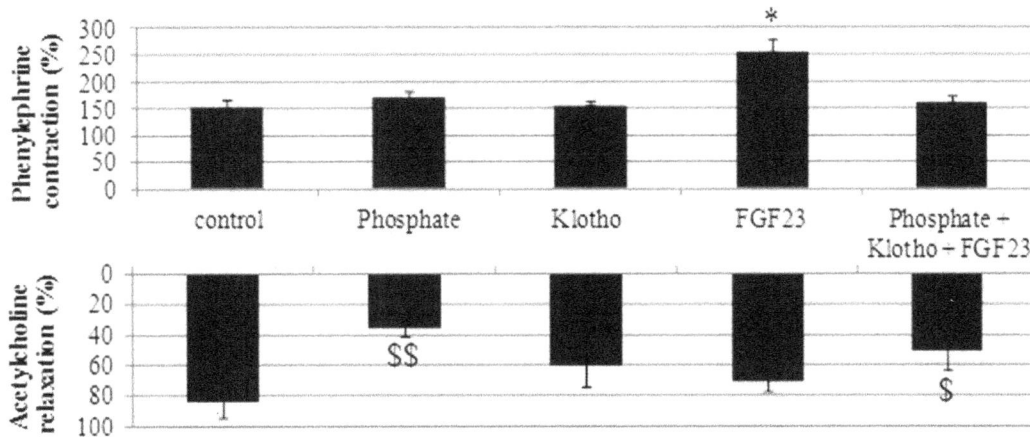

Figure 5. Vascular effects of phosphate (2.0 mM) associated with FGF23 (10–400 ng/ml) (A) and contraction obtained with phenylephrine and relaxation obtained with acetylcholine after incubation of aortic rings in presence of phosphate (2.0 mM), Klotho (1.6 nM), FGF23 (10 ng/ml) or the three combined (B). * $p < 0.005$ vs. all other groups, \$ $p < 0.05$ or \$\$ $p < 0.001$ vs control group.

Thus the vascular action of Klotho appears to reflect a balance between its effects on ROS and NO concentration. In single Klotho exposure experiments the decrease of vasoconstriction appeared to be mainly linked to NO stimulation. In contrast, incubation with increasing Klotho concentrations induced vasoconstriction, probably due to NO degradation by ROS and the longer half-life of ROS compared to NO. A subtle balance between NO and ROS effects could be one of the explanations for the present controversy on the vascular effects of Klotho.

A previous report showed a positive association between high FGF23 serum concentrations and vascular dysfunction [16]. In line with this finding, we show for the first time a direct, acute vascular effect of FGF23 at serum concentrations observed in uremic patients [25]. As previously suspected, but not proven so far, FGF23 alone exerted a marked vasoconstrictor effect in aortic rings. In contrast, Lindberg et al failed to observe an FGF23 effect on aorta reactivity [27]. The discrepancy could be explained by their use of small resistance vessels and lower FGF23 concentrations. In our study, the FGF23 vasoconstrictor effect was found to be related to ROS concentration in HVSMC and associated with ERK1/2 activation in aortic tissue. The activation of ROS appeared to be the only contribution of FGF23 to vascular dysfunction. In contrast to Klotho, the vasoconstrictive effect in response to increasing concentrations of FGF23 was similar to that obtained with a unique concentration and there was no effect on NO. Taken together, our findings are compatible with the hypothesis that in vascular tissues, FGF23 exerts Klotho-independent effects, and that the mechanism of action of FGF23 may differ from one type of tissue to another. The importance of the

cardiovascular effects of FGF23 excess and their independence of the Klotho coreceptor have recently been questioned in a study done in patients with a broad range of kidney function impairment [28].

Strikingly, the exposure of phosphate pre-contracted vessels to increasing levels of FGF23 further increased aortic constriction and ROS concentration, suggesting a synergistic effect. Thus in contrast to Klotho, FGF23 was unable to reverse the contractile effects of phosphate. Moreover, FGF23 at physiological concentration (10 ng/ml) exerted vasoconsctrictive, Klotho independent vascular effects.

When Klotho was associated with FGF23, the vasoconstriction induced by FGF23 could be abolished by Klotho, probably via enhanced NO production. Interestingly, Klotho also mitigated the direct effects of combined phosphate and FGF23 on aortic contractility, thereby protecting the vessel wall. Similar complex interactions between Klotho and FGF23 at the site of the VSMC have recently been observed by Lim et al, although they examined longer time periods [7]. In the setting of CKD, ROS excess may trigger signalling events that further exacerbate VSMC proliferation and vascular remodelling. However, in physiological condition ROS such as H_2O_2 play an essential role in signal transduction and regulation of vascular function.

Finally, when studying the combined effects of phosphate, Klotho and FGF23, we observed no direct change in vascular function despite the vasoconstriction induced by each substance separately.

After incubation in presence of phosphate or Klotho or FGF23, the response to phenylephrine was increased by FGF23 and endothelium dependent relaxation was decreased by phosphate. The combined stimulation with phosphate and Klotho and FGF23 did not change the contraction induced by phenylephrine, but this combination decreased the endothelium dependent vasorelaxation induced by acetylcholine

Moreover, the combined exposure of these three compounds led to enhanced ROS concentration by HUVECs. As to eNOS activation, it was comparable when HUVEC were exposed to Klotho alone or in association with phosphate and/or FGF23. Thus with triple exposure there is an imbalance between the contraction effect mediated by smooth muscle generated ROS and the relaxation effect mediated by endothelial NO. The predominant phenomenon appears to be endothelial ROS generation opposing the endothelial NO effect. This observation is in accordance with the partial inhibition of endothelium dependent relaxation in response to acetylcholine.

The present study has some limitations. We did not test the different compounds in vivo. Moreover, in contrast to the study of Faul et al [15], we did not explore the role of FGF receptors in the observed FGF23 effects. In a subsequent study, it will be interesting to test the effect of FGF receptor inhibitors on arterial contraction induced by FGF23.

In conclusion, although separate in vitro exposure to phosphate, soluble Klotho, or FGF23 stimulates aorta contraction directly, Klotho mitigates the vasoconstrictive effects of phosphate and FGF23 and thereby protects the vessel wall against potentially excessive vasoconstrictive effects of high phosphate and FGF23 concentrations. Our findings support the theory that Klotho deficiency in CKD is noxious whereas Klotho sufficiency is protective against the negative effects of high phosphate and FGF23 concentrations, which are additive. Since both Klotho deficiency and FGF23 excess appear to be deleterious one could speculate about the relative merits of potential therapeutic effects of Klotho stimulation versus FGF23 suppression. Since high phosphate, Klotho and FGF23 concentrations combined can induce endothelial cell dysfunction the correction of Klotho deficiency alone may not be sufficient.

Author Contributions

Conceived and designed the experiments: IS HO. Performed the experiments: IS HO PG JC CB. Analyzed the data: IS HO PG JC CB JM TBD ZAM. Contributed reagents/materials/analysis tools: IS HO. Wrote the paper: IS HO TBD ZAM.

References

1. Keith DS, Nichols GA, Gullion CM, Brown JB, Smith DH (2004) Longitudinal follow-up and outcomes among a population with chronic kidney disease in a large managed care organization. Arch Intern Med 164:659–663.
2. Stam F, van Guldener C, Becker A, Dekker JM, Heine RJ, et al. (2006) Endothelial dysfunction contributes to renal function-associated cardiovascular mortality in a population with mild renal insufficiency: the Hoorn study. J Am Soc Nephrol 17:537–545.
3. Recio-Mayoral A, Banerjee D, Streather C, Kaski JC (2011) Endothelial dysfunction, inflammation and atherosclerosis in chronic kidney disease—a cross-sectional study of predialysis, dialysis and kidney-transplantation patients. Atherosclerosis 216:446–451
4. Montezano AC, Touyz RM (2012) Reactive oxygen species and endothelial function—role of nitric oxide synthase uncoupling and Nox family nicotinamide adenine dinucleotide phosphate oxidases. Basic Clin Pharmacol Toxicol 110:87–94.
5. Matsumura Y, Aizawa H, Shiraki-Iida T, Nagai R, Kuro-o M, et al. (1998) Identification of the human klotho gene and its two transcripts encoding membrane and secreted klotho protein. Biochem Biophys Res Commun 242:626–630.
6. Prié D, Ureña Torres P, Friedlander G (2009) Latest findings in phosphate homeostasis. Kidney Int 75:882–889.
7. Lim K, Lu TS, Molostvov G, Lee C, Lam FT, et al. (2012) Vascular Klotho deficiency potentiates the development of human artery calcification and mediates resistance to fibroblast growth factor 23. Circulation 125:2243–2255.
8. Quarles LD (2008) Endocrine functions of bone in mineral metabolism regulation. J Clin Invest 118:3820–3828.
9. Nakai K, Komaba H, Fukagawa M (2010) New insights into the role of fibroblast growth factor 23 in chronic kidney disease. J Nephrol 23:619–625.
10. Saito T, Fukumoto S (2009) Fibroblast Growth Factor 23 (FGF23) and Disorders of Phosphate Metabolism. Int J Pediatr Endocrinol 2009:496514.
11. Kuro-o M, Matsumura Y, Aizawa H, Kawaguchi H, Suga T, et al. (1997) Mutation of the mouse klotho gene leads to a syndrome resembling ageing. Nature 390:45–51.
12. Shimada T, Kakitani M, Yamazaki Y, Hasegawa H, Takeuchi Y, et al. (2004) Targeted ablation of Fgf23 demonstrates an essential physiological role of FGF23 in phosphate and vitamin D metabolism. J Clin Invest 113:561–568.
13. Galitzer H, Ben-Dov IZ, Silver J, Naveh-Many T (2010) Parathyroid cell resistance to fibroblast growth factor 23 in secondary hyperparathyroidism of chronic kidney disease. Kidney Int 77:211–218.
14. Canalejo R, Canalejo A, Martinez-Moreno JM, Rodriguez-Ortiz ME, Estepa JC, et al. (2010) FGF23 fails to inhibit uremic parathyroid glands. J Am Soc Nephrol 21:1125–1135.
15. Faul C, Amaral AP, Oskouei B, Hu MC, Sloan A, et al. (2011) FGF23 induces left ventricular hypertrophy. J Clin Invest 121:4393–4408.
16. Mirza MA, Larsson A, Lind L, Larsson TE (2009) Circulating fibroblast growth factor-23 is associated with vascular dysfunction in the community. Atherosclerosis 205:385–390.
17. Saito Y, Yamagishi T, Nakamura T, Ohyama Y, Aizawa H, et al. (1998) Klotho protein protects against endothelial dysfunction. Biochem Biophys Res Commun 248:324–329.
18. Saito Y, Nakamura T, Ohyama Y, Suzuki T, Iida A, et al. (2000) In vivo klotho gene delivery protects against endothelial dysfunction in multiple risk factor syndrome. Biochem Biophys Res Commun 276:767–772.
19. Six I, Maizel J, Barreto FC, Rangrez AY, Dupont S, et al. (2012) Effects of phosphate on vascular function under normal conditions and influence of the uraemic state. Cardiovasc Res 96:130–139.
20. Rakugi H, Matsukawa N, Ishikawa K, Yang J, Imai M, et al. (2007) Anti-oxidative effect of Klotho on endothelial cells through cAMP activation. Endocrine 31(1):82–87.
21. Yang K, Nie L, Huang Y, Zhang J, Xiao T, et al. (2012) Amelioration of uremic toxin indoxyl sulfate-induced endothelial cell dysfunction by Klotho protein. Toxicol Lett 215:77–83.
22. Carracedo J, Buendía P, Merino A, Madueño JA, Peralbo E, et al. (2012) Klotho modulates the stress response in human senescent endothelial cells. Mech Ageing Dev 133:647–654.
23. Nakamura T, Saito Y, Ohyama Y, Masuda H, Sumino H, et al. (2002) Production of nitric oxide, but not prostacyclin, is reduced in klotho mice. Jpn J Pharmacol 89:149–156.
24. Izquierdo MC, Perez-Gomez MV, Sanchez-Niño MD, Sanz AB, Ruiz-Andres O, et al. (2012) Klotho, phosphate and inflammation/ageing in chronic kidney disease. Nephrol Dial Transplant 27 Suppl 4:iv6–10.
25. Hu MC, Shi M, Zhang J, Quiñones H, Griffith C, et al. (2011) Klotho deficiency causes vascular calcification in chronic kidney disease. J Am Soc Nephrol 22:124–136.
26. Nagano N, Miyata S, Abe M, Kobayashi N, Wakita S, et al. (2006) Effect of manipulating serum phosphorus with phosphate binder on circulating PTH and FGF23 in renal failure rats. Kidney Int 69:531–537.
27. Lindberg K, Olauson H, Amin R, Ponnusamy A, Goetz R, et al. (2013) Arterial Klotho Expression and FGF23 Effects on Vascular Calcification and Function. PLoS One 8(4):e60658.
28. Agarwal I, Ide N, Ix JH, Kestenbaum B, Lanske B, et al. (2014) Fibroblast growth factor-23 and cardiac structure and function. J Am Heart Assoc 3(1):e000584.

16

Glomerular Filtration Rate and Proteinuria: Association with Mortality and Renal Progression in a Prospective Cohort of a Community-Based Elderly Population

Se Won Oh[1], Sejoong Kim[2], Ki Young Na[2,3], Ki Woong Kim[4], Dong-Wan Chae[2,3], Ho Jun Chin[2,3]*

1 Department of Internal Medicine, Inje University College of Medicine, Goyang City, Gyeonggi-do, Korea, 2 Department of Internal Medicine, Seoul National University Bundang Hopsital, Seong-Nam, Korea, 3 Department of Internal Medicine, Seoul National University College of Medicine, Seoul, Korea, 4 Department of Psychiatry, Seoul National University College of Medicine, Seoul, Korea

Abstract

Limited prospective data are available on the importance of estimated glomerular filtration rate (GFR) and proteinuria in the prediction of all-cause mortality (ACM) in community-based elderly populations. We examined the relationship between GFR or proteinuria and ACM in 949 randomly selected community-dwelling elderly subjects (aged ≥65 years) over a 5-year period. A spot urine sample was used to measure proteinuria by the dipstick test, and GFR was estimated using the chronic kidney disease-epidemiology collaboration (CKD-EPI) equation. Information about mortality and causes of death was collected by direct enquiry with the subjects and from the national mortality data. Compared to subjects without proteinuria, those with proteinuria of grade ≥1+ had a 1.725-fold (1.134–2.625) higher risk of ACM. Compared to subjects with GFR ≥90 ml/min/1.73 m^2, those with GFR<45 ml/min/1.73 m^2 had a 2.357 -fold (1.170–4.750) higher risk for ACM. Among the 403 subjects included in the analysis of renal progression, the annual rate of GFR change during follow-up period was −0.52±2.35 ml/min/1.73 m^2/year. The renal progression rate was 7.315-fold (1.841–29.071) higher in subjects with GFR<60 ml/min/1.73 m^2 than in those with GFR ≥60 ml/min/1.73 m^2. Among a community-dwelling elderly Korean population, decreased GFR of <45 ml/min/1.73 m^2 and proteinuria were independent risk factors for ACM.

Editor: Valquiria Bueno, UNIFESP Federal University of São Paulo, Brazil

Funding: This work was supported by an independent Research Grant (IRG) from Pfizer Global Pharmaceuticals (grant number 06-05-039) and a Grant for developing Seongnam Health Promotion Program for the Elderly from Seongnam City Government in Korea (grant number 800-20050211. The funders had no role in study design, data collection and analysis, decision to publish, or preparation of the manuscript.

Competing Interests: This study was supported by Pfizer Global Pharmaceuticals. There are no patents, products in development or marketed products to declare.

* E-mail: mednep@snubh.org

Introduction

The prevalence of chronic kidney disease (CKD) has been increasing, causing concern both worldwide and in Korea [1]. Age is one of the most important risk factors related to the prevalence of CKD. The prevalence of a glomerular filtration rate (GFR) of < 60 ml/min/1.73 m^2 is 0.9% in subjects aged <60 years but increases to 51.2% among those aged ≥80 years in the USA [2]. The prevalence of albuminuria has been reported as 32.7% among a population of subjects aged ≥80 years [2]. However, studies evaluating the association of age with incident CKD among community-dwelling elderly populations in a prospective cohort are limited [2]. Studies on GFR changes with aging have shown that GFR declines steadily at a rate of 0.96 ml/min/1.73 m^2 annually after 30–40 years of age and decreased more rapidly after the age of 60 years [3,4]. Therefore, it is debatable whether mildly decreased GFR without definite evidences of renal damage, such as proteinuria or azotemia-related complications, should be considered as a "disease" in the elderly population [5]. In older populations, the prevalence of some of the CKD-related complications in subjects with GFR of 45–59 ml/min/1.73 m^2

was not higher than that in subjects with GFR ≥60 ml/min/1.73 m^2 [6]. A recent meta-analysis by the CKD prognosis consortium showed that the risks for mortality and renal progression were high in older populations with mildly decreased GFR [7]. However, there were several points to be cleared, which were reported in community-based prospective cohort studies. GFR has not been found to be a risk factor for all-cause mortality (ACM) [8], and the criterion of decreased renal function, in terms of GFR<60 ml/min/1.73 m^2, has been found to be less suitable for the prediction of cardiovascular mortality (CVM) [9] and ACM [10]. Furthermore, albuminuria, rather than GFR, has been found to be a risk factor for incident cardiovascular disease [11]. Another issue is that Korean data included in the consortium were obtained from participants who underwent health examination in 2 selected centers and did not represent the community population [12]. Therefore, we sought to prospectively analyze the decline in the GFR, incidence of renal progression, and the effect of GFR and proteinuria on ACM in a randomly selected, community-based, elderly population residing in a Korean city, over a 5-year follow-up period.

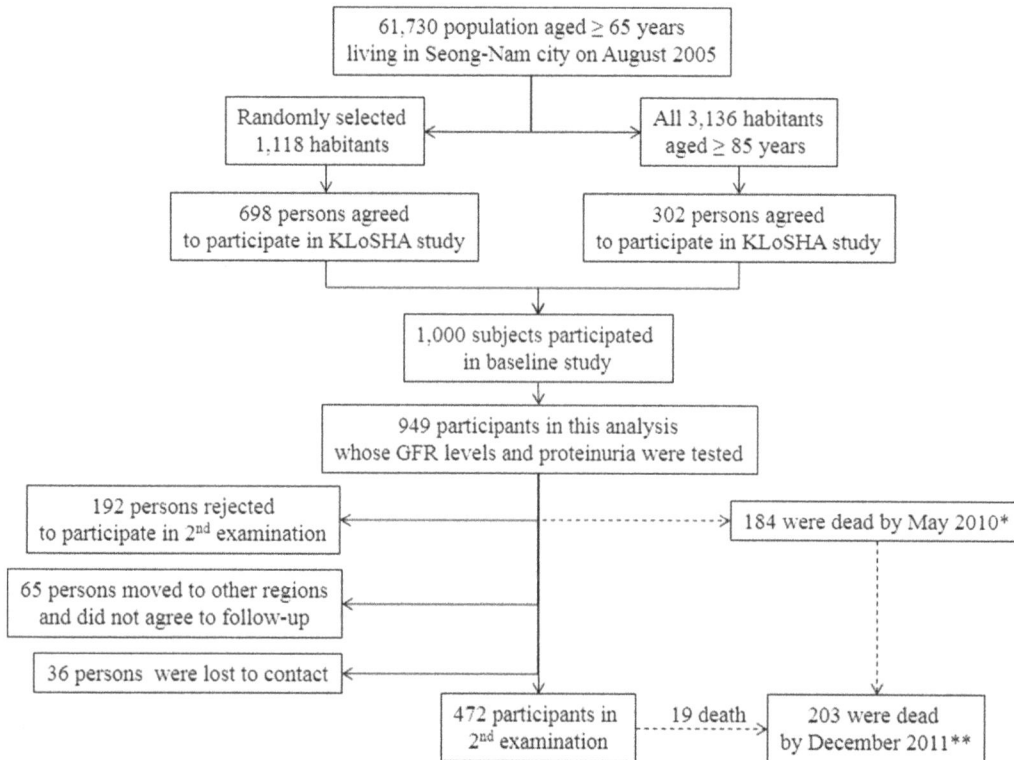

Figure 1. Participants in KLoSHA study. *Mortality was detected by direct contact and the national database. **Mortality was identified by the national database.

Materials and Methods

Design of KLoSHA and Study Population

This study was conducted as a part of the Korean Longitudinal Study on Health and Aging (KLoSHA), which included a randomly selected, community-based, elderly population. The detailed design of the KLoSHA has been described in our previous report [13]. This study protocol was reviewed and approved by the institutional review board of the Seoul National University Bundang Hospital (B-0508/023-003). The study was conducted in accordance with the Declaration of Helsinki. The baseline study was conducted from September 2005 to September 2006; the follow-up study, from May 2010 to March 2012. After obtaining written informed consent from all participants, the assessments were performed at SNUBH. Among 1,000 subjects originally included in the KLoSHA, 949 subjects with baseline serum creatinine and proteinuria, as determined by the dipstick test (Figure 1) were enrolled in the current study.

Demographic and Clinical Characteristics

Blood pressure values considered for the analysis were the means of 3 measurements. All medications taken by the participants were gathered and identified. Diabetes mellitus (DM) was defined by the use of anti-diabetic medicines, a serum fasting glucose level ≥126 mg/dl, or hemoglobin A1c (HbA1c) level ≥6.5%. Hypertension was defined as systolic blood pressure (SBP) ≥140 mmHg, diastolic blood pressure (DBP) ≥90 mmHg, or the use of anti-hypertensive medication. Proteinuria was defined as protein ≥1+, as determined by a dipstick urine test, while hematuria was defined as a red blood cell (RBC) count ≥5 per high-power field, as examined by a light microscopic examination of a urine sample. Serum creatinine level was

measured by the alkaline picrate Jaffe kinetic method using an automatic analyzer (Toshiba 200FR, Tokyo, Japan). Serum creatinine levels were calibrated to an assay traceable on an isotope dilution mass spectrometry (IDMS) device (Roche diagnostics). GFR was calculated using the CKD-epidemiology collaboration (CKD-EPI) equation [14]. The participants were categorized into 4 groups on the basis of the GFR. Proteinuria was determined by the urine dipstick test, using an automated urine analyzer (CLINITEK ATLAS, Siemens Healthcare Diagnostics, Deerfield, IL, USA). Anemia was defined by hemoglobin levels < 12 g/dL and <13 g/dL in women and men, respectively.

Outcomes

We obtained information about the survival status of the subjects participating in the baseline study via contact through telephone, cellular phone, and/or mail. This information was then confirmed by comparison against the mortality data maintained by the National Statistical Office (NSO) of Korea for the period between September 2005 and December 2011, using each individual's unique identification number. The estimated GFR decline rate for the participants who were examined a second time was determined using covariate analysis (ANCOVA). We defined renal progression as an annual decrease rate in GFR of ≥2.5 ml/min/1.73 m^2/year during the follow-up period and GFR<45 ml/min/1.73 m^2 at the second examination [15].

Statistical Analyses

All analyses were performed using SPSS (SPSS version 20.0, Chicago, IL). We compared the cumulative incidences of ACM among the participants by using the log-rank test. Cox's hazard proportional analysis was used to estimate the hazard ratios (HRs) for mortality. HRs for ACM was adjusted for age, gender, habit of

Table 1. Basal characteristics of elderly population at baseline study according to age.

	All	Age<75 years	Age≥75 years	p-value
Number	949	534	415	
Age (years)	75.8±9.0	68.8±2.9	84.8±5.6	<0.001
Gender (Male, %)	45.4	45.5	45.3	0.950
BMI (kg/m²)	24.0±3.3	24.6±3.2	22.9±3.2	<0.001
DBP (mmHg)	82.7±10.6	83.5±10.3	81.5±10.9	0.003
SBP (mmHg)	132.3±17.9	132.3±16.8	132.3±19.2	0.973
Smoking (%)				0.202
Never	58.9	59.9	57.6	
Ex-smoker	29.6	27.5	32.3	
Current smoker	11.5	12.5	10.1	
Diabetes mellitus (%)	24.2	25.7	22.4	0.328
Hypertension (%)	73.8	72.6	75.4	0.279
Hemoglobin (g/dL)	13.7±1.5	14.0±1.4	13.3±1.5	<0.001
Anemia (%)	8.6	4.3	14.3	<0.001
Creatinine (mg/dL)	0.93±0.37	0.89±0.35	0.98±0.40	0.001
GFR (ml/min/1.73 m²)	72.2±17.0	78.1±14.5	64.6±17.0	<0.001
≥90	15.2	24.2	3.6	<0.001
60–89	60.5	64.6	55.2	
45–59	16.5	8.2	27.2	
<45	7.8	3.0	14.0	
Proteinuria by dipstick (%)				0.012
none	83.6	86.7	79.5	
trace	8.2	6.6	10.4	
1+ or more	8.2	6.7	10.1	
Hematuria (%)	10.5	9.7	11.6	0.363
Medication (%)				
ACEI or ARB	14.4	12.7	16.6	0.091
Anti-platelet agent	21.1	20.6	21.7	0.686
Statin	8.1	9.4	6.5	0.110
No of AntiHTN (%)				0.196
0	53.5	55.4	51.1	
1	28.9	28.5	29.4	
2	10.7	9.4	12.5	
≥3	6.9	7.7	7.0	

GFR: Calculated by CKD-EPI equation, BMI: body mass index, Proteinuria: measured by dipstick test, Anemia: defined in female with hemoglobin less than 12 g/dL and, in male, less than 13 g/dL. Hematuria: RBC≥5/HPF, Anti-platelet agent: aspirin 100 mg, triflusal, sarpogrelate, or clopidogrel, No of AntiHTN: number of antihypertensive medication.

smoking, CRP, cholesterol, triglyceride, albumin, platelet, and hemoglobin. We selected these adjusting factors which showed significant associations with mortality in the univariate analysis. Formal tests for multiplicative interactions were conducted by comparing −2 log likelihood in regression models, including the full population, with and without interaction terms (for example, risk factor 1 * risk factor 2). We compared the incidence of renal progression in the different groups using logistic regression analysis. The number of subjects with renal progression was small, and we grouped the subjects according to the GFR level of 60 ml/min/1.73 m². P-values of 0.05 were considered statistically significant.

Results

Baseline Characteristics

The mean age of the participants was 75.8±9.0 years. DM was present in 24.2% of the subjects; hypertension, in 73.8%. The GFR was ≥90 ml/min/1.73 m² in 15.2% of the subjects; 60–89 ml/min/1.73 m², in 60.5%; 45–59 ml/min/1.73 m², in 16.5%; and <45 ml/min/1.73 m², in 7.8%. Proteinuria of grade ≥1+was noted in 8.2% of the population. The proportion of subjects with GFR<60 ml/min/1.73 m² was higher in the oldest old group, aged ≥75 years, than in the group of subjects aged 65–74 years (41.2% vs. 11.2%) (Table 1).

Table 2. The event rate of all-cause mortality according to basal characteristics.

	N	ACM rate /100 PY	(95% CI)	p*
All	949	4.05	3.98–4.11	
Gender				0.005
Male	431	4.92	4.80–5.06	
Female	518	3.34	3.27–3.41	
Age (years)				<0.001
<75	534	1.27	1.25–1.28	
≥75	415	8.48	8.20–8.77	
DM				0.825
no	719	4.10	4.02–4.18	
yes	230	3.90	3.78–4.03	
Hypertension				0.576
no	248	3.81	3.69–3.94	
yes	700	4.14	4.06–4.22	
DBP (mmHg)				0.246
<80	196	5.03	4.82–5.27	
80–89	492	3.67	3.62–3.78	
≥90	259	4.03	3.92–4.15	
SBP (mmHg)				0.707
<130	397	4.30	4.18–4.42	
130–149	350	3.73	3.64–3.83	
≥150	200	4.15	4.02–4.30	
BP (mmHg)				0.895
<130/80	165	4.23	4.04–4.44	
≥130/80	782	4.02	3.95–4.09	
GFR (ml/min/1.73 m^2)				<0.001
≥90	144	1.47	1.43–1.51	
60–89	574	3.32	3.26–3.38	
45–59	157	7.10	6.74–7.50	
<45	74	10.23	9.36–11.29	
Proteinuria				0.001
none	793	3.61	3.55–3.67	
trace	78	5.79	5.44–6.20	
≥1+	78	7.14	6.63–7.75	

*ACM: all-cause mortality, p-value: calculated by Pearson's Chi-square test, 100 PY: 100 person-years.

All-cause Mortality

The follow-up duration for mortality was 63.4±16.4 months after the baseline visit. Overall, there were 203 cases of ACM and 4.05 deaths/100 person-years (Table 2). The estimated 5-year survival rates were 91.5% in GFR group 1, 89.7% in GFR group 2, 66.9% in GFR group 3, and 52.5% in GFR group 4 (p<0.001; Figure 2). The estimated 5-year survival rates were 92.4% in subjects with no proteinuria, 70.5% in subjects with trace proteinuria, and 65.4% in subjects with proteinuria ≥1+ (p = 0.001; Figure 2). In the estimation of mortality, no interactions were noted between the GFR group and proteinuria group, age group, or gender and between proteinuria group and age group or gender. Subjects with proteinuria of grade ≥1+ had a 1.725-fold higher risk for ACM than those without proteinuria (p = 0.011), and subjects with GFR<45 ml/min/1.73 m^2 had a 2.357-fold

higher risk for ACM than those with GFR ≥90 ml/min/1.73 m^2 (p = 0.016; Table 3).

GFR Decline and Renal Progression

The follow-up study was conducted 59.4±6.9 months after the baseline visit. Among the 472 subjects who underwent the follow-up examination, 403 were included in the analysis of renal progression. The annual rate of GFR change during the follow-up period was −0.52±2.35 ml/min/1.73 m^2/year. Compared to participants without DM or lower GFR, those with DM or lower GFR showed a more rapid decline in GFR during the follow-up period (Table 4). The proportion of subjects with renal progression was 11/403 (2.7%). There was no interaction between GFR group and age or DM for renal progression. Negative interactions were found between gender and GFR group (p-interactions = 0.047).

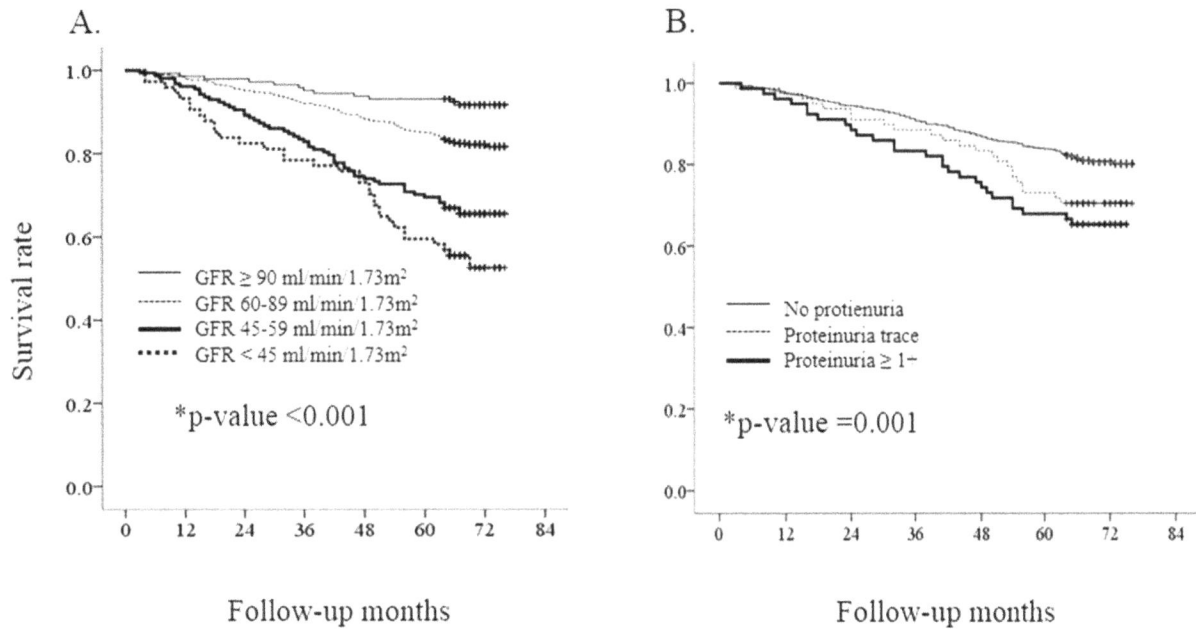

Figure 2. The survival rate according to GFR and proteinuria. A. GFR group for all-caused mortality. B. Proteinuria group for all-caused mortality *p-value by Log-rank test.

Multiple logistic regression analysis revealed that the renal progression rate was 7.315-fold (1.841–29.071) higher in subjects with GFR<60 ml/min/1.73 m^2 than in those with GFR $\geq$ 60 ml/min/1.73 m^2.

Discussion

In this community-based elderly cohort, the grade of GFR was found to be an independent risk factor for ACM. However, subjects with a GFR of 45–59 ml/min/1.73 m^2 did not have higher risk for ACM than those with GFR $\geq$90 ml/min/1.73 m^2. Proteinuria was an independent risk factor for ACM. The annual rate of GFR decline was 0.52 ml/min/1.73 m^2. GFR<60 ml/min/1.73 m^2 was an important risk factor for renal progression.

Studies analyzing the relationships between GFR or proteinuria and outcomes in the elderly have shown variable results depending on the characteristics of the enrolled population. Recent meta-

analyses have shown that the HRs of low GFR (<60 ml/min/1.73 m^2) with ACM [7,16,17], CVM[16], and end stage renal disease (ESRD) [7] were similar meanings irrespective of patient age. The studies included all of community populations, high-risk populations for CKD, and CKD populations and showed differences compared to community-based studies. The relationship between serum creatinine level and mortality was most evident in populations with traditional cardiovascular risk factors or renal insufficiency, and not in community-based cohorts [18]. Among patients (age, >55 years) who had documented vascular disease or diabetes with symptoms of end organ damage, the HRs for ACM according to GFR levels increased in proportion to the severity of the traditional risk factors for cardiovascular disease [19]. A study on patients visiting the outpatient clinics showed a less evident relationship between mild-to-moderately decreased GFR and outcomes. O'Hara et al. reported that, compared to elderly patients with GFR $\geq$60 ml/min/1.73 m^2, those with a

Table 3. The significant effect on mortality of proteinuria and GFR.

	HR for ACM*
Proteinuria group	
None	1.000 (ref.)
trace	1.235 (0.777–1.963)
$\geq$1+	1.725 (1.134–2.625)
GFR group	
$\geq$90	1.000 (ref.)
60–89	1.370 (0.746–2.517)
45–59	1.654 (0.841–3.254)
<45	2.357 (1.170–4.750)

*Cox's hazard proportional model adjusted with age, gender, habit of smoking, CRP, cholesterol, triglyceride, albumin, platelet, and hemoglobin.
ACM: all-cause mortality, ref.: reference group, HR: Hazard ratio, CI: confidence interval, NC: cannot be calculated.

Table 4. GFR decline according to baseline characteristics in participants followed up 2nd examination.

	N	GFR decline * Mean (95% CI)	p-value		N	GFR decline * Mean (95% CI)	p-value
All	403	0.52 (0.31–0.73)		SBP (mmHg)			0.510
Gender			0.237	<130	164	0.42 (0.07–0.76)	
Male	206	0.64 (0.35–0.93)		130–149	158	0.49 (0.16–0.82))	
Female	197	0.15 (0.09–0.69)		≥150	81	0.77 (0.29–1.26)	
Age (years)			0.677	BP (mmHg)			0.068
<75	308	0.47 (0.15–0.78)		<130/80	67	0.08 (***0.44**–0.59*)	
≥75	75	0.68 (***0.11**–1.47*)		≥130/80	336	0.61 (0.38–0.83)	
DM			<0.001	GFR (ml/min/1.73 m²)			0.012
no	304	0.29 (0.05–0.53)		≥90	84	0.29 (***0.40**–0.96*)	
yes	99	1.21 (0.79–1.63)		60–89	260	0.38 (0.11–0.64)	
HTN			0.084	45–59	41	1.22 (0.33–2.10)	
no	112	0.22 (0.18–0.62)		<45	18	2.88 (1.41–4.35)	
yes	291	0.63 (0.39–0.88)		Proteinuria			0.892
DBP (mmHg)			0.589	none	357	0.53 (0.31–0.75)	
<80	75	0.28 (0.21–0.78)		trace	24	0.56 (***0.30**–1.42*)	
80–89	216	0.57 (0.28–0.86)		≥1+	22	0.31 (***0.59**–1.21*)	
≥90	112	0.57 (0.15–0.99)					

GFR decline: GFR decline rate (ml/min/1.73 m²/year) estimated by covariate analysis adjusted for age, gender, DM, HTN, GFR, and proteinuria by dipstick test at baseline study.
**The number with bold character indicates GFR increase rate.

GFR of 50–59 ml/min/1.73 m^2 did not have an increased risk for death [20]. A prospective cohort study of community-dwelling persons aged ≥65 years showed that GFR was not a risk factor for ACM and CVM [8]. Therefore, a randomly sampled community-based cohort with representativeness is more suitable for determining the effect of changes of GFR with aging on outcomes.

In this respect, the KLoSHA protocol offered several advantages in the evaluation of the relationship between renal parameters and outcomes. The majority of these data were sampled by random selection from non-institutionalized habitants. A prospective study provides higher quality of evidences than those provided by a cross-sectional study. We were able to contact almost all the participants for confirmation of mortality and verified this information against the data maintained by the National Statistical Office of Korea. All Koreans have a unique identifier, which is the primary key to obtain individualized data. Finally, serum creatinine was measured in a single institution throughout the study period and represented as IDMS-traceable value, which was suitable for application of the CKD-EPI equation.

The definition of GFR for the assessment of increased risk of mortality in elderly population can also vary with the nature of the included population. Several prospective community-based cohort studies showed that a GFR value of 60 ml/min/1.73 m^2 was not a suitable cut-off for the prediction of ACM [8,9,20] or CVM [9,10] among the elderly population. Other studies, including those on community populations, showed no relationship between CVM and GFR in populations of subjects aged ≥65 years [8,18,21] or ≥ 70 years [17]. The other issue is the effect of albuminuria among participants with decreased GFR on mortality. In elderly patients aged ≥60 years, GFR<60 ml/min/1.73 m^2 estimated by serum creatinine was found to be a risk factor in participants with albuminuria, but not for those without albuminuria [22]. Albuminuria has been reported as a risk factor for ACM and CVM in elderly populations with high risk(s) [11,16] and in community-based elderly cohorts [11,23,24,25]. For example, in the PREVEND study, albuminuria, but not GFR, was found to be associated with CVM and ACM [11].

A few prospective studies have evaluated the association of age with the decline in estimated GFR with aging [2]. A longitudinal study on an elderly cohort (60–93 years) in Sweden revealed that the GFR estimated by the CKD-EPI equation declined at an annual rate of 1.042 ml/min/1.73 m^2 in men and 0.970 ml/min/1.73 m^2 in women [26]; these rates are higher than those noted in this study. Imai et al. reported that the annual decline in GFR

using the MDRD equation in an elderly population (60–79 years) followed for 10 years [27] was 0.32–0.39 ml/min/1.73 m^2 per year, which is similar to that obtained in our study. Ethnic differences in the rate of decline in GFR should be accounted for in a well-designed study. We used the criteria for renal progression used in the KDIGO controversy conferences [15]. Our study revealed that a GFR<60 ml/min/1.73 m^2 was the most important risk factor of renal progression, as observed in other studies [8,28].

There are several limitations in the interpretation of this study's results. The CKD-EPI equation has not been fully validated in elderly Koreans, although our colleagues have reported that the ethnic coefficients of the CKD-EPI equations were close to "1," on the basis of a study on 131 CKD patients and healthy volunteers [29]. We followed the participants over 5 years but 29.3% of initial population was not followed up at the second examination. The significant percent of dropout rate is an important limitation of this study. Especially, renal progression was evaluated in only subjects who completed follow up examination. Several criteria for renal outcomes have been proposed thus far, and we used the criteria defined at the KDIGO controversies conference [15]. In addition, we evaluated a relatively small numbers of subjects with severely decreased renal function and proteinuria. The results should be carefully interpreted in subjects with eGFR<45 ml/min/1.73 m^2 or proteinuria. We evaluate the renal outcome on the basis of the difference of serum creatinine at baseline and at the end of the follow up study, and we did not confirm the sustained decline in eGFR during follow up period. Finally, this study is based on a city population, and the generalization of the results for a nationwide population or for all Asians is debatable.

In conclusion, we found that in a community-dwelling elderly Korean population, a decreased GFR<45 ml/min/1.73 m^2 and proteinuria were independent risk factors for ACM. With aging, the annual rate of decrease in GFR was 0.52 ml/min/1.73 m^2/year and the baseline GFR was the most important risk factor for renal progression.

Author Contributions

Conceived and designed the experiments: HJC SWO SK KYN KWK DWC. Performed the experiments: HJC SWO. Analyzed the data: HJC SWO. Contributed reagents/materials/analysis tools: HJC SWO. Wrote the paper: HJC SWO. Revised the paper for important intellectual content and have seen and approved the final version: SWO SK KYN KWK DWC HJC.

References

1. Kim S, Lim CS, Han DC, Kim GS, Chin HJ, et al. (2009) The prevalence of chronic kidney disease (CKD) and the associated factors to CKD in urban Korea: a population-based cross-sectional epidemiologic study. J Korean Med Sci 24: S11–S21.
2. Bowling CB, Muntner P (2012) Epidemiology of chronic kidney disease among older adults: a focus on the oldest old. J Gerontol A Biol Sci Med Sci 67: 1379–1386.
3. Davies DF, Shock NW (1950) Age changes in glomerular filtration rate, effective renal plasma flow, and tubular excretory capacity in adult males. J Clin Invest 29: 496–507.
4. Lindeman RD, Tobin J, Shock NW(1985) Longitudinal studies on the rate of decline in renal function with age. J Am Geriatr Soc 33: 278–285.
5. Glassock RJ, Winearls C (2009) Ageing and the glomerular filtration rate: truths and consequences. Trans Am Clin Climatol Assoc 120: 419–428.
6. Bowling CB, Inker LA, Gutiérrez OM, Allman RM, Warnock DG, et al. (2011) Age-specific associations of reduced estimated glomerular filtration rate with concurrent chronic kidney disease complications. Clin J Am Soc Nephrol 6: 2822–2888.
7. Hallan SI, Matsushita K, Sang Y, Mahmoodi BK, Black C, et al. (2012) Chronic Kidney Disease Prognosis Consortium: Age and association of kidney measures with mortality and end-stage renal disease. JAMA 308: 2349–2360.
8. Dalrymple LS, Katz R, Kestenbaum B, Shlipak MG, Sarnak MJ, et al. (2011) Chronic kidney disease and the risk of end-stage renal disease versus death. J Gen Intern Med 26: 379–385.
9. Stengel B, Metzger M, Froissart M, Rainfray M, Berr C, et al. (2011) Epidemiology and prognostic significance of chronic kidney disease in the elderly–the Three-City prospective cohort study. Nephrol Dial Transplant 26: 3286–3295.
10. Nerpin E, Ingelsson E, Risérus U, Sundström J, Larsson A, et al. (2011) The combined contribution of albuminuria and glomerular filtration rate to the prediction of cardiovascular mortality in elderly men. Nephrol Dial Transplant 26: 2820–2827.
11. Smink PA, Lambers Heerspink HJ, Gansevoort RT, de Jong PE, Hillege HL, et al. (2012) Albuminuria, estimated GFR, traditional risk factors, and incident cardiovascular disease: the PREVEND (Prevention of Renal and Vascular Endstage Disease) study. Am J Kidney Dis 60: 804–811.
12. Kimm H, Yun JE, Jo J, Jee SH (2009) Low serum bilirubin level as an independent predictor of stroke incidence: a prospective study in Korean men and women. Stroke 40: 3422–3427.
13. Chin HJ, Song YR, Lee JJ, Lee SB, Kim KW, et al. (2008) Moderately decreased renal function negatively affects the health-related quality of life among the elderly Korean population: a population-based study. Nephrol Dial Transplant 23: 2810–2817.

14. Levey AS, Stevens LA, Schmid CH, Zhang YL, Castro AF 3rd, et al. (2009) A new equation to estimate glomerular filtration rate. Ann Intern Med 150: 604–612.

15. Levey AS, de Jong PE, Coresh J, El Nahas M, Astor BC, et al. (2011) The definition, classification, and prognosis of chronic kidney disease: a KDIGO Controversies Conference report. Kidney Int 80: 17–28.

16. Chronic Kidney Disease Prognosis Consortium, Matsushita K, van der Velde M, Astor BC, Woodward M, et al. (2010) Association of estimated glomerular filtration rate and albuminuria with all-cause and cardiovascular mortality in general population cohorts: a collaborative meta-analysis. Lancet 375: 2073–2081.

17. Tonelli M, Wiebe N, Culleton B, House A, Rabbat C, et al. (2006) Chronic kidney disease and mortality risk: a systematic review. J Am Soc Nephrol 17: 2034–2047.

18. Garg AX, Clark WF, Haynes RB, House AA (2002) Moderate renal insufficiency and the risk of cardiovascular mortality: results from the NHANES I. Kidney Int 61: 1486–1494.

19. Clase CM, Gao P, Tobe SW, McQueen MJ, Grosshennig A, et al. ONTARGET (ONgoing Telmisartan Alone and in combination with Ramipril Global Endpoint Trial) and TRANSCEND (Telmisartan Randomized Assessment Study in Angiotensin-Converting-Enzyme-Inhibitor Intolerant Subjects with Cardiovascular Disease) (2011) Estimated glomerular filtration rate and albuminuria as predictors of outcomes in patients with high cardiovascular risk: a cohort study. Ann Intern Med 154: 310–318.

20. O'Hare AM, Bertenthal D, Covinsky KE, Landefeld CS, Sen S, et al. (2006) Mortality risk stratification in chronic kidney disease: one size for all ages? J Am Soc Nephrol 17: 846–853.

21. Culleton BF, Larson MG, Wilson PW, Evans JC, Parfrey PS, et al. (1999) Cardiovascular disease and mortality in a community-based cohort with mild renal insufficiency. Kidney Int 56: 2214–2219.

22. van der Velde M, Bakker SJ, de Jong PE, Gansevoort RT (2010) Influence of age and measure of eGFR on the association between renal function and cardiovascular events. Clin J Am Soc Nephrol 5: 2053–2059.

23. Muntner P, Bowling CB, Gao L, Rizk D, Judd S, et al. (2011) Age-specific association of reduced estimated glomerular filtration rate and albuminuria with all-cause mortality. Clin J Am Soc Nephrol 6: 2200–2207.

24. Hallan S, Astor B, Romundstad S, Aasarød K, Kvenild K, et al. (2007) Association of kidney function and albuminuria with cardiovascular mortality in older vs younger individuals: The HUNT II Study. Arch Intern Med 167: 2490–2496.

25. Rifkin DE, Katz R, Chonchol M, Fried LF, Cao J, et al. (2010) Albuminuria, impaired kidney function and cardiovascular outcomes or mortality in the elderly. Nephrol Dial Transplant 25: 1560–1567.

26. Christensson A, Elmståhl S (2011) Estimation of the age-dependent decline of glomerular filtration rate from formulas based on creatinine and cystatin C in the general elderly population. Nephron Clin Pract 117: c40–c50.

27. Imai E, Horio M, Yamagata K, Iseki K, Hara S, et al. (2008) Slower decline of glomerular filtration rate in the Japanese general population: a longitudinal 10-year follow-up study. Hypertens Res 31: 433–441.

28. Fox CS, Larson MG, Leip EP, Culleton B, Wilson PW, et al. (2004) Predictors of new-onset kidney disease in a community-based population. JAMA 291: 844–850.

29. Lee CS, Cha RH, Lim YH, Kim H, Song KH, et al. (2010) Ethnic coefficients for glomerular filtration rate estimation by the Modification of Diet in Renal Disease study equations in the Korean population. J Korean Med Sci 25: 1616–1625.

17

Development of an Adverse Drug Reaction Risk Assessment Score among Hospitalized Patients with Chronic Kidney Disease

Fatemeh Saheb Sharif-Askari[1]*, Syed Azhar Syed Sulaiman[1], Narjes Saheb Sharif-Askari[1], Ali Al Sayed Hussain[2]

1 Discipline of Clinical Pharmacy, School of Pharmaceutical Science, Universiti Sains Malaysia, Penang, Malaysia, **2** Pharmacy Department, Dubai Health Authority, Dubai, United Arab Emirates

Abstract

Background: Adverse drug reactions (ADRs) represent a major burden on the healthcare system. Chronic kidney disease (CKD) patients are particularly vulnerable to ADRs because they are usually on multiple drug regimens, have multiple comorbidities, and because of alteration in their pharmacokinetics and pharmacodynamic parameters. Therefore, one step towards reducing this burden is to identify patients who are at increased risk of an ADR.

Objective: To develop a method of identifying CKD patients who are at increased risk for experiencing ADRs during hospitalisation.

Materials and Methods: Factors associated with ADRs were identified by using demographic, clinical and laboratory variables of patients with CKD stages 3 to 5 (estimated glomerular filtration rate, 10–59 ml/min/1.73 m^2) who were admitted between January 1, 2012, and December 31, 2012, to the renal unit of Dubai Hospital. An ADR risk score was developed by constructing a series of logistic regression models. The overall model performance for sequential models was evaluated using Akaike Information Criterion for goodness of fit. Odd ratios of the variables retained in the best model were used to compute the risk scores.

Results: Of 512 patients (mean [SD] age, 60 [16] years), 62 (12.1%) experienced an ADR during their hospitalisation. An ADR risk score included age 65 years or more, female sex, conservatively managed end-stage renal disease, vascular disease, serum level of C-reactive protein more than 10 mg/L, serum level of albumin less than 3.5 g/dL, and the use of 8 medications or more during hospitalization. The C statistic, which assesses the ability of the risk score to predict ADRs, was 0.838; 95% CI, 0.784–0.892).

Conclusion: A score using routinely available patient data can be used to identify CKD patients who are at increased risk of ADRs.

Editor: Paola Romagnani, University of Florence, Italy

Funding: The authors have no support or funding to report.

Competing Interests: The authors have declared that no competing interests exist.

* E-mail: dr.fatemeh.askari@gmail.com

Introduction

Adverse drug reactions (ADRs) represent a major burden on the healthcare system, and are a common cause of hospital admission as well as of in-hospital morbidity and mortality [1–3]. Chronic kidney disease (CKD) patients are particularly vulnerable to ADRs because they are usually on multiple drug regimens, have different comorbid conditions [4], and because of alteration in their pharmacokinetics and pharmacodynamic parameters [5]. Therefore, one important step towards reducing ADRs is to identify those patients who are at increased risk of an ADR and to address their individual risk factors.

Differences in individual genome can be considered as predictors for an ADR [6], however high cost and lack of laboratory facilities limit their applicability in daily clinical practice. Another method is to develop a clinical tool or a risk assessment scale for identifying high-risk patients. Some risk factors for ADRs that have been suggested to date include age, gender, number of drugs the patient is receiving, alcohol intake, comorbidity, and factors that alter drug distribution or metabolism, such as renal or hepatic insufficiency, heart failure and anemia [7–13].

Although renal insufficiency is found to be a potential risk factor for ADRs in previous studies [9,14,15], there are no methods for identifying and stratifying CKD patients regarding their likelihood of developing an ADR. Hence, based on these considerations, the main aim of this study was to develop a comprehensive and easy applicable method of identification of hospitalized adult patients with CKD stages 3 to 5 who are at increased risk of developing an

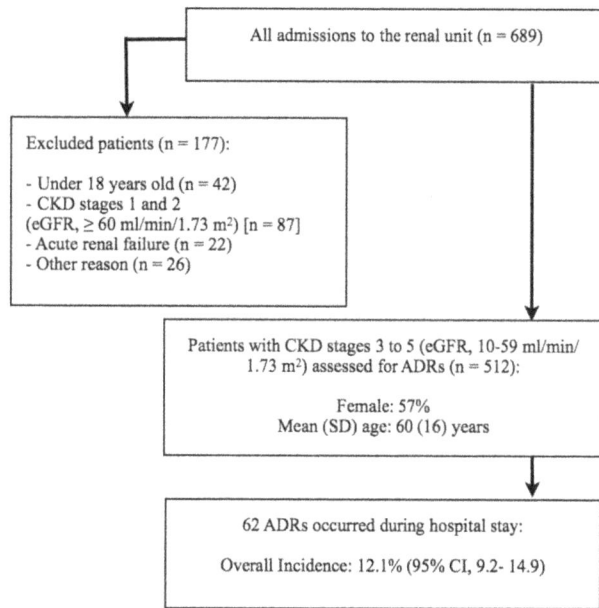

Figure 1. The flow chart of the study. Abbreviations:ADR, adverse drug reaction; CKD, chronic kidney disease; eGFR, estimated glomerular filtration rate; SD, standard deviation; CI, confidence interval.

ADR. The aim was also to create a risk score by using routinely obtained data from hospitalized patients with CKD that can be easily applied in clinical practice.

Materials and Methods

Study Design and Participants

This was a prospective, observational study conducted at the renal unit of Dubai Hospital in the United Arab Emirates. Consecutive adult patients with CKD stages 3 to 5 (estimated glomerular filtration rate [eGFR], 10–59 ml/min/1.73 m^2) who were admitted to the renal unit, between January 1, 2012, and December 31, 2012 were included. Exclusion criteria were: patients aged less than 18 years; patients who were admitted with acute renal failure; and patients who were discharged within 24 hours of admission. Prior to data collection, ethics approval was obtained from the Medical Research Committee of Dubai Health Authority, reference number MRC-SR-10/2011-01. The Medical Research Committee did not required a written informed consent from each study participant, however in case further information were required regarding identification or assessment of each ADR, a verbal informed consent was taken from the respective patient.

Variables

Independent Variables. The principal researcher (F.S.A) used a standardized form to collect patients data at their admission. Patients independent variables included demographic characteristics, such as age and sex; physical examination results, such as blood pressure and weight; comorbid conditions, such as diabetes, hypertension, vascular disease, heart failure, atrial fibrillation and anemia; laboratory tests, such as serum and biochemical parameters; and drugs taken during hospital stay. Drugs were coded according to the Anatomical and Therapeutic Chemical (ATC) classification [16], and categorized with a cutoff of 8. Diagnoses were coded according to the International Classification of Diseases, Tenth Revision, Clinical Modification,

codes [17]. Patients comorbid conditions were categorized as present or absent at the time of admission. The estimated glomerular filtration rate (eGFR) was computed using the Modification of Diet and Renal Disease (MDRD) equation [18]:

$$170 \times (\text{Serum Creatinine})^{-0.999} \times (\text{Age})^{-0.176} \times (\text{Serum Urea Nitrogen})^{-0.170} \times (\text{Serum Albumin})^{0.318}$$

For females, the result was multiplied by 0.762. Based on National Kidney Foundation (NKF), patients with eGFR 30 to 59 ml/min/1.73 m^2 were at stage 3, those with eGFR 15 to 29 ml/min/1.73 m^2 were at stage 4, and those with eGFR < 15 ml/min/1.73 m^2 were at (ESRD) end-stage renal disease. Based on the type of renal replacement therapy, patients with ESRD were divided further into the hemodialysis, peritoneal dialysis and conservative management groups [19].

Dependent Variables. The outcome of interest was the occurrence of ADR, which was defined according to the Edwards and Aronson [20] definition as: "Any appreciably harmful or unpleasant reaction, resulting from the use of a medicinal product, which predicts hazards from future administration and warrants prevention or specific treatment, or alteration of the dosage regimen, or withdrawal of the product". Only ADRs that developed during hospital stay were included, while ADRs that caused hospital admission were excluded. All ADRs were identified based on the reported evidences of adverse events in either previously published studies [21,22] and/or the British National Formulary [23]. For each suspected ADR, detailed information about; causative drug(s), such as administered dosage and frequency; objective data, such as physical examination and laboratory results; subjective data, such as dizziness and rash were collected by principal researcher. The drug related causality was assessed by using Naranjo algorithm [24]. ADRs were classified into definite (score, 9–12 points), probable (score, 5–8 points), possible (score, 1–4 points), or doubtful (score, 0 point). Only definite and probable ADRs taking place during hospital stay were considered for this study. All suspected ADRs were reviewed by a second independent reviewer (N.S.A). In cases where the two reviewers disagreed in the scoring of any ADR, they met to reach an agreement, or the case was referred to a senior researcher for review.

Statistical Analysis

For the purpose of descriptive analysis, patient's demographic data, physical examination results, comorbid conditions, laboratory tests and medication usage data were compared in according to the presence of ADRs. We used the t-test or Mann-Whitney U test, depending on the skewness of data, for continuously distributed variables and the chi-square (x^2) test for categorical variables. Continuous variables were first analyzed without categorization, but a different cutoff value was used in multivariate analysis.

Model Development. To meet the objective of the study, a sequential series of logistic regression models was developed using ADR as the dependent variable. We used a combination of medical literature guidance and forward selection method to determine variable selection [25]. At the univariate analysis, variables with a probability value of P<0.05 were entered in the multivariate logistic regression analysis. To prevent model over fitting, the maximum number of variables entered in the multivariate regression models was one variable for every eight ADR events [26]. All selected variables were tested for multi-collinearity to avoid any strong correlation between the variables. The presence of collinearity was examined by the evaluation of variance inflation factors and magnitude of standard errors. Variables with more than 10% missing values were not included in

Development of an Adverse Drug Reaction Risk Assessment Score among Hospitalized Patients with Chronic...

145

Table 1. Medication most commonly implicated in causing the ADRs.

Drug category	No. (%)[a]	Implicated medicines (n)	Adverse Reaction
Cardiovascular agents			
	2 (3)	ACEI/ARB	Hyperkalemia
	2 (3)	Furosemide	Hypokalemia
	1 (2)	Propranolol	Dermatitis
Analgesics			
	1 (2)	Acetaminophen	Vasovagal attack
Psychotropics			
	2 (3)	Benzodiazepine	Drawziness
Anti-diabetic agents			
	4 (6)	Sulfonylurea	Hypoglycemia
Anticoagulants			
	8 (13)	Warfarin	Bleeding
	16 (26)	Enoxaparin	Bleeding
	11 (17)	Heparin	Bleeding
	7 (11)	Heparin	Thrombocytopenia
	2 (3)	Foundaparinux	Bleeding
Antithrombotics			
	1 (2)	Alteplase	Skin bruits
Antiplatelets			
	3 (4)	Antiplatelets	Bleeding
Others			
	1 (2)	Mycophenolate moftil	Bone marrow suppression
	1 (2)	Darboepoetin	Gastrointestinal disorders

Abbreviations: ACEIs/ARBs, Angiotensin-converting enzyme inhibitors/angiotensin receptor blockers.
[a]The total number of definite or probable ADRs, n = 62.

the analysis. All other missing data were imputed using the multiple imputation technique with 5 imputations.

Models were developed in accordance with the chronology in which patient data are available in clinical practice. Models were consecutively extended with data from patient demographic, physical examination, comorbid conditions, laboratory test and medications used during hospital stay. In each model, variables with probability value of P>0.10 were excluded from further analysis. All models were adjusted for age, sex and estimated GFR. Results from the multivariate logistic regression were expressed in terms of the odd ratio for a particular variable with accompanying 95% confidence interval.

Model Performance. Improvement in model performance was tested using measures for calibration and discrimination. For each model, the calibration was measured using the Hosmer and Lemeshow goodness of fit test [27]. Calibration determines the differences between observed and predicted outcomes for groups of patients, with better model having smaller differences between predicted and observed outcomes [28]. The discriminatory power of each model was assessed using the concordance statistics (C statistics). Discrimination refers to the ability of a model to clearly distinguish between 2 groups of outcomes (discriminate between those patients with and those patients without the risk of developing an ADR) and can range from 0.5 (no discrimination) to 1.0 (perfect discrimination) [29,30]. The overall model fit for sequential models was compared using the Akaike Information Criterion (AIC), which takes into account both the statistical goodness of fit and the number of variables required to achieve this

particular degree of fit, by imposing a penalty for increasing the number of variables. The optimal fitted model was selected by the minimum value of AIC [30].

Model Validation. In our study, bootstrapping was used to assess the internal validation of the model [31,32]. Bootstrapping is a resampling process that enable one to make conclusions about the population that the data originated from by drawing with replacement from the original data set [30]. We drew 1000 bootstrap resamples to evaluate the reliability of the regression coefficients. The standard errors were used to calculate 95% bootstrap confidence interval of odd ratios.

All statistical analysis were performed using SPSS (version 21; SPSS, Inc., Chicago, IL) and STATA 12 statistical software (StataCorp, College station, TX). Two-sided P values of less than 0.05 were considered statistically significant.

Development of an ADR Risk Score. To obtain an easily applicable prediction rule, odd ratios of the variables retained in the best model were used to compute the risk scores. For example, a point of 1 was given to variables associated with an ADR with an odd ratio between 1.00 and 1.99; a point of 2, to those with an odd ratio between 2.00 and 2.99; a point of 3, to those with an odd ratio between 3.00 and 3.99; a point of 4, to those with an odd ratio between 4.00 and 4.99. For each patients, the score was calculated by an arithmetic sum of points for the variables present. Patients were classified into various cutoff points according to their risk score. Differences in the event rate for increasing ADR risk score values were assessed using the chi-square test for trend [33].

Table 2. Comparison of Patients Characteristics According to the Occurrence of an ADR.

Characteristics	No. (%) of Participants		
	No ADR (n = 450)	ADR (n = 62)	P Value
Demographics			
Age, mean (SD), y	60 (16)	65 (14)	0.023
Female sex	188 (42)	32 (52)	0.142
Male sex	262 (58)	30 (48)	0.142
Current or previous smoking	99 (22)	20 (32)	0.073
Physical examination, mean (SD)			
Systolic BP, mm Hg	142 (33)	128 (37)	0.065
Diastolic BP, mm Hg	75 (21)	71 (23)	0.215
Comorbid conditions			
Diabetes	324 (72)	51 (82)	0.087
Vascular disease[a]	187 (42)	42 (68)	<0.001
Heart failure	92 (20)	16 (26)	0.332
Atrial fibrillation	34 (8)	9 (14)	0.064
Anemia	209 (46)	34 (55)	0.215
History of gastrointestinal bleeding	64 (14)	14 (23)	0.086
Renal replacement therapy			
Hemodialysis	205 (46)	21 (34)	0.082
Peritoneal dialysis	30 (7)	2 (3)	0.294
Conservative management	79 (18)	21 (34)	0.002
Laboratory data			
GFR, mL/min/1.73 m^2			
Baseline, median (IQR)	9.00 (14.00)	10.50 (8.50)	0.234
30–59	58 (13)	6 (10)	0.473
15–29	78 (17)	12 (20)	0.695
<15	314 (70)	44 (71)	0.848
Serum creatinine, median (IQR), mg/dL	5.70 (6.70)	3.95 (4.08)	0.016
Hemoglobin, mean (SD), g/dL	10.22 (2.07)	9.55 (1.97)	0.081
Serum albumin, mean (SD), g/dL	3.56 (0.62)	3.17 (0.81)	<0.001
Serum calcium, mean (SD), mg/dL	8.31 (0.96)	8.41 (0.90)	0.416
Serum phosphate, mean (SD), mg/dL	5.53 (2.23)	4.95 (2.56)	0.083
Serum bicarbonate, mean (SD), mEq/L	20.31 (5.13)	18.85 (5.96)	0.071
C-reactive protein, median (IQR), mg/L	22.50 (94.75)	53.50 (134)	<0.001
Medication use			
No. of medications, mean (SD)	7 (2)	11 (2)	<0.001

Abbreviations: ADR, adverse drug reaction; BP, blood pressure; GFR, glomerular filtration rate; IQR, interquartile range; SD, standard deviation.
SI conversions: To convert serum creatinine to μmol/L, multiply by 88.4.
[a]Vascular disease is defined as presence of coronary artery disease or peripheral vascular disease.

Finally, the predictive ability of the score was evaluated by using the C statistic.

Results

During the study period, a total of 512 patients with CKD stages 3 to 5 (eGFR, 10–59 ml/min/1.73 m^2) were admitted to the renal unit. The mean (SD) age of the participants was 60 (16) years, and 57% of patients were female. Out of 512 patients, 62 (12.1%) experienced a probable or definite ADR during hospital stay (Figure 1). The majority of ADRs were caused by anticoagulant drugs (n = 44; 70% of all ADRs), with heparin

(n = 18; 28%), enoxaparin (n = 16; 26%) and warfarin (n = 8; 13%) were the most implicated medications (Table 1).

Univariate Analysis

The main characteristics of patients grouped according to the occurrence of ADRs are reported in Table 2. Compared with patients without ADR, those with an ADR were older, with the mean (SD) age of 65 (14) years in the ADR group, compered with 60 (16) years in the non-ADR group (P = 0.023); had more comorbid conditions, with the prevalence of vascular disease (P< 0.001); were among conservatively managed ESRD patients (P = 0.002); and were prescribed more medications during hospital

Table 3. Odd Ratios and Goodness of Fit for Sequential Models of Prediction of an ADR.

| | Models | | | |
| | 1 | 2 | 3 | 4 |
Variable	Demographics	Demographics + Comorbid conditions	Demographics + Comorbid conditions + Laboratory data	Demographics + Comorbid conditions + Laboratory data + Medication use
GFR, per ml/min/1.73 m²	0.99 (0.97–1.01)	0.99 (0.97–1.02)	1.00 (0.97–1.02)	1.00 (0.97–1.03)
Age, ≥65 y	1.90 (1.09–3.31)	1.34 (0.75–2.41)	1.23 (0.67–2.24)	1.16 (0.62–2.17)
Female sex	1.37 (0.80–2.36)	1.45 (0.83–2.52)	1.50 (0.85–2.66)	1.33 (0.73–2.41)
ESRD, Conservative management		2.29 (1.23–4.27)	1.88 (0.98–3.62)	2.39 (1.21–4.74)
Vascular disease[a]		2.73 (1.50–4.97)	2.40 (1.30–4.45)	2.36 (1.25–4.46)
Serum albumin<3.5 g/dL			2.37 (1.31–4.27)	2.24 (1.21–4.14)
>10 mg/L serum C-reactive protein			2.57 (1.44–4.56)	2.41 (1.33–4.37)
≥ 8 No. of medications				4.64 (2.51–8.59)
C statistic[b]	0.587 (0.507–0.669)	0.689 (0.617–760)	0.761 (0.696–0.826)	0.813 (0.760–0.867)
Akaike Information Criterion[b]	378.49	363.94	344.60	323.23
p Value	<0.001	<0.001	<0.001	<0.001

Abbreviation: ESRD, end-stage renal disease; GFR, glomerular filtration rate.
Data are presented as odd ratios (95% confidence interval) unless otherwise specified.
[a]Vascular disease is defined as presence of coronary artery disease or peripheral vascular disease.
[b]Higher values for C statistic and lower values for Akaike Information Criterion indicate better models.

stay, with the mean (SD) of 11 (2) medications for patient with an ADR, compared to 7 (2) medications for non-ADR patients (P< 0.001). Moreover, patients with an ADR were more hypoalbuminemic, with the mean (SD) serum level of albumin of 3.17 (0.81) g/dL in an ADR group, versus 3.56 (0.62) g/dL in non-ADR group (P<0.001); and had higher serum level of C-Reactive protein (CRP), with the median (IQR) serum level of CRP of 53.50 (134) mg/dL in an ADR group, versus 22.50 (94.75) g/dL in non-ADR group (P<0.001).

Model Performance

The odd ratios for the variables and values for discrimination and goodness of fit for successive models are shown in Table 3.

Model 1, including age, female sex and eGFR, performed poorly (C statistic, 0.587; 95% CI, 0.507–0.669, and AIC 378.49; P< 0.001). However, the C statistic and AIC did improve with the inclusion of conservatively managed ESRD and vascular disease in model 2 (0.689; 95% CI, 0.617–0.760, and 363.94; P<0.001), laboratory values in model 3 (0.761; 95% CI, 0.696–0.826, and 344.60; P<0.001) and the use of 8 or more medications in model 4 (0.813; 95% CI, 0.760–0.867, and 323.23; P<0.001). The Hosmer-Lemeshow statistic was 0.874 for the best model (model 4).

Table 4. Logistic Regression and Bootstrapping Model for an ADR.

| | Logistic Regression | | | |
Variable	SE	OR (95% CI)	Bootstrap SE	Bootstrap (95% BootCI)
GFR, per ml/min/1.73 m²	0.014	1.00 (0.97–1.03)	0.014	(0.97–1.03)
Age, ≥65 y	0.317	1.16 (0.62–2.17)	0.338	(0.60–2.26)
Female sex	0.302	1.33 (0.73–2.41)	0.323	(0.70–2.52)
ESRD, Conservative management	0.348	2.39 (1.21–4.74)	0.370	(1.12–5.09)
Vascular disease[a]	0.325	2.36 (1.24–4.46)	0.357	(1.16–4.77)
Serum albumin<3.5 g/dL	0.313	2.24 (1.21–4.14)	0.323	(1.18–4.27)
>10 mg/L serum C-reactive proteins	0.304	2.41 (1.33–4.37)	0.340	(1.26–4.62)
≥ 8 No. of medications	0.314	4.64 (2.51–8.59)	0.342	(2.39–9.01)

Abbreviation: BootCI, bootstrap confidence interval; CI, confidence interval; ESRD, end- stage renal disease; GFR, glomerular filtration rate; SE, standard error; OR, odd ratio.
[a]Vascular disease is defined as presence of coronary artery disease or peripheral vascular disease.

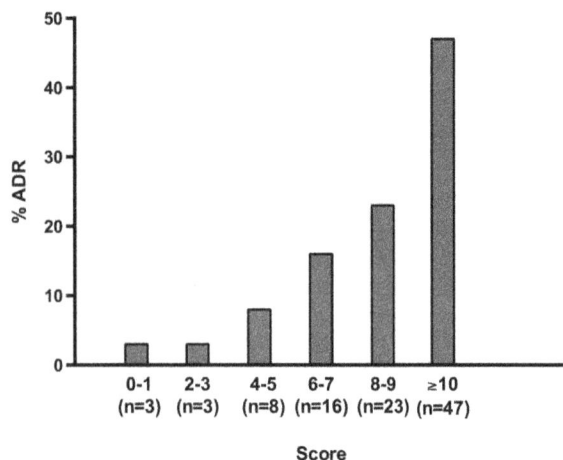

Figure 2. Adverse Drug Reaction (ADR) Rate According to ADR Risk Score Derived From Model 4.

Model Validation

Table 4, presents the results of the logistic regression of the best model along with the bootstrap results. The bootstrap procedure did not change significant variables.

Adverse Drug Reaction Risk Score

As shown in Table 5, the use of 8 or more medications was the variable most strongly associated with ADRs, and scored 4 points, followed by the presence of conservatively managed ESRD and vascular disease, each which scored 2 points. Among laboratory data, serum level of CRP more than 10 mg/L and serum level of albumin less than 3.5 g/dL, each scored 2 points. Female sex was given a score of 1 point and patients aged 65 years or more were scored as 1 point. The score was calculated for each patient by assigning points for each of the variables present and then adding these points. In our data, the score ranged from 0 to 15; the mean (SD) was 4.60 (3.40); the median was 4.00; and the C statistic, which assesses the ability of the risk score to predict ADRs, was 0.838 (95% CI, 0.784–0.892). Table 6, shows the incidence of

occurrence of ADRs among patients across various score categories.

Figure 2, shows that there was a progressive, significant pattern of increasing rate in ADRs as the risk score increased (P<0.001 by chi-square test for trend).

Discussion

The present study developed a practical and efficient method for identifying CKD patients who are at increased risk for ADR. This method uses patient characteristics data that can be obtained routinely on hospital admission, and that can be incorporated into the clinical practice as a tool to identify CKD patients who are at a high risk of ADRs. Numerous studies have tried to identify and stratify hospitalized patients who are at increased risk for experiencing ADRs [9,11,34], however, this study might be the first to incorporate patient laboratory data in the prediction model and thus, this ADR risk score is more representative of every-day clinical practice.

In this study, several risk factors for the development of ADRs in hospitalized patients with CKD were identified. As confirmed by past findings [7,9,14], the strongest independent factor was the number of concurrently used medications. Patients with CKD may, of course, have concurrent comorbid conditions that require complex medical regimens [4], and the coadminstration of multiple medications can lead to drug-drug interactions, that increases their possibility of developing ADRs [35].

The current study found that in hospitalized patients with CKD, the rate of developing ADRs increased exponentially with decreasing renal function, with more than two-thirds of ADRs occurring in patients with ESRD. This result is in agreement with a study by Corsonello and colleagues [36] who found an association between patient renal function and the risk of ADRs in elderly hospitalized patients. However, we also found that among ESRD, non-dialysis dependent patients were more than two times more susceptible to develop ADRs compared to hemodialysis patients. This could be because renal impairment related pharmacokinetic and pharmacodynamic changes such as a decrease in the elimination of the parent drug or of toxic metabolites, alteration in drug distribution or protein binding, metabolic abnormalities, or possibly increased target organ susceptibility in uremic patients [5]. This finding emphasizes the

Table 5. Regression Coefficient and Score of Each Variable Included in Predictive Model.

Variable	OR (95% CI)	Score
Demographics		
Age, ≥65 y	1.16 (0.62–2.17)	+1
Female sex	1.33 (0.73–2.41)	+1
Comorbid conditions		
ESRD, Conservative management	2.39 (1.21–4.74)	+2
Vascular disease[a]	2.36 (1.24–4.46)	+2
Laboratory data		
Serum albumin<3.5 g/dL	2.24 (1.21–4.14)	+2
>10 mg/L serum C-reactive proteins	2.41 (1.33–4.37)	+2
Medication use		
≥ 8 No. of medications	4.64 (2.51–8.59)	+4

Abbreviation: CI, confidence interval; ESRD, end-stage renal disease; OR, odd ratio.
[a]Vascular disease is defined as presence of coronary artery disease or peripheral vascular disease.

Table 6. Distribution of Patients According to the Risk Score Derived From Model 4.

Risk score	Total[a]	No. patients with ADRs; n (%)	Incidence of patients with No ADRs; n (%)
0–1	99	2 (3)	97 (22)
2–3	132	2 (3)	130 (29)
4–5	103	5 (8)	98 (22)
6–7	65	10 (16)	55 (12)
8–9	56	14 (23)	42 (9)
≥10	57	29 (47)	28 (6)
Total	512	62	450

Abbreviations: ADR, adverse drug reaction.
[a]Total number of patients per score category.

need to triage patients for decision regarding the initiation of renal replacement therapy.

In this study, patients with a lower serum level of albumin were at increased risk of experiencing ADRs during hospital stay. This is in line with the Corsonello and colleague [37] study, that showed an association between hypoalbuminemia in patients with concealed renal failure and ADRs. These can also be explained by the decreased binding of albumin-bound drugs, and the accumulation of the unbound fraction in plasma [5].

In addition, patients with vascular disease experienced more ADRs during in hospital stay. Noticeably, patients with CKD are often excluded from coronary artery disease trials; therefore, the safety profile of cardiovascular medications in these patients is mostly based upon knowledge of postmarketing rather than controlled trials [38]. Moreover, in our study, patients who developed ADRs had a higher serum level of CRP, and both CRP value and vascular disease remained significant predictors of developing ADRs when included simultaneously in the regression model. Possible mechanisms include a role for CRP as an inflammatory marker and the formation of atherosclerosis, and its role in the vascular diseases [39].

The ADR risk score has important implications for clinical practice and research. For example, by using this score, lower-risk patients could be managed less extensively, whereas, higher-risk patients could receive more intensive interventions aimed at reducing drug-related adverse outcomes and improving the cost-

effectiveness of CKD therapy. Also, by using this score, different risk levels could be used to triage patients for a decision regarding the initiation of renal replacement therapy. Furthermore, the score could be used to identify higher-risk patients who could be enrolled in clinical trials and be evaluated for risk-treatment interactions [40].

The strength of this study is in its development of an ADR risk score for hospitalized patients with moderate to severe CKD. The score is practical because all the variables included can be obtained routinely in a hospital setting. However, the limitation of our study is that the ADR risk score was developed based on hospitalized CKD patients. Thus, it may not be confidently applied in the ambulatory care. Hence, we recommend future studies to evaluate its validity and applicability in ambulatory care.

In conclusion, the current study has developed a practical and efficient risk score for identifying CKD patients who are at increased risk for experiencing ADRs during hospital stay. The score uses routinely available patient data.

Author Contributions

Conceived and designed the experiments: FSA SAS NSA. Performed the experiments: FSA SAS NSA AA. Analyzed the data: FSA SAS NSA. Contributed reagents/materials/analysis tools: FSA SAS NSA AA. Wrote the paper: FSA SAS NSA.

References

1. Pirmohamed M, James S, Meakin S, Green C, Scott AK, et al. (2004) Adverse drug reactions as cause of admission to hospital: prospective analysis of 18 820 patients. BMJ 329: 15–19.

2. Lazarou J, Pomeranz BH, Corey PN (1998) Incidence of adverse drug reactions in hospitalized patients: A meta-analysis of prospective studies. JAMA 279: 1200–1205.

3. Wester K, Jonnson AK, Sigset O, Druid H, Hagg S (2008) Incidence of fatal adverse drug reactions: a population based study. Br J Clin Pharmacol 65: 573–579.

4. Manley HJ, McClaran ML, Overbay DK, Wright MA, Reid GM, et al. (2003) Factors associated with medication-related problems in ambulatory hemodialysis patients. Am J Kidney Dis 41: 386–393.

5. Verbeeck RK, Musuamba FT (2009) Pharmacokinetics and dosage adjustment in patients with renal dysfunction. Eur J Clin Pharmacol 65: 757–773.

6. Wilke RA, Lin DW, Roden DM, Watkins PB, Flockhart D, et al. (2007) Identifying genetic risk factors for serious adverse drug reactions: current progress and challenges. Nat Rev Drug Discov 6: 904–916.

7. Field TS, Gurwitz JH, Avorn J, McCormick D, Jain S, et al. (2001) Risk factors for adverse drug events among nursing home residents. Arch Intern Med 161: 1629–1634.

8. Onder G, Landi F, Della Vedova C, Atkinson H, Pedone C, et al. (2002) GIFA Study. Moderate alcohol consumption and adverse drug reactions among older adults. Pharmacoepidemiology and Drug Saf 11: 385–392.

9. Onder G, Petrovic M, Tangiisuran B, Meinardi MC, Markito-Notenboom WP, et al. (2010) Development and validation of a score to assess risk of adverse drug reactions among in-hospital patients 65 years or older: the GerontoNet ADR risk score. Arch Intern Med 170: 1142–1148.

10. Catananti C, Liperoti R, Settanni S, Lattanzio F, Bernabei R, et al. (2009) Heart failure and adverse drug reactions among hospitalized older adults. Clin Pharmacol Ther 86: 307–310.

11. Bates DW, Miller EB, Cullen DJ, Burdick L, Williams L, et al. (1999) Prevention Study Group. Patient risk factors for adverse drug events in hospitalized patients. Arch of Intern Med 159: 2553–2560.

12. Steel K, Gertman PM, Crescenzi C, Anderson J (2004) Iatrogenic illness on a general medical service at a university hospital. Qual Saf Health Care 13: 76–80.

13. Gurwitz JH, Rochon P (2002) Improving the quality of medication use in elderly patients: a not-so-simple prescription. Arch Intern Med 162:1670–1672.

14. Corsonello A, Pedone C, Corica F, Mussi C, Carbonin P, et al. (2005) Gruppo Italiano di Farmacovigilanza nell' Anziano (GIFA) Investigators. Concealed renal insufficiency and adverse drug reactions in elderly hospitalized patients. Arch Intern Med 165:790–795.

15. Helldén A, Bergman U, von Euler M, Hentschke M, Odar-Cederlöf I, et al. (2009) Adverse drug reactions and impaired renal function in elderly patients admitted to the emergency department. Drugs Aging 26: 595–606.

16. Pahor M, Chrischilles EA, Guralnik JM, Brown SL, Wallace RB, et al. (1994) Drug data coding and analysis in epidemiologic studies. Eur J Epidemiol 10: 405–411.

17. World Health Organization (2004) International Classification of Diseases, Tenth Revision (ICD-10). Geneva, Switzerland. World Health Organization.

18. Levey AS, Bosch JP, Lewis JB, Greene T, Rogers N, et al. (1999) Modification of Diet in Renal Disease Study Group: A more accurate method to estimate glomerular filtration rate from serum creatinine: a new prediction equation. Ann Intern Med 130: 461–470.

19. National Kidney Foundation (2002) K/DOQI clinical practice guidelines for chronic kidney disease: evaluation, classification, and stratification. Am J Kidney Dis 39 (Suppl 1):S1–S266.

20. Edwards IR, Aronson JK (2000) Adverse drug reactions: definitions, diagnosis, and management. Lancet 356: 1255–1259.

21. Rozich JD, Haraden CR, Resar RK (2003) Adverse drug event trigger tool: a practical methodology for measuring medication related harm. Qual Saf Health Care 12: 194–200.

22. Morimoto T, Gandhi TK, Seger AC, Hsieh TC, Bates DW (2004) Adverse drug events and medication errors: detection and classification methods. Qual Saf Health Care 13: 306–314.

23. British Medical Association, Royal Pharmaceutical Society of Great Britain (2012) British National Formulary. London: BMA, RPS, (No 64).

24. Naranjo CA, Busto U, Sellers EM, Sandor P, Ruiz I, et al. (1981) A method for estimating the probability of adverse drug reactions. Clin Pharmacol Ther 30: 239–245.

25. Steyerberg EW, Eijkemans MJC, Harrell FE, Habbema JDF (2001) Prognostic modeling with logistic regression analysis in search of a sensible strategy in small data sets. Med Decis Making 21: 45–56.

26. Vittinghoff E, McCulloch CE (2007) Relaxing the rule of ten events per variable in logistic and cox regression. Am J Epidemiol 165: 710–718.

27. Lemeshow S, Hosmer DW (1982) A review of goodness of fit statistics for use in the development of logistic regression models. Am J Epidemiol 115: 92–106.

28. Steyerberg EW, Vickers AJ, Cook NR, Gerds T, Gonen M, et al. (2010) Assessing the performance of prediction models: a framework for traditional and novel measures. Epidemiology 21: 128–138.

29. Pencina MJ, D' Agostino RB, D' Agostino RB, Vasan RS (2008) Evaluating the added predictive ability of a new marker: from area under the ROC curve to reclassification and beyond. Stat Med 27: 157–172.

30. Steyerberg EW (2009) Clinical Prediction Models: A Practical Approach to Development, Validation, and Updating. New York, NY: Springer.

31. Efron B, Tibshirani R (1993) An Introduction to the Bootstrap. London: Chapman and Hall.

32. Steyerberg EW, Harrell FE Jr, Borsboom GJJM, Eijkemans MJC, Vergouwe Y, et al. (2001) Internal validation of predictive models: efficiency of some procedures for logistic regression analysis. J Clin Epidemiol 54: 774–781.

33. Antman EM, Cohen M, Bernink PJ, McCabe CH, Horacek T, et al. (2000) The TIMI risk score for unstable angina/non–ST elevation MI: a method for prognostication and therapeutic decision making. JAMA 284: 835–842.

34. Johnston PE, France DJ, Byrne DW, Murff HJ, Lee B, et al. (2006) Assessment of adverse drug events among patients in a tertiary care medical center. Am J Health Syst Pharm 63: 2218–2227.

35. Hohl CM, Dankoff J, Colacone A, Afilalo M (2001) Polypharmacy, adverse drug-related events, and potential adverse drug interactions in elderly patients presenting to an emergency department. Ann Emerg Med 38: 666–671.

36. Corsonello A, Pedone C, Lattanzio F, Onder G, Incalzi R (2011) Association between glomerular filtration rate and adverse drug reactions in elderly hospitalized patients. Drugs Aging 28: 379–390.

37. Corsonello A, Pedone C, Corica F, Mazzei B, Di Iorio A, et al. (2005) Concealed renal failure and adverse drug reactions in older patients with type 2 diabetes mellitus. J Gerontol A Biol Sci Med Sci 60: 1147–1151.

38. Charytan D, Kuntz RE (2006) The exclusion of patients with chronic kidney disease from clinical trials in coronary artery disease. Kidney Int 70: 2021–2030.

39. Matsushita K, van der Velde M, Astor BC, Woodward M, Levey AS, et al. (2010) Association of estimated glomerular filtration rate and albuminuria with all-cause and cardiovascular mortality in general population cohorts: a collaborative meta-analysis. Lancet 375: 2073–2081.

40. Kent DM, Hayward RA (2007) Limitations of applying summary results of clinical trials to individual patients: The need for risk stratification. JAMA 298: 1209–1212.

18

Screening for Decreased Glomerular Filtration Rate and Associated Risk Factors in a Cohort of HIV-Infected Patients in a Middle-Income Country

Patrícia Santiago[1,2], Beatriz Grinsztejn[1], Ruth Khalili Friedman[1], Cynthia B. Cunha[1], Lara Esteves Coelho[1], Paula Mendes Luz[1], Albanita Viana de Oliveira[3], Ronaldo Ismério Moreira[1], Sandra W. Cardoso[1], Valdilea G. Veloso[1], José H. Rocco Suassuna[2]*

1 STD/AIDS Clinical Research Laboratory, Instituto de Pesquisa Clínica Evandro Chagas-Fundação Oswaldo Cruz, Rio de Janeiro, Brazil, **2** Clinical and Academic Unit of Nephrology, Hospital Universitário Pedro Ernesto, Faculdade de Ciências Médicas, Universidade do Estado do Rio de Janeiro, Rio de Janeiro, Brazil, **3** Department of Pathology, Faculdade de Ciências Médicas, Universidade do Estado do Rio de Janeiro, Rio de Janeiro, Brazil

Abstract

With the introduction of combined active antiretroviral therapy and the improved survival of HIV-infected patients, degenerative diseases and drug toxicity have emerged as long-term concerns. We studied the prevalence of decreased glomerular filtration rate (GFR) and associated risk factors in a cohort of HIV-infected patients from a middle-income country. Our cross-sectional study included all adult patients who attended an urban outpatient clinic in 2008. GFR was estimated using the CKD-EPI equation. The prevalence ratio (PR) of decreased GFR (defined as <60 mL/min/1.73 m^2) was estimated using generalizing linear models assuming a Poisson distribution. We analyzed data from 1,970 patients, of which 82.9% had been exposed to ART. A total of 249 patients (12.6%) had a GFR between 60 and 89 mL/min/1.73 m^2, 3.1% had a GFR between 30 and 59, 0.3% had a GFR between 15 and 29, and 0.4% had a GFR <15. Decreased GFR was found in only 74 patients (3.8%). In the multivariate regression model, the factors that were independently associated with a GFR below 60 mL/min/1.73 m^2 were as follows: age ≥ 50 years (PR = 3.4; 95% CI: 1.7–6.8), diabetes (PR = 2.0; 95% CI: 1.2–3.4), hypertension (PR = 2.0; 95% CI: 1.3–3.2), current CD4+ cell count <350 cells/mm3 (PR = 2.1; 95% CI: 1.3–3.3), past exposure to tenofovir (PR = 4.7; 95% CI: 2.3–9.4) and past exposure to indinavir (PR = 1.7; 95% CI: 1.0–2.8). As in high-income countries, CKD was the predominant form of kidney involvement among HIV-infected individuals in our setting. The risk factors associated with decreased glomerular filtration were broad and included virus-related factors as well as degenerative and nephrotoxic factors. Despite the potential for nephrotoxicity associated with some antiretroviral drugs, in the short-term, advanced chronic renal disease remains very rare.

Editor: Emmanuel A. Burdmann, University of Sao Paulo Medical School, Brazil

Funding: The authors have no support or funding to report.

Competing Interests: The authors have declared that no competing interests exist.

* E-mail: jsuassuna@alternex.com.br

Introduction

The introduction of combined active antiretroviral therapy (cART) for HIV infection was followed by a significant decline in the number of deaths attributable to opportunistic infections. As the survival of chronically HIV-infected individuals increased, so did the prevalence of major chronic degenerative disorders, including metabolic, cardiovascular, renal, and bone-related conditions. For example, the widespread use of cART caused a marked drop in the incidence of rapidly progressive HIV-associated nephropathy (HIVAN), but HIV infection is now associated with indolently developing chronic kidney disease (CKD) [1,2]. Currently, renal disease risk in patients with HIV infection appears to be compounded by ethnicity, chronic comorbidities, concurrent viral infections, and the use of antiretroviral drugs with nephrotoxic potential [2,3]. Regardless of the underlying cause, CKD is considered a significant independent risk factor for mortality among HIV-infected patients in both developed and resource-limited settings [4–7]. Given these adverse associations, all HIV-infected persons are advised to undergo kidney function evaluation [8].

In 1991, the Brazilian Ministry of Health launched a pioneer program to provide free access to antiretroviral treatment for all HIV-infected individuals as needed. A marked drop in morbidity and mortality rewarded Brazil's unique position of a middle-income economy with more than 200.000 patients receiving cART [9]. While successful, increasing patient life expectancy and HIV infection prevalence is anticipated to place a growing burden on limited local specialized human resources and health care logistics. Because the first step toward preparation and planning involves collecting evidence, the objectives of this study were to screen for decreased glomerular filtration rate (GFR) and associated risk factors in an outpatient cohort of HIV-infected patients followed at Instituto de Pesquisa Clinica Evandro Chagas (IPEC)/Fiocruz, a referral center for HIV care and research in the city of Rio de Janeiro, Brazil.

Methods

Ethics Statement

The project was submitted to the Institutional Review Board of Instituto de Pesquisa Clínica Evandro Chagas - Fundação Oswaldo Cruz and approved on Sept 13, 2010 as # 044/2010. A translation of the conclusion of the board is read as follows: "In substitution to written informed consent, following declaration #196 of 1996 from the Brazilian National Health Council, the investigators in charge (PS and BG) subscribed to a term of agreement pledging confidentiality and anonymity of the participants of the study". The project was not specifically funded.

Cohort Identification and Study Design

The IPEC clinical HIV service has been providing patient care since 1986. The HIV cohort database was started in 1998. Longitudinal data are updated regularly using clinic and inpatient clinical documentation, laboratory results, and pharmacy records. Medical providers and support staff record clinical information, including prescriptions for antiretroviral drugs. Trained data abstractors collect relevant information onto standardized forms for further processing.

We performed a cross-sectional study including all patients aged 18 years or older who attended the IPEC outpatient clinic and had at least one serum creatinine evaluation during the calendar year of 2008. HIV infection was diagnosed according to the Brazilian Ministry of Health criteria [10]: either two ELISA tests or two rapid tests followed by a confirmatory test, either a Western blot or immunofluorescence assay. Creatinine was measured with the Roche enzymatic assay at the IPEC Safety Laboratory, which is certified by the American College of Pathology. We excluded patients with missing ethnicity data and those whose creatinine results were obtained during or up to six weeks after admission to a hospital. The outcome of interest was the estimated glomerular filtration rate (eGFR), calculated from a single fasting creatinine measurement using the CKD-EPI equation. The GFR results were stratified according to the NKF-K/DOQI staging system. All of the patients classified in stages 3 through 5 (i.e., with a GFR < 60 mL/min/1.73 m^2) were considered to have a decreased GFR.

The data that were obtained concurrently with the assessment of renal function and evaluated as explanatory variables for reduced GFR included gender, age, ethnicity, HIV transmission group, AIDS defining illness (according to the 1993 AIDS CDC definition), time since the HIV infection diagnosis, co-infection with the hepatitis B (HBV) virus (defined as a positive HBsAg test), co-infection with the hepatitis C (HCV) virus (defined as positive anti-HCV serology), diabetes (defined as the use of anti-diabetic drugs or a record in the patient's chart), hypertension (defined as a record in the chart or the use of antihypertensive therapy), hyperlipidemia (defined by the prescription of lipid-lowering drugs or documentation in the chart), current HIV1-RNA plasma viral load, current CD4+ cell count, nadir CD4+ cell count, past and current ARV exposure, and exposure to selected nephrotoxins in the three years prior to the GFR assessment (aciclovir, valaciclovir, ganciclovir, gentamicin, amikacin, amphotericin B, and meglumine antimoniate).

Statistical Analysis

The prevalence ratio (PR) of decreased GFR was estimated with generalizing linear models created assuming a Poisson distribution with logarithmic link function and robust variance. The covariates that were significantly associated with renal dysfunction in the univariate analysis (p<0.10) were entered in the multivariate models. Given the low prevalence of the study outcome, the variables were retained if they met the condition p≤0.10 in a backward elimination strategy and if they were considered potential confounders (e.g., when removed, a change equal to or greater than 20% in the prevalence ratio of any other variable of the model was observed). All of the analyses were performed using STATA/SE version 10.1.

Results

Study Population

Between January 1 and December 31, 2008, 2,345 patients were seen at the IPEC outpatient clinic. A total of 375 patients (16%) were excluded from further analyses for the following reasons: lack of serum creatinine testing (310), creatinine testing performed exclusively during hospitalization or within 6 weeks after hospital discharge (to prevent the inclusion of patients with acute kidney injury) (63), and lack of ethnicity data (thus interfering with the estimation of GFR by the CKD-EPI equation) (2). We analyzed data from 1,970 patients. The median age was 41.6 (interquartile range [IQR] 34.0–48.2) years; 63.6% were male and 57.1% were white (Table 1). The patients were followed at IPEC for 10,456 person-years.

Hyperlipidemia, hypertension, and diabetes mellitus were present in 46.9%, 26.6%, and 9.3% of the patients, respectively. The median time since the diagnosis of HIV infection was 78.5 (IQR 29.1–136.2) months, and 42.8% met the clinical definition for AIDS. The median nadir and current CD4+ cell counts were 189 (IQR 78–308) and 460 (IQR 307–650) cells/mm^3, respectively. The plasma viral load was undetectable in 70.5% of the subjects.

Overall, 1,634 patients (82.9%) had been exposed to ART, with a mean cumulative exposure (MCE) of 67.7 months (SE: 1.3) and a total of 9206 person-years of follow up. Of the patients, 807 (41.0%) had been exposed to tenofovir (MCE 25.0±19.3 months), 305 (15.5%) had been exposed to indinavir (MCE 31.8±26.5 months), 490 (24.9%) had been exposed to atazanavir (MCE: 25.7±18.8 months), and 516 (26.2%) had been exposed to lopinavir (MCE: 27.4±21.3 months).

At the time of evaluation, 744 patients were on tenofovir (TDF), and 67.5% (n = 502) had been exposed for at least one year. Among the patients exposed to TDF in the past (n = 63), 52.4% had been exposed for more than one year. A total of 860 patients were exposed to atazanavir and/or lopinavir (ATVLPV); 546 were currently using one of these drugs, and of these patients, 77.7% (n = 424) had at least one year of exposure. Among the patients exposed to ATVLPV in the past (n = 314), 72.9% had been exposed for at least one year. Prior exposure to potentially nephrotoxic non-ARV drugs was recorded in 345 subjects (17.5%) as follows: aciclovir, 13.2%; valaciclovir, 4.9%; ganciclovir, 0.6%; amikacin, 0.2%; gentamicin, 0.1%; amphotericin B preparations, 0.1%; and meglumine antimoniate, 0.1%.

The median eGFR for the entire cohort was 111.4 mL/min/ 1.73 m^2. Table 2 presents the categories of eGFR prevalence according to the NKF-K/DOQI stages. Of the 1,970 patients, 1,647 (83.6%) had an eGFR above 90 mL/min/1.73 m^2, 249 patients (12.6%; 95% CI: 11.2–14.2) had an eGFR between 60 and 89 mL/min/1.73 m^2, 61 patients (3.1%; 95% CI: 2.4–4.0) had an eGFR between 30 and 59 mL/min/1.73 m^2, six patients (0.3%; 95% CI: 0.1–0.7) had an eGFR between 15 and 29 mL/ min/1.73 m^2, and seven patients (0.4%; 95% CI: 0.1–0.7) had an eGFR below 15 mL/min/1.73 m^2. Notably, 74 patients (3.8%; 95% CI: 3.0–4.7) fulfilled the primary outcome criterion of an eGFR below 60 mL/min per 1.73 m^2.

Table 1. Demographic and clinical characteristics of the study patients.

Characteristic		Total Cohort n (%)	eGFR ≥60 n (%)	eGFR <60 n (%)
Gender	Male	1252 (63.6%)	1203 (63.4%)	49 (66.2%)
	Female	718 (36.4%)	693 (36.6%)	25 (33.8%)
Ethnic origin	Non white	845 (42.9%)	815 (43.0%)	30 (40.5%)
	White	1125 (57.1%)	1081 (57.0%)	44 (59.5%)
Age (years)	<40	879 (44.6%)	867 (45.7%)	12 (16.2%)
	40–50	698 (35.4%)	674 (35.5%)	24 (32.4%)
	>50	393 (19.9%)	355 (18.7%)	38 (51.4%)
Diabetes mellitus	Present	182 (9.3%)	162 (8.6%)	20 (27.0%)
Hypertension	Present	523 (26.6%)	483 (25.5%)	40 (54.1%)
Hyperlipidemia	Present	913 (46.9%)	870 (46.4%)	43 (58.9%)
Hepatitis B surface antigen	Detectable	58 (2.9%)	56 (3.0%)	2 (2.7%)
Hepatitis C antibody	Detectable	119 (6.0%)	111 (5.9%)	8 (11.0%)
Time since first HIV-positive serology (IQR)	Months	78.5 (29.1–136.2)	77.1 (28.9–134.2)	117.7 (50.7–158.7)
AIDS defining illness	Present	843 (42.8%)	804 (42.4%)	39 (52.7%)
Nadir CD4+ count <200 cells/mm^3	Present	1008 (51.7%)	961 (51.1%)	47 (67.1%)
CD4+ count <350 cells/mm^3 within 6 months of index creatinine	Present	610 (31.9%)	574 (31.2%)	36 (50.7%)
HIV viral load within 6 months of index creatinine	Detectable	558 (29.5%)	535 (29.5%)	22 (31.9%)
Exposure to tenofovir	Never	1162 (59.0%)	1133 (59.8%)	29 (39.7%)
	Prior	63 (3.2%)	50 (2.6%)	13 (17.8%)
	Current	744 (37.8%)	713 (37.6%)	31 (42.5%)
Exposure to atazanavir and/or lopinavir	Never	1111 (56.4%)	1088 (57.4%)	23 (31.5%)
	Prior	312 (15.8%)	298 (15.7%)	14 (19.2%)
	Current	546 (27.7%)	510 (26.9%)	36 (49.3%)
Exposure to indinavir	Prior	305 (15.5%)	278 (14.7%)	27 (37.0%)
Exposure to non-ARV nephrotoxic drugs*	Present	338 (17.5%)	324 (17.4%)	14 (19.7%)

*Patients to whom it was prescribed one of these in the last three years: guanosine analogue antiviral drugs (aciclovir, ganciclovir, valaciclovir), aminoglycosides (amikacin, gentamicin), amphotericin B preparations, and meglumine antimoniate.

Table 1 also shows that in comparison with the patients with GFR ≥60 mL/min per 1.73 m^2, the patients with decreased GFR were more frequently aged 50 years or older (51.4% vs. 18.7%) and had higher prevalence rates of hyperlipidemia (58.9% vs. 46.6%), hypertension (54.1% vs. 25.5%), diabetes (27.0% vs. 8.6%), and positive anti-HCV serology (11.0% vs. 5.9%). These patients also had been diagnosed with HIV for a longer time, with a median time of 117.7 (IQR 50.7–158.7) vs. 77.1 (IQR 28.9–134.2) months, and they were more likely to have an AIDS

diagnosis (52.7% vs. 42.4%) and a current CD4+ count below 350 cells/mm^3 (50.7% vs. 31.2%).

Exposure to TDF (60.3% vs. 40.2%), current (42.5% vs. 37.6%) and previous use of TDF (17.8% vs. 2.6%), and exposure for at least one year (43.0% vs. 26.5%) were more common among the patients with decreased GFR. The same trend was observed for exposure to ATVLPV (68.5% vs. 42.6%), current use of ATVLPV (49.3% vs. 26.9%), and exposure to these drugs for at least one year (58.9% vs. 32.2%). Past exposure to indinavir was also more common among the patients with reduced GFR (37% vs. 14.7%).

Table 2. Prevalence of estimated GFR (eGFR) categories in the IPEC/FIOCRUZ cohort of HIV-infected patients.

Glomerular filtration rate (mL/min per 1.73 m^2)*	n	% (95% CI)
≥90	1647	83.6 (81.9–85.2)
60–89	249	12.6 (11.2–14.2)
30–59	61	3.1 (2.4–4.0)
15–29	6	0.3 (0.1–0.7)
<15	7	0.4 (0.1–0.7)

*Estimated by the CKD-EPI equation.

Exposure to potentially nephrotoxic non-ARV drugs was observed in 19.7% of the patients with GFR <60 mL/min/1.73 m² vs. 17.4% of the patients with GFR ≥60 mL/min/1.73 m² (Table 1).

In the univariate analysis, age, diabetes, hypertension, hyperlipidemia, hepatitis C, time since the HIV diagnosis, opportunistic diseases, current CD4+ count, indinavir exposure, and past and current exposure to TDF and ATVLPV were significantly and positively associated with the primary outcome (Table 3).

In the multivariate adjusted Poisson regression model, the following factors were significantly associated (p<0.05) with a GFR <60 mL/min per 1.73 m²: age ≥50 years (PR = 3.4; 95% CI: 1.7–6.8), diabetes (PR = 2.0; 95% CI: 1.2–3.4), hypertension (PR = 2.0; 95% CI: 1.3–3.2), current CD4+ cell count <350 cells/

mm³ (PR = 2.1; 95% CI: 1.3–3.3), and past exposure to TDF (PR = 4.7; 95% CI: 2.3–9.4) and IDV (PR = 1.7; 95% CI: 1.0–2.8). Among the patients using ATV or LPV at the time of creatinine evaluation, the prevalence of decreased GFR was higher than the prevalence of those never exposed to such drugs, although this association was not statistically significant (PR = 1.7; 95% CI: 0.9–3.1; p = 0.09) (Table 3).

Discussion

The main findings of our study were as follows: (1) as far as we know, our study investigated the prevalence of decreased GFR in the largest cohort of HIV patients highly exposed to antiretroviral

Table 3. Factors associated with decreased GFR (<60 mL/min per 1.73 m²) in HIV-infected patients of the IPEC/FIOCRUZ Cohort.

Characteristic		Crude PR (95% CI)	p-value	Adjusted PR (95% CI)	p-value
Gender	Male	1.00			
	Female	0.89 (0.55–1.43)	0.628	–	–
Ethnic origin	Non white	1.00			
	White	0.91 (0.58–1.43)	0.677	–	–
Age (years)	<40	1.00		1.00	
	40–50	2.52 (1.27–5.00)	0.008	1.5 (0.7–2.9)	0.287
	>50	7.08 (3.74–13.41)	<0.001	3.4 (1.7–6.8)	0.001
Diabetes mellitus	No	1.00		1.00	
	Yes	3.63 (2.23–5.93)	<0.001	2.0 (1.2–3.4)	0.009
Hypertension	No	1.00		1.00	
	Yes	3.25 (2.08–5.08)	<0.001	2.0 (1.3–3.2)	0.004
Hyperlipidemia	No	1.00			
	Yes	1.62 (1.03–2.57)	0.038	–	–
Hepatitis B surface antigen	No	1.00			
	Yes	0.92 (0.23–3.64)	0.901	–	–
Hepatitis C antibody	No	1.00			
	Yes	1.91 (0.94–3.89)	0.074	–	–
Months since first HIV-positive serology (IQR)		1.06 (1.02–1.1)	0.002	–	–
AIDS defining illness	No	1.00			
	Yes	1.49 (0.95–2.33)	0.081	–	–
Nadir CD4+ count (cells/mm³)	≥200	1.00			
	<200	1.91 (1.17–3.12)	0.01	–	–
CD4+ count within 6 months of index creatinine (cells/mm³)	≥350	1.00		1.00	
	<350	2.19 (1.39–3.46)	0.001	2.1 (1.3–3.3)	0.003
HIV viral load within 6 months of index creatinine	Detectable	1.00			
	Undetectable	0.89 (0.54–1.47)	0.658	–	–
Exposure to tenofovir	Never	1.00		1.00	
	Prior	8.27 (4.52–15.11)	<0.001	4.7 (2.3–9.4)	<0.001
	Current	1.67 (1.01–2.75)	0.044	1.1 (0.6–2.0)	0.713
Exposure to atazanavir and/or lopinavir	Never	1.00		1.00	
	Prior	2.17 (1.13–4.16)	0.020	0.9 (0.4–2.0)	0.746
	Current	3.18 (1.91–5.32)	<0.001	1.7 (0.9–3.1)	0.090
Prior exposure to indinavir	No	1.00		1.00	
	Yes	3.20 (2.02–5.07)	<0.001	1.7 (1.0–2.8)	0.054
Exposure to non-ARV nephrotoxic drugs	No	1.00			
	Yes	1.16 (0.65–2.06)	0.614	–	–

drugs from a middle-income country; (2) we found that only 3.8% of the participants had a GFR below 60 mL/min per 1.73 m^2 as estimated by the CKD-EPI equation; and (3) the results indicate that a decreased GFR was positively and independently associated with markers of the severity of HIV infection as well as with other chronic degenerative diseases and exposure to nephrotoxic antiretroviral drugs.

Large cohort studies (i.e., with more than one thousand members) investigating the prevalence of CKD in HIV-infected individuals have been conducted with either cART-treated patients from high-income countries [11–22] or predominantly treatment-naïve subjects from low-income settings [23–25]. Healthcare in middle-income countries fits between these two extremes. While low-income countries still struggle to meet the needs of their people, middle-income economies have already developed the ability to deliver basic health services but face hurdles regarding coverage, priority setting, financing, and efficiency. With regard to HIV treatment, despite undeniable progress, middle-income countries exhibit marked differences in access to cART and treatment consistency [26]. The epidemiological features of our cohort, including the prevalence of CKD risk factors, are akin to those in higher-income countries (e.g., the predominance of urban white males in early middle age (median age 41.6 years), access to cART, and a moderate prevalence of chronic comorbidities).

Decreased GFR was uncommon (3.8%) among the HIV-infected patients in our cohort. Differences in the baseline sociodemographic data, the cohort inclusion criteria and the accrual period as well as exposure to different antiretroviral medications preclude exact comparisons among published reports. Nevertheless, data from the high-income country cohorts mentioned above show that the median ages and prevalence rates of CKD (defined by GFR <60 mL/min/1.73 m^2) for the three main creatinine-based GFR estimation methods were as follows: an age of 42.8 years and a CKD prevalence of 4.2% for CG [17,19], an age of 39.3 years and a CKD prevalence of 4.5% for MDRD [11–16,20,27], and an age of 41.3 years and a CKD prevalence of 4.5% for CKD-EPI GFR [18,19,21,22].

Notably, 16.4% of the members of the cohort had estimated GFRs below 90 mL/min/1.73 m^2. Previously, similar double figure rates have been highlighted as an indication of a high burden of CKD in HIV-infected cohorts [19,28,29]. However, a sizable proportion of healthy normal adults have eGFR values within the range of 60 to 89 mL/min/1.73 m^2. Consequently, it is feared that such a high cut-off inappropriately inflates the prevalence of CKD [30,31]. In any case, even this threshold has been shown as an independent risk factor for cardiovascular mortality in apparently healthy adults [32].

Concerns about the over-diagnosis of CKD are extensive for our chosen eGFR cut-off of 60 mL/min/1.73 m^2 [33,34]. Nevertheless, this boundary is widely used for screening purposes [35,36]. More importantly, a single eGFR value under 60 mL/min/1.73 m^2 is independently associated with an increased risk of cardiovascular [32,37–40] and all-cause mortality [37,39]. Furthermore, most cases of false-positive CKD labeling involve older individuals, mostly females with low muscle mass. We studied a targeted group of young to middle-aged men with known risk factors for chronic kidney damage, therefore enhancing the positive predictive value and minimizing the negative predictive value of the eGFR test [30,31].

Cross-sectional studies in healthy individuals show that directly measured glomerular filtration rated are lower in older adults than younger adults [41] and that this gap is magnified when GFR is estimated with creatinine-based equations [42]. We, like others

[11,15,16,19,21,27], did find that a lower eGFR was independently associated with increasing age. This finding was particularly relevant given the rising incidence of HIV infection in older adults [43,44] and the remarkable success of cART, which is allowing younger infected adults to age [45]. In addition, HIV-associated inflammation, exposure to potentially toxic antiretroviral drugs, accelerated aging, and chronic comorbidities contribute to the premature occurrence of "non-AIDS" degenerative diseases, including CKD [46,47]. With regard to this matter and in agreement with previous reports [3,15,17,22,48], we noted that both diabetes and hypertension were significantly and independently associated with a low eGFR.

Previous studies have provided evidence that cART controls kidney cell damage and preserves renal function [49] and that its withdrawal is associated with HIVAN and kidney function deterioration [50]. In our cohort, 18.1% of the patients receiving cART had detectable viral loads, and 32% had a current CD4+ cell count below 350, indicating some degree of uncontrolled infection, due to either viral resistance or non-adherence. Overall, our patients had fairly advanced HIV disease, as shown by the median nadir of 189 CD4+ cells/mm^3 and by the fact that 42.8% had a previous AIDS defining illness. Against this background, we did not find an association between reduced GFR and either of these variables, but we noticed that a reduced GFR was significantly associated with a current CD4+ count below 350 cells/mm^3, a marker of incomplete immune reconstitution.

The rationale behind cART is to administer multiple drugs targeting different stages of HIV cell entry and the cell life cycle to achieve long-lasting viral suppression. This strategy exposes patients to multiple potential drug interactions and entails a lifelong risk of drug toxicity, including nephrotoxicity [51]. We observed that the past use of tenofovir and indinavir was associated with a decreased glomerular filtration rate. An association between current atazanavir and/or lopinavir use and decreased glomerular filtration rate was also observed but it did not reach statistical significance (p = 0.09).

Tenofovir was used by 41% of our patients, and 84.8% of those patients were still using the drug. Even after accounting for demographics, HIV-related factors, comorbidities, and other antiretroviral drugs, past TDF use remained independently associated with low GFR compared with those with no previous exposure. This result suggests that kidney damage and dysfunction do not quickly reverse after the exposure ends. In fact, among the patients who discontinue TDF because of renal impairment, only a minority returns to their pre-TDF GFR [52]. Furthermore, data from a large cohort in the US showed that past users of TDF remained at an increased risk of proteinuria and rapid renal function decline compared with those never exposed to TDF [2]. Because TDF is a first-line treatment for HIV infection that is increasingly used in all antiretroviral regimens and in pre-exposure prophylaxis, attention to the early signs of renal toxicity, perhaps even above the 60 mL/min/1.73 m^2 cutoff, is necessary [52].

Contrary to previous use, the current use of TDF was not associated with a decreased GFR. This finding differs from other reports that did find such an association [19,20]. Several possible underlying explanations can be given for this result, including differences in study definitions, in the background characteristics of the study populations, and in the length of exposure to tenofovir, among others. Nevertheless, we believe that the broadly reported association between TDF and renal dysfunction [2,53] led to careful and repeated measurements of serum creatinine, resulting in earlier withdrawal and prevention of unchecked toxic exposure to TDF. In fact, recent data from the D:A:D study showed that decreased GFR was associated with a significant rate of TDF discontinuation, which prevented further deterioration of renal function. Interestingly, this behavior was not replicated when the GFR declined in patients exposed to other antiretroviral agents [54].

Both indinavir and atazanavir have been associated with crystalluria, crystal nephropathy, nephrolithiasis, and CKD in previous studies [17,55]. In our cohort, past users of indinavir had a higher risk of GFR decline that reached borderline significance (PR = 1.7; 95% CI: 1.0–2.8). In recent years, the newer protease inhibitors, particularly atazanavir and lopinavir, have replaced indinavir. Contrary to the above mentioned studies, past or current use of atazanavir or lopinavir was not significantly associated with a GFR below 60 mL/min/1.73 m^2. However, in the multivariate regression model, there was a trend toward an association of current use of ATVLPV and low GFR (PR = 1.7; 95% CI: 0.9–3.1). It is possible that the low prevalence of the decreased GFR end-point in the cohort contributed to this negative finding. Further investigation is necessary to delineate the impact of these drugs on kidney function.

This study does have several limitations. First, as in all cohorts, the sample includes adherent individuals with extensive and complicated medical histories that may obscure the associations of interest [56]. Second, because of the cross-sectional design, we can draw associations between events but cannot establish temporal sequences. Third, the diagnosis of low GFR was based on an isolated creatinine measurement. In spite of this, as discussed above, this strategy has been used widely in screening investigations related to CKD and associated risk factors [35,36,57,58], and a single eGFR below 60 mL/min/1.73 m^2 is associated with cardiovascular [32,37–40] and non-vascular mortality [37,39]. We were also particularly careful to exclude patients who developed acute kidney injury by excluding any creatinine measurement obtained during a period of hospitalization or up to six weeks thereafter. Fourth, given the low prevalence of the low GFR outcome in our cohort, we may have missed factors associated with renal disease. Finally, kidney disease in subjects with eGFR values above 60 mL/min/1.73 m^2 may have been underestimated because we lacked data on proteinuria and renal tubular involvement, both early and significant indicators of renal disease in HIV patients.

This study also had multiple strengths. It was conducted at a referral center for HIV/AIDS care and research in one of the epicenters of the Brazilian AIDS epidemic on a very well characterized cohort with mixed ethnic background and universal access to first-line NNRTI-based regimens, as well as free access to PI-based regimens for subsequent treatment steps after first- and second-line virological failure. Additionally, we employed the recently developed CKD-EPI equation, which provides a more accurate estimate of GFR than other creatinine-based equations [59], an observation that was also confirmed in patients with HIV infection [60].

In summary, in this well-characterized cohort of Brazilian patients with HIV/AIDS with long-term exposure to cART, an age over 50 years, a current CD4 count less than 350 cells/mm^3, diabetes, hypertension, previous use of tenofovir, and previous use of indinavir were associated with a decreased glomerular filtration rate (p<0.05). The current use of atazanavir or lopinavir showed a weaker association with the outcome (p = 0.09), and this result may be related to the low prevalence of the outcome and the study population size. We were able to confirm that the current risk factors for CKD in HIV-infected individuals are broad and include virus-related factors as well as degenerative and nephrotoxic factors. With long-term exposure to cART, within the context of premature aging and cumulative chronic comorbidities, cumulative exposure to even low-grade nephrotoxins may eventually prove to have deleterious effects. Nevertheless, it is reassuring that despite the potential for nephrotoxicity from some pivotal antiretroviral drugs, in the short-term, advanced renal disease remains very rare.

Author Contributions

Conceived and designed the experiments: BG RKF AVO RIM SWC VGV JHRS. Performed the experiments: PS CBC LEC. Analyzed the data: PS BG RKF CBC RIM SWC VGV JHRS. Contributed reagents/materials/analysis tools: AVO CBC. Wrote the paper: PS BG RKF SWC PML JHRS.

References

1. Phair J, Palella F (2011) Renal disease in HIV-infected individuals. Curr Opin HIV AIDS 6: 285–289.
2. Scherzer R, Estrella M, Li Y, Choi AI, Deeks SG, et al. (2012) Association of tenofovir exposure with kidney disease risk in HIV infection. AIDS 26: 867–875.
3. Fernando S (2008) Prevalence Chronic Kidney Disease in an Urban HIV infected Population. Am J Med Sci 335: 89–94.
4. Szczech LA, Hoover DR, Feldman JG, Cohen MH, Gange SJ, et al. (2004) Association between renal disease and outcomes among HIV-infected women receiving or not receiving antiretroviral therapy. Clin Infect Dis 39: 1199–1206.
5. Gardner LI, Holmberg SD, Williamson JM, Szczech LA, Carpenter CC, et al. (2003) Development of proteinuria or elevated serum creatinine and mortality in HIV-infected women. J Acquir Immune Defic Syndr 32: 203–209.
6. Wyatt CM, Arons RR, Klotman PE, Klotman ME (2006) Acute renal failure in hospitalized patients with HIV: risk factors and impact on in-hospital mortality. AIDS 20: 561–565.
7. Mulenga LB, Kruse G, Lakhi S, Cantrell RA, Reid SE, et al. (2008) Baseline renal insufficiency and risk of death among HIV-infected adults on antiretroviral therapy in Lusaka, Zambia. AIDS 22: 1821–1827.
8. Gupta S, Eustace J, Winston J (2005) Guidelines for the management of chronic kidney disease in HIV-infected patientes: recomendations of the HIV Medicine Association of the infectious diseases society of America. Clinical Infectious Diseases 40: 1559–1585.
9. WHO' UNAIDS and UNICEF Global HIV/AIDS response: epidemic update and health sector progress towards universal access: progress report 2011. Geneva: WHO.
10. Brasil. Ministério da Saúde. Secretaria de Vigilância em Saúde. (2009) *Portaria SVS/MS No 151, de 14 de outubro de 2009*.: Available from: http://www.aids.gov.br/sites/default/files/portaria151_2009.pdf [Accessed 9th September 2013].
11. Wyatt C (2007) Chronic Kidney Disease in HIV infection: an urban epidemic. AIDS 21: 2101–2110.
12. Choi AI, Rodriguez RA, Bacchetti P, Bertenthal D, Volberding PA, et al. (2007) Racial Differences in End-Stage Renal Disease Rates in HIV Infection versus Diabetes. Journal of the American Society of Nephrology 18: 2968–2974.
13. Lucas GM, Lau B, Atta MG, Fine DM, Keruly J, et al. (2008) Chronic kidney disease incidence, and progression to end-stage renal disease, in HIV-infected individuals: a tale of two races. J Infect Dis 197: 1548–1557.
14. Roe J, Campbell Lucy J, Ibrahim F, Hendry Bruce M, Post Frank A (2008) HIV Care and the Incidence of Acute Renal Failure. Clinical Infectious Diseases 47: 242–249.
15. Campbell LJ, Ibrahim F, Fisher M, Holt SG, Hendry BM, et al. (2009) Spectrum of chronic kidney disease in HIV-infected patients. HIV Medicine 10: 329–336.
16. Colson AW, Florence E, Augustijn H, Verpooten GA, Lynen L, et al. (2010) Prevalence of chronic renal failure stage 3 or more in HIV-infected patients in Antwerp: an observational study. Acta Clin Belg 65: 392–398.
17. Mocroft A, Kirk O, Reiss P, De Wit S, Sedlacek D, et al. (2010) Estimated glomerular filtration rate, chronic kidney disease and antiretroviral drug use in HIV-positive patients. AIDS 24: 1667–1678.
18. Alves TP, Hulgan T, Wu P, Sterling TR, Stinnette SE, et al. (2010) Race, Kidney Disease Progression, and Mortality Risk in HIV-Infected Persons. Clinical Journal of the American Society of Nephrology 5: 2269–2275.
19. Déti EK, Thiébaut R, Bonnet F, Lawson-Ayayi S, Dupon M, et al. (2010) Prevalence and factors associated with renal impairment in HIV-infected patients, ANRS C03 Aquitaine Cohort, France. HIV Medicine 11: 308–317.
20. Flandre P, Pugliese P, Cuzin L, Bagnis CI, Tack I, et al. (2011) Risk Factors of Chronic Kidney Disease in HIV-infected Patients. Clinical Journal of the American Society of Nephrology.
21. Ibrahim F, Hamzah L, Jones R, Nitsch D, Sabin C, et al. (2012) Baseline kidney function as predictor of mortality and kidney disease progression in HIV-positive patients. Am J Kidney Dis 60: 539–547.

22. Medapalli RK, Parikh CR, Gordon K, Brown ST, Butt AA, et al. (2012) Comorbid diabetes and the risk of progressive chronic kidney disease in HIV-infected adults: data from the Veterans Aging Cohort Study. J Acquir Immune Defic Syndr 60: 393–399.

23. Reid A, Stohr W, Walker AS, Williams IG, Kityo C, et al. (2008) Severe renal dysfunction and risk factors associated with renal impairment in HIV-infected adults in Africa initiating antiretroviral therapy. Clin Infect Dis 46: 1271–1281.

24. Lucas GM, Clarke W, Kagaayi J, Atta MG, Fine DM, et al. (2010) Decreased Kidney Function in a Community-based Cohort of HIV-Infected and HIV-Negative Individuals in Rakai, Uganda. JAIDS Journal of Acquired Immune Deficiency Syndromes 55: 491–494.

25. Gupta SK, Ong'or WO, Shen C, Musick B, Goldman M, et al. (2011) Reduced renal function is associated with progression to AIDS but not with overall mortality in HIV-infected Kenyan adults not initially requiring combination antiretroviral therapy. J Int AIDS Soc 14: 31.

26. Ramos Jr AN, Matida LH, Hearst N, Heukelbach J (2011) Mortality in Brazilian Children with HIV/AIDS: The Role of Non-AIDS-Related Conditions After Highly Active Antiretroviral Therapy Introduction. AIDS Patient Care and STDs 25: 713–718.

27. Mocroft A, Kirk O, Gatell J, Reiss P, Gargalianos P, et al. (2007) Chronic renal failure among HIV-1-infected patients. AIDS 21: 1119–1127.

28. Overton ET, Nurutdinova D, Freeman J, Seyfried W, Mondy KE (2009) Factors associated with renal dysfunction within an urban HIV-infected cohort in the era of highly active antiretroviral therapy. HIV Med 10: 343–350.

29. Sorlí ML, Velat M, Guelar AM, Montero M, Villar J, et al. (2008) Subclinical kidney disease in HIV-infected patients. Journal of the International AIDS Society 11: P130.

30. Glassock RJ, Winearls C (2008) Screening for CKD with eGFR: doubts and dangers. Clin J Am Soc Nephrol 3: 1563–1568.

31. Jaar BG, Khatib R, Plantinga L, Boulware LE, Powe NR (2008) Principles of screening for chronic kidney disease. Clin J Am Soc Nephrol 3: 601–609.

32. Van Biesen W, De Bacquer D, Verbeke F, Delanghe J, Lameire N, et al. (2007) The glomerular filtration rate in an apparently healthy population and its relation with cardiovascular mortality during 10 years. Eur Heart J 28: 478–483.

33. Coresh J, Selvin E, Stevens LA, Manzi J, Kusek JW, et al. (2007) Prevalence of chronic kidney disease in the United States. JAMA 298: 2038–2047.

34. Giles PD, Fitzmaurice DA (2007) Formula estimation of glomerular filtration rate: have we gone wrong? BMJ 334: 1198–1200.

35. Hallan SI, Dahl K, Oien CM, Grootendorst DC, Aasberg A, et al. (2006) Screening strategies for chronic kidney disease in the general population: follow-up of cross sectional health survey. BMJ 333: 1047.

36. White SL, Polkinghorne KR, Atkins RC, Chadban SJ (2010) Comparison of the prevalence and mortality risk of CKD in Australia using the CKD Epidemiology Collaboration (CKD-EPI) and Modification of Diet in Renal Disease (MDRD) Study GFR estimating equations: the AusDiab (Australian Diabetes, Obesity and Lifestyle) Study. Am J Kidney Dis 55: 660–670.

37. Astor BC, Hallan SI, Miller ER, Yeung E, Coresh J (2008) Glomerular Filtration Rate, Albuminuria, and Risk of Cardiovascular and All-Cause Mortality in the US Population. American Journal of Epidemiology 167: 1226–1234.

38. Matsushita K, van der Velde M, Astor BC, Woodward M, Levey AS, et al. (2010) Association of estimated glomerular filtration rate and albuminuria with all-cause and cardiovascular mortality in general population cohorts: a collaborative meta-analysis. Lancet 375: 2073–2081.

39. Di Angelantonio E, Chowdhury R, Sarwar N, Aspelund T, Danesh J, et al. (2010) Chronic kidney disease and risk of major cardiovascular disease and non-vascular mortality: prospective population based cohort study. Bmj 341: c4986–c4986.

40. Yahalom G, Kivity S, Segev S, Sidi Y, Kurnik D (2013) Estimated glomerular filtration rate in a population with normal to mildly reduced renal function as predictor of cardiovascular disease. European Journal of Preventive Cardiology.

41. Davies DF, Shock NW (1950) Age changes in glomerular filtration rate, effective renal plasma flow, and tubular excretory capacity in adult males. J Clin Invest 29: 496–507.

42. O'Hare AM, Choi AI, Bertenthal D, Bacchetti P, Garg AX, et al. (2007) Age affects outcomes in chronic kidney disease. J Am Soc Nephrol 18: 2758–2765.

43. Deeks SG (2011) HIV infection, inflammation, immunosenescence, and aging. Annu Rev Med 62: 141–155.

44. Effros RB, Fletcher CV, Gebo K, Halter JB, Hazzard WR, et al. (2008) Aging and infectious diseases: workshop on HIV infection and aging: what is known and future research directions. Clin Infect Dis 47: 542–553.

45. Myers JD (2009) Growing old with HIV: the AIDS epidemic and an aging population. JAAPA 22: 20–24.

46. Guaraldi G, Orlando G, Zona S, Menozzi M, Carli F, et al. (2011) Premature age-related comorbidities among HIV-infected persons compared with the general population. Clin Infect Dis 53: 1120–1126.

47. Hasse B, Ledergerber B, Furrer H, Battegay M, Hirschel B, et al. (2011) Morbidity and aging in HIV-infected persons: the Swiss HIV cohort study. Clin Infect Dis 53: 1130–1139.

48. Crum-Cianflone N, Ganesan A, Teneza-Mora N, Riddle M, Medina S, et al. (2010) Prevalence and Factors Associated with Renal Dysfunction Among HIV-Infected Patients. AIDS Patient Care and STDs 24: 353–360.

49. Atta MG, Gallant JE, Rahman MH, Nagajothi N, Racusen LC, et al. (2006) Antiretroviral therapy in the treatment of HIV-associated nephropathy. Nephrol Dial Transplant 21: 2809–2813.

50. Scialla JJ, Atta MG, Fine DM (2007) Relapse of HIV-associated nephropathy after discontinuing highly active antiretroviral therapy. AIDS 21: 263–264.

51. Atta MG, Deray G, Lucas GM (2008) Antiretroviral Nephrotoxicities. Seminars in Nephrology 28: 563–575.

52. Wever K (2010) Incomplete Reversibility of Tenofovir-Related Renal Toxicity in HIV-Infected Men. J Acquir Immune Defic Syndr 00: 1–4.

53. Cooper RD, Wiebe N, Smith N, Keiser P, Naicker S, et al. (2010) Systematic Review and Meta-analysis: Renal Safety of Tenofovir Disoproxil Fumarate in HIV-Infected Patients. Clinical Infectious Diseases 51: 496–505.

54. Ryom L, Mocroft A, Kirk O, Worm SW, Kamara DA, et al. (2013) Association between antiretroviral exposure and renal impairment among HIV-positive persons with normal baseline renal function: the D:A:D study. J Infect Dis 207: 1359–1369.

55. Kalyesubula R, Perazella MA (2011) Nephrotoxicity of HAART. AIDS Res Treat 2011: 562790.

56. Holmberg SD (2008) Chapter One: Background. In: Holmberg SD, editor. Scientific Errors and Controversies in the U5 HIV/AIDS Epidemic: How They Slowed Advances and Were Resolved. Westport, CT: Praeger. 1–20.

57. Matsushita K, Selvin E, Bash LD, Astor BC, Coresh J (2010) Risk Implications of the New CKD Epidemiology Collaboration (CKD-EPI) Equation Compared With the MDRD Study Equation for Estimated GFR: The Atherosclerosis Risk in Communities (ARIC) Study. American Journal of Kidney Diseases 55: 648–659.

58. US Renal Data System (2011) USRDS 2011 Annual Data Report: Atlas of Chronic Kidney Disease and End-Stage Renal Disease in the United States. In: National Institutes of Health NIoDaDaKD, editor. Bethesda, MD.

59. Earley A, Miskulin D, Lamb EJ, Levey AS, Uhlig K (2012) Estimating equations for glomerular filtration rate in the era of creatinine standardization: a systematic review. Ann Intern Med 156: 785–795.

60. Inker LA, Wyatt C, Creamer R, Hellinger J, Hotta M, et al. (2012) Performance of creatinine and cystatin C GFR estimating equations in an HIV-positive population on antiretrovirals. J Acquir Immune Defic Syndr 61: 302–309.

19

A New Modified CKD-EPI Equation for Chinese Patients with Type 2 Diabetes

Xun Liu[1][9][¤a], Xiaoliang Gan[2][9], Jinxia Chen[1][¤b], Linsheng Lv[3], Ming Li[1], Tanqi Lou[1]*

1 Division of Nephrology, Department of Internal Medicine, The Third Affiliated Hospital of Sun Yat-sen University, Guangzhou, China, 2 Department of Anesthesiology, Zhongshan Ophthalmic Center, Sun Yat-sen University, Guangzhou, China, 3 Operating Room, The Third Affiliated Hospital of Sun Yat-sen University, Guangzhou, China

Abstract

Objective: To improve the performance of glomerular filtration rate (GFR) estimating equation in Chinese type 2 diabetic patients by modification of the CKD-EPI equation.

Design and patients: A total of 1196 subjects were enrolled. Measured GFR was calibrated to the dual plasma sample ^{99m}Tc-DTPA-GFR. GFRs estimated by the re-expressed 4-variable MDRD equation, the CKD-EPI equation and the Asian modified CKD-EPI equation were compared in 351 diabetic/non-diabetic pairs. And a new modified CKD-EPI equation was reconstructed in a total of 589 type 2 diabetic patients.

Results: In terms of both precision and accuracy, GFR estimating equations all achieved better results in the non-diabetic cohort comparing with those in the type 2 diabetic cohort (30% accuracy, $P \leq 0.01$ for all comparisons). In the validation data set, the new modified equation showed less bias (median difference, 2.3 ml/min/1.73 m^2 for the new modified equation vs. ranged from -3.8 to -7.9 ml/min/1.73 m^2 for the other 3 equations [$P < 0.001$ for all comparisons]), as was precision (IQR of the difference, 24.5 ml/min/1.73 m^2 vs. ranged from 27.3 to 30.7 ml/min/1.73 m^2), leading to a greater accuracy (30% accuracy, 71.4% vs. 55.2% for the re-expressed 4 variable MDRD equation and 61.0% for the Asian modified CKD-EPI equation [$P = 0.001$ and $P = 0.02$]).

Conclusion: A new modified CKD-EPI equation for type 2 diabetic patients was developed and validated. The new modified equation improves the performance of GFR estimation.

Editor: Zhanjun Jia, University of Utah School of Medicine, United States of America

Funding: This work was supported by the National Natural Science Foundation of China (Grant No. 81070612 and 81370866), the China Postdoctoral Science Foundation (Grant No. 201104335), Guangdong Science and Technology Plan (Grant No. 2011B031800084 and 2013B021800190), the Fundamental Research Funds for the Central Universities (Grant No. 11ykpy38), the National Project of Scientific and Technical Supporting Programs Funded by Ministry of Science & Technology of China (Grant No. 2011BAI10B05) and China Scholarship Council (Grant No. 201308440060). The funders had no role in study design, data collection and analysis, decision to publish, or preparation of the manuscript.

Competing Interests: The authors have declared that no competing interests exist.

* Email: liuxun@medmail.com.cn

¤a Current address: Division of Nephrology, Tufts Medical Center, Boston, Massachusetts, United States of America
¤b Current address: Institute of Nephrology, Affiliated Hospital of Guangdong Medical College, Zhanjiang, China

[9] These authors contributed equally to this work.

Introduction

Diabetic nephropathy is the leading cause of end stage renal disease and is associated with significantly high risk of cardiovascular events [1]. Glomerular filtration rate (GFR) is the best index of kidney function.[2]. American Diabetes Association standards highlight GFR screening for nephropathy in diabetic patients [3]. The Modification of Diet in Renal Disease (MDRD) equation and the Chronic Kidney Disease Epidemiology Collaboration (CKD-EPI) equation are most frequently used and favored in North America, Europe and Australia [4]. However, when either equation was applied to type 2 diabetic patients, both have imperfections [5–8], because of the intrinsic factors such as serum glucose status [9] and body mass index [10] in diabetic subjects that could affect the

accuracy of GFR estimates. Recently, a four-level race variable (Black, Asian, Native American and Hispanic, and White and other) CKD-EPI equation [11] was developed. In order to know whether the most frequently used equations really performed worse in diabetic subjects, a well-designed paired cohort was set up in this study to exclude other impact factors. And if this hypothesis was confirmed, a new equation was reconstructed later by modification of the original GFR estimating equation in a cohort of type 2 diabetic patients.

Subjects, Materials and Methods

Participant selection

This study enrolled participants consequently from Jan 2010 to Dec 2012 in the Third Affiliated Hospital of Sun Yat-sen

Table 1. CKD-EPI equation, asian modified CKD-EPI equation and the new equation.

Basis of equation and sex	Serum creatinine	Equation for estimating GFR
CKD-EPI equation		
Female	≤ 0.7 mg/dl	$144 \times (SC \div 0.7)^{-0.329} \times 0.993^{Age}[\times 1.159 \ \textit{if black}]$
Female	> 0.7 mg/dl	$144 \times (SC \div 0.7)^{-1.209} \times 0.993^{Age}[\times 1.159 \ \textit{if black}]$
Male	≤ 0.9 mg/dl	$141 \times (SC \div 0.9)^{-0.411} \times 0.993^{Age}[\times 1.159 \ \textit{if black}]$
Male	> 0.9 mg/dl	$141 \times (SC \div 0.9)^{-1.209} \times 0.993^{Age}[\times 1.159 \ \textit{if black}]$
Asian modified CKD-EPI equation		
Female	≤ 0.7 mg/dl	$151 \times (SC \div 0.7)^{-0.328} \times 0.993^{Age}$
Female	> 0.7 mg/dl	$151 \times (SC \div 0.7)^{-1.210} \times 0.993^{Age}$
Male	≤ 0.9 mg/dl	$149 \times (SC \div 0.9)^{-0.412} \times 0.993^{Age}$
Male	> 0.9 mg/dl	$149 \times (SC \div 0.9)^{-1.210} \times 0.993^{Age}$
New modified CKD-EPI equation		
Female	≤ 0.7 mg/dl	$94 \times (SC \div 0.7)^{-0.511} \times 0.998^{Age}$
Female	> 0.7 mg/dl	$128 \times (SC \div 0.7)^{-0.543} \times 0.992^{Age}$
Male	≤ 0.9 mg/dl	$117 \times (SC \div 0.9)^{-0.277} \times 0.994^{Age}$
Male	> 0.9 mg/dl	$102 \times (SC \div 0.9)^{-0.558} \times 0.994^{Age}$

University, China. Participants were excluded if they had any of the following: 1) younger than 18 years, or 2) type 1 diabetes, or 3) type 2 diabetes with known non-diabetic renal disease. The other exclusion criteria were described elsewhere [12]. GFR category was classified according to the National Kidney Foundation Disease Outcomes Quality Initiative clinical practice guidelines [13]. A total of 1196 subjects were enrolled, including 589 type 2 diabetic patients and 607 non-diabetic participants. The study protocol was approved by the institutional review board at the Third Affiliated Hospital of Sun Yat-sen University. Written informed consent was obtained from each participant.

Laboratory methods

GFR was measured by the 99mTc-diethylene triamine pentaacetic acid ($^{99\ m}$Tc-DTPA) renal dynamic imaging method [14–15], as described previously [16]. The minimum sample size was determined to be as 36 based in the findings in a previous study [17]. The calibration equation form DTPA renal dynamic imaging GFR to dual plasma sample DTPA-GFR in this study was as the following: dual plasma sample DTPA-GFR (ml/min/1.73 m^2) = 0.167+1.057* DTPA renal dynamic imaging-GFR (ml/min/1.73 m^2) (R^2 = 0.767, P<0.001). Serum creatinine (SC) level was measured by the enzymatic method on a Hitachi 7180 autoanalyzer (Hitachi, Tokyo, Japan; reagents from Roche Diagnostics, Mannheim, Germany), and recalibrated to isotope dilution mass spectrometry.

Statistical analysis

We used a stratified random sampling method based on age, body mass index (BMI) and GFR categories to obtain paired samples of participants represented either the type 2 diabetes or the non-diabetic cohorts. The bias between mGFR and estimated GFR (eGFR) was defined as mGFR minus eGFR. Precision was measured as the interquartile range (IQR) for difference. Accuracy was determined as the percentage of eGFR not deviating more the 30% from the mGFR. Confidence intervals for all metrics were calculated by means of bootstrap methods [18]. A Wilcoxon

Mann-Whitney test was used for bias. In comparison between two data sets, independent samples t test was used for quantitative variables, and two independent samples test for accuracy. In comparison within a data set, McNemar test was used for accuracy. GFR was estimated by using the following equations: re-expressed 4-variable MDRD equation ($GFR = 175 \times SC^{-1.154} \times Age^{-0.203} \times [0.742 \ \textit{if patient is female}] \times [1.212 \ \textit{if patient is black}]$) [19], CKD-EPI equation (Table 1) [20] and Asian modified CKD-EPI equation (Table 1) [11]. All analyses were performed using SPSS software (version 11.0 SPSS, Chicago IL, USA) and Matlab software (version 2011b The Mathworks, Boston MA, USA).

Results

Performance of the equations between diabetic and non-diabetic cohorts

Study population in this part of study. Three hundred and fifty-one pair of participants were selected from the total population of this study. In the type 2 diabetic cohort, the mean (±SD) mGFR was 62.8±28.1 ml/min/1.73 m^2. The mean mGFR was similar in the non-diabetic cohort (60.7±27.9 ml/min/1.73 m^2), as were the mean age, BMI, body-surface area, SC and gender (Table 2).

Comparison of the performances between diabetic and non-diabetic cohorts. Bias of both the CKD-EPI equation and the Asian modified CKD-EPI equation in the non-diabetic cohort were less than those in the type 2 diabetic cohort (median difference, 2.9 and 0.3 ml/min/1.73 m^2 vs. −3.7 and −7.3 ml/min/1.73 m^2 [P<0.001 for both comparisons]). In terms of both precision and accuracy, GFR estimating equations all achieved better results in the non-diabetic cohort comparing with those in the type 2 diabetic cohort (IQR for difference, ranged from 20.5 to 22.2 ml/min/1.73 m^2 for all 3 equations vs. ranged from 28.0 to 31.5 ml/min/1.73 m^2; 30% accuracy, ranged from 64.4% to 66.7% vs. ranged from 53.0% to 57.3% [P≤0.01 for all comparisons]). However, Bias of re-expressed 4 variable MDRD

Table 2. Participant characteristic.*

Subjects (n)	Participant group		P value
	Non-diabetics (n = 351)	**Diabetics (n = 351)**	
Age (year)	58.3±13.3	60.3±12.5	0.2
Male sex [n (%)]	209(59.5)	208(59.3)	0.5
Body mass index (kg/m^2)	23.9±3.3	24.1±3.6	0.8
Body-surface area (m^2)	1.7±0.2	1.7±0.2	0.1
Serum creatinine (mg/dl)	1.9±1.7	1.8±1.7	0.9
Measured GFR (ml/min/1.73 m^2)	60.7±27.9	62.8±28.1	0.7

*: Plus-minus values are means±SD.
Abbreviations: GFR, glomerular filtration rate.

equation in the non-diabetic cohort was greater than that in the type 2 diabetic cohort (median difference, 5.1 ml/min/1.73 m^2 vs. -2.2 ml/min/1.73 m^2 [P<0.001]) (Table 3).

Performances of the equations in the type 2 diabetic cohort. Both the re-expressed 4 variable MDRD equation and the CKD-EPI equation appeared unbiased (median difference, -2.2 ml/min/1.73 m^2 for the re-expressed 4 variable MDRD equation vs. -3.7 ml/min/1.73 m^2 for the CKD-EPI equation [P=0.5]). However, precision was improved with the CKD-EPI equation (IQR for the difference, 28.0 ml/min/1.73 m^2), as compared with the re-expressed 4 variable MDRD equation and with the Asian modified CKD-EPI equation (IQR for the difference, 31.2 and 31.5 ml/min/1.73 m^2), as was accuracy (30% accuracy, 57.3% vs. 51.3% and 53.0% [P=0.004 and P=0.01]) (Table 3).

Development of a new modified equation to estimate GFR for type 2 diabetic patients

Patient's characteristics in this part of study. The general characteristics of type 2 diabetic patients are presented in Table 4. The diabetic cohort here enrolled the participants in the analyses for the first result in this paper. A total of 589 patients

were enrolled, including 327 men and 260 women, and the mean age was 61.0±12.7 yr, with body mass index 24.9±4.1 kg/m^2, fasting plasma glucose 160.4±77.0 mg/dL, glycated hemoglobin 9.3±11.9%, SC 1.4±1.5 mg/dL, and mGFR 74.4±31.0 ml/min/1.73 m^2. We randomly selected 379 subjects (the development data set) from the entire study population, and the remaining 210 patients were included in the validation data set.

Development of the new modified equation. We reconstructed a new modified equation using data from the development data set of this part of study by the generalized additive model. The new modified equation used the same three variables (age, gender and SC), the same knot points for SC and the same forms of smooth functions as the CKD-EPI equation. mGFR and SC were transformed to natural logarithms. The development data set was divided in to four categories according to gender and the knot points for SC. And four linear regression models were developed. The coefficients were estimated by the least-square error method (Table 1).

Overall performance of the predicting models

In the validation data set, the new modified equation showed less bias (median difference, 2.3 ml/min/1.73 m^2 for the new

Table 3. Performance between measured GFR and estimated GFR.

Variable	CKD group	
	Non-diabetics	**Diabetics**
Bias - median difference (ml/min/1.73 m^2, 95% CI)		
Re-expressed 4 variable MDRD equation	5.1(3.2, 7.6)	$-2.2(-6.8, 0.8)$
CKD-EPI equation	2.9(1.3, 4.6)	$-3.7(-6.7, 0.5)$
Asian modified CKD-EPI equation	0.3((−1.8, 1.8)	$-7.3(-10.9, -2.2)$
Precision - IQR of the difference (ml/min/1.73 m^2, 95% CI)		
Re-expressed 4 variable MDRD equation	21.2(18.4, 24.1)	31.2(25.3, 30.9)
CKD-EPI equation	20.5(17.9, 23.1)	28.0(25.3, 30.9)
Asian modified CKD-EPI equation	22.2(19.5, 25.3)	31.5(27.7, 34.1)
Accuracy - 30% accuracy (%, 95% CI)		
Re-expressed 4 variable MDRD equation	64.4(60.0, 69.2)	51.3(45.9, 56.4)
CKD-EPI equation	66.7(61.8, 71.5)	57.3(52.1, 62.1)
Asian modified CKD-EPI equation	65.0(60.1, 69.8)	53.0(47.9, 58.1)

Abbreviations: GFR, glomerular filtration rate; CKD, chronic kidney disease; MDRD, Modification of Diet in Renal Disease; CKD-EPI, Chronic Kidney Disease Epidemiology Collaboration; CI, confidence interval; IQR, interquartile range.

Table 4. Patient's characteristic.

Characteristic (N = 589)	Mean (standard deviation) or number (percentage)
Age (year)	61.0(12.7)
Male sex [n (%)]	327(55.5)
Body mass index (kg/m²)	24.9(4.1)
Body-surface area (m²)	1.7(0.2)
Serum albumin, mean (g/dL)	3.8(0.8)
Serum urea nitrogen (mg/dL)	24.0(18.0)
Serum creatinine (mg/dL)	1.4(1.5)
Serum uric acid (mg/dL)	6.4(2.3)
Serum total cholesterol (mg/dL)	199.1(85.2)
Serum triglycerides (mg/dL)	215.5(197.1)
Serum high-density lipoprotein (mg/dL)	67.2(70.5)
Serum low-density lipoprotein (mg/dL)	99.8(53.9)
Fasting plasma glucose (mg/dL)	160.4(77.0)
Glycated haemoglobin (%)	9.3(11.9)
Urine albumin to creatinine ratio (mg/mg)	57.8(132.3)
Measured GFR (ml/min/1.73 m²)	70.9(29.1)
GFR categories [n (%)]	
<15 (ml/min/1.73 m²)	13(2.2)
15–29 (ml/min/1.73 m²)	40(6.8)
30–59 (ml/min/1.73 m²)	151(25.6)
60–89 (ml/min/1.73 m²)	191(32.4)
>90 (ml/min/1.73 m²)	194(32.9)

Abbreviations: GFR, glomerular filtration rate.

modified equation vs. ranged -3.8 to -7.9 ml/min/1.73 m² for the other 3 equations [P<0.001 for all comparisons]), as was precision (IQR of the difference, 24.5 ml/min/1.73 m² vs. ranged from 27.3 to 30.7 ml/min/1.73 m²), leading to a greater accuracy (30% accuracy, 71.4% vs. 55.2% for the re-expressed 4 variable MDRD equation and 61.0% for the Asian modified CKD-EPI equation [P = 0.001 and P = 0.02], 62.9% for the CKD-EPI equation [P = 0.4] (Table 5).

Discussions

In the present study, we first confirmed the hypothesis that GFR estimating equations all achieved better results in the non-diabetic cohort comparing with those in the type 2 diabetic cohort by paired samples study. Then, we developed a new equation in a cohort of type 2 diabetic patients by modification of the CKD-EPI equation which performed the best in diabetic subjects. In the validation data set, the new modified equation achieved less bias, higher precision and greater accuracy compared with all three original equations. These results were consistent with the previous findings [15,21–26] that modification of the original equation in a local cohort which was quiet different to the original one may improve the performance of GFR estimation in the same population. And our results will help clinicians to make suitable clinical decision for diabetic patients and avoid unnecessary examination and treatment.

Why the modified CKD-EPI equation outperformed all three original equations? There are several reasons. First, the development data set in this study was mainly type 2 diabetic patients, which was differed to the other original equations. Obesity is common in diabetic patients [27], leading to a relative low body muscle mass [28], influenced the generation of creatinine in the body. And hyperglycemia status in diabetic patients influences the measurement of GFR [29]. Second, GFR measurement method in this study was calibrated to the dual sample DTPA clearance. However, the development data sets of the other original

Table 5. Performance of bias, precision and accuracy between measured GFR and estimated GFR in the validation data set.

Variable	Measured GFR (ml/min/1.73 m²)		
	Overall (n = 210)	<60 (n = 86)	≥60 (n = 124)
Bias – median difference (ml/min/1.73 m², 95% CI)			
Re-expressed 4 variable MDRD equation	−4.4(−8.3, −1.0)	2.3(−1.8, 5.8)	−10.7(−16.4, −6.8)
CKD-EPI equation	−3.8(−6.9, −0.2)	2.1(−1.8, 5.8)	−8.1(−11.4, −3.9)
Asian modified CKD-EPI equation	−7.9(−11.5, −3.6)	0.3(−4.1, 4.2)	−13.2(−17.1, −8.3)
New modified equation	2.3(−1.3, 5.7)	−6.5(−9.5, −4.8)	12.9(8.5, 16.4)
Precision – IQR of the difference (ml/min/1.73 m², 95% CI)			
Re-expressed 4 variable MDRD equation	30.7(26.3, 36.4)	20.2(13.8, 28.6)	37.1(27.6, 49.3)
CKD-EPI equation	27.3(22.3, 30.8)	21.2(14.8, 30.2)	28.3(22.3, 33.2)
Asian modified CKD-EPI equation	29.9(25.0, 33.7)	23.4(16.8, 32.5)	29.9(23.0, 34.3)
New modified equation	24.5(21.0, 28.4)	13.6(10.2, 17.5)	23.4(18.8, 32.3)
Accuracy - 30% accuracy (%, 95% CI)			
Re-expressed 4 variable MDRD equation	55.2(48.1, 61.9)	41.9(31.4, 52.3)	64.5(56.5, 72.6)
CKD-EPI equation	62.9(56.2, 69.5)	44.2(33.7, 54.7)	75.8(68.6, 83.1)
Asian modified CKD-EPI equation	61.0(54.3, 67.8)	46.5(36.1, 57.0)	71.0(62.9, 79.0)
New modified equation	71.4(65.2, 77.1)	58.1(47.7, 68.6)	80.6(73.4, 87.1)

Abbreviations: GFR, glomerular filtration rate; MDRD, Modification of Diet in Renal Disease; CKD-EPI, Chronic Kidney Disease Epidemiology Collaboration; CI, confidence interval; IQR, interquartile range.

equations used urinary clearance of iothalamate instead. Third, the validation cohort in this study had similar characters as those in the development cohort. Systematic differences generally lead to bias, whereas variation in populations' characteristics leads to imprecision.

There are limitations in our study. First, the new modified equation needs further external validations. Second, the study population in this study was restricted to Chinese patients with type 2 diabetes. Third, difference in the method to measure GFR between different equations would lead to systemic error in comparison with each other. Forth, the sample size of the validation data set in this study was relatively small. Fifth, there is not suitable statistic method for the comparison of IQR of difference between different GFR predicting models up till now.

In conclusion, we confirmed that the performances of GFR estimating equations in type 2 diabetic patients were worse than

those in non-diabetic participants. And a new modified CKD-EPI equation for type 2 diabetic patients was developed and validated. The new modified equation improves the performance of GFR estimation, which may help physician to evaluate the kidney function in diabetic patients. Extensive external validations will be the next step before broadly applications.

Acknowledgments

Thanks to the patients for their good cooperation.

Author Contributions

Conceived and designed the experiments: XL TQL. Performed the experiments: XL JXC LSL ML. Analyzed the data: XL JXC XLG LSL. Contributed reagents/materials/analysis tools: XL XLG. Wrote the paper: XL XLG.

References

1. Tonelli M, Muntner P, Lloyd A, Manns BJ, Klarenbach S, et al (2012) Risk of coronary events in people with chronic kidney disease compared with those with diabetes: a population-level cohort study. Lancet 380:807–814.

2. Levey AS, Coresh J (2012) Chronic kidney disease. Lancet 379:165–180.

3. American Diabetes Association. Standards of medical care in diabetes–2013 (2013) Diabetes Care 36:S11–66.

4. Earley A, Miskulin D, Lamb EJ, Levey AS, Uhlig K (2012) Estimating equations for glomerular filtration rate in the era of creatinine standardization: a systematic review. Ann Intern Med 156:785–795, W–270, W–271, W–272, W–273, W–274, W–275, W–276, W–277, W–278.

5. Silveiro SP, Araújo GN, Ferreira MN, Souza FD, Yamaguchi HM, et al (2011) Chronic Kidney Disease Epidemiology Collaboration (CKD-EPI) equation pronouncedly underestimates glomerular filtration rate in type 2 diabetes. Diabetes Care 34:2353–2355.

6. Rognant N, Lemoine S, Laville M, Hadj-Aïssa A, Dubourg L (2011) Performance of the chronic kidney disease epidemiology collaboration equation to estimate glomerular filtration rate in diabetic patients. Diabetes Care 34:1320–1322.

7. Rigalleau V, Lasseur C, Perlemoine C, Barthe N, Raffaitin C, et al (2005) Estimation of glomerular filtration rate in diabetic subjects: Cockcroft formula or modification of Diet in Renal Disease study equation? Diabetes Care.28:838–843.

8. Nair S, Mishra V, Hayden K, Lisboa PJ, Pandya B, et al (2011) The four-variable modification of diet in renal disease formula underestimates glomerular filtration rate in obese type 2 diabetic individuals with chronic kidney disease. Diabetologia 54:1304–1307.

9. Rigalleau V, Lasseur C, Raffaitin C, Perlemoine C, Barthe N, et al (2006) Glucose control influences glomerular filtration rate and its prediction in diabetic subjects. Diabetes Care 29:1491–1495.

10. Kawamoto R, Kohara K, Tabara Y, Miki T, Ohtsuka N, et al (2008) An association between body mass index and estimated glomerular filtration rate. Hypertens Res 31:1559–1564.

11. Stevens LA, Claybon MA, Schmid CH, Chen J, Horio M, et al (2011) Evaluation of the Chronic Kidney Disease Epidemiology Collaboration equation for estimating the glomerular filtration rate in multiple ethnicities. Kidney Int 79:555–562.

12. Xun Liu, Huijuan Ma, Hui Huang, Cheng Wang, Hua Tang, et al (2013) Is the Chronic Kidney Disease Epidemiology Collaboration creatinine-cystatin C equation useful for glomerular filtration rate estimation in the elderly? Clinical Interventions in Aging 8: 1387–1391.

13. National Kidney Foundation (2002) K/DOQI clinical practice guidelines for chronic kidney disease: evaluation, classification, and stratification. Am J Kidney Dis 39: S1–266.

14. Heikkinen JO, Kuikka JT, Ahonen AK, Rautio PJ et al (2001) Quality of dynamic radionuclide renal imaging: multicentre evaluation using a functional renal phantom. Nucl Med Commun 22:987–995.

15. Pei X, Yang W, Wang S, Zhu B, Wu J, et al (2013) Using mathematical algorithms to modify glomerular filtration rate estimation equations. PLoS One 8:e57852.

16. Liu X, Pei X, Li N, Zhang Y, Zhang X, et al (2013) Improved glomerular filtration rate estimation by an artificial neural network. PLoS One 8:e58242.

17. Xun Liu, Yanni Wang, Cheng Wang, Chenggang Shi, Cailian Cheng, et al (2013) A New Equation to Estimate Glomerular Filtration Rate in Chinese Elderly Population. PLOS ONE 8: e79675.

18. Efron B, Tibshirani RJ (1993) An introduction to the bootstrap. New York: Chapman and Hall.

19. Levey AS, Coresh J, Greene T, Stevens LA, Zhang YL, et al (2006) Chronic Kidney Disease Epidemiology Collaboration. Using standardized serum creatinine values in the modification of diet in renal disease study equation for estimating glomerular filtration rate. Ann Intern Med 145:247–254.

20. Levey AS, Stevens LA, Schmid CH, Zhang YL, Castro AF 3rd, et al (2009) A New Equation to Estimate Glomerular Filtration Rate. Ann Intern Med 150:604–612.

21. Teo BW, Xu H, Wang D, Li J, Sinha AK, et al (2011) GFR estimating equations in a multiethnic Asian population. Am J Kidney Dis 58:56–63.

22. Lee CS, Cha RH, Lim YH, Kim H, Song KH, et al (2010) Ethnic coefficients for glomerular filtration rate estimation by the Modification of Diet in Renal Disease study equations in the Korean population. J Korean Med Sci25:1616–1625.

23. Matsuo S, Imai E, Horio M, Yasuda Y, Tomita K, et al (2009) Revised Equations for Estimating Glomerular Filtration Rate (GFR) form Serum Creatinine in Japan. Am J Kidney Dis 53:982–992.

24. Praditpornsilpa K, Townamchai N, Chaiwatanarat T, Tiranathanagul K, Katawatin P, et al (2011) The need for robust validation for MDRD-based glomerular filtration rate estimation in various CKD populations. Nephrol Dial Transplant 26:2780–2785.

25. Horio M, Imai E, Yasuda Y, Watanabe T, Matsuo S et al (2010) Modification of the CKD epidemiology collaboration(CKD-EPI) equation for Japanese: accuracy and use for population estimates. Am J Kidney Dis 56:32–38.

26. van Deventer HE, George JA, Paiker JE, Becker PJ, Katz IJ (2008) Estimating glomerular filtration rate in black South Africans by use of the modification of diet in renal disease and Cockcroft-Gault equations. Clin Chem 54:1197–1202.

27. de Boer IH, Sibley SD, Kestenbaum B, Sampson JN, Young B, Cleary PA et al (2007) Central obesity, incident microalbuminuria, and change in creatinine clearance in the epidemiology of diabetes interventions and complications study. J Am Soc Nephrol.18: 235–43.

28. Kim TN, Park MS, Kim YJ, Lee EJ, Kim MK, et al (2014) Association of low muscle mass and combined low muscle mass and visceral obesity with low cardiorespiratory fitness. PLoS One.9: e100118.

29. Bjornstad P, McQueen RB, Snell-Bergeon JK, Cherney D, Pyle L, et al (2014) Fasting blood glucose—a missing variable for GFR-estimation in type 1 diabetes? PLoS One.9: e96264.

20

Determinants of Renal Tissue Oxygenation as Measured with BOLD-MRI in Chronic Kidney Disease and Hypertension in Humans

Menno Pruijm[1], Lucie Hofmann[2], Maciej Piskunowicz[3], Marie-Eve Muller[1], Carole Zweiacker[1], Isabelle Bassi[1], Bruno Vogt[2], Matthias Stuber[4], Michel Burnier[1]*

1 Department of Nephrology, University Hospital, Lausanne, Switzerland, 2 Department of Nephrology and Hypertension, Bern University Hospital, Bern, Switzerland, 3 Department of Radiology, Medical University of Gdansk, Gdansk, Poland, 4 Department of Radiology, University Hospital, Lausanne, Switzerland

Abstract

Experimentally renal tissue hypoxia appears to play an important role in the pathogenesis of chronic kidney disease (CKD) and arterial hypertension (AHT). In this study we measured renal tissue oxygenation and its determinants in humans using blood oxygenation level-dependent magnetic resonance imaging (BOLD-MRI) under standardized hydration conditions. Four coronal slices were selected, and a multi gradient echo sequence was used to acquire T2* weighted images. The mean cortical and medullary R2* values ($=1/T2^*$) were calculated before and after administration of IV furosemide, a low R2* indicating a high tissue oxygenation. We studied 195 subjects (95 CKD, 58 treated AHT, and 42 healthy controls). Mean cortical R2 and medullary R2* were not significantly different between the groups at baseline. In stimulated conditions (furosemide injection), the decrease in R2* was significantly blunted in patients with CKD and AHT. In multivariate linear regression analyses, neither cortical nor medullary R2* were associated with eGFR or blood pressure, but cortical R2* correlated positively with male gender, blood glucose and uric acid levels. In conclusion, our data show that kidney oxygenation is tightly regulated in CKD and hypertensive patients at rest. However, the metabolic response to acute changes in sodium transport is altered in CKD and in AHT, despite preserved renal function in the latter group. This suggests the presence of early renal metabolic alterations in hypertension. The correlations between cortical R2* values, male gender, glycemia and uric acid levels suggest that these factors interfere with the regulation of renal tissue oxygenation.

Editor: Jaap A. Joles, University Medical Center Utrecht, Netherlands

Funding: This study was supported by research grants from the Swiss National Science Foundation (FN 32003B-132913 and 149309) and by the Centre d'Imagerie BioMédicale (CIBM) of the University of Lausanne (UNIL). The funders had no role in study design, data collection and analysis, decision to publish, or preparation of the manuscript.

Competing Interests: The authors have declared that no competing interests exist.

* E-mail: michel.burnier@chuv.ch

Introduction

Numerous experimental studies have suggested that disturbed oxygenation plays a role in the development and progression of kidney disease including hypertensive nephropathy[1–3].Thus, using micro-electrodes for direct pO2 measurements, low cortical O2 levels have been found in spontaneous hypertensive rats and in rats with streptozotocine-induced diabetes or in the subtotal nephrectomy model [4,5].

Until recently, human data were largely lacking mainly due to the lack of non-invasive methods to estimate renal tissue oxygenation. Over the last decade, blood oxygenation level-dependent magnetic resonance imaging (BOLD-MRI) has become a powerful tool to estimate renal tissue oxygenation non-invasively in humans. The basic principle of BOLD-MRI is that changes in renal tissue desoxyhemoglobin concentrations involve generation of phase incoherence of magnetic spins, leading to an increase in apparent relaxation rate R2* (expressed in $\sec^{-1}$). Under the assumption that blood pO2 is in equilibrium with tissue pO2, R2* values provide estimates of tissue oxygenation, a low R2* indicating a high tissue oxygenation [6]. Using post-processing programs, several circles - called regions of interest (ROI's) - are placed manually per slice in the cortex and in the medulla. This allows the assessment of the average cortical and medullary R2* value, per kidney or for both kidneys together, without the need to administer contrast product [7].

Several studies have used BOLD-MRI in humans to investigate renal oxygenation in different forms of chronic kidney disease (CKD) [8,9]. The largest study which assessed renal oxygenation at different degrees of kidney dysfunction was published by Michaely et al and included 400 patients [10]. Interestingly, no correlation was found between cortical and medullary R2* values and the estimated glomerular filtration rate (eGFR, according to the MDRD-formula) in this study. However this evaluation had several limitations: renal function was not measured in all patients (280 with measured creatinine levels), no information was collected on medication intake or baseline characteristics such as blood pressure or underlying renal disease, and BOLD-MRI was not performed under standardized conditions of fluid and sodium intake which are known to have a strong influence on renal oxygenation measured by BOLD-MRI [11,12].

Changes in renal tissue oxygenation may also contribute to the development of ischemic and hypertensive nephropathies [5]. For these reasons, most studies performed in hypertensive patients so far have been conducted in patients with renal artery stenosis [13,14]. Other studies in patients with essential hypertension have focused on the role of sodium, angiotensin II or race on cortical and medullary oxygenation [12,15,16]. These studies were performed in a relatively small number of participants, or did not include a control group. Whether or not essential hypertension is characterized by chronic hypoxia in humans remains therefore an open question.

The aim of the present study was therefore to assess renal tissue oxygenation at baseline and after an acute administration of furosemide in patients with various levels of renal function as well as in patients with essential hypertension and a normal renal function and in control subjects. Moreover, we analyzed the potential determinants of renal cortical and medullary tissue oxygenation in these patient groups.

Methods

This research project was approved by the local institutional review committee (Ethical Committee of the Canton de Vaud, Switzerland) and conducted according to the principles expressed in the Declaration of Helsinki. Written informed consent was obtained from each participant.

Subjects

Patients with CKD stage 1–5, or with hypertension without CKD were eligible for this study. CKD was defined as an estimated glomerular filtration rate (eGFR) $\leq$60 ml/min/1.73 m^2, or the presence of structural or functional abnormalities for at least three months [17]. Arterial hypertension (AHT) was defined as mean office blood pressure (BP) $\geq$140/90 mmHg measured at more than one occasion, or an office BP <140/90 mmHg while taking one or more antihypertensive drugs. Other inclusion criteria were: age $\geq$18 years and the ability to understand the study protocol and to sign an informed consent. Controls were normotensive, untreated healthy individuals without a history of kidney disease or hypertension or any other concomitant disease. Exclusion criteria for all participants were: a contra-indication to MR-imaging such as claustrophobia or the presence of a pacemaker or other implanted metallic device.

Study protocol

Patients were recruited at the outpatient nephrology and hypertension clinic of the university hospital in Lausanne (CHUV). Controls were recruited by local advertisement. Participants were maintained on their regular diet. Salt intake, proteinuria, and creatinine clearance were measured before BOLD-MRI by a 24 h urine collection. On the day of each BOLD-MRI measurement, an identical oral hydration protocol was followed by each participant at home (loading dose of 5 ml/kg of water at 8am, followed by 3 ml/kg every hour till 12am), see extended methods for further details and justification of this hydration protocol. Subjects joined our research unit at 11.30 am. BP was measured three times by an experienced research nurse using an automated Omron 705IT oscillometric device according to the recommendations of the European Society of Hypertension [18]. Peripherical oxygen saturation was measured using a fingertip pulse oxymeter (Oxy, Medair AB, Delsbo Sweden), and blood was drawn by a catheter inserted into an antecubital vein.

BOLD-MRI

BOLD-MRI was performed between 1 and 2 pm in the radiology department. Magnetic resonance measurements were carried out on a 3T whole-body MR system (MAGNETOM Trio, Siemens Medical Systems, Erlangen, Germany), as described previously [12,19,20]. Briefly, four coronal slices with good cortico-medullary differentiation obtained in expiration were selected from morphological images for functional evaluation with BOLD-MRI. Twelve T_2*-weighted images were recorded within a single breath-hold of 12.4 seconds with a modified Multi Echo Data Image Combination sequence (MEDIC) with the following parameters: repetition time (TR) 68 ms, echo time (TE) 6–52.2 ms (equidistant echo time spacing 4.2 ms), flip angle 20°, field of view (FOV) 400×400 mm^2, voxel size 1.6×1.6×5 mm^3, bandwidth 700 Hz/pixel, matrix 256×256 (interpolation to 512×512). All images were exported for analysis with a home-built IDL program (Interactive Data Language, Boulder, CO, USA). R_2* maps were calculated voxel by voxel using a Levenberg-Marquardt least-squares algorithm to fit an exponential function to the signal intensities measured for each echo time. ROIs were traced in the form of circles of equal size (containing approximately 20 voxels each) in the medulla and the cortex (two in the cortex and two in the medulla in each kidney), as illustrated in Figure 1. The reported R_2* value was the mean value of four slices (16 ROIs) for the medulla and the cortex. This technique has been shown to have a good reproducibility [7,20]. Medullary-cortical R_2*ratio (MCR2*), as a marker of metabolic workload, was calculated for each participant by dividing the mean medullary R_2* by cortical R_2* levels [21]. The procedure was repeated for all four coronal series obtained fifteen minutes after the administration of 20 mg furosemide intravenously.

Statistics

Clinical data were analyzed using STATA 11.0 (StataCorp, College Station, Texas, USA). Quantitative variables were expressed as mean $\pm$ standard deviation, or as median (25th–75th percentile range), as appropriate. Qualitative variables were expressed as number of patients and percentage. Comparisons between baseline characteristics of study groups were analyzed with ANOVA. Distribution of variables was also expressed using the probability density function according to Kernel. In case of non-normal distribution, variables were log-transformed. Multivariable logistic regression, adjusting for the predefined variables age, sex, current smoking, body mass index, diabetes, hemoglobin, and 24 h urinary sodium excretion, was used to determine the independent association of cortical and medullary R2* values with CKD status. These variables were selected based on their known association with CKD (body mass index, diabetes, age), or because of a theoretical association with renal tissue oxygenation (hemoglobin, 24 h urinary sodium excretion, smoking).

Similarly, in order to determine the independent association of each independent variable of interest with the dependent variables cortical and medullary R2* values, multivariate linear regression was performed, adjusted for the same predefined covariates.

Associations between the eGFR slope and R2* values were examined with Spearman's rank correlation and multivariable linear regression analysis. Results of the logistic multivariate analysis are presented as Odds-ratio (OR) and 95% confidence interval (95% CI). Results of all linear multivariate analyses are presented as beta-coefficients (β) and their 95% confidence intervals. P values were derived from maximum likelihood ratio tests. Statistical significance was considered for a two-sided P< 0.05.

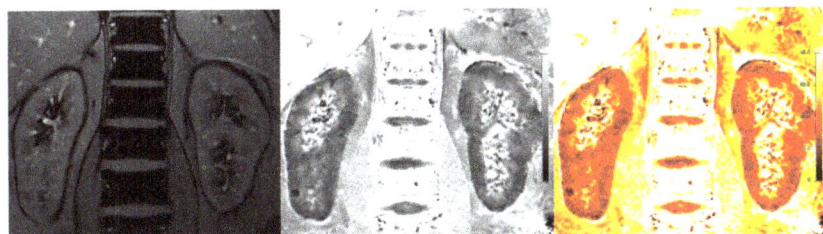

Figure 1. Illustration of BOLD image analysis. Anatomical templates are shown on the left, R2* maps in the middle, and color maps on the right (low R2* levels corresponding to higher tissue oxygenation in red, high R2* levels in yellow). Two regions of interest (ROIs) are traced in the form of circles (20 voxels each) in the cortex and medulla of each kidney; this procedure is repeated on four different slices.

Results

Clinical characteristics of the patients and controls

Details of the screening procedure are provided in the 'extended Methods and Results S1' section. Baseline clinical characteristics of patients with CKD and hypertension and of controls are shown in Table 1. Patients in the CKD-and hypertensive group were well-matched for age, sex and other baseline characteristics. Healthy volunteers were significantly younger, and more often female. Medical treatments of subjects according to group are shown in Table 2 and across different stages of CKD in Table S1.

R2* levels in hypertension and CKD as compared with healthy controls

There were no differences in mean or median cortical and medullary R2* levels between the right and left kidney in all groups (cortex (median (range)) respectively 17.4 (16.1; 18.6) and 17.6 (16.3; 18.8) sec^{-1}, $p = 0.29$; and medulla (mean$\pm$SD): 28.7 ± 4.2 vs 28.7 ± 2.5 sec^{-1}, $p = 0.94$). Therefore, only the mean cortical and medullary R2* values of both kidneys are shown and used for statistical analysis. The distribution of medullary R2* was comparable in all groups, but that of cortical R2* values differed markedly between groups (Figure 2A and B). A bimodal cortical distribution was observed in controls and AHT patients, yet not in CKD patients (Figure 2B). The bimodality of the probability density function of cortical R2* values was partly explained by gender (Figure 3); no gender-differences were seen in the distribution of medullary R2* values (Figure S1). The mean medullary and cortical R2* values and medullary-cortical ratio's of each group were comparable between the CKD, hypertensive and control group (Table 3). No differences were seen in cortical and

Table 1. Baseline characteristics of patients and controls enrolled in the study.

	Control (n = 42)	CKD (n = 95)	AHT (n = 58)
Age (years)	46±13*	56±15	57±11
Sex (% female)	52*	30	32
Currently smoking (%)	7*	27	35
Body Mass Index (kg/m2)	26±5	27±5	29±5
Systolic BP (mmHg)	122±13*	135±19	142±16**
Diastolic BP (mmHg)	73±10	76±12	82±10**
eGFR (CKD-EPI, ml/min/1.73 m²)	97±14*	57±31	91±15**
eGFR (MDRD, ml/min/1.73 m²)	94±15*	57±29	91±16**
Hemoglobin (g/dl)	136±11	130±18	138±13**
Blood glucose (mmol/l)	5.6±0.9*	6.5±2.1	6.1±1.2
Diabetes (%)	0*	23	17
Blood potassium (mmol/l)	3.9±0.2*	4.2±0.6	3.8±0.3**
Venous bicarbonate (mmol/l)	27(20;30)*	25 (14;32)	27 (23;32)**
Blood uric acid (μmol/l)	289 (130;450)*	391 (168;662)	342 (163;548)**
Oxygen saturation (%)	97±2.0	96±1.9	96±1.6
24 h Urinary volume (ml)	1731 (694;5008)	2068 (585;4356)	1812 (780;3945)
24 h Urinary sodium excretion (mmol)	156±72	173±92	174±87
24 h Urinary protein excretion (g)	0.06 (0;0.12)	0.3 (0;9.4)	0.07 (0;0.17)
24 h Urinary albumin excretion (mg)	4.7 (0;23)	100 (1;6131)	10 (0;29)
24 h Urinary creatinine clearance (ml/min)	125 (83;213)	68 (14; 170)	115 (73;249)

Values are expressed as mean±SD, or as median (min; max) as appropriate. CKD = chronic kidney disease; AHT = arterial hypertension.
* $p<0.05$: control group versus CKD;
** $p<0.05$ AHT versus CKD.

Table 2. Drug treatment of participants.

	CKD (n = 95)	AHT (n = 58)	Controls (n = 42)
Antihypertensive medication (%)			
Beta blocker	34.9	39.6	0
Alpha blocker	2.3	0	0
ACE-inhibitor	17.4	11.5	0
AT-II type 1 receptor blocker	52.3	26.4	0
Calcium channel blockers	32.6	35.9	0
Thiazide diuretic	27.9	20.8	0
Loop diuretic	17.4	3.9	0
Cholesterol lowering medication			
Statine	57	33	5
Fibrate	1.2	0	0
Ezetimibe	5.8	9.6	0
Antiplatelet agent			
Aspirin	31.4	41.5	2.4
Uric acid lowering medication			
Allopurinol	17.4	3.9	0
Vitamin D	23.3	3.9	0
Antidiabetic medication			
Oral antidiabetics	8.1	11.5	0
Insuline	17.4	3.8	0

All values are expressed as the percentage of patients of each group treated with the drug in question; CKD: chronic kidney disease (CKD), AHT: arterial hypertension AHT.

medullary R2* levels between stage I–V of CKD (Figure 4 and Figure S2 for results by gender).

In addition, within the CKD group no significant difference was observed according to the renal diagnosis (Figure 5).

Changes in R2* after furosemide in hypertension or CKD patients as compared with controls

The situation was different in acute conditions, since the response to furosemide differed significantly between groups. Medullary R2* but not cortical values decreased significantly (suggesting an increase in medulla oxygenation) in the three groups, both in men and women (Table 3) but the reduction was significantly smaller in the CKD and AHT groups (Figure 6). Although there was a trend towards larger furosemide-induced decreases in medullary R2* in men, this difference was not statistically significant. In age-and gender adjusted multivariable linear regression analysis the furosemide-induced change in medullary R2* (f-R2*) correlated significantly with eGFR$_{mdrd}$ (adjusted β per ml/min/1.73 m^2: −0.03 (95% CI 0.01; 0.05), p = 0.003); the latter association persisted when intake of loop diuretics was introduced in the model (see extended Methods and Results S1).

The difference in furosemide-induced change between the AHT and control group was not explained by a difference in eGFR. In multivariate logistic regression adjusted for age, sex, and eGFR$_{mdrd}$, the furosemide-induced change in medullary change in R2* level remained significantly smaller in the presence of AHT (OR 0.81; 0.64–0.98, p = 0.047).

Associations between renal tissue R2* levels, CKD status, hypertension, and kidney function

In multivariate logistic regression, adjusted for age, sex, body mass index, hemoglobin, current smoking and urinary sodium excretion, with CKD status as dichotomized dependent variable (CKD compared with healthy controls and hypertensive subjects pooled together), medullary R2* levels were not associated with CKD status (OR(95% CI): 1.01 (0.86;1.18), p = 0.92). Medullary R2* levels were also not associated with CKD status when comparing the CKD group separately with healthy controls (CKD vs controls, OR: 0.95 (0.79; 1.15), p = 0.59), or with the hypertensive group (CKD vs. AHT, OR: 1.1 (0.91;1.35), p = 0.3).

Although cortical R2* levels were higher in CKD patients, this difference was not statistically significant in adjusted models (CKD versus non-CKD, OR: 1.20 (0.95; 1.51, p = 0.14)). The same trend was seen when comparing the CKD group separately with healthy controls (OR: 1.10 (0.85; 1.41), p = 0.49).

The determinants of renal cortical and medullary oxygenation were also analyzed in the entire population using linear models. There was no association between medullary R2* levels and eGFR or any of the other predefined variables in the adjusted multivariable linear regression analysis (Table 4A). No significant difference was observed when antihypertensive treatment (renin-angiotensin system (RAAS) blockers or antihypertensive treatment in general) was added to the model. Similar results were found for the association between medullary R2* values and creatinine clearance as measured by 24 h urinary collection (adjusted β per ml/min: −0.01, p = 0.96).

Results for cortical R2* levels and its associations with predefined variables were also largely negative (Table 4A). There was a positive association between gender and R2* levels (adjusted

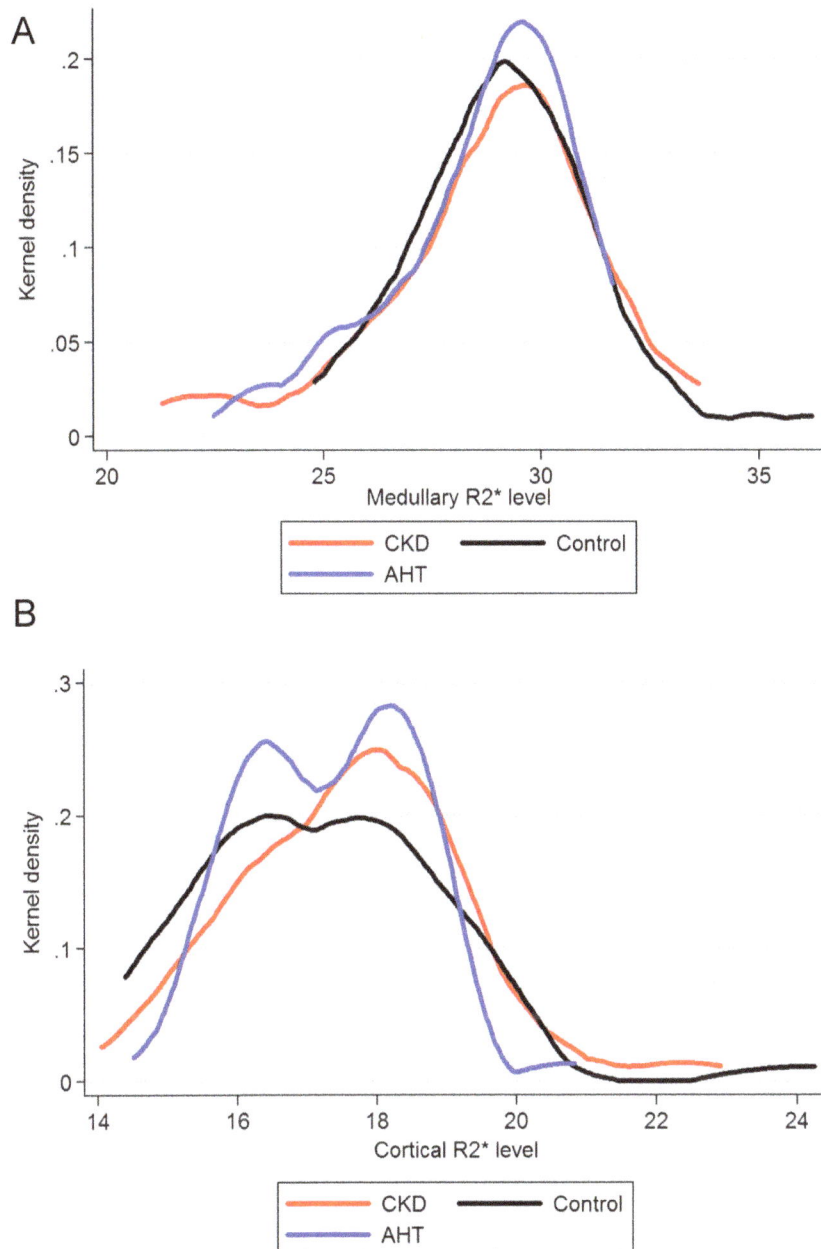

Figure 2. Probability density function (Kernel density) of renal R2* values. A/medullary R2* values and B/cortical R2* values.

β −1.8, p = 0.01). Hence, male participants had higher cortical R2* levels, corresponding to lower cortical oxygenation.

Since only a small proportion of the variability in R2* levels was explained by the predefined variables, some additional analyses were performed on the entire population. Thus, a negative correlation was found between medullary R2* levels and mean arterial blood pressure (Table 4B). However, the correlation between mean arterial pressure (MAP) and medullary R2* values was weak and disappeared when including antihypertensive treatment in the model (β −0.04 per mmHg, p = 0.043 before, and β −0.03, p = 0.13 after adjustment for antihypertensive treatment). Results of multivariable linear regression analysis are shown in more detail in Table S2, S3, S4. Diabetic subjects (n = 32) had higher cortical R2* values than non-diabetic subjects (mean R2* 18.7±5.9 vs 17.5±1.6 sec^{-1}, p = 0.05), yet diabetes

was not associated with cortical oxygenation in adjusted logistic regression models (Table S3). In contrast, cortical R2* levels correlated positively and significantly with circulating glucose levels as measured just before BOLD-MRI (Table 4B and Table S4). Including antidiabetic treatments in the multivariate regression model did not alter this result.

The positive correlation found between uric acid and cortical R2* levels did not change after the inclusion of allopurinol and diuretic treatments, or mean arterial blood pressure in the model. Results for cortical R2* levels stratified by sex are shown in Table 5. Similar positive associations were found between cortical R2* levels and uric acid; the association between cortical R2* levels and glycemia were only present in men, whereas there was a positive association between cortical R2* and age in women yet not in men.

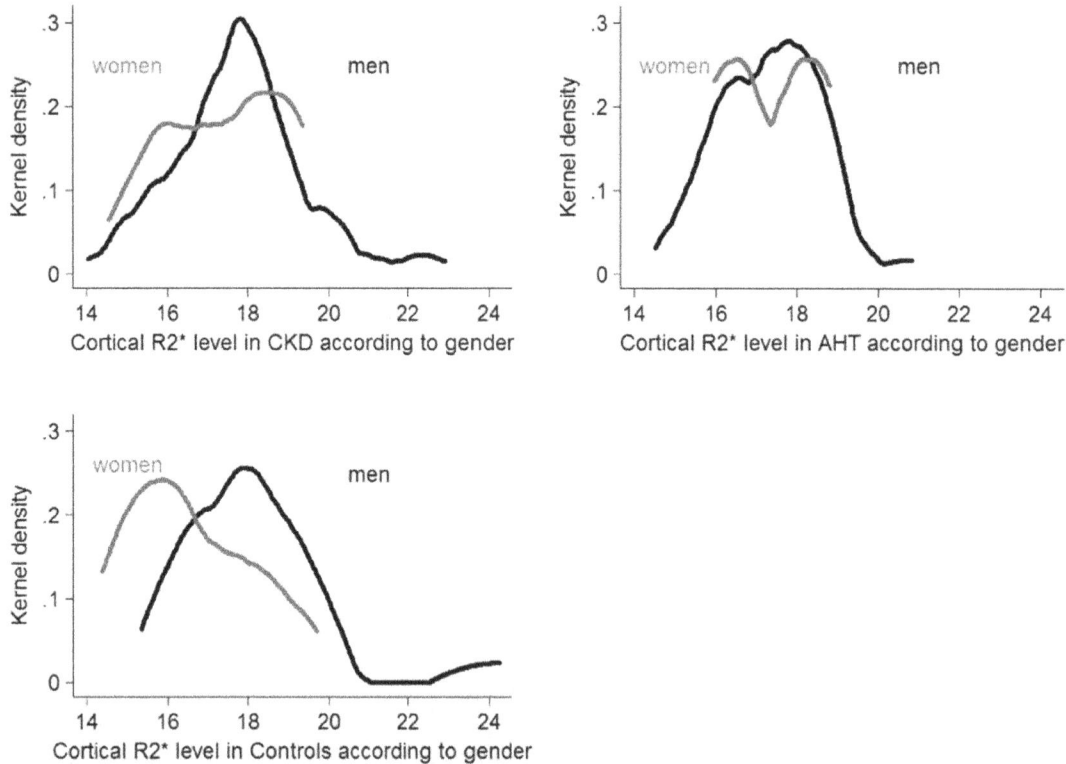

Figure 3. Probability density function (Kernel density) of cortical R2* values by gender, according to group.

Table 3. Baseline medullary and cortical R2*values and medullary cortical ratio's (MCR), overall and by gender.

	Control	CKD	AHT	p (ANOVA)
Baseline Medullary R2*	**29.3±2.4**	**28.8±2.6**	**28.6±2.1**	**0.44**
men	29.5±2.7	29.1±2.6	28.7±2.1	0.53
women	29.0±1.7	28.3±2.7	28.4±2.2	0.50
Furosemide-induced Change medullary R2*	**−6.1±2.9**	**−3.7±2.4**	**−4.7±2.1**	**<0.001**
men	−6.8±3.3	−3.7±2.5	−4.9±2.1	0.001
women	−5.4±2.2	−3.7±2.1	−4.2±2.1	0.02
Baseline Cortical R2*	**17.1 (15.9;18.7)**	**17.6 (16.5;18.6)**	**17.4 (16.3;18.3)**	**0.27**
men	17.8 (16.9;19.0)	17.8 (17.0;18.5)	17.4 (16.4;18.2)	0.36
women	16.2 (15.3;17.8)*	17.5 (16.1;18.7)	17.4 (16.0;18.6)	0.18
Furosemide-induced Change cortical R2*	**−1.2 (−0.83;−1.52)**	**−1.2 (−0.58;−1.8)**	**−1.3 (−0.86;−1.92)**	**0.36**
men	−1.0 (−0.88;−2.2)	−1.2 (−0.55;−1.8)	−1.3 (−1.0;−1.78)	0.81
women	−1.2 (−0.52;−1.5)	−1.5 (−0.59;−2.0)	−1.9 (−0.9;−2.4)	0.08
Baseline MCR ratio R2*	**1.70±0.2**	**1.62±0.2**	**1.65±0.1**	**0.11**
men	1.64±0.2	1.62±0.2	1.66±0.1	0.71
women	1.76±0.1	1.63±0.16	1.64±0.13	0.01
MCR ratio R2* after furosemide	**1.44±0.2**	**1.51±0.2**	**1.50±0.1**	**0.21**
men	1.35±0.2	1.51±0.2	1.48±0.11	0.06
women	1.54±0.2*	1.52±0.1	1.55±0.16	0.98

All values are shown before and after the administration of intravenous furosemide. Subjects on loop diuretics (n = 2 in the AHT group and n = 15 in the CKD group) are not included in the furosemide-induced changes.
Values expressed in sec^{-1}, as mean±SD or as median (25th–75th percentile), as appropriate. CKD = chronic kidney disease; AHT = arterial hypertension. * P<0.05 concerning within-group differences between men and women.

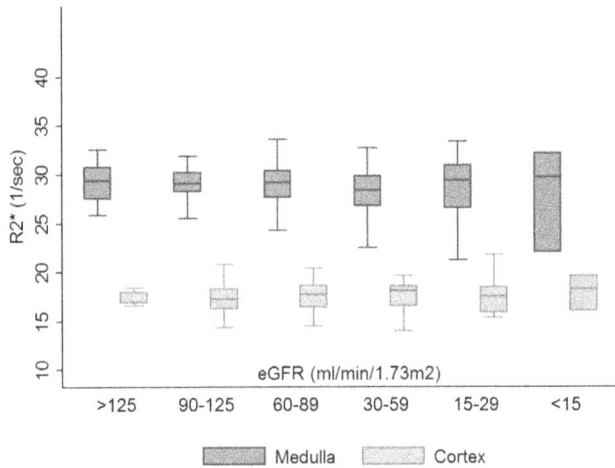

Figure 4. Medullary and cortical R2* values over decreasing eGFR$_{mdrd}$ values. The number of subjects was n = 10 (for the eGFR> 125 ml/min/1.73 m² category), 64 (eGFR 90–125), 65 (60–89), 36 (30–59), 15 (15–29) and 5 (<15), respectively.

In order to assess whether some of the results were linked to an over-representation of young women in the control group, sensitivity analyses were performed in a subgroup excluding healthy women <40 years (n = 13) and men aged >75 years suffering from CKD (n = 5). The main results of the study remained unchanged (see Methods and Results S1).

Discussion

The main findings of this study are that: 1) mean cortical and medullary R2* values as a proxy for renal tissue oxygenation are similar in hypertensive patients, CKD patients and healthy controls; however, the distribution of cortical R2* values differs markedly between groups, 2) the medullary R2* response to

furosemide is blunted in hypertensive patients and markedly reduced in CKD patients, 3) baseline renal tissue oxygenation appears to be remarkably stable over different degrees of kidney dysfunction, independently of the cause of kidney disease and 4) cortical R2* levels are positively associated with male gender, glycemia and uric acid levels.

The first interesting observation of this paper is that although mean cortical and medullary R2* look identical in hypertensive and CKD patients and controls, the distribution of cortical R2* differs between groups with a clear bimodal distribution in controls and AHT and a unimodal shape of the distribution in CKD. As found in our population, part of the bimodal distribution is linked to the male/female ratio. However, this ratio is similar in hypertensives and CKD patients suggesting other mechanisms explaining the differences in distribution, which should be the subject of further study.

The second finding of our study is that renal cortical and medullary oxygenation as measured by BOLD-MRI appears to be extremely well maintained in patients with CKD. Indeed, in contrast to what has been observed experimentally we did not find any decrease in cortical or medullary oxygenation even in advanced CKD; the nature of the underlying renal disease does not appear to play a major role. In this respect, our data are in accordance with the study by Michaely et al [10], although the latter study could be criticized for some methodological issues. Despite the fact that our study has been performed under very standardized hydration conditions, and detailed information was available on possible confounders such as medication, sodium intake and the type of underlying kidney disease we were not able to demonstrate a reduction of tissue oxygenation as renal disease progressed. In addition, this study also found no alterations in renal R2* values in persons with essential hypertension in comparison with healthy controls, despite the fact that numerous previous animal studies have reported renal tissue hypoxia in AHT [5].

The discrepancy between animal studies and BOLD-studies in humans regarding oxygenation can be interpreted in different ways. First of all, it might be that BOLD-MRI is not sensitive enough or simply not as good a tool to assess renal tissue oxygenation in CKD-patients as is direct invasive measurements using microelectrodes. Nonetheless, early animal studies performed to validate the BOLD-MRI technique have reported linear

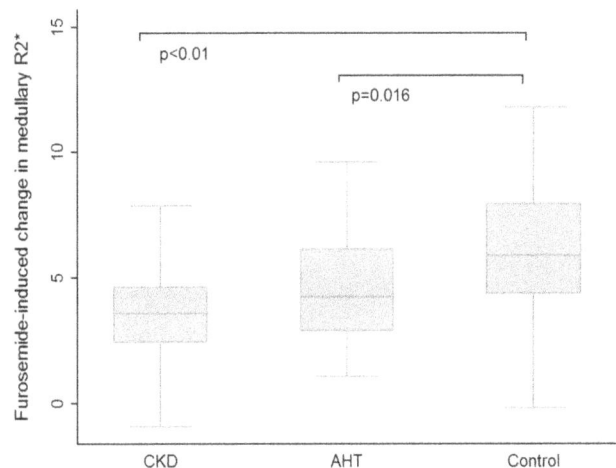

Figure 5. Cortical and medullary R2* values according to the cause of CKD. Values shown as boxplots; No (no CKD, n = 100), DM (diabetic nephropathy, n = 20), AHT (hypertensive nephropathy, n = 31), GN(glomerulonephritis, n = 17), reflux (reflux nephropathy, n = 6), one (solitary kidney, n = 7), IF (interstitial nephritis, n = 6), other (other cause of kidney disease, n = 8). There were no differences between cortical and medullary R2* levels between the groups (ANOVA p = 0.10 and p = 0.99, respectively)

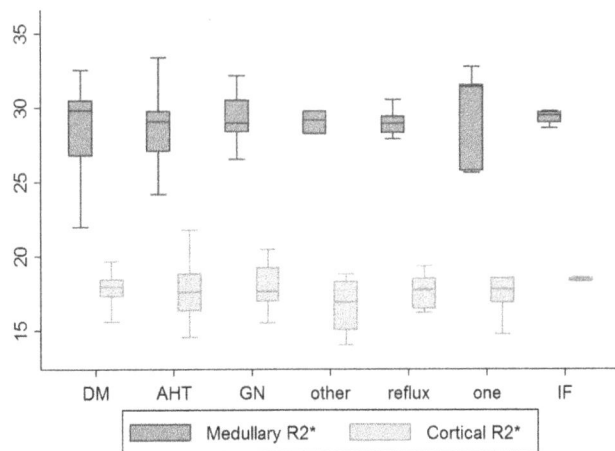

Figure 6. Furosemide-induced change in medullary R2* values according to group.

Table 4. Multivariate linear regression analysis examining correlations between baseline characteristics and medullary and cortical R2* levels.

	Medullary R2*		Cortical R2*	
A/	**β[1]**	**P**	**β[1]**	**p**
Sex (female vs. male)	−0.43	0.49	−1.8	0.01
Age (per year)	−0.01	0.72	−0.01	0.7
BMI (per kg/m2)	−0.03	0.61	−0.04	0.58
eGFR (MDRD)	−0.003	0.75	−0.01	0.29
Smoking (yes vs. no)	0.28	0.77	1.04	0.16
Urinary 24 h sodium excretion (mmol)	0.002	0.52	0.004	0.13
Diabetes (yes vs. no)	−1.01	0.41	1.67	0.07
B/	**β[1]**	**P**	**β[1]**	**p**
Mean Arterial BP (per mmHg)	−0.04	0.036	0.003	0.91
Urinary 24 h protein excretion (per g)	−0.18	0.58	−0.39	0.32
RAAS-blocker (yes vs.no)	−0.86	0.11	0.34	0.6
Serum glycemia (per mmol/l)	−0.11	0.54	0.91	<0.001
Serum uric acid (per μmol/l)	−0.0001	0.76	0.014	<0.001

Correlations are expressed as regression coefficient β. Correlations between R2* levels and predefined factors are shown under (A). The analysis including the additional variables glycemia, serum uric acid level and 24 h urinary proteinuria in the model is shown under (B).
[1] adjusted for gender, age, BMI, eGFR, smoking, urinary sodium excretion, Hemoglobin, and diabetes.

relationships between directly measured renal pO2 values and the BOLD signal [22]. Alternatively, the ROI-technique used to analyze BOLD-images might be less applicable in CKD patients, where loss of cortico-medullary differentiation hampers manual placement of ROIs. This might play a role in the interpretation of medullary R2* values, but cortical R2* values are expected to be reliable, thanks to its anatomic proximity with the kidney capsula. Besides, the majority of subjects in the present study had less advanced stage I–III kidney disease, and largely maintained cortico-medullary differentiation; in patients with preserved differentiation, BOLD-MRI is a reliable, reproducible method. Nevertheless, it remains an open question if studies using different methods of analysis such as the recently described compartmental model [23] would obtain similar results. Assuming that BOLD-MRI is able to correctly estimate tissue oxygenation in humans, our findings together with those of Michaely et al put into question whether 'chronic renal hypoxia' truly exists in humans. In conditions of acute hypoxia, hypoxia-inducible factors (HIF) are stabilized, which stimulates erythropoietin production, angiogenesis and metabolic reprogramming, offering protection and increasing survival of renal tubular cells under hypoxic conditions [2,24]. In contrast, chronic HIF stabilization stimulates interstitial fibrosis, a process that is generally believed to compress peritubular capillaries, which further decreases local tissue oxygenation and leads to a vicious circle of HIF-stabilization, increased formation of interstitial fibrosis, glomerulosclerosis and renal function decline [3,25]. However, hypoxia-induced fibrosis may not be a vicious circle that further worsens oxygenation, but merely a way to maintain renal oxygenation by adapting oxygen consumption to the demand. Identical mechanisms might operate in animals. Animal models reporting hypoxia in CKD such as the 5/6 nephrectomy model may not have been carried out long

Table 5. Multivariate linear regression analysis examining correlations between baseline characteristics and cortical R2* levels, stratified by gender.

Cortical R2*	Men		Women	
	β°	**p**	**β°**	**p**
Age (per year)	−0.05	0.17	0.049	0.02
BMI (per kg/m2)	−0.07	0.57	−0.03	0.54
eGFR (MDRD)	−0.03	0.11	−0.002	0.81
Smoking (yes vs. no)	1.69	0.1	−1.06	0.16
Urinary 24 h sodium excretion (mmol)	−0.007	0.11	0.001	0.65
Diabetes (yes vs. no)	2.47	0.06	−0.63	0.46
Glycemia (per mmol/l)	1.13	<0.001	0.31	0.15
Uric acid (per mmol/l)	0.015	0.004	0.01	0.001

°adjusted for age, BMI, eGFR, smoking, urinary sodium excretion, Hb, and diabetes.

enough to simulate the long-term adaptive changes in the kidney that might occur after several decades of chronic kidney disease or hypertension in humans. In line with this hypothesis, Priardarshy et al [26] evaluated renal oxygenation six to eight weeks after remnant kidney creation (instead of the 2 weeks applied by Manotham et al.)[1], and found that renal oxygenation was not decreased, but rather increased in the remnant kidney. A similar observation was made in renal artery stenosis with a reduction of renal tissue oxygenation acutely but a good maintenance of tissue oxygenation in the chronically stenotic kidney [14].

A role of renal handling of sodium in mediating oxygen consumption is supported by our observation that the medullary R2* response to furosemide differs between controls and hypertensives with a blunted response in hypertension and an even more marked reduction in CKD patients. In CKD, the markedly reduced response to furosemide can be explained by the reduced renal function leading to lower concentrations of furosemide within the kidney. However, this cannot be the explanation for hypertensive patients who had a comparable renal function as controls. Pratt et al have previously demonstrated ethnic differences in the response to furosemide [27]; to the best of our knowledge, differences in response to furosemide between normo-and hypertensive white subjects have not been reported previously. The blunted response to furosemide observed in hypertensive patients may be an indirect marker of the alterations in renal sodium handling in hypertension. Persons with essential hypertension have an increased proximal tubular reabsorption and a reduced distal delivery of sodium, which might blunt the effect of furosemide [28]. Alternatively, there might be differences in mitochondrial metabolism and oxygen consumption in the thick ascending limb of Henle between hypertensive and normotensive subjects, in analogy with recently described differences between Dahl salt-sensitive rats and salt-resistant control strains [29].

Our multivariate analysis enabled us to identify several new factors associated with renal tissue oxygenation. Thus, cortical R2* levels was positively and strongly associated with male gender. The relationship with male gender was robust and persisted in sensitivity analyses, and suggests that cortical oxygenation might be regulated differently in men and women. It may also provide some clues why renal function declines faster in men. However, our data do not offer any explanation for the higher R2* values in men, and studies measuring simultaneously renal perfusion and tubular sodium handling are necessary to clarify this issue.

Renal tissue hypoxia has been a consistent finding in mouse and rat models of diabetic nephropathy [4,30]. The reason why this occurs is less certain, but oxydative stress and glomerular hyperfiltration leading to increased tubular sodium load and oxygen consumption have been proposed as the main mechanisms [31,32]. BOLD-MRI studies in humans have shown mixed results, some studies reporting higher, others lower R2* values in patients with diabetes [8,9,33]. In this study, DM2 patients had slightly higher cortical R2* levels than controls, suggesting lower tissue oxygenation, yet this association was not maintained in adjusted models. Interestingly, cortical oxygenation correlated linearly and positively with glucose levels as measured just before the MRI exam, suggesting that glycemia directly or indirectly (via sodium transport) influences cortical oxygenation. In a study assessing the influence of renin-angiotensin blockers on renal oxygenation in patients with type 2 DM, we have recently reported similar results [19]. These data suggest that episodes of hyperglycemia might induce transient increases in oxygen consumption due to hyperfiltration which increases sodium transport in the proximal tubule [34]. The pre-MRI glycemia has not been systematically reported in previous studies, which might partly explain previous

mixed results. The herein described association offers an alternative explanation in humans for to the relationship between badly controlled diabetes mellitus and adverse renal outcome [35]. However, the described relationship is based on a cross-sectional analysis which limits causal inferences, and needs confirmation in interventional studies.

Our observation that circulating uric acid levels correlate positively with cortical R2* levels adds information to the ongoing debate about the role of uric acid in cardiovascular disease. Hyperuricemia-induced cortical vasoconstriction could be partly responsible for the herein described correlation between uric acid and cortical hypoxia [36], but more studies are necessary to clarify this.

This study has some limitations. Firstly, no information was acquired on renal perfusion. We therefore cannot determine whether changes in oxygenation were the result of alterations in oxygen delivery. Nevertheless, Textor and colleagues have shown previously that renal tissue oxygenation is largely independent of renal blood flow, and that cortical (but not medullary) oxygenation only falls in case of severe renal artery stenosis occluding more than 90% of the lumen [13]. Another limitation of our study is its cross-sectional design. Finally, all measurements were performed without stopping concomitant medication, which might have weakened eventual underlying differences in R2* levels between the groups

Conclusion

Our data suggest that renal tissue oxygenation at rest is comparable in controls, treated hypertensives and CKD patients. However, the response to furosemide differs between groups providing some insights on the mechanisms linking renal tubular function, oxygen consumption and renal function in hypertension and/or chronic kidney diseases. Our data do not support the concept that chronic kidney disease is associated with decreased renal tissue oxygenation in humans, as repeated observed in animal models. However, acute changes in oxygenation most likely occur in humans, as illustrated by the changes in R2* in response to furosemide. Future interventional studies should clarify the role of renal sodium handling, blood glucose and serum uric acid in the regulation of renal tissue oxygenation as newly described in this study. The differences in cortical R2* levels between men and women suggest that renal oxygenation is possibly regulated differently in men and women; this point also needs further study. Although no correlation was found between R2* values and (previous) kidney function, it is still possible that renal tissue R2* values predict kidney function decline but this is to be demonstrated in prospective studies.

Supporting Information

Figure S1   Probability density function (Kernel density) of medullary R2* values by gender, according to group.

Figure S2   Medullary and cortical R2* values over decreasing eGFR$_{mdrd}$ values, by gender. The number of subjects was n = 44 (for the eGFR>90 ml/min/1.73 m^2 category), 41 (eGFR 60–90), 25 (eGFR 30–60), 15 (eGFR <30) in men and respectively 30,24,11, and 5 in women.

Table S1   Drug treatment of patients across different stages of chronic kidney disease (CKD).

Table S2   Multivariate linear regression analysis examining associations between baseline characteristics and medullary R2* levels. Associations between medullary R2* levels and baseline characteristics are expressed as regression coefficient β (95% CI).

Table S3   Multivariate linear regression analysis examining associations between baseline characteristics and cortical R2* levels. Associations between cortical R2* levels and baseline characteristics are expressed as regression coefficient β (95% CI).

Table S4   Multivariate linear regression analysis examining correlations between baseline characteristics and medullary and cortical R2* levels. This analysis includes the

additional variables glycemia, serum uric acid level and 24 h urinary proteinuria.

Methods and Results S1   Extended methods and results. - Screening. -Methods: Justification hydration protocol. -Results: * Furosemide-induced change in R2* in patients already on diuretics. * Sensitivity analysis in subgroup excluding healthy women <40 years and male CKD patients >75 years.

Author Contributions

Conceived and designed the experiments: M. Pruijm BV LH MS MB. Performed the experiments: M. Pruijm M. Piskunowicz CZ MM IB. Analyzed the data: M. Pruijm M. Piskunowicz LH IB MM BV MB. Wrote the paper: M. Pruijm MB.

References

1. Manotham K, Tanaka T, Matsumoto M, Ohse T, Miyata T, et al. (2004) Evidence of tubular hypoxia in the early phase in the remnant kidney model. J Am Soc Nephrol 15: 1277–1288.

2. Haase VH (2013) Mechanisms of Hypoxia Responses in Renal Tissue. J Am Soc Nephrol.

3. Higgins DF, Kimura K, Bernhardt WM, Shrimanker N, Akai Y, et al. (2007) Hypoxia promotes fibrogenesis in vivo via HIF-1 stimulation of epithelial-to-mesenchymal transition. J Clin Invest 117: 3810–3820.

4. dos Santos EA, Li LP, Ji L, Prasad PV (2007) Early changes with diabetes in renal medullary hemodynamics as evaluated by fiberoptic probes and BOLD magnetic resonance imaging. Invest Radiol 42: 157–162.

5. Welch WJ, Baumgartl H, Lubbers D, Wilcox CS (2001) Nephron pO2 and renal oxygen usage in the hypertensive rat kidney. Kidney Int 59: 230–237.

6. Prasad PV (2006) Evaluation of intra-renal oxygenation by BOLD MRI. Nephron Clin Pract 103: c58–c65.

7. Simon-Zoula SC, Hofmann L, Giger A, Vogt B, Vock P, et al. (2006) Non-invasive monitoring of renal oxygenation using BOLD-MRI: a reproducibility study. NMR Biomed 19: 84–89.

8. Inoue T, Kozawa E, Okada H, Inukai K, Watanabe S, et al. (2011) Noninvasive evaluation of kidney hypoxia and fibrosis using magnetic resonance imaging. J Am Soc Nephrol 22: 1429–1434.

9. Yin WJ, Liu F, Li XM, Yang L, Zhao S, et al. (2011) Noninvasive evaluation of renal oxygenation in diabetic nephropathy by BOLD-MRI. Eur J Radiol.

10. Michaely HJ, Metzger L, Haneder S, Hansmann J, Schoenberg SO, et al. (2012) Renal BOLD-MRI does not reflect renal function in chronic kidney disease. Kidney Int 81: 684–689.

11. Prasad PV, Epstein FH (1999) Changes in renal medullary pO2 during water diuresis as evaluated by blood oxygenation level-dependent magnetic resonance imaging: effects of aging and cyclooxygenase inhibition. Kidney Int 55: 294–298.

12. Pruijm M, Hofmann L, Maillard M, Tremblay S, Glatz N, et al. (2010) Effect of sodium loading/depletion on renal oxygenation in young normotensive and hypertensive men. Hypertension 55: 1116–1122.

13. Gloviczki ML, Glockner JF, Crane JA, McKusick MA, Misra S, et al. (2011) Blood oxygen level-dependent magnetic resonance imaging identifies cortical hypoxia in severe renovascular disease. Hypertension 58: 1066–1072.

14. Rognant N, Guebre-Egziabher F, Bacchetta J, Janier M, Hiba B, et al. (2011) Evolution of renal oxygen content measured by BOLD MRI downstream a chronic renal artery stenosis. Nephrol Dial Transplant 26: 1205–1210.

15. Schachinger H, Klarhofer M, Linder L, Drewe J, Scheffler K (2006) Angiotensin II decreases the renal MRI blood oxygenation level-dependent signal. Hypertension 47: 1062–1066.

16. Textor SC, Gloviczki ML, Flessner MF, Calhoun DA, Glockner J, et al. (2012) Association of filtered sodium load with medullary volumes and medullary hypoxia in hypertensive African Americans as compared with whites. Am J Kidney Dis 59: 229–237.

17. Levey AS, Eckardt KU, Tsukamoto Y, Levin A, Coresh J, et al. (2005) Definition and classification of chronic kidney disease: a position statement from Kidney Disease: Improving Global Outcomes (KDIGO). Kidney Int 67: 2089–2100.

18. O'Brien E, Asmar R, Beilin L, Imai Y, Mallion JM, et al. (2003) European Society of Hypertension recommendations for conventional, ambulatory and home blood pressure measurement. J Hypertens 21: 821–848.

19. Pruijm M, Hofmann L, Zanchi A, Maillard M, Forni V, et al. (2012) Blockade of the renin-angiotensin system and renal tissue oxygenation as measured with BOLD-MRI in patients with type 2 diabetes. Diabetes Res Clin Pract.

20. Hofmann L, Simon-Zoula S, Nowak A, Giger A, Vock P, et al. (2006) BOLD-MRI for the assessment of renal oxygenation in humans: acute effect of nephrotoxic xenobiotics. Kidney Int 70: 144–150.

21. Djamali A, Sadowski EA, Muehrer RJ, Reese S, Smavatkul C, et al. (2007) BOLD-MRI assessment of intrarenal oxygenation and oxidative stress in patients with chronic kidney allograft dysfunction. Am J Physiol Renal Physiol 292: F513–F522.

22. Pedersen M, Dissing TH, Morkenborg J, Stodkilde-Jorgensen H, Hansen LH, et al. (2005) Validation of quantitative BOLD MRI measurements in kidney: application to unilateral ureteral obstruction. Kidney Int 67: 2305–2312.

23. Ebrahimi B, Gloviczki M, Woollard JR, Crane JA, Textor SC, et al. (2012) Compartmental analysis of renal BOLD MRI data: introduction and validation. Invest Radiol 47: 175–182.

24. Kojima I, Tanaka T, Inagi R, Kato H, Yamashita T, et al. (2007) Protective role of hypoxia-inducible factor-2alpha against ischemic damage and oxidative stress in the kidney. J Am Soc Nephrol 18: 1218–1226.

25. Fine LG, Norman JT (2008) Chronic hypoxia as a mechanism of progression of chronic kidney diseases: from hypothesis to novel therapeutics. Kidney Int 74: 867–872.

26. Priyadarshi A, Periyasamy S, Burke TJ, Britton SL, Malhotra D, et al. (2002) Effects of reduction of renal mass on renal oxygen tension and erythropoietin production in the rat. Kidney Int 61: 542–546.

27. Chun TY, Bankir L, Eckert GJ, Bichet DG, Saha C, et al. (2008) Ethnic differences in renal responses to furosemide. Hypertension 52: 241–248.

28. Burnier M, Bochud M, Maillard M (2006) Proximal tubular function and salt sensitivity. Curr Hypertens Rep 8: 8–15.

29. Zheleznova NN, Yang C, Ryan RP, Halligan BD, Liang M, et al. (2012) Mitochondrial proteomic analysis reveals deficiencies in oxygen utilization in medullary thick ascending limb of Henle in the Dahl salt-sensitive rat. Physiol Genomics 44: 829–842.

30. Prasad P, Li LP, Halter S, Cabray J, Ye M, et al. (2010) Evaluation of renal hypoxia in diabetic mice by BOLD MRI. Invest Radiol 45: 819–822.

31. Baines A, Ho P (2002) Glucose stimulates O2 consumption, NOS, and Na/H exchange in diabetic rat proximal tubules. Am J Physiol Renal Physiol 283: F286–293.

32. Hansell P, Welch WJ, Blantz RC, Palm F (2013) Determinants of kidney oxygen consumption and their relationship to tissue oxygen tension in diabetes and hypertension. Clin Exp Pharmacol Physiol 40: 123–137.

33. Wang ZJ, Kumar R, Banerjee S, Hsu CY (2011) Blood oxygen level-dependent (BOLD) MRI of diabetic nephropathy: preliminary experience. J Magn Reson Imaging 33: 655–660.

34. Vallon V, Schroth J, Satriano J, Blantz RC, Thomson SC, et al. (2009) Adenosine A(1) receptors determine glomerular hyperfiltration and the salt paradox in early streptozotocin diabetes mellitus. Nephron Physiol 111: 30–38.

35. Holman RR, Paul SK, Bethel MA, Matthews DR, Neil HA (2008) 10-year follow-up of intensive glucose control in type 2 diabetes. N Engl J Med 359: 1577–1589.

36. Messerli FH, Frohlich ED, Dreslinski GR, Suarez DH, Aristimuno GG (1980) Serum uric acid in essential hypertension: an indicator of renal vascular involvement. Ann Intern Med 93: 817–821.

21

Multicenter Epidemiological Study to Assess the Population of CKD Patients in Greece: Results from the PRESTAR Study

Konstantinos Sombolos[1], **Demitrios Tsakiris**[2], **John Boletis**[3], **Demetrios Vlahakos**[4], **Kostas C. Siamopoulos**[5], **Vassilios Vargemezis**[6], **Pavlos Nikolaidis**[7], **Christos Iatrou**[8], **Eugene Dafnis**[9], **Konstantinos Xynos**[10], **Christos Argyropoulos**[11]*

1 Nephrology Clinic, Papanikolaou Hospital, Thessaloniki, Greece, **2** Nephrology Clinic, Papageorgiou Hospital, Thessaloniki, Greece, **3** Nephrology Clinic, Laiko Hospital, Athens, Greece, **4** Nephrology Clinic, ATTIKON University Hospital, Athens, Greece, **5** Nephrology Clinic, Ioannina University Hospital, Ioannina, Greece, **6** Nephrology Clinic, Alexandroupoli University Hospital, Alexandroupoli, Greece, **7** Nephrology Clinic, AHEPA Hospital, Thessaloniki, Greece, **8** Center for Nephrology, G Papadakis, Nikea Hospital, Athens, Greece, **9** Nephrology Clinic, PE.PA.G.N.I, Crete University Hospital, Iraklio, Greece, **10** AbbVie Pharmaceuticals, Chicago, Illinois, United States of America, **11** AbbVie Pharmaceuticals SA, Athens, Greece

Abstract

Background: Chronic Kidney Disease (CKD) is a relatively common condition not only associated with increased morbidity and mortality but also fuelling End Stage Renal Disease (ESRD). Among developed nations, Greece has one of the highest ESRD incidence rates, yet there is limited understanding of the epidemiology of earlier stages of CKD.

Methods: Cross-sectional survey of pre-dialysis CKD outpatients in nephrology clinics in the National Health Care system between October 2009 and October 2010. Demographics, cause of CKD, blood pressure, level of renal function, duration of CKD and nephrology care, and specialty of referral physician were collected and analyzed. Different methods for estimating renal function (Cockroft-Gault [CG], CKD-Epi and MDRD) and staging CKD were assessed for agreement.

Results: A total of 1,501 patients in 9 centers were enrolled. Diabetic nephropathy was the most common nephrologist assigned cause of CKD (29.7%). In total, 36.5% of patients had self-referred to the nephrologist; patients with diabetes or serum creatinine above 220 μmol/l (eGFR<40 ml/min/1.73 m^2) were more likely to have been referred by a physician. Agreement between MDRD and CKD-Epi, but not between CG, the other estimating equations, was excellent. There was substantial heterogeneity with respect to renal diagnoses, referral patterns and blood pressure among participating centers.

Conclusions: In this first epidemiologic assessment of CKD in Greece, we documented delayed referral and high rates of self-referral among patients with CKD. eGFR reporting, currently offered by a limited number of laboratories, may facilitate detection of CKD at an earlier, more treatable stage.

Editor: Emmanuel A. Burdmann, University of Sao Paulo Medical School, Brazil

Funding: The PRESTAR (PRospective Epidemiology STudy Aiming to Register CKD Patients Stage 3, 4, and 5 not on Hemodialysis Followed by Nephrologists) study was designed and funded by the Greek Affiliate of Abbott Laboratories. AbbVie reviewed the manuscript for potential issues pertaining to Intellectual Property rights protection and for scientific content. Abbott and AbbVie Laboratories Sales and Marketing personnel did not influence the content development of this manuscript in any way, including through discussions with the external authors (SK, DT, JB, DV, KS, VV, PV, CI, ED). The funder provided support in the form of salaries for authors CA & KX, designed the study and provided funding for data collection and analysis and participated in the decision to publish and the preparation of the manuscript. The specific roles of these authors are articulated in the "author contributions" section.

Competing Interests: Drs. SK, DT, JB, DV, KS, VV, PV, CI, and ED are clinician investigators responsible for enrolling patients and collecting the data; they all received investigator fees for their participation in PRESTAR. Dr. KX is a former Abbott (now AbbVie) employee and may own Abbott/AbbVie stock, while Dr. CA was an Abbott Laboratories Hellas (now AbbVie Pharmaceuticals SA) Medical Affairs contractor. Abbott Laboratories funded this study.

* Email: argchris@hotmail.com

Introduction

Chronic Kidney Disease (CKD) is a relatively common condition associated with increased morbidity and mortality, mainly due to cardiovascular causes [1,2]. The increasing prevalence of risk factors for CKD such as obesity, diabetes and hypertension appears to fuel an emergent CKD epidemic on a global scale [3]. Contrary to patients with End Stage Renal Disease (ESRD), the care of patients with pre-dialysis CKD is primarily being overseen by general medicine, primary care physicians (PCPs), with specialist (nephrologist) input provided for patients with advanced stages of CKD [4–6]. These practice patterns translate to substantial missed opportunities to optimize care of patients with CKD in terms of disease education, selection of dialysis modality, pre-emptive transplantation, and implementing plans for the timely creation and maturation of dialysis access [7–9]. Furthermore, referral and [10–12] treatment in nephrology clinics has been shown to decrease the rate of progression of CKD and optimize the treatment of CKD complications [13].

In spite of these advantages, our understanding of how patients are referred for pre-dialysis nephrology consultation is limited, especially in settings in which formal partnerships between PCPs and nephrologists and referral recommendations for patients with CKD are not in place [14]. Furthermore, such information is rarely available on a country-wide basis, limiting the possibility of linking pre-dialysis practices to dialysis treatment pattern and outcomes in national registries. This is particularly important in settings characterized by high incidence of ESRD, given the toll the disease exacts on patients, caregivers and healthcare systems. Greece has one of the highest ESRD incidence rates [15] among industrialized nations, yet there is limited understanding of the epidemiology of earlier stages of CKD at the national level. In this cross-sectional, multicenter assessment, we describe the patient characteristics, causes of CKD and distribution of renal function in outpatients of nephrology clinics in the Greek National Healthcare System. Additionally, we characterize the referral patterns in relation to diagnosis of renal disease and the level of renal function, and describe center specific variations in these parameters. Finally, we examine the relative performance of different equations for estimated Glomerular Filtration Rate (eGFR) in the Greek CKD population.

Subjects and Methods

Design and Participants

This is a multicentre, observational, cross-sectional epidemiological study conducted in 9 outpatient Nephrology Clinics of the National Health System from across the different regions of Greece from October 2009 to October 2010. Centers were selected for participation based on previous workload and catchment area that included both urban and rural segments of the population. The sample size for the study was selected to ensure that the percentage of CKD 3–5 patients will be estimated with a degree of error of 2.3% when the expected percentage is 70%. Patients were eligible to participate in the study if they were older than 18 years, able to give informed consent, established patients of the clinic, not currently receiving renal replacement therapy. Patients with acute kidney injury/acute renal failure and patients with neoplasms or any other serious disease with projected life expectancy of less than 12 months were excluded from the study to ensure that only medically stable outpatients could be observed. During the course of the study the following data were collected from consecutive patients: demographics, cause of CKD assigned by the treating consultant nephrologist, day of first diagnosis of CKD and first nephrology visit, intervening period between first diagnosis and the study visit and between first nephrology visit and the study visit, specialty of referring physician, blood pressure, weight and height and laboratory values of blood urea nitrogen, creatinine and PTH available for physician review during the study visit. Field collected data were used to derive body mass index (BMI) and different estimates of renal function (estimated creatinine clearance by Cockroft-Gault (CG), CG normalized to Body Surface Area (CG-BSA) and estimated glomerular filtration rate (eGFR) according to the CKD-Epi and the MDRD equations (the latter modified to use standardized creatinine values which was almost invariably used by Greek clinical laboratories during the study). For this study, renal function was classified by CKD stage according to the numerical cutoffs in the NKF classification system for estimates normalized to BSA (MDRD, CKD-Epi, CG-BSA) as well as the CG equation. This study was conducted in accordance with a pre-

specified protocol and applicable local regulations and guidelines. The protocol was prospectively registered with the National Medicines Organization (registration code EE 25/01-09/09) and approved by the Institutional Review Board of each participating center (Hospital Scientific Committee of Papanikolaou General Hospital Decision of the 3rd Meeting/31-3-2009, Hospital Scientific Committee of Papageorgiou General Hospital Decision of the 131th Meeting/25-05-2009, Hospital Scientific Committee of Laiko Hospital Decision: 114/3-6-09, Hospital Scientific Committee of Attikon University Hospital Decision of the 2nd Meeting/16-03-2009, Hospital Scientific Committee of University Hospital of Ioannina Decision: 196/30-6-2009, Hospital Scientific Committee of University Hospital of Alexandroupoli Decision: 378/9-06-2009, Hospital Scientific Committee of AHEPA Hospital Decision: 257/6-5-2009, Hospital Scientific Committee of Crete University Hospital Decision: 3564/5-5-2009), and each participant provided written informed consent before patient enrollment.

Statistical Methods

Descriptive statistical methods were used to summarize the distribution of all variables: for continuous variables the mean and the standard deviation, and for categorical variables the frequencies of responses at each level were reported. Unadjusted assessments were carried out with the Kruskal Wallis test (continuous responses) and the chi-square test (discrete responses). The pair-wise agreement between estimating equations for renal function was examined by means of Bland Altman plots [16]. We assessed agreement between CKD stages based on all other estimating equations compared to the CKD-Epi with the Spearman correlation coefficient. Regression methods were used to examine the relationship between renal function at the time of the study visit and other covariates, using when appropriate, penalized splines for semi-parametric modeling [17]. Center wise comparisons were carried out by random effect models and portrayed as forest plots, while model heterogeneity was assessed by means of the I^2 statistic. All analyses were performed with SAS v9.1 (table generation) and R v2.12.1 (meta-analyses and figures).

Results

Patient Characteristics and Comparison of Renal Function Estimating Equations

The study included 1501 patients from 9 outpatient nephrology clinics, with a range of 80–300 patients per clinic. Patients on average were older (mean age 66.2 ± 14.6 years, median: 69.6 years), predominantly male (54. 9%), slightly overweight (median BMI: 27.8 kg/m^2). The three most commonly assigned causes of CKD were: diabetic nephropathy (29.7%), hypertensive vascular disease (25.3%) and glomerular diseases (16.3%). The average time interval since the initial diagnosis of CKD was 4.4 ± 5.5 years, while the average time interval since the initial nephrology consultation was 3.0 ± 3.7 years. Other patient characteristics are shown in Table 1.

Average eGFR (by CKD-Epi) was 40.9 ± 23.9 ml/min/ 1.73 m^2, similar to the MDRD estimate (39.9 ± 22.1 ml/min/ 1.73 m^2). Estimating renal function by CG, or GC normalized to BSA (CGBSA) resulted in higher numerical values (Figure 1A) than either MDRD or CKD-Epi. Agreement was best between CKD-Epi and MDRD (Figure 1B, average bias 1 ml/min/ 1.73 m^2, although MDRD yielded lower estimates for values> 60 ml/min/1.73 m^2) and worse between CG and CKD-Epi (Figure 1C); normalization of CG to BSA (CGBSA) improved agreement (Figure 1D, average bias -3.7 ml/min/1.73 m^2).

Table 1. Patient characteristics.

Age (yrs)	66.2 (14.6)
Gender (Male)	824 (55%)
Time since initial diagnosis of renal disease (yrs)	4.4±5.5
Time since initial nephrology consultation (yrs)	3.0±3.7
Systolic Blood Pressure (mmHg)	137.1±17.8
Diastolic Blood Pressure (mmHg)	80.5±10.4
Cause of CKD	
Diabetic Nephropathy	445 (29.7)
Hypertensive Vascular Disease	380 (25.3)
Glomerular Disease	244 (16.3)
Interstitial Nephropathy	75 (5.0)
Solitary kidney post nephrectomy	61 (4.1)
Arterial Hypertension – Congestive Heart Failure	56 (3.7)
Obstructive Nephropathy	38 (2.5)
Polycystic Kidney Disease	35 (2.3)
Autoimmune Disease	29 (1.9)
Nephrolithiasis	28 (1.9)
Dysplastic/Hypoplastic Disease	21 (1.4)
Malignancy	12 (0.8)
Post infectious	7 (0.5)
Drug Related	4 (0.3)
Others	115 (7.7)
Weight (kg)	77.9±15.5
Height (cm)	164.7±9.4
Body Mass Index (BMI, kg/m^2)	28.8±5.5
Body Surface Area (BSA, m^2)	1.84±0.20
Blood Urea Nitrogen (mmol/l)	80.9±45.8
Serum creatinine (μmol/l)	176.8±97.2
eGFR (by CKD-Epi, ml/min/1.73 m^2)	40.9±23.9

Data are given as Mean ±SD or n (%) unless stated otherwise.

Approximately 44% of all patients would be classified as having CKD Stage 3 irrespective of the estimating equation used, while CG and CGBSA classification led to higher prevalence estimates of stages 1–2 in the study population (Figure 2). The correlation between CKD stages based on different estimating equations was highest between MDRD and CKD-Epi (Spearman's ρ 0.96) and lowest between MDRD and CG (Spearman's ρ 0.82).

Renal Function, Cause of CKD and Referral Patterns

The level of renal function (eGFR) in nephrology outpatients appeared to differ according to the renal diagnosis, with diabetic patients having lower eGFR, while patients with glomerular disease having higher eGFR (Table 2). Overall, 63.2% (948/1501) of all CKD patients had been referred to a nephrologist by a physician, most commonly an internist (48.0% of referred patients), a diabetologist or a cardiologist in the overall population and across the different CKD stages (Table 3).

The likelihood of a patient being referred to a nephrologist were assessed as a function of serum creatinine concentration (Figure 3A) and eGFR (Figure 3B) adjusted for the time the patient had spent under nephrology care. The odds ratio of a referral increased as serum creatinine increased above 88.4 μmol/l (1 mg/dl) and peaked around 150 μmol/l and remained

relatively stable until 220 μmol/l, to increase thereafter. Stated in other terms, the patients were much more likely to be referred for a creatinine concentration exceeding 220 μmol/l (~2.5 mg/dl) than at lower creatinine values. Viewed as a function of eGFR, the odds of a nephrology referral were a monotonic (decreasing) function of the estimated GFR, so that patients with eGFR< 40 ml/min/1.73 m^2 were more likely to have been referred to a specialist than to have self-referred.

In unadjusted analyses examining renal diagnosis and likelihood of referral, patients with diabetes were more likely to had been referred to a nephrologist by another physician (Odds Ratio 1.82, 95% CI 1.61–2.06, p<0.001), while patients with glomerular and interstitial disease were less likely to have been referred (Table 4). In analyses adjusting for age, gender, SBP, DBP, eGFR (CKD-Epi), center, and time spent under nephrology care, patients with diabetes were more likely to have been referred to a nephrologist (OR: 1.73, 95% CI: 1.25–2.38, p = 0.036), while patients with polycystic kidney disease were less likely to have been referred (OR: 0.69, 95% CI: 0.48–0.97, p = 0.032). Age was not independently associated with lower odds of nephrology referral (p>0.10).

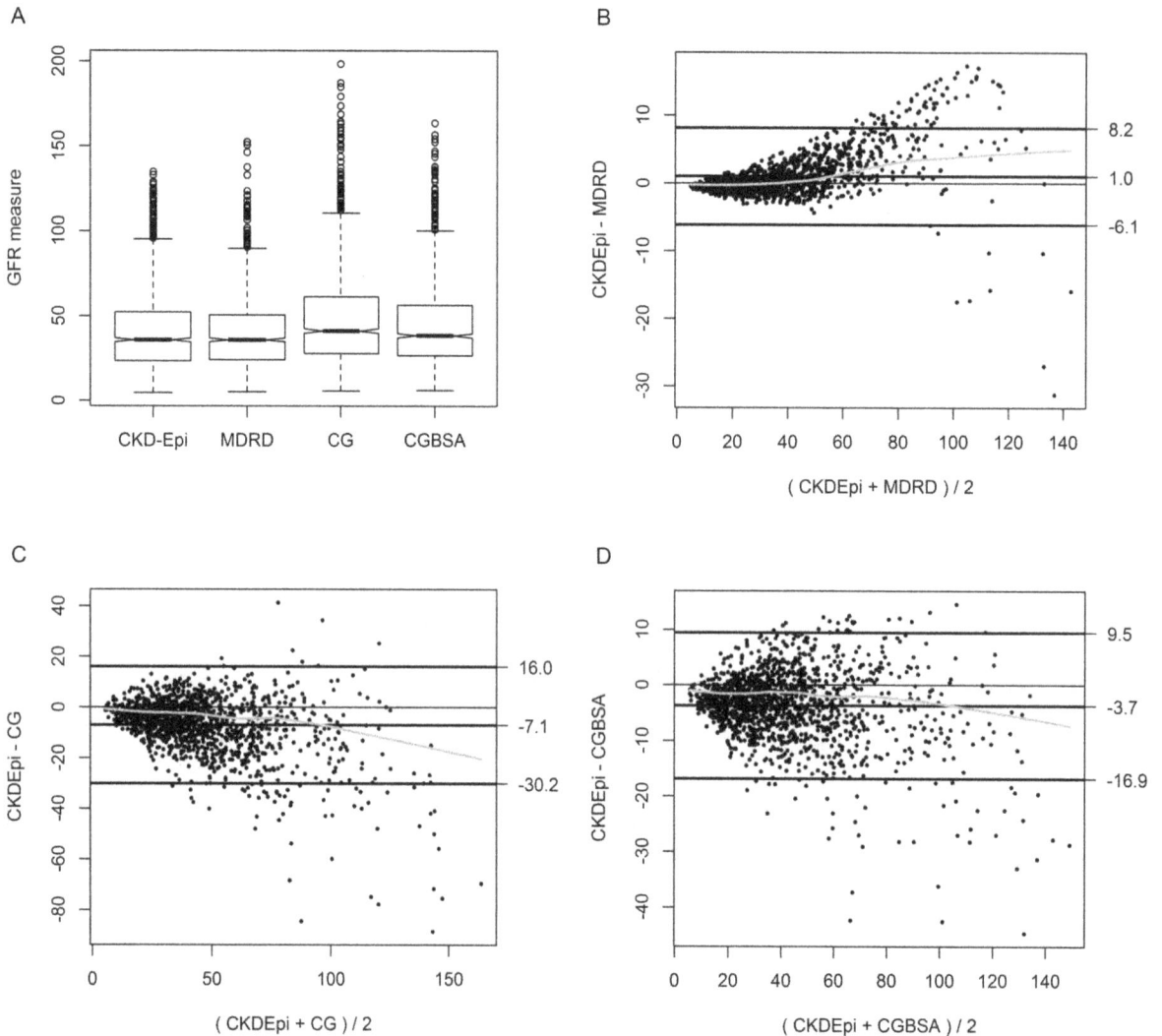

Figure 1. Estimating equations for renal function in the PreSTAR study (A) Box whisker plots of individual estimates based on the CKD Epi (CKD-Epi), MDRD, Cockroft Gault (CG) and Cockroft Gault normalized to Body Surface Area (CGBSA). The thick horizontal line is the median estimate, the bottom and top of each box are the 25th and 75th percentiles, the thin horizontal lines are the most extreme data points within 1.5 times the interquartile range, while the outliers are shown as circles. (B–D) Bland Altman (BA) plot of the MDRD (B), CG(C) and CGBSA against CKD-Epi (D). Each BA plot shows the difference between the two levels of renal function (y-axis) against their average (x-axis) for each patient. The three thick black lines demarcate the bias and the upper and lower limits of agreement, while the thin horizontal line is the zero bias line. In each plot, the gray line is a non-parametric estimate of the constancy of the bias across the range of possible values.

Center level variations

Large center-wise variations and heterogeneity were observed in a number of characteristics of the outpatients attending nephrology clinics (Figure 4): percentage of patients with diabetes (I^2: 89.19%, p<0.001), CKD-Epi eGFR (I^2: 95.74%, p<0.001) SBP (I^2: 88.58%, p<0.001), DBP (I^2: 93.56%, p<0.001), BMI (I^2: 90.4%, p<0.001), percentage of patients referred by a physician (I^2: 97.62%, p<0.001), and time under care in the nephrology clinic(I^2: 96.16%, p<0.001).

Discussion

The purpose of this research was to report for the first time the characteristics of the outpatients attending the nephrology clinics of the Greek National Health System (GHNS). We found that a large proportion of patients had referred themselves to nephrologists, with the likelihood of self-referral increasing with higher eGFR levels. Diabetic patients were more likely to have been referred by a physician, even after adjusting for eGFR and other factors. There appears to be some heterogeneity at the center level with respect to the proportion of diabetic patients and self-referrals and the level of blood pressure.

The findings of this report need to be interpreted in light of several factors operating in the Greek healthcare system: a) patients have direct access to laboratory results, irrespective of the public or private ownership of the laboratory, b) lack of automatic eGFR reporting by the laboratories, c) lack of consensus guidelines for referrals to specialists, and finally d) extremely low barriers limiting patient access to specialty care in the outpatient clinics of the GNHS.

Direct patient access to laboratory results, along with their reference range, probably explains the large percentage of self-referrals in this study. Under this scenario, it is very likely that small changes in serum creatinine levels or dipstick positive

Distribution of Patients per Stage

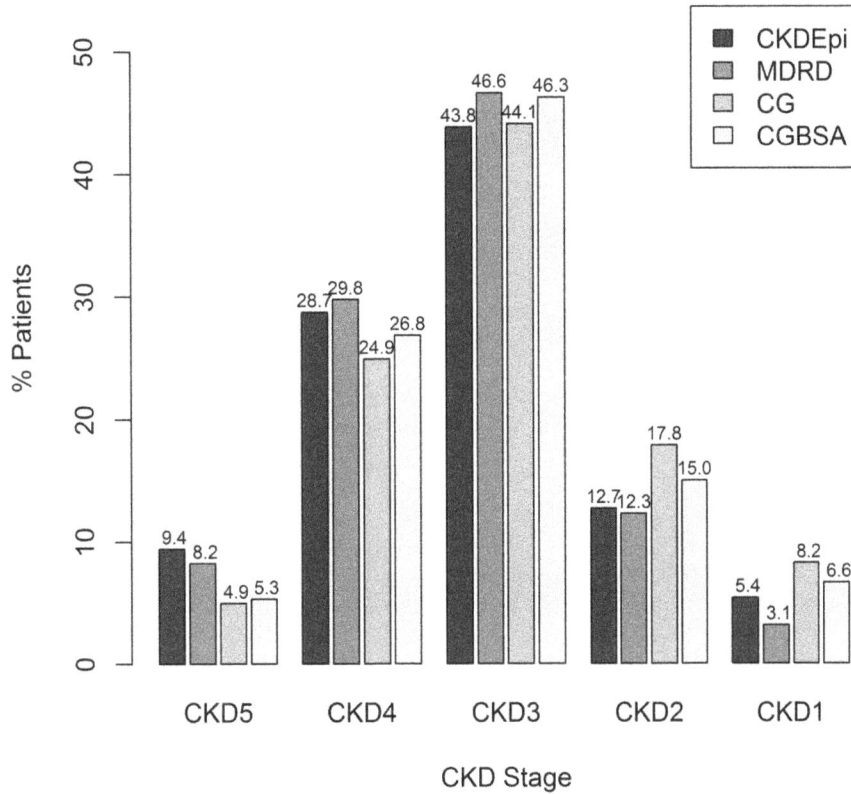

Figure 2. Distribution of stages of CKD in PRESTAR according to different estimating equations, CKD-Epi, MDRD, Cockroft Gault (CG), CG normalized to Body Surface Area (CGBSA).

albuminuria are interpreted by patients as indicating a potential problem with their kidneys. This in turn will prompt them to seek specialty evaluation in the GHNS, which by design does not have a gatekeeper mechanism to restrict access and only commissions a small fee for specialty evaluation. Hence many patients with relatively preserved renal function, but some form of renal pathology, will end up being evaluated by a nephrologist. From this perspective, direct patient access to creatinine test results may provide a less costly alternative to screening programs [9,18] for the identification of patients who may benefit from specialty care [19].

On the other hand, patients referred to a nephrologist by another physician had lower levels of eGFR, implying that either renal disease is under-recognized or some form of filtering of

patients by referring physicians is taking place. Such a filtering has been observed in other settings, in which only a small minority (27%) of patients with CKD would be identified as such by their primary providers [20], while large increases in serum creatinine (36%) are used as triggers for patient referral. As very few laboratories currently report eGFR in Greece, we postulate that recognition of renal impairment by non-nephrologists is largely based on serum creatinine concentration, which is an insensitive marker of renal dysfunction [21]. This hypothesis is supported by our finding that the odds of referral as a function of serum creatinine level exceeds parity only when serum creatinine increases above the upper limit of normal ($\sim$110 μmol/l) but substantially increases only when creatinine is higher than 220 μmol/l ($\sim$2.5 mg/dl), or approximately two times the upper

Table 2. Renal function (eGFR by CKD-Epi in ml/min/1.73 m^2) according to presence or absence of renal diagnosis.

Renal Diagnosis	Present	Absent	P-value
Diabetic Nephropathy	34±18	45±28	<0.001
Hypertensive Vascular Disease	38±19	43±27	0.089
Glomerular Disease	52±29	40±24	<0.001
Interstitial Nephropathy	42±26	42±26	0.830
Polycystic Kidney Disease	48±24	42±26	0.047

Table 3. Specialty of physicians referring patients to Greek National Health System Outpatient Nephrology Clinics.

Referring Specialty	Stage 1 51 (100%)	Stage 2 106 (100%)	Stage 3 425 (100%)	Stage 4 265 (100%)	Stage 5 101 (100%)	All 948 (100%)
Internal Medicine	26 (51.0)	47 (44.3)	194 (45.6)	138 (52.1)	50 (49.5)	455 (48.0)
Diabetology	1 (2.0)	12 (11.3)	43 (10.1)	30 (11.3)	10 (9.9)	96 (10.1)
Cardiology	0 (0.0)	2 (1.9%)	50 (11.8)	23 (8.7)	9 (8.9)	84 (8.9)
Urology	4 (7.8)	9 (8.5)	31 (7.3)	17 (6.4)	4 (4.0)	65 (6.9)
Endocrinology	1 (2.0)	9 (8.5)	26 (6.1)	15 (5.7)	7 (6.9)	58 (6.1)
General Surgery	2 (3.9)	4 (3.8)	18 (4.2)	8 (3.0)	1 (1.0)	33 (3.5)
Rheumatology	2 (3.9)	5 (4.7)	10 (2.4)	6 (2.3)	3 (3.0)	26 (2.7)
Hematology	3 (5.9)	3 (2.8)	12 (2.8)	2 (0.8)	2 (2.0)	22 (2.3)
GP/Family Medicine	0 (0.0)	2 (1.9)	5 (1.2)	7 (2.6)	2 (2.0)	16 (1.7)
Nephrology	1 (2.0)	3 (2.8)	9 (2.1)	2 (0.8)	1 (1.0)	16 (1.7)
Pulmonary Medicine	0 (0.0)	3 (2.8)	5 (1.2)	4 (1.5)	1 (1.0)	13 (1.4)
Neurology	0 (0.0)	1 (0.9)	3 (0.7)	2 (0.8)	2 (2.0)	8 (0.8)
Vascular Surgery	0 (0.0)	1 (0.9)	3 (0.7)	3 (1.1)	1 (1.0)	8 (0.8)
All others	11 (21.5)	5 (4.7)	16 (3.8)	8 (3.0)	8 (7.9)	48 (4.8)

The number of patients (N = 948) in this table differs from the total number of patients in the study (N = 1501), because N = 1501–948 = 553 patients were self-referrals. Data are given as n(%).

limit of normal. This level, clearly understood to warrant specialty evaluation in the pre-eGFR days [22], coincides with the putative "point of no return" of many renal diseases [23,24] suggesting that some patients may in fact receive sub-optimal care due to such filtering. In contrast, self-referring patients do not seem to apply such filtering, seeking specialty evaluation even when creatinine has increased just above the range of normal values reported by the laboratory. This finding is no different from previous reports showing that non nephrologists will refer late, i.e. after creatinine is higher than 177 μmol/l($\sim$2.0 mg/dl) [25], a pattern which may be due to limited awareness of the need for early specialty evaluation and care [25–31]. Alternatively such late referrals can be due to perceptions of the nephrologist role as one of

transitioning the patient with advanced CKD towards a plan for ESRD management when eGFR declines below 30 ml/min/1.73 m^2 [32]. In that regards, automatic eGFR reporting, which has been shown to aid the identification of subtle renal impairment [33–35], increase the prescription rate of nephro-protective ACEis/ARBs [33,36,37] and the probability of specialty referral [38], may be viewed as an important tool for the management of CKD patients by primary care practitioners. On the other hand, eGFR reporting may increase the number of inappropriate evaluations and the nephrologist workload [39], as patients are seen at higher levels of eGFR. Nevertheless, recent evaluations have shown that although consults increase [36,40], the proportion of inappropriate consults does not invariably go up [40,41],

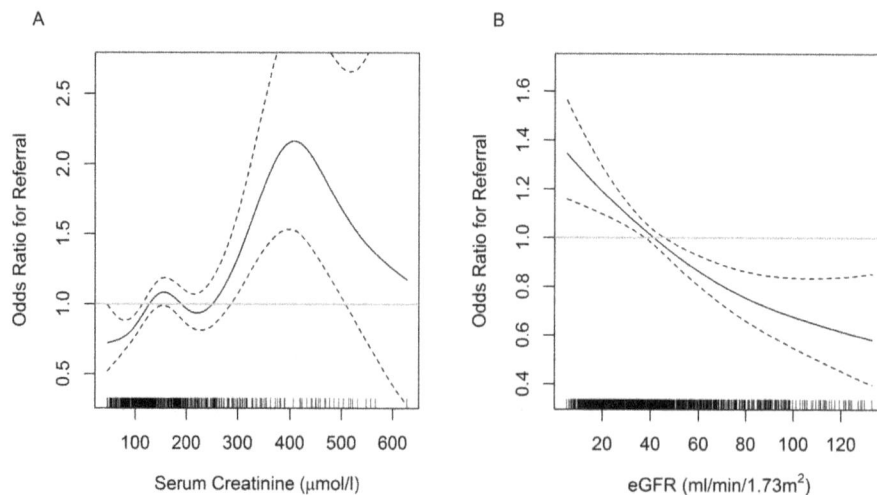

Figure 3. Adjusted odds of a patient having been referred to a nephrologist by a specialist in relation to serum creatinine (A) and eGFR (CKD-Epi), (B) during the study visit. Models were adjusted for age, gender, race, presence of diabetic renal disease, center, systolic and diastolic blood pressure and time the patient had been under nephrology care. Solid black line: estimated adjusted odds ratio, dashed black lines: associated pointwise 95% confidence internal, gray horizontal line: corresponds to an odds ratio of one.

Table 4. Likelihood of a physician referral to a nephrologist by renal diagnosis.

Renal Diagnosis	Unadjusted Analyses			Adjusted Analyses		
	OR	95% CI	P	OR	95% CI	P
Diabetic Nephropathy	1.82	1.43–2.32	<0.001	1.73	1.25–2.39	<0.001
Hypertensive Vascular Disease	0.82	0.65–1.05	0.12	0.40	0.16–1.00	0.051
Glomerular Disease	0.46	0.35–0.61	<0.001	0.73	0.50–1.07	0.10
Interstitial Nephropathy	0.57	0.36–0.91	0.02	0.97	0.52–1.81	0.92
Polycystic Kidney Disease	0.60	0.31–1.18	0.14	0.69	0.49–0.97	0.032

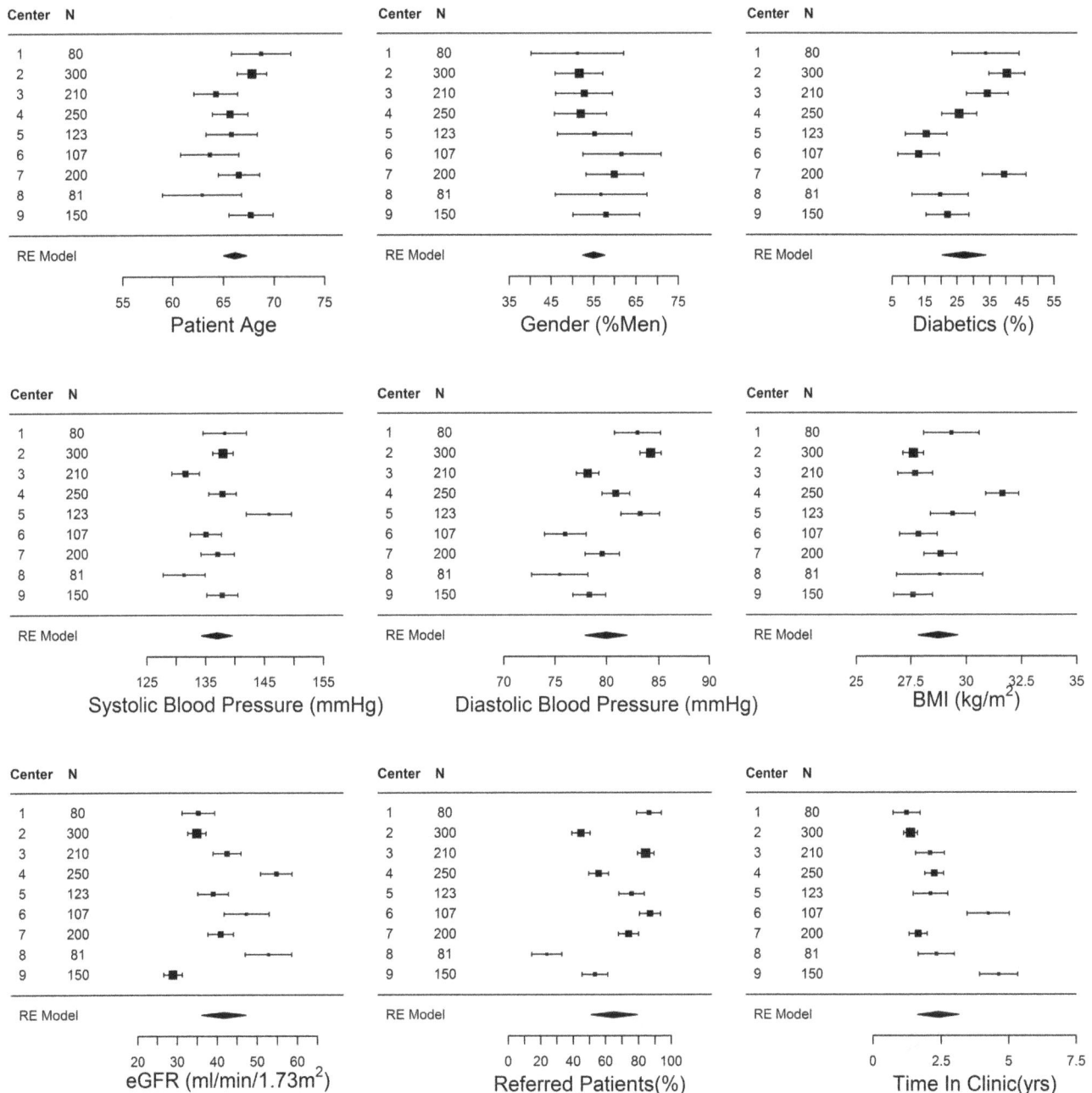

Figure 4. Center wise variations in patient demographics, blood pressure, renal function, diabetes and percentage of referred patients (Could number of patients in each center be added as a footnote?).

the reported eGFR does not influence the rate of consults among patients without CKD, and the additional workload is modest (23 additional consults per nephrologist per year) [42].

Early nephrology referral has been associated with slower disease progression and a 45% reduction in the risk of death [43], and is thus an important aspect of a comprehensive CKD population health care program. Furthermore, patients referred late have inferior control of risk factors for CKD progression, CKD complications, uremic cardiomyopathy and worse patient survival [44,45] when they reach dialysis [7,46]. On the other hand, specialty referral has been shown to lead to higher rates of prescriptions for ACEis/ARBs [47], NSAID avoidance [48], stabilization or improvement in renal function decline CKD [12,43,49] and improved survival among patients with consistent nephrology follow-up [50,51].

Since eGFR reporting may be a valuable component for the optimization of pre-dialysis CKD care and it is currently not implemented on a large scale in the Greek health care system, we explored the utility of different estimating equations for either GFR or creatinine clearance. Assuming the CKD-Epi equation as the emerging gold standard [52,53], our analyses highlight potential pitfalls of the other methods including the imprecision of the MDRD at higher levels of eGFR, the large bias of the CG (moderated somewhat by scaling the result to BSA) and the potential for misclassification at earlier CKD stages. This is particularly important from the perspective of public health expenditure in Greece, as therapies targeting complications of CKD stages 3–5 are currently fully reimbursed without any patient copayment (currently standing at 25% of the price of non CKD related therapies) Hence accurate staging of CKD is important for both early identification and public health budget optimization, goals that can be attained by widespread adoption of the CKD-Epi equation in the GNHS.

In this report, we also observed center variations in a number of characteristics relating to diagnosis, pathway to specialty evaluation, and blood pressure levels of CKD patients under nephrology care. Since the participating centers in this study cover both rural and urban segments of the Greek population, it is possible that some of these differences directly reflect some heterogeneity in the distribution of risk factors for CKD, local practice patterns of referring physicians and nephrologists and models of cooperation between them. Nevertheless, the fact that such differences do exist, suggest a missed opportunity for standardizing care at a national level by e.g. CKD diagnosis and treatment educational programs aiming at non-specialists and promotion and adoption of guidelines specifying thresholds for appropriate referral and blood pressure targets.

The findings and interpretations in this report should be interpreted in light of certain limitations. First, the cross-sectional design of the study precludes drawing conclusions about the rate of renal function decline over time among study participants. Second, we did not have access to referring physicians' records so we cannot explain the apparent channeling bias in referring patients with diabetes to a nephrologist. This pattern may reflect the limited understanding of the subtle manifestations of a wide spectrum of renal pathology by non-specialists, the sensitization of non-nephrologists to the renal complications of diabetes [54], or possibly a skewed view by non-specialists about the benefits of nephrologist co-management [13,49,55–57]. A study of referring physicians could help us understand these referral patterns, suggesting one possible way for filling this knowledge gap. Third, even though the MDRD and CKD-Epi equations have been evaluated in a number of different populations and cohorts, no direct validation exists for the Greek population, so that the comparison between these equations should not be viewed as one of a method against a gold standard. Finally our study was conducted before the 2012 KDIGO classification of CKD stages along the two dimensions of eGFR and albuminuria categories, and thus we did not collect data about abnormal urinary biomarkers (proteinuria, albuminuria or even hematuria) in our patients. Hence, we cannot exclude the likelihood that such abnormalities drive nephrology referrals at higher levels of eGFR especially for patients with glomerular disease who are more likely to manifest proteinuria and/or hematuria.

In summary, we have undertaken the first national cross-sectional evaluation of non-dialysis dependent CKD patients in outpatient nephrology clinics of the Greek National Health System. We found that many patients appear to be referred late by physicians, while self-referred patients consult a nephrologist at a higher level of renal function possibly due to direct access to test results. To reduce the burden of ESRD in Greece, with the 8th highest incidence rate in the world [15], which during the current financial crisis bears the cost of providing unfunded dialysis services to a large number of uninsured individuals including illegal immigrants future initiatives should focus on the adoption of eGFR reporting in order to facilitate early detection, appropriate confirmatory testing, and prescription of reno-protective medications in order to reduce the progression to dialysis dependency.

Acknowledgments

We would like to thank the patients and the staff in the hospital centers for their participation as well as Abbott Laboratories Hellas clinical research staff for their valuable contribution during the execution of this study.

Author Contributions

Conceived and designed the experiments: KX. Performed the experiments: KS DT JB DV KCS VV PN CI ED. Analyzed the data: CA. Wrote the paper: KS DT JB DV KCS VV PN CI ED KX CA.

References

1. Yang M, Fox CH, Vassalotti J, Choi M (2011) Complications of progression of CKD. Adv Chronic Kidney Dis 18: 400–405. doi: 10.1053/j.ackd.2011.10.001.

2. Locatelli F, Vecchio LD, Pozzoni P (2002) The importance of early detection of chronic kidney disease. Nephrol Dial Transplant 17 Suppl 11: 2–7.

3. Stenvinkel P (2010) Chronic kidney disease: a public health priority and harbinger of premature cardiovascular disease. J Intern Med 268: 456–467. doi: 10.1111/j.1365-2796.2010.02269.x.

4. Campbell KH, Smith SG, Hemmerich J, Stankus N, Fox C, et al. (2011) Patient and provider determinants of nephrology referral in older adults with severe chronic kidney disease: a survey of provider decision making. BMC Nephrol 12: 47. doi: 10.1186/1471-2369-12-47.

5. Kinchen KS, Sadler J, Fink N, Brookmeyer R, Klag MJ, et al. (2002) The timing of specialist evaluation in chronic kidney disease and mortality. Ann Intern Med 137: 479–486.

6. Richards N, Harris K, Whitfield M, O'Donoghue D, Lewis R, et al. (2008) The impact of population-based identification of chronic kidney disease using estimated glomerular filtration rate (eGFR) reporting. Nephrol Dial Transplant 23: 556–561. doi: 10.1093/ndt/gfm839.

7. De Jager DJ, Voormolen N, Krediet RT, Dekker FW, Boeschoten EW, et al. (2011) Association between time of referral and survival in the first year of dialysis in diabetics and the elderly. Nephrol Dial Transplant 26: 652–658. doi: 10.1093/ndt/gfq438.

8. Lenz O, Mekala DP, Patel DV, Fornoni A, Metz D, et al. (2005) Barriers to successful care for chronic kidney disease. BMC Nephrol 6: 11. doi: 10.1186/1471-2369-6-11.

9. Stolk M, McCoy C (2011) Chronic kidney disease: screening, follow-up and referral. Med Health R I 94: 63–65.

10. Gøransson LG, Bergrem H (2001) Consequences of late referral of patients with end-stage renal disease. J Intern Med 250: 154–159.

11. Levin A (2000) Consequences of late referral on patient outcomes. Nephrol Dial Transplant 15 Suppl 3: 8–13.

12. Black C, Sharma P, Scotland G, McCullough K, McGurn D, et al. (2010) Early referral strategies for management of people with markers of renal disease: a systematic review of the evidence of clinical effectiveness, cost-effectiveness and economic analysis. Health Technol Assess 14: 1–184. doi: 10.3310/hta14210.

13. Orlando LA, Owen WF, Matchar DB (2007) Relationship between nephrologist care and progression of chronic kidney disease. N C Med J 68: 9–16.

14. Abdel-Kader K, Fischer GS, Li J, Moore CG, Hess R, et al. (2011) Automated clinical reminders for primary care providers in the care of CKD: a small cluster-randomized controlled trial. Am J Kidney Dis 58: 894–902. doi: 10.1053/j.ajkd.2011.08.028.

15. U S Renal Data System (2011) International Comparisons. USRDS 2011 Annual Data Report: Atlas of Chronic Kidney Disease and End-Stage Renal Disease in the United States. Bethesda, MD: National Institutes of Health, National Institute of Diabetes and Digestive and Kidney Diseases.

16. Bland JM, Altman DG (1986) Statistical methods for assessing agreement between two methods of clinical measurement. Lancet 1: 307–310.

17. Ruppert D, Wand MP, Carroll RJ (2009) Semiparametric regression during 2003-2007. Electron J Stat 3: 1193–1256. doi: 10.1214/09-EJS525.

18. Jurkovitz CT, Elliott D, Li S, Saab G, Bomback AS, et al. (2012) Physician utilization, risk-factor control, and CKD progression among participants in the Kidney Early Evaluation Program (KEEP). Am J Kidney Dis 59: S24–S33. doi: 10.1053/j.ajkd.2011.11.019.

19. Cheung CK, Bhandari S (2009) Perspectives on eGFR reporting from the interface between primary and secondary care. Clin J Am Soc Nephrol 4: 258–260. doi: 10.2215/CJN.05151008.

20. Aakre KM, Thue G, Svarstad E, Skadberg Ø, Sandberg S (2011) Laboratory investigation and follow-up of chronic kidney disease stage 3 in primary care. Clin Chim Acta 412: 1138–1142. doi: 10.1016/j.cca.2011.03.004.

21. Swedko PJ, Clark HD, Paramsothy K, Akbari A (2003) Serum creatinine is an inadequate screening test for renal failure in elderly patients. Arch Intern Med 163: 356–360.

22. Mendelssohn DC, Barrett BJ, Brownscombe LM, Ethier J, Greenberg DE, et al. (1999) Elevated levels of serum creatinine: recommendations for management and referral. CMAJ 161: 413–417.

23. Maschio G, Oldrizzi L, Rugiu C (1991) Is there a "point of no return" in progressive renal disease? J Am Soc Nephrol 2: 832–840.

24. Komatsu H, Fujimoto S, Sato Y, Hara S, Yamada K, et al. (2005) "Point of no return (PNR)" in progressive IgA nephropathy: significance of blood pressure and proteinuria management up to PNR. J Nephrol 18: 690–695.

25. Tamba K, Kusano E, Tabei K, Kajii E, Asano Y (2009) Physicians make different decisions from nephrologists at serum creatinine 2.0 mg/dl. Clin Exp Nephrol 13: 447–451. doi: 10.1007/s10157-009-0176-4.

26. Agrawal V, Ghosh AK, Barnes MA, McCullough PA (2009) Perception of indications for nephrology referral among internal medicine residents: a national online survey. Clin J Am Soc Nephrol 4: 323–328. doi: 10.2215/CJN.03510708.

27. Boulware LE, Troll MU, Jaar BG, Myers DI, Powe NR (2006) Identification and referral of patients with progressive CKD: a national study. Am J Kidney Dis 48: 192–204. doi: 10.1053/j.ajkd.2006.04.073.

28. Diamantidis CJ, Powe NR, Jaar BG, Greer RC, Troll MU, et al. (2011) Primary care-specialist collaboration in the care of patients with chronic kidney disease. Clin J Am Soc Nephrol 6: 334–343. doi: 10.2215/CJN.06240710.

29. Lenz O, Fornoni A (2006) Chronic kidney disease care delivered by US family medicine and internal medicine trainees: results from an online survey. BMC Med 4: 30. doi: 10.1186/1741-7015-4-30.

30. Navaneethan SD, Kandula P, Jeevanantham V, Nally JV Jr, Liebman SE (2010) Referral patterns of primary care physicians for chronic kidney disease in general population and geriatric patients. Clin Nephrol 73: 260–267.

31. Finkelstein FO, Story K, Firanek C, Barre P, Takano T, et al. (2008) Perceived knowledge among patients cared for by nephrologists about chronic kidney disease and end-stage renal disease therapies. Kidney Int 74: 1178–1184. doi: 10.1038/ki.2008.376.

32. Coritsidis GN, Linden E, Stern AS (2011) The role of the primary care physician in managing early stages of chronic kidney disease. Postgrad Med 123: 177–185. doi: 10.3810/pgm.2011.09.2473.

33. Wyatt C, Konduri V, Eng J, Rohatgi R (2007) Reporting of estimated GFR in the primary care clinic. Am J Kidney Dis 49: 634–641. doi: 10.1053/j.ajkd.2007.02.258.

34. Phillips LA, Donovan KL, Phillips AO (2009) Renal quality outcomes framework and eGFR: impact on secondary care. QJM 102: 415–423. doi: 10.1093/qjmed/hcp030.

35. Akbari A, Swedko PJ, Clark HD, Hogg W, Lemelin J, et al. (2004) Detection of chronic kidney disease with laboratory reporting of estimated glomerular filtration rate and an educational program. Arch Intern Med 164: 1788–1792. doi: 10.1001/archinte.164.16.1788.

36. Kagoma YK, Weir MA, Iansavichus AV, Hemmelgarn BR, Akbari A, et al. (2011) Impact of estimated GFR reporting on patients, clinicians, and health-care systems: a systematic review. Am J Kidney Dis 57: 592–601. doi: 10.1053/j.ajkd.2010.08.029.

37. Jain AK, Cuerden MS, McLeod I, Hemmelgarn B, Akbari A, et al. (2012) Reporting of the estimated glomerular filtration rate was associated with increased use of angiotensin-converting enzyme inhibitors and angiotensin-II receptor blockers in CKD. Kidney Int 81: 1248–1253. doi: 10.1038/ki.2012.18.

38. Jain AK, McLeod I, Huo C, Cuerden MS, Akbari A, et al. (2009) When laboratories report estimated glomerular filtration rates in addition to serum creatinines, nephrology consults increase. Kidney Int 76: 318–323. doi: 10.1038/ki.2009.158.

39. Jain A, Hemmelgarn BR (2011) Impact of estimated glomerular filtration rate reporting on nephrology referrals: a review of the literature. Curr Opin Nephrol Hypertens 20: 218–223. doi: 10.1097/MNH.0b013e3283446193.

40. Noble E, Johnson DW, Gray N, Hollett P, Hawley CM, et al. (2008) The impact of automated eGFR reporting and education on nephrology service referrals. Nephrol Dial Transplant 23: 3845–3850. doi: 10.1093/ndt/gfn385.

41. Akbari A, Grimshaw J, Stacey D, Hogg W, Ramsay T, et al. (2012) Change in appropriate referrals to nephrologists after the introduction of automatic reporting of the estimated glomerular filtration rate. CMAJ 184: E269–E276. doi: 10.1503/cmaj.110678.

42. Hemmelgarn BR, Zhang J, Manns BJ, James MT, Quinn RR, et al. (2010) Nephrology visits and health care resource use before and after reporting estimated glomerular filtration rate. JAMA 303: 1151–1158. doi: 10.1001/jama.2010.303.

43. Jones C, Roderick P, Harris S, Rogerson M (2006) Decline in kidney function before and after nephrology referral and the effect on survival in moderate to advanced chronic kidney disease. Nephrol Dial Transplant 21: 2133–2143. doi: 10.1093/ndt/gfl198.

44. Herget-Rosenthal S, Quellmann T, Linden C, Hollenbeck M, Jankowski V, et al. (2010) How does late nephrological co-management impact chronic kidney disease? - an observational study. Int J Clin Pract 64: 1784–1792. doi: 10.1111/j.1742-1241.2010.02535.x.

45. Shin SJ, Kim HW, Chung S, Chung HW, Lee SJ, et al. (2007) Late referral to a nephrologist increases the risk of uremia-related cardiac hypertrophy in patients on hemodialysis. Nephron Clin Pract 107: c139–c146. doi: 10.1159/000110034.

46. Hasegawa T, Bragg-Gresham JL, Yamazaki S, Fukuhara S, Akizawa T, et al. (2009) Greater first-year survival on hemodialysis in facilities in which patients are provided earlier and more frequent pre-nephrology visits. Clin J Am Soc Nephrol 4: 595–602. doi: 10.2215/CJN.03540708.

47. Chen S-C, Chang J-M, Chou M-C, Lin M-Y, Chen J-H, et al. (2008) Slowing renal function decline in chronic kidney disease patients after nephrology referral. Nephrology (Carlton) 13: 730–736. doi: 10.1111/j.1440-1797.2008.01023.x.

48. Abdel-Kader K, Fischer GS, Johnston JR, Gu C, Moore CG, et al. (2011) Characterizing pre-dialysis care in the era of eGFR reporting: a cohort study. BMC Nephrol 12: 12. doi: 10.1186/1471-2369-12-12.

49. Meran S, Don K, Shah N, Donovan K, Riley S, et al. (2011) Impact of chronic kidney disease management in primary care. QJM 104: 27–34. doi: 10.1093/qjmed/hcq151.

50. Tseng C-L, Kern EFO, Miller DR, Tiwari A, Maney M, et al. (2008) Survival benefit of nephrologic care in patients with diabetes mellitus and chronic kidney disease. Arch Intern Med 168: 55–62. doi: 10.1001/archinternmed.2007.9.

51. Chen S-C, Hwang S-J, Tsai J-C, Liu W-C, Hwang S-C, et al. (2010) Early nephrology referral is associated with prolonged survival in hemodialysis patients even after exclusion of lead-time bias. Am J Med Sci 339: 123–126. doi: 10.1097/MAJ.0b013e3181c0678a.

52. O'Callaghan CA, Shine B, Lasserson DS (2011) Chronic kidney disease: a large-scale population-based study of the effects of introducing the CKD-EPI formula for eGFR reporting. BMJ Open 1: e000308. doi: 10.1136/bmjopen-2011-000308.

53. Stevens LA, Padala S, Levey AS (2010) Advances in glomerular filtration rate-estimating equations. Curr Opin Nephrol Hypertens 19: 298–307. doi: 10.1097/MNH.0b013e32833893e2.

54. Davis Giardina T, Singh H (2011) Should patients get direct access to their laboratory test results? An answer with many questions. JAMA 306: 2502–2503. doi: 10.1001/jama.2011.1797.

55. Campbell GA, Bolton WK (2011) Referral and comanagement of the patient with CKD. Adv Chronic Kidney Dis 18: 420–427. doi: 10.1053/j.ackd.2011.10.006.

56. Bayliss EA, Bhardwaja B, Ross C, Beck A, Lanese DM (2011) Multidisciplinary team care may slow the rate of decline in renal function. Clin J Am Soc Nephrol 6: 704–710. doi: 10.2215/CJN.06610810.

57. Mondry A, Zhu A-L, Loh M, Vo TD, Hahn K (2004) Active collaboration with primary care providers increases specialist referral in chronic renal disease. BMC Nephrol 5: 16. doi: 10.1186/1471-2369-5-16.

22

A Propensity-Score Matched Comparison of Perioperative and Early Renal Functional Outcomes of Robotic versus Open Partial Nephrectomy

Zhenjie Wu[1◊], Mingmin Li[2◊], Le Qu[1◊], Huamao Ye[1], Bing Liu[1], Qing Yang[1], Jing Sheng[2], Liang Xiao[1], Chen Lv[1], Bo Yang[1], Xu Gao[1], Xiaofeng Gao[1], Chuanliang Xu[1], Jianguo Hou[1], Yinghao Sun[1*], Linhui Wang[1*]

1 Department of Urology, Changhai Hospital, Second Military Medical University, Shanghai, P. R. China, 2 Department of Radiology, Changhai Hospital, Second Military Medical University, Shanghai, P. R. China

Abstract

Objectives: To compare the perioperative and early renal functional outcomes of RPN with OPN for kidney tumors.

Materials and Methods: A total of 209 RPN or OPN patients with availability of preoperative cross-sectional imaging since 2009 at our center were included. To adjust for potential baseline confounders propensity-score matching was performed, which resulted in 94 OPNs matched to 51 RPNs. Perioperative and early renal functional outcomes were compared.

Results: In propensity-score matched analysis, RPN procedures were well tolerated and resulted in significant decreases in postoperative analgesic time (24 vs. 48 hr, $p<0.001$) and visual analog pain scale (3 vs. 4, $p<0.001$). Besides, the RPN patients had a significantly shorter LOS (9 vs. 11 days, $p=0.008$) and less EBL (100 vs. 200 ml, $p<0.001$), but median operative time was significantly longer (229 vs. 182 min, $p<0.001$). Ischemia time, transfusion rates, complication rates, percentage eGFR decline and CKD upstaging were equivalent after RPN versus OPN. In multivariable logistic regression analysis, RPN patients were less likely to have a prolonged LOS (odds ratio [OR]: 0.409; $p=0.016$), while more likely to experience a longer operative time (OR: 4.296; $p=0.001$). However, the statistical significance for the protective effect of RPN versus OPN in EBL was not confirmed by examining the risk of EBL$\geq$400 ml (OR: 0.488; $p=0.212$).

Conclusions: When adjusted for potential selection biases, RPN offers comparable perioperative and early renal functional outcomes to those of OPN, with the added advantage of improved postoperative pain control and a shorter LOS.

Editor: Domenico Coppola, H. Lee Moffitt Cancer Center & Research Institute, United States of America

Funding: This study has been supported by National Natural Science Foundation of China (81272817, 81172447), the Talents Project of Shanghai Health System (XBR2011027), the Scientific and Technological Talents Project of Shanghai (13XD1400100), Natural Science Foundation of Shanghai (11ZR1447800), The "Leading Talent" Project of Shanghai (2013046), and Hospital "1255" Discipline Construction Projects (CH125520300), Hospital's Youth Initiation Fund. The funders had no role in study design, data collection and analysis, decision to publish, or preparation of the manuscript.

Competing Interests: The authors have declared that no competing interests exist.

* E-mail: sunyh@medmail.com.cn (YHS); wlhui_chh@163.com (LHW);

◊ These authors contributed equally to this work.

Introduction

Partial nephrectomy (PN) has become the established standard treatment for most localized small renal tumors in that it yields equivalent long-term oncological outcomes and better preservation of renal function compared to those of radical nephrectomy (RN) [1–3]. Moreover, a large population-based analysis by Tan et al revealed that cancer-specific survival rates following PN and RN in patients with early-stage kidney cancer are comparable and PN is associated with an improved overall survival rate [4].

Of currently available PN techniques, open surgery remains a standard of care for PN [1]. While in areas other than PN, laparoscopic surgery appears to have definite advantages in reduced surgical invasiveness and postoperative recovery which would not be offset by worse function outcomes of the organ operated or increased perioperative complication profiles relative to open surgery [5–7]. Despite its mini-invasiveness and excellent results in experienced hands, laparoscopic PN (LPN) is reported to be associated with a prolonged warm ischemia time and a higher complication rate than with OPN [8,9]. It is the increased technical difficulty as well as the steep learning curve that limits the diffusion of LPN. In contrast, robotic PN (RPN) appears to be a more reproducible approach with improved dexterity, magnified three-dimensional visualization and better ergonomics, which may bridge the gap between the LPN and OPN. A recently published meta-analysis on RPN vs. LPN showed a significantly decreased warm ischemia time with RPN and comparable outcomes in terms of operative time, estimated blood loss, length of stay, complication or positive margins. As RPN is increasingly gaining popularity, a rigorous comparison against the gold standard of

OPN is desperately needed. Even though several observational studies comparing RPN and OPN have been recently reported, most are significantly suffering from the confounding of salient baseline covariates with conflicting results [10–13]. Therefore, we aimed to evaluate the effects of RPN on perioperative and early renal functional outcomes relative to OPN based on a propensity-score matched cohort.

Materials and Methods

Patient and Measurement

Following the approval of our Institutional Review Board (IRB) of Changhai hospital (Second Military Medical University, SMMU), the electronic medical record system and the radiological database (Picture Archiving and Communication Systems, PACS) were queried to identify all patients with preoperative cross-sectional imaging (enhanced computerized tomography or magnetic resonance imaging) who underwent RPN or OPN from 2009 to 2013 at a tertiary reference center. All radiological images were reviewed and evaluated electronically by a senior radiologist (MML) and an experienced urologist (ZJW) who were blinded to the surgical approaches and outcomes. Tumor size was recorded as the largest diameter on the axial plane. For each renal tumor a diameter-axial-polar (DAP) score ranging from 3 to 9 points was assigned according to the reported methodology [14]. Hilar lesions were determined according to the definition in the R.E.N.A.L. nephrometry system [15].

Surgical approach and technique, eg. OPN or RPN, were chosen according to the primary surgeon's judgment instead of randomization. All procedures were performed by surgeons with advanced training in open and minimally invasive surgery. RPN operations were conducted with the da Vinci Si Surgical System (Intuitive Surgical, Inc., Sunnyvale, CA, USA) by one of four surgeons with substantial experience in partial nephrectomy. Patients were placed in flank position. A standard three-arm approach with one or two trocars for the assistant, and an optional robotic port as needed was used. After the Gerota's fascia was opened, the renal vessels were dissected and the tumor was identified with the assistance of intraoperative ultrasonography as needed. Most of the hilar controlled RPN procedures were performed with renal artery-only clamping. Tumor resection was performed with a tumor-free parenchymal margin of 0.5–1 cm in thickness. Standard OPN procedures were done, with flank incisions between the 10th or 11th interspace. The renal pedicle was usually controlled en bloc with a vascular clamp. Cold ischemia with ice slush was used. In all open and robotic cases, opened calices and bleeding sites were repaired carefully. The parenchymal defect was closed using a combination of sliding-clip (Hem-o-lok) renorrhaphy and a running suture. Additional absorbable hemostatic agents were used when necessary. When necessary, patients received continuous intravenous analgesics for a maximum of 48 hours after surgery. For the pain assessment, the visual analog scale (VAS) was used, which ranges from 0 (no pain) to 10 (excruciating pain).The pain scale was self-administered on first three postoperative days by the nurse during the morning round. The highest pain score was included for analysis.

Perioperative data analyzed included patient age, gender, body mass index (BMI), American Society of Anesthesiologists (ASA) classification, age-weighted Charlson Comorbidity Index (CCI) score, DAP nephrometry score as well as tumor size, operative duration, estimated blood loss (EBL), ischemia time, proportion of patients with intraoperative collecting system entry, hemostatic agent use, perioperative transfusions and complications, conversions to radical nephrectomy, postoperative analgesic time, pain

scale, length of hospital stay (LOS), surgical margin status and eGFR change. Positive surgical margin was defined as cancer cells at the level of inked parenchymal excision surface. The eGFR was calculated using the Modification of Diet in Renal Disease 2 equation [16]. For baseline eGFR the SCr value prior to surgery (generally within one week before surgery) was used. The last eGFR measurement was within 3 months after surgery. The follow-up SCr value for the last eGFR measurement was obtained by searching the lab testing system with the patient name, patient identity number or inpatient number, and otherwise the SCr most immediately preceding discharge was used. For each patient, chronic kidney disease (CKD) was defined according to the National Kidney Foundation Kidney Disease Outcome Quality Initiative classification [17]. The upstaging of CKD was considered as a change in one class of CKD or more. Percentage eGFR change was defined as (last eGFR-baseline eGFR)/baseline eGFR. Postoperative complications were graded according to the Clavien scale. The PACS database was queried for the oncological outcome analysis. Patients who had stopped follow-up at our institution were contacted by telephone to inquiry their latest imaging results. For those who did not respond, the most recent follow-up images within the PACS were used.

Statistical Analysis

Prior to analysis, patient information was anonymized and de-identified. Categorical variables were shown as the frequency and percentage, and continuous variables were presented as the median and interquartile range (IQR). Frequency distributions between categorical variables were compared using χ^2 test or Fisher's exact test while continuous variables were compared using the nonparametric Mann-Whitney test. Due to inherent differences between patients who underwent RPN and OPN in terms of baseline characteristics, we performed a propensity score matched analysis to adjust for these differences. Exclusion criteria for propensity score analysis of the RPN versus OPN groups were as follows (numbers represent counts of patients): solitary kidney patients (2, 6), multiple ispilateral tumors (0, 8), history of partial nephrectomy in the contralateral kidney (0, 4), "zero ischemia" (off-clamp or segmental branches clamped) patients (1, 1), missing ischemia time (0, 6), and missing postoperative eGFR measurement (0, 2).

The probability to undergo a RPN procedure in the current study was estimated. The propensity score was generated by way of a multivariable logistic model considering the following variables: patient demographics (age, gender, BMI); ASA score; CCI; hilar tumor; DAP sum score; and preoperative eGFR level. Based on the resulting propensity score, one case was matched to one or multiple controls using a caliper of 0.01. Subsequently, covariate balance and surgical outcomes between the matched groups were examined. Finally, backward stepwise logistic multivariable regression analysis were conducted for prediction of several outcomes, namely, the odds of operative time of 4 hr or more, EBL of 400 ml or greater, ischemia time of 20 min or longer, a prolonged LOS (≥10 d), any postoperative complication during hospital stay, postoperative eGFR decrease ≥10% and any CKD upstaging. All statistical analyses were performed using the IBM SPSS Statistics v.20. The null hypothesis was rejected for all analyses at $p < 0.05$, and all p values were 2-tailed.

Results

Overall, 209 patients were included, of which 123 (58.9%) and 86 (41.1%) patients were treated by OPN or RPN, respectively. There was one intraoperative conversion of RPN to OPN due to hemorrhage and one conversion to radical nephrectomy in the OPN group for oncological reason (report of malignance in the frozen section analysis). There was no death (Clavien 5) from surgical complication in either group. No patients had positive surgical margin. The median percentage decrease in eGFR at a median of 3 months was 6% (IQR: -20-4) and no patients required dialysis. The median oncological follow-up was 12 months (IQR: 6–24). One patient (0.8%) of OPN with clear cell renal cell carcinoma (Fuhrman III) had local recurrence at three years after surgery and underwent radical nephrectomy. There were no metastatic diseases developed in the study cohort.

Prior to matching, more patients in the OPN group had a hilar tumor (16.3% vs 7%, $p = 0.045$) and a higher DAP nephrometry score (7 vs 6.5, $p = 0.037$) compared with that of the RPN group. No differences according to age, gender, BMI, ASA, age-adjusted CCI and preoperative eGFR were detected between the two groups. Propensity-score matching was subsequently performed, which resulted in a cohort including 51 RPN and 94 OPN patients. As expected, differences in patient characteristics between the two groups were all non-significant, indicating a high degree of similarity in the distribution of potential confounders (Table 1).

Within the propensity-score matched cohort (Table 2), RPN procedures were well tolerated and resulted in significant decreases in postoperative analgesic time (24 vs. 48, $p<0.001$) and visual analog pain scale (3 vs. 4, $p<0.001$). Besides, RPN patients had less EBL and a shorter LOS, whereas the OR time was significantly longer (229 vs. 182, $p<0.001$) and more patients encountering delayed bleeding (7.8% vs. 5.5%, $p = 0.030$) than that of OPN patients. The differences between the two groups were not statistically significant with regard to ischemia time, proportion of patients with intraoperative collecting system entry, hemostatic agent use, transfusion rates, overall complication rate, the rate of urine leak, postoperative eGFR decrease in percentage or CKD upstaging. The propensity-score adjusted multivariable logistic regression analysis showed that relative to OPN patients, RPN patients were less likely to have a prolonged LOS (≥ 10 d) following surgery (odds ratio [OR]: 0.409; 95% confidence interval [CI]: 0.198–0.845; $p = 0.016$), while more likely to experience a longer operative time (≥ 4 h) (OR: 4.296; 95% CI: 1.870–9.871; $p = 0.001$). However, the statistical significance for the protective effect of RPN versus OPN in EBL was not confirmed by examining the risk of EBL≥ 400 ml (OR: 0.488; 95% CI: 0.158–1.506; $p = 0.212$) and the higher risk of delayed bleeding for RPN did not reach statistical significance(OR: 1.834; 95% CI: 0.440–7.643; $p = 0.405$). Finally, no statistically significant differences were detected regarding ischemia time of 20 min or longer (OR: 0.954; $p = 0.905$), postoperative complication rate (OR: 1.654; $p = 0.247$), eGFR decline≥ 10% (OR: 1.002; $p = 0.996$), or CKD upstaging (OR: 0.977; $p = 0.954$) (Table 3).

Discussion

The present study yielded some important findings. In comparison with OPN, RPN provided comparable perioperative and functional outcomes with the added benefits of better postoperative pain control and a shorter postoperative hospital length of stay. Specifically, RPN patients are 40.9% less likely to experience a prolonged LOS and have a marginal advantage in EBL without compromising surgical success relative to OPN, albeit with a four-fold risk of operative time over 4 hours.

Four other reported studies evaluated surgical outcomes after RPN versus OPN [10–13]. In those series, the treatment-selection bias was not balanced, although two of them announced

prospective design and data collection. For example, percentage of imperative indication for PN [10,13], CCI [10], BMI [11], tumor size [10], or tumor anatomic complexity [12] significantly differed between the two groups. The crude comparison might reflect a "real world" scenario that more patients with complex renal tumors underwent open surgery, as showed in our unmatched series. However, the heterogeneity in baseline characteristics would mix the impact of treatment on outcomes. Many studies reported that differences in tumor complexity, BMI, or CCI may account for the observed differences in outcomes [18–21], which reinforces the necessity that statistical methods must be used to adjust for systematic differences.

The current data with propensity-score adjustment to achieve a minimum inherent selection bias according to treatment type may help to address the controversy on ischemia time with RPN versus OPN. Lee et al reported a longer ischemia time in the RPN group (23 vs. 19 min, $p<0.001$) [11]. In accordance with our results, the study by Simhan et al demonstrated comparable ischemia time following RPN and OPN [13], which was also confirmed in two prospective non-randomized comparative studies [10,12]. In this regard, surgeons' experience in RPN also contributes to the reduction in intraoperative ischemia time. In several recently reported series of RPN for complex renal tumors (a higher nephrometry score, multifocal, or completely endophytic, etc.), the ischemia time can still be controlled at about 20 min [22–24]. Regarding the postoperative renal functional outcome, a large tertiary-care center series comparing RPN and OPN revealed that there was no significant difference in eGFR change at a mean follow-up of 21.3 months. In that study, however, more patients with solitary kidney were treated with OPN (12.1 vs 0%, $p<0.001$), which can intrinsically influence the estimation of eGFR in the OPN group. Similarly, Lee et al and Masson-Lecomte et al proved the equipoise between RPN and OPN [11,12]. In our study, the comparable early renal functional outcome was confirmed and no increased risk of CKD upstaging was associated with RPN. Recently, a novel method for renal hypothermia during RPN that recapitulates the open approach has been under further evaluation, which would contribute to a better functional preservation [25].

More recently, Ficarra et al reported a multicenter matched-pair analysis comparing robotic versus open PN, in which 200 RPNs and 200 OPNs were examined [26]. In that series, EBL and LOS were more favorable after RPN than OPN, and no differences were recorded regarding intraoperative complications (1 vs. 3, $p = 0.31$), blood transfusions (21 vs. 20, $p = 0.78$), high grade (Clavien 3–4) postoperative complications (9 vs. 9, $p = 1.000$), and absolute eGFR decline at 3 months after surgery (16.6 vs. 16.4 ml/min, $p = 0.28$). These data are in perfect agreement with our findings, but the protective effect of RPN in EBL (100 vs. 150 ml, $p<0.001$ in their cohort; 100 vs. 200 ml, $p<0.001$ in our series) is marginal. What's more, in the procedure of RPN the amount of blood loss could be underestimated for blood loss might not be fully recognized due to gravity effects on the blood into more dependent abdominal compartments that go unrecognized and "unsuctioned" from the body cavity. This effect may be of little clinical significance for it is not predictive of EBL$\geq$ 400 ml in multivariable analysis. In this regard, it may be better to assess the change in perioperative hemoglobin or hematocrit. However, there could be differences in hydration status in the perioperative setting that might affect accurate measurement.

It is equally interesting to note that there was no significant differences between the two approaches in operative time but a significantly longer warm ischemia time with RPN than with OPN in Ficarra et al's study. Actually, in their series the OPN patients

Table 1. Distribution of potential confounders used in the propensity-score model in patients before and after matching.

Median (Q$_1$–Q$_3$) or n(%)	Entire sample				Propensity-score matched groups			
	Total	RPN	OPN	p value	Total	RPN	OPN	p value
No. of pts	209	86	123	-	145	51	94	-
Age, yr	50	52	49	0.141	52	53	52	0.750
	(42–59)	(43–60)	(41–59)		(46–60)	(45–59)	(46–60)	
Gender				0.155				0.744
Male	129(61.7)	58(67.4)	71(57.7)		97(66.9)	35(68.6)	62(66)	
Female	80(38.3)	28(32.6)	52(42.3)		48(33.1)	16(31.4)	32(34)	
BMI, kg/m^2	24.6 (22.3–26.2)	24.7 (22.9–26.2)	24.2 (21.3–26.3)	0.341	24.9 (22.8–26.4)	24.8 (22.8–26.2)	25.1 (22.9–26.6)	0.762
ASA				0.705				1.000
1–2	196(93.8)	80(93)	116(94.3)		136(93.8)	48(94.1)	88(93.6)	
3–4	13(6.2)	6(7)	7(5.7)		9(6.2)	3(5.9)	6(6.4)	
Age-adjusted CCI				0.830				0.305
0–1	181(86.6)	75(87.2)	106(86.2)		125(86.2)	46(90.2)	79(84)	
≥2	28(13.4)	11(12.8)	17(13.8)		20(13.8)	5(9.8)	15(16)	
Hilar tumor	26(12.4)	6(7)	20 (16.3)	**0.045**	10(6.9)	3(5.9)	7(7.4)	1.000
DAP sum score	7 (6–7)	6.5(5–7)	7(6–8)	**0.037**	7 (5–7)	6 (5–7)	7 (5–7)	0.370
Preoperative eGFR (ml/min per 1.73 m^2)	98 (86.6–110.3)	96.5 (86.1–108.7)	98.4 (87.5–112.1)	0.425	97 (86.4–106.5)	95.5 (88.3–104.5)	97.5 (85.0–109.1)	0.828

IQR = interquartile range; RPN = robotic partial nephrectomy; OPN = open partial nephrectomy; ASA = American Society of Anesthesiologists; CCI = Charlson Comorbidity Index; DAP = diameter-axial-polar.

Table 2. Propensity-score adjusted comparison of surgical outcomes for RPN and OPN.

Median (Q$_1$–Q$_3$) or n(%)	RPN (n = 51)	OPN (n = 94)	p value
OR time, min	229 (203–268)	182(161–223)	**<0.001**
EBL, ml	100 (100–200)	200(113–300)	**<0.001**
Ischemia time, min	21 (15–27)	20 (17–27)	0.899
LOS, d	9 (8–12)	11 (9–13)	**0.008**
Blood transfusion	3 (5.9)	4 (4.3)	0.697
Collecting system entry	14(27.5)	27(29.7)	0.871
Hemostatic agent use[*]	42(82.4)	73(77.7)	0.505
Intraoperative complication	1 (2)	1 (1.1)	1.000
Conversion to radical nephrectomy	0 (0)	1 (1.1)	1.000
VAPS (0–10)	3 (3–4)	4 (4–6)	**<0.001**
Postoperative Analgesic time, hr	24 (19–24)	48 (24–48)	**<0.001**
Postoperative complication			
Overall	13 (25.5)	17 (18.1)	0.293
Clavien 1–2	12 (23.5)	16 (17)	0.343
Clavien 3–5	1 (2)	1 (1.1)	1.000
Delayed bleeding[#]	4(7.8)	5(5.5)89	**0.030**
Urine leak[ξ]	1(2)	2(2.1)	0.613
Positive surgical margin	0 (0)	0 (0)	-
Last eGFR, ml/min per 1.73 m^2	92.4 (76.7–102.5)	88.5 (74.9–100.5)	0.561
Percentage change in eGFR	−6 (−18–3)	−8 (−21–2)	0.744
Preoperative CKD 1–2	50 (98)	91 (96.8)	0.666
Postoperative CKD 1–2	46 (90.2)	87 (92.6)	0.754
CKD upstaging	15 (29.4)	29 (30.9)	0.857

IQR = interquartile range; RPN = robotic partial nephrectomy; OPN = open partial nephrectomy; OR = operative room; EBL = estimated blood loss; LOS = length of stay; VAPS = visual analog pain scale; CKD = chronic kidney disease.
*SURGICEL.
#defined as a decreased level of Hb requiring blood transfusion or surgical/endoscopic/radiologic intervention 24 hr after surgery or later.
ξdefined as extra-renal urine extravasation that required prolonged maintenance of a drain, re-insertion of a drain, insertion of a ureteral stent or other surgical intervention. All leaks were verified by drain fluid chemical analysis. Cases of urinary leak in both RPN and OPN groups were managed expectantly.

were collected from 19 different Italian centers while most RPN patients were captured from databases abroad. The resulted heterogeneity in surgical experience and technique could lead to biased estimates of treatment effects. The majority of our series were performed by the consultant surgeon of the kidney tumor specialized group at our institution, although RPN is considered to have a short learning curve in the hands of a surgeon with extensive minimally invasive surgery experience [27]. The longer operative room time with RPN in our series might be explained by

Table 3. Propensity-score adjusted multivariable stepwise logistic regression analysis for surgical outcomes of RPN versus OPN.

Dependent variable	RPN vs OPN: odds ratio (95% CI)[*]	p value
OR time ≥4 hr	4.296 (1.870–9.871)	**0.001**
EBL ≥400 ml	0.488 (0.158–1.506)	0.212
Ischemia time ≥20 min	0.954 (0.439–2.074)	0.905
LOS ≥10 d	0.409 (0.198–0.845)	**0.016**
Postoperative complication	1.654 (0.706–3.876)	0.247
Delayed bleeding	1.834(0.440–7.643)	0.405
eGFR decrease ≥10%	1.002 (0.491–2.045)	0.996
CKD upstaging	0.977 (0.453–2.110)	0.954

RPN = robotic partial nephrectomy; OPN = open partial nephrectomy; OR = operative room; EBL = estimated blood loss; LOS = length of stay; CKD = chronic kidney disease.
*Models adjusted for age, gender, baseline Charlson comorbidity index, BMI, ASA, and DAP score.

the inclusion of the time for preparation and docking of the robot [12].

The current study highlights the non-inferiority of RPN to OPN with regard to intraoperative ischemia time, postoperative complications and early functional outcomes and the additional benefits of a shorter LOS as well as less EBL using propensity-score matched comparison and prediction analysis. In spite of its strengths, our report has limitations inherent in its retrospective nature. Some unmeasured data which were not retrospectively retrievable may be of paramount importance, especially with regard to time off take-in, drainage, time required for patients return to their occupations, etc., which may favor one approach over another. There may also have been some unobserved bias amongst the groups such as surgeons' background or intraoperative technique that we were not able to adjust for. The differences in the ischemia type between the two groups, and utilization of the Modification in Diet Renal Disease 2 equation for eGFR which is affected by diet would cause potential bias in the evaluation of renal functional impairment. Besides, missing data fields which led to further exclusion of cases could decrease the power of our study. Also, the few events of major postoperative complications may eliminate the potential differences between the two groups. Finally, the oncological outcomes were not compared directly because the follow-up duration between RPN and OPN were significantly different.

Conclusions

When adjusted for potential selection biases, RPN offers comparable perioperative and early renal functional outcomes to those of OPN, with the added advantage of improved postoperative pain control and a shorter length of hospital stay. However, these results should be interpreted with caution, given that statistical adjustment is not a substitute for an awaited randomized trial. A long-term follow-up is needed to confirm the oncological safety and efficacy of RPN.

Author Contributions

Conceived and designed the experiments: ZJW MML LQ HMY YHS LHW. Performed the experiments: ZJW MML LQ HMY BL QY LX CL BY XG XFG CLX JGH YHS. Analyzed the data: ZJW MML LQ HMY BL QY JS LX. Contributed reagents/materials/analysis tools: ZJW MML LQ HMY BL QY JS LX. Wrote the paper: ZJW MML.

References

1. Ljungberg B, Bensalah K, Bex A, Canfield S, Dabestani S, et al. Guidelines on Renal Cell Carcinoma. Uroweb 2013. Available: http://www.uroweb.org/gls/pdf/10_Renal_Cell_Carcinoma_LRV2.pdf. Accessed 2014 Jan 28.
2. MacLennan S, Imamura M, Lapitan MC, Omar MI, Lam TB, et al. (2012) Systematic review of oncological outcomes following surgical management of localised renal cancer. Eur Urol 61: 972–993.
3. Sun M, Bianchi M, Hansen J, Trinh QD, Abdollah F, et al. (2012) Chronic kidney disease after nephrectomy in patients with small renal masses: a retrospective observational analysis. Eur Urol 62: 696–703.
4. Tan HJ, Norton EC, Ye Z, Hafez KS, Gore JL, et al. (2012) Long-term survival following partial vs radical nephrectomy among older patients with early-stage kidney cancer. JAMA 307: 1629–1635.
5. Hemal AK, Kumar A, Kumar R, Wadhwa P, Seth A, et al. (2007) Laparoscopic versus open radical nephrectomy for large renal tumors: a long-term prospective comparison. J Urol 177: 862–866.
6. Agabiti N, Stafoggia M, Davoli M, Fusco D, Barone AP, et al. (2013) Thirty-day complications after laparoscopic or open cholecystectomy: a population-based cohort study in Italy. BMJ Open 3.
7. Ng SS, Leung KL, Lee JF, Yiu RY, Li JC, et al. (2008) Laparoscopic-assisted versus open abdominoperineal resection for low rectal cancer: a prospective randomized trial. Ann Surg Oncol 15: 2418–2425.
8. Gill IS, Kavoussi LR, Lane BR, Blute ML, Babineau D, et al. (2007) Comparison of 1,800 laparoscopic and open partial nephrectomies for single renal tumors. J Urol 178: 41–46.
9. Gong EM, Orvieto MA, Zorn KC, Lucioni A, Steinberg GD, et al. (2008) Comparison of laparoscopic and open partial nephrectomy in clinical T1a renal tumors. J Endourol 22: 953–957.
10. Vittori G (2014) Open versus robotic-assisted partial nephrectomy: a multicenter comparison study of perioperative results and complications. World J Urol 32: 287–293.
11. Lee S, Oh J, Hong SK, Lee SE, Byun SS (2011) Open versus robot-assisted partial nephrectomy: effect on clinical outcome. J Endourol 25: 1181–1185.
12. Masson-Lecomte A, Yates DR, Hupertan V, Haertig A, Chartier-Kastler E, et al. (2013) A prospective comparison of the pathologic and surgical outcomes obtained after elective treatment of renal cell carcinoma by open or robot-assisted partial nephrectomy. Urol Oncol 31: 924–929.
13. Simhan J, Smaldone MC, Tsai KJ, Li T, Reyes JM, et al. (2012) Perioperative outcomes of robotic and open partial nephrectomy for moderately and highly complex renal lesions. J Urol 187: 2000–2004.
14. Simmons MN, Hillyer SP, Lee BH, Fergany AF, Kaouk J, et al. (2012) Diameter-axial-polar nephrometry: integration and optimization of R.E.N.A.L. and centrality index scoring systems. J Urol 188: 384–390.
15. Kutikov A, Uzzo RG (2009) The R.E.N.A.L. nephrometry score: a comprehensive standardized system for quantitating renal tumor size, location and depth. J Urol 182: 844–853.
16. Levey AS, Bosch JP, Lewis JB, Greene T, Rogers N, et al. (1999) A more accurate method to estimate glomerular filtration rate from serum creatinine: a new prediction equation. Modification of Diet in Renal Disease Study Group. Ann Intern Med 130: 461–470.
17. Levey AS, Coresh J, Balk E, Kausz AT, Levin A, et al. (2003) National Kidney Foundation practice guidelines for chronic kidney disease: evaluation, classification, and stratification. Ann Intern Med 139: 137–147.
18. Wang L, Li M, Chen W, Wu Z, Cai C, et al. (2013) Is diameter-axial-polar scoring predictive of renal functional damage in patients undergoing partial nephrectomy? An evaluation using technetium Tc 99 m ((9)(9)Tcm) diethylene-triamine-penta-acetic acid (DTPA) glomerular filtration rate. BJU Int 111: 1191–1198.
19. Ficarra V, Bhayani S, Porter J, Buffi N, Lee R, et al. (2012) Predictors of warm ischemia time and perioperative complications in a multicenter, international series of robot-assisted partial nephrectomy. Eur Urol 61: 395–402.
20. Isac WE, Autorino R, Hillyer SP, Hernandez AV, Stein RJ, et al. (2012) The impact of body mass index on surgical outcomes of robotic partial nephrectomy. BJU Int 110: E997–e1002.
21. Roscigno M, Ceresoli F, Naspro R, Montorsi F, Bertini R, et al. (2013) Predictive Accuracy of Nephrometric Scores Can Be Improved by Adding Clinical Patient Characteristics: A Novel Algorithm Combining Anatomic Tumour Complexity, Body Mass Index, and Charlson Comorbidity Index to Depict Perioperative Complications After Nephron-sparing Surgery. Eur Urol.
22. Autorino R, Khalifeh A, Laydner H, Samarasekera D, Rizkala E, et al. (2013) Robotic Partial Nephrectomy for Completely Endophytic Renal Masses: a Single Institution Experience. BJU Int.
23. Laydner H, Autorino R, Spana G, Altunrende F, Yang B, et al. (2012) Robot-assisted partial nephrectomy for sporadic ipsilateral multifocal renal tumours. BJU Int 109: 274–280.
24. White MA, Haber GP, Autorino R, Khanna R, Hernandez AV, et al. (2011) Outcomes of robotic partial nephrectomy for renal masses with nephrometry score of >/ = 7. Urology 77: 809–813.
25. Rogers CG, Ghani KR, Kumar RK, Jeong W, Menon M (2013) Robotic partial nephrectomy with cold ischemia and on-clamp tumor extraction: recapitulating the open approach. Eur Urol 63: 573–578.
26. Ficarra V, Minervini A, Antonelli A, Bhayani S, Guazzoni G, et al. (2013) A Multicenter Matched-Pair Analysis Comparing Robot-Assisted Versus Open Partial Nephrectomy. BJU Int.
27. Mottrie A, De Naeyer G, Schatteman P, Carpentier P, Sangalli M, et al. (2010) Impact of the learning curve on perioperative outcomes in patients who underwent robotic partial nephrectomy for parenchymal renal tumours. Eur Urol 58: 127–132.

23

Radiologic and Clinical Bronchiectasis Associated with Autosomal Dominant Polycystic Kidney Disease

Teng Moua[1]*, Ladan Zand[2], Robert P. Hartman[3], Thomas E. Hartman[3], Dingxin Qin[2], Tobias Peikert[1], Qi Qian[2]

1 Division of Pulmonary/Critical Care, Mayo Clinic Rochester, Rochester, Minnesota, United States of America, 2 Division of Nephrology, Mayo Clinic Rochester, Rochester, Minnesota, United States of America, 3 Department of Radiology, Mayo Clinic Rochester, Rochester, Minnesota, United States of America

Abstract

Background: Polycystin 1 and 2, the protein abnormalities associated with autosomal dominant polycystic kidney disease (ADPKD), are also found in airway cilia and smooth muscle cells. There is evidence of increased radiologic bronchiectasis associated with ADPKD, though the clinical and functional implications of this association are unknown. We hypothesized an increased prevalence of both radiologic and clinical bronchiectasis is associated with APDKD as compared to non-ADPKD chronic kidney disease (CKD) controls.

Materials and Methods: A retrospective case-control study was performed at our institution involving consecutive ADPKD and non-ADPKD chronic kidney disease (CKD) patients seen over a 13 year period with both chest CT and PFT. CTs were independently reviewed by two blinded thoracic radiologists. Manually collected clinical data included symptoms, smoker status, transplant history, and PFT findings.

Results: Ninety-two ADPKD and 95 non-ADPKD CKD control patients were compared. Increased prevalence of radiologic bronchiectasis, predominantly mild lower lobe disease, was found in ADPKD patients compared to CKD control (19 vs. 9%, $P = 0.032$, OR 2.49 (CI 1.1–5.8)). After adjustment for covariates, ADPKD was associated with increased risk of radiologic bronchiectasis (OR 2.78 (CI 1.16–7.12)). Symptomatic bronchiectasis occurred in approximately a third of ADPKD patients with radiologic disease. Smoking was associated with increased radiologic bronchiectasis in ADPKD patients (OR 3.59, CI 1.23–12.1).

Conclusions: Radiological bronchiectasis is increased in patients with ADPKD particularly those with smoking history as compared to non-ADPKD CKD controls. A third of such patients have symptomatic disease. Bronchiectasis should be considered in the differential in ADPKD patients with respiratory symptoms and smoking history.

Editor: Emmanuel A. Burdmann, University of Sao Paulo Medical School, Brazil

Funding: These authors have no support or funding to report.

Competing Interests: The authors have declared that no competing interests exist.

* E-mail: moua.teng@mayo.edu

Introduction

Autosomal dominant polycystic kidney disease (ADPKD) characteristically manifests with progressive fluid filled renal cysts leading to end-stage renal disease in approximately 50% of patients [1,2]. The contributing genetic defects are found in polycystin-1 and 2, two transmembrane regulatory proteins responsible for mechanoreception, cell polarization, and orientation [3,4].

Multiple non-pulmonary extra-renal manifestations of ADPKD have been described [5,6,7]. Interestingly, polycystins are expressed in the cilia of both human airway epithelial [8] and airway smooth muscle cells [9]. Consequently, functional abnormalities in polycystins may result in radiological bronchiectasis due to decreased mucociliary clearance or impaired airway injury repair [8]. The functional and clinical significance of this radiologic association remains mostly unexplored.

In the current study we investigated the possible association of radiologic bronchiectasis with abnormal PFT and increased clinical pulmonary disease in a retrospective review of consecutive ADPKD patients seen at our institution as case patients compared to non-ADPKD CKD controls.

Materials and Methods

IRB approval was obtained (Mayo Clinic IRB#: 09-002623) regarding study of patients giving written consent to have their stored medical records reviewed for the purposes of research. Clinical records of consecutive adult ADPKD patients seen at Mayo Clinic, Rochester, who underwent both high resolution chest computed tomography (HRCT) and pulmonary function testing (PFT) between 1998 and 2011, were reviewed. Patients were excluded if they had a known secondary etiology for clinical or radiologic bronchiectasis as reviewed in the available record, specifically cystic fibrosis (CF), prior mechanical airway obstruction, chest trauma or surgery resulting in focal lung injury, recurrent or severe pneumonia, or clinical immunodeficiencies such as common variable immunodeficiency (CVID) resulting in proclivity towards recurrent infection. Patients who underwent transplantation of any organ other than lung (solid and hematological) were included in the study. Non-ADPKD chronic kidney disease (CKD) patients who also underwent chest CT and PFT during the same study period were selected as consecutive unmatched controls. The most recent chest CT in the record was used if multiple studies were completed.

Collected demographics were manually obtained from the primary medical record for both study groups including age, gender, smoker status (active, former, and non-smoker), pack years, and transplant history. Laboratory data included stable GFR and creatinine within one year of the selected study CT. Clinical pulmonary diagnoses or symptoms of individual study patients at the time of CT were categorized in the following manner: Group 0 = None or no longstanding clinical pulmonary disease, Group 1 = idiopathic clinical bronchiectasis defined as presenting symptoms of chronic productive cough, dyspnea, and/ or other constitutional symptoms such as fever, weight loss, not explained by a secondary or underlying pulmonary diagnosis, Group 2 = All other airways disease (COPD, asthma, bronchial or small airways disease), and Group 3 = All other parenchymal, pleural, or pulmonary vascular disease (acute infection, interstitial lung disease or fibrosis, granulomatous disease, malignant and non-malignant nodules or masses, pulmonary emboli, vasculitis, and pleural disease). For patients with multiple pulmonary diagnoses, idiopathic clinical bronchiectasis (Group 1) was selected first as a primary categorization if present followed by all other airways disease (Group 2), then all other parenchymal/pleural/ pulmonary vascular disease (Group 3). Our rationale was to categorize or capture existing clinical bronchiectasis or airways disease in the setting of radiologic findings.

CT criteria for radiologic bronchiectasis included one or more of the following: 1) an enlarged bronchial diameter greater than that of the accompanying blood vessel (Signet ring sign), 2) failure of airway tapering at least 2 cm beyond the last branch point, or 3) visible airway within one centimeter of the lung periphery [10,11,12]. All selected CT scans were independently reviewed by two experienced thoracic radiologists (RH & TH) who were blinded to the presence of ADPKD and CKD with agreement on presence and severity of radiologic bronchiectasis by consensus.

Pulmonary function testing done within one year of the selected chest CT was categorized based on standard criteria [13,14,15] into one of four diagnostic findings: 1) Normal, 2) Obstructive, 3) Restrictive, or 4) Other (mixed restrictive and obstructive, non-specific pattern, and isolated low diffusing capacity for carbon monoxide (DLCO)); interpreted previously in the record by an experienced non-study pulmonologist. No further revision or reinterpretation of PFT findings was done by study investigators. If PFT was not available within one year of the selected scan, the most recent PFT in the clinical record was reviewed. Selected PFT measurements, including pre-bronchodilator percent predicted forced expiratory volume in 1 second (FEV_1) and forced vital capacity (FVC), total lung capacity (TLC), forced expiratory flow at 25–75% of the FVC (FEF $_{25-75}$), FEV1/FVC ratio, and diffusing capacity for carbon monoxide (DLCO) were also collected and compared between the two cohorts.

Statistical analysis was performed using JMP Software Version 9.4 (Cary, NC) with Chi-square or Fisher's exact test applied to proportional or categorical data, and a Two Sample T-test with 2-sided P value used for comparison of continuous or mean data. Chi-square and ANOVA were used to compare proportion and means among multiple groups. For predictors of a dichotomous outcome, univariable and multivariable logistic regression was applied adjusting for a priori selected covariates of age, gender, GFR, smoker status, and transplant history. Two-tailed P values<0.05 were considered statistically significant.

No external funding was involved in the hypothesis, study design, data collection, or analysis, of this work.

Results

Ninety-two consecutive ADPKD patients and 95 consecutive non-ADPKD CKD patients underwent both chest CT and PFT and were ultimately included in the study and control groups, respectively. Comparison baseline demographic and clinical characteristics are presented in Table 1. Of the initial screening cohort fitting radiologic criteria for bronchiectasis, two were excluded from the ADPKD group secondary to history of prior severe pneumonia as likely causes of radiologic findings, and one was excluded from the CKD group due to concomitant cystic fibrosis diagnosis.

Compared to ADPKD there were more men in the consecutively selected CKD control group (67% vs. 46%, P = 0.003). Mean FEV_1, FVC, and DLCO were statistically lower in the CKD group compared to ADPKD, though smoking status and summary PFT findings were not statistically different (P = 0.35 and P = 0.121, respectively). Frequency of organ transplantation of both solid and hematological origin was similar (P = 0.123). The majority of CT scans in both groups was obtained for assessment of clinical respiratory symptoms or previously established pulmonary disease, with none obtained for incidental findings found initially on lower lung cuts of abdominal CTs. In those whom underwent organ transplantation, 25% of reviewed CTs occurred prior to transplantation. The median time from date of transplant to CT was 35.4 (range −121 to 291) months, with no statistical difference between the two groups (P = 0.62).

Subgroup comparison data for baseline clinical features among APDKD patients with and without radiologic bronchiectasis is presented in Table 2. Smoking history was more prevalent in ADPKD patients with radiological bronchiectasis (74% vs. 44%, P = 0.04) without difference in other baseline characteristics.

Radiologic changes of bronchiectasis were more frequent in ADPKD patients (19 (21%) vs. 9 (9%); P = 0.032, OR 2.49 (CI 1.1–5.8)), with no difference in prevalence of clinically symptomatic disease (6 (7%) vs. 3 (3%), P = 0.32) (Table 1.) Univariate logistic regression for selected covariates is presented in Table 3 for the whole cohort and Table 4 for subgroup analysis of the ADPKD group. The presence of ADPKD was associated with radiologic bronchiectasis, even after adjusting for age, gender, GFR, transplant history, and smoking by multivariate regression (OR 2.78, CI 1.16–7.12). Smoking history among ADPKD patients after adjustment for age, gender, GFR, and transplant history, was associated with increased risk of radiologic bronchiectasis (OR 4.79, CI 1.43–19.58) despite similar rates of smoking between ADPKD and CKD patients. Smoking was not associated with increased clinical disease among the two groups (ADPKD 5/ 6 (83%) vs. 41/86 (47%), P = 0.09 vs. Control 1/3 (33%) vs. 53/92 (57%), P = 0.40).

Distribution of summary PFT patterns and frequency of clinical pulmonary diagnoses were similar among ADPKD patients and controls (Table 5). Statistically lower percent predicted mean FEV_1, FVC, and DLCO were noted in CKD controls (Table 1) despite increased prevalence of active smokers in ADPKD patients. Abnormal FEF 25–75 was primarily associated with concomitant obstructive physiology in those clinically diagnosed with COPD or emphysema followed by advanced restriction seen in interstitial lung disease. There were no isolated low FEF 25–75

Table 1. Demographics and baseline characteristics.

Characteristic	ADPKD (N = 92)	Control (N = 95)	P value
Age, mean (SD)	59.84 (12.6)	61.59 (12.9)	0.35
Gender, M/F (%)	42/50 (46/54)	64/31 (67/33)	**0.003**
BMI, mean (SD)	29.21 (6.9)	30.06 (6.1)	0.37
Smoker Status;			0.35
Non-smoker N (%)	46 (50)	41 (43)	
Former N (%)	38(41)	52 (55)	
Active N (%)	8(9)	2(2)	
Pack years, mean (SD)	31.41 (20.7)	37.32 (29.5)	0.26
Creatinine, mean (SD)	2.10 (1.9)	1.93 (1.2)	0.47
GFR, mean (SD)	50.1 (28.7)	46.92 (25.4)	0.43
Radiologic bronchiectasis, N (%)	19 (21)	9 (9.1)	**0.032**
Clinical bronchiectasis, N (%)	6 (7)	3 (3)	0.32
Summary PFT dx			0.121
Normal, N (%)	42 (46)	29 (31)	
Obstructive, N (%)	26 (28)	30 (31)	
Restrictive, N (%)	6 (6)	13 (14)	
Other, N (%)	18 (20)	23 (24)	
FEV1 % predicted, mean (SD), range	79.28 (21.5), (36–119)	71.96 (24), (22–121)	**0.032**
FVC % predicted, mean (SD), range	86.78 (18.7), (36–134)	77.15 (22.6), (24–119)	**0.003**
FEV1/FVC, mean (SD), range	72.2 (10.1), (35.2–88.5)	72.3 (10.2), (33.9–95.2)	0.98
FEF 25-75 % predicted, mean (SD), range	67.2 (33.1), (13–152)	61 (36.8), (6–174)	0.23
TLC % predicted, mean (SD), range	96.25 (22.4), (53–164) (N = 52)	89.64 (20.1), (47–130) (N = 56)	0.112
DLCO % predicted, mean (SD), range	76.11 (19.3), (34–134) (N = 85)	68.24 (23.4), (17–125) (N = 80)	**0.022**
Transplant of any kind, N (%)	37 (40)	28 (29)	0.123
Time from Transplant to Study CT, months, median (range)	35.4 (−121–291) (N = 37)	31.4 (−30–163.5) (N = 28)	0.63

values with normal FEV1/FVC and TLC to suggest early or small airways disease. Indications for PFT testing were no different between those with APDKD and CKD, primarily done for assessment of acute or chronic respiratory symptoms or those with known pulmonary disease (63%) followed by perioperative assessment for surgical clearance or related pulmonary complications of organ transplantation (37%). There was no difference in final clinical pulmonary diagnoses.

All ADPKD patients with clinical bronchiectasis (6 patients) had at least one or more years (range 14–60 months) of symptoms by the time of their CT assessment. Symptoms included productive cough, recurrent rhinosinusitis, and intermittent dyspnea. Chronic rhinosinusitis was seen in two APDKD patients with clinical bronchiectasis and none without radiologic disease, while occurring in only one patient from the CKD cohort who did not have radiologic disease. No other etiologies for bronchiectasis were evident at the time of clinical assessment. All were treated with various antibiotic and/or inhaler regimens previously or at the time of reviewed CT.

ADPKD-associated bronchiectasis most commonly represented mild bilateral lower lobe radiologic disease as opposed to more focal disease (Table 6) observed in control patients. Cylindrical bronchiectasis was the predominant radiological pattern in both groups (Figure 1).

Discussion

Our study confirms previously reported [8,16] increased prevalence of radiologic bronchiectasis associated with ADPKD (21% vs. 9%, P = 0.032). We observed similarly mild bilateral lower lobe disease using only chest CT studies. In the majority of cases, such radiologic findings were not identified during initial CT interpretation. Approximately one third of ADPKD patients with radiologic bronchiectasis (6 of 19, 32%) also had clinical idiopathic bronchiectasis however there was no difference in PFT pattern or prevalence of other pulmonary diagnoses. Finally, in ADPKD patients, smoking was associated with an increased risk of radiologic bronchiectasis (OR 4.79, CI 1.43–19.58) in our cohort even after adjustment for a priori covariates.

In the US, prevalence of clinically diagnosed bronchiectasis increases with age and ranges between 4.2 per 100,000 (age 18–34) and 271.8 cases per 100,000 individuals (age 75 and older) [17]. A recent trend analysis based on Medicare ICD-9 claims data between 2000 and 2007, found bronchiectasis prevalence to be 8.7% per year (period prevalence of 1,106 cases per 100,000 people) [18]. However, in the absence of universally accepted clinical and radiologic disease definitions, reliable prevalence studies are lacking [19,20]. Kwak and colleagues [21] investigated the prevalence of radiologic bronchiectasis in 1409 Korean adult patients who underwent CT scanning as part of general health assessment. They reported radiologic disease in 129 (9.1%) and

Table 2. Subgroup Analysis of ADPKD with and without radiologic bronchiectasis.

	ADPKD Bronchiectasis (N = 19)	ADPKD No Bronchiectasis (N = 73)	P value
Characteristic			
Age, mean (SD)	62.63 (12.2)	59.1 (12.7)	0.28
Gender, M/F (%)	11/8 (58/42)	31/42 (42/58)	0.23
BMI, mean (SD)	27.52 (5.4)	29.66 (7.3)	0.24
Smoker status;			**0.021**
Non-smoker N (%),	5 (26)	41 (56)	
Former N (%)	12 (63)	26 (36)	
Active N (%)	2 (11)	6 (8)	
Creatinine, mean (SD)	1.62 (1.1)	2.23 (2.1)	0.24
GFR, mean (SD)	52.26 (22.7)	49.53 (30.2)	0.71
PFT dx			0.52
Normal, N (%)	8 (42)	34 (47)	
Obstructive, N (%)	6 (32)	20 (27)	
Restrictive, N (%)	0 (0)	6 (8)	
Other, N (%)	5 (26)	13 (18)	
FEV1 % predicted, mean (SD), range	81.42 (19.9), (39–108)	78.73 (22.1), (36–119)	0.63
FVC % predicted, mean (SD), range	87.68 (14.6), (53–105)	86.55 (19.7), (36–134)	0.81
FEV1/FVC (SD), range	72.32 (9.9), (55.6–86.5)	72.22 (10.3), (35.2–88.5)	0.96
FEF 25–75 % predicted (SD), range	60.5 (33.2), (15–136)	68.9 (33.1), (13–152)	0.33
TLC % predicted, mean (SD), range	99.7 (13.6), (79–122) (N = 10)	95.43 (24.1), (53–164) (N = 42)	0.59
DLCO % predicted, mean (SD), range	71.83 (19), (45–107) (N = 18)	77.25 (19.4), (34–134) (N = 67)	0.29
Transplant of any kind (N, %)	10 (53)	27 (37)	0.22
Time from Transplant to study CT, months, median (range)	67. 4 (−37–268)	22.8 (−120–292)	0.27

more than half were clinically symptomatic (53.7%) [21]. Female gender, increased age, and history of prior tuberculosis were risk factors for the presence of radiologic disease in the study. Despite comprehensive medical evaluation the cause of bronchiectasis frequently remained unidentified and such cases were subsequently classified as idiopathic. While we used a non-ADPKD CKD control cohort in our study, currently available evidence does not suggest a higher risk of radiological or clinical bronchiectasis in such patients. We did find a similar rate of radiologic bronchiectasis (9%) in our control patients as compared to the general population studied by Kwak et al.

Table 3. Univariate logistic regression analysis for predictors of radiologic bronchiectasis for the entire cohort (N = 187).

	Odds Ratio	95% Confidence Intervals	P value
Age	0.98	0.94–1.01	0.202
Gender	1.21	0.54–2.83	0.64
Smoker status	1.69	0.75–4.0	0.21
Presence of ADPKD	2.49	1.1–6.1	**0.031**
Creatinine	0.98	0.73–1.24	0.88
GFR	1.0	0.98–1.01	0.92
FEV1	1.42	0.25–8.32	0.69
FVC	1.0	0.99–1.02	0.52
TLC	1.0	0.98–1.03	0.50
DLCO	0.99	0.97–1.01	0.161
Transplant Hx	1.25	0.54–2.85	0.59
Time from Transplant to Study CT	1.01	0.99–1.02	0.141

Table 4. Subgroup univariate logistic regression analysis for predictors of radiologic bronchiectasis in patients with ADPKD (N = 92).

	Odds Ratio	95% Confidence Intervals	P value
Age	1.02	0.98–1.07	0.27
Gender	1.86	0.68–5.33	0.23
Smoker status	3.59	1.23–12.1	**0.026**
Creatinine	0.80	0.51–1.10	0.185
GFR	1.0	0.99–1.02	0.71
FEV1	1.0	0.98–1.03	0.62
FVC	1.0	0.98–1.03	0.81
TLC	1.0	0.97–1.04	0.59
DLCO	0.98	0.95–1.01	0.28
Transplant Hx	1.89	0.68–5.34	0.22
Time from Transplant to Study CT	1.0	0.99–1.01	0.26

Jain et al. recently reviewed the clinical and radiologic features of ADPKD associated bronchiectasis in 163 transplanted and non-transplanted patients [16]. They found older age as predictive of radiologic disease using a modified scoring system with the majority of presenting radiologic features similarly mild in nature. Although demographic data was not available in all studied patients, only older age was again seen as a significant risk factor for bronchiectasis based on multivariable analysis. There was also noted increased frequency and severity of radiologic disease among those with renal transplantation compared to non-transplanted patients (52.4% vs 31.4%, P = 0.02). In contrast, our study noted significant correlation of radiologic bronchiectasis with active and prior smoking history, without difference in age distribution among our more highly selected cohort using chest CT and PFT findings. Including both solid (excluding lung transplant) and hematologic organ transplants in both case and control cohorts, we noted no difference in frequency of both radiologic and clinical bronchiectasis.

The spectrum of clinical disease among those with radiologic bronchiectasis was mild to moderate at most and not statistically different between the two groups in our study. Although symptoms were reported on average greater than a year prior to selected study CT, none had history of significant weight loss, recurrent fevers, or hemoptysis. Even among those with persistent clinical symptoms, severity of radiologic disease was not advanced, with

the majority of all patients with radiologic disease presenting as mild cylindrical bilateral lower lobe disease.

While the overall rate of smoking was similar between ADPKD and control patients, subgroup analysis revealed that radiologic bronchiectasis occurred more frequently in ADPKD smokers than non-smokers. This association is intriguing in the setting of known airway epithelial injury with exposure to cigarette smoke including impaired mucociliary clearance, stunned ciliary function, and decreased ciliary growth [22,23,24,25,26]. Smoking may further hasten these effects in patients with ADPKD whom perhaps have intrinsic ciliary dysfunction as compared to CKD controls whom did not see an association of radiologic bronchiectasis with smoking history in our study. Further work is needed to confirm this association while smoking cessation should be generally encouraged in all patients.

Interestingly we observed statistically lower mean FEV_1, FVC, and DLCO among CKD patients compared to ADPKD despite comparable smoking status. As CKD patients were consecutively allocated based on presence of HRCT and PFT without matching, such findings were unlikely explained by smoking having a protective effect on PFT findings in ADPKD patients or a much more severe effect in CKD. Smoking over the entire cohort was not associated with increased radiologic or clinical bronchiectasis, but again with subgroup analysis of ADPKD patients, significantly associated with radiologic disease even after correction for a priori covariates. Summary PFT findings (normal, obstructive,

Table 5. Frequency and distribution of summary respiratory diagnoses.

	No Clinical Respiratory Disease (Group 0)	Idiopathic clinical bronchiectasis (Group 1)	All Other Airways Diseases (Group 2)	Other Respiratory (Group 3)
ADPKD¶				
Radiologic Bronchiectasis (N = 19)	2	6	5	6
No bronchiectasis (N = 73)	15	0	22	36
Control¶				
Radiologic Bronchiectasis (N = 9)	2	3	0	4
No bronchiectasis (N = 86)	22	0	20	44

¶P values were not significant for distribution of clinical respiratory diagnoses between ADPKD cohort and control.

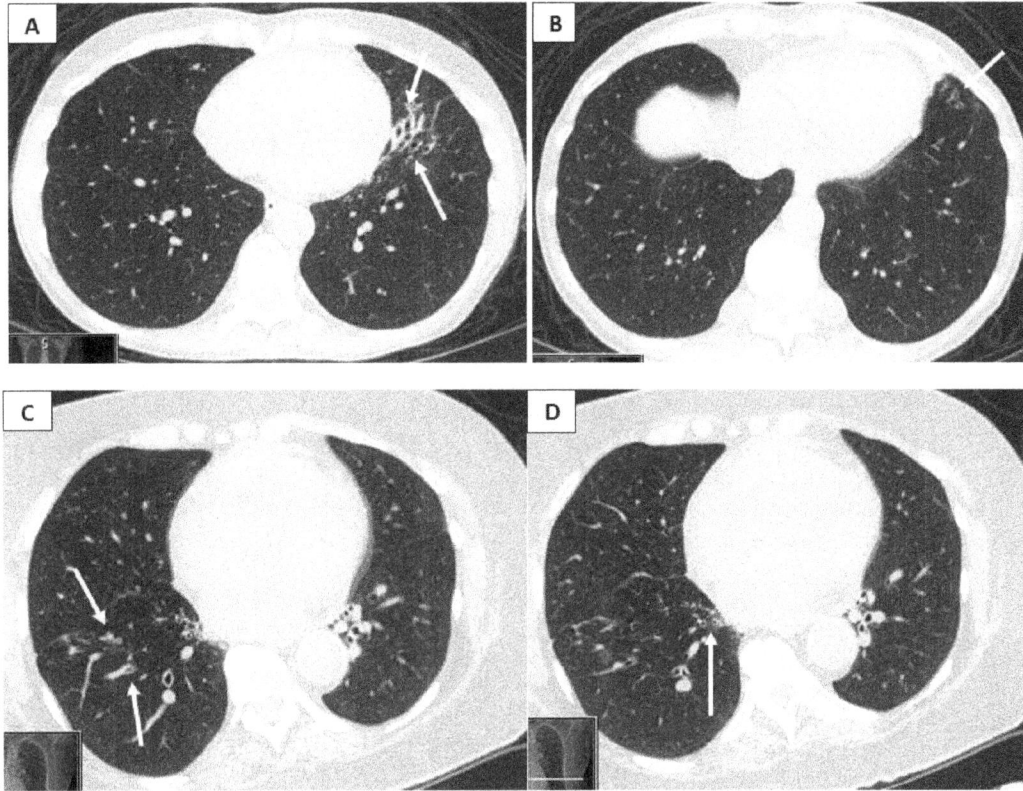

Figure 1. Radiologic and clinical bronchiectasis associated with ADPKD. Top panels (A and B) represent bronchiectasis in a 65 yo ADPKD female with productive cough and dyspnea on exertion, without a known secondary etiology. Panel B delineates enlarged airways visible within 1 cm of the lung periphery. Second panels (C and D) represent radiologic bronchiectasis manifesting predominantly in the right lower lobe of a 70 yo ADPKD female without clinical disease.

restrictive, and other) were not statistically different between ADPKD and CKD patients, or among ADPKD patients with or without radiologic or clinical bronchiectasis.

A proposed mechanism for the development of bronchiectasis in patients with ADPKD may be linked to abnormalities in polycystin-1 and 2, the gene products of PKD1 and PKD 2 located on chromosomes 16 and 4 respectively. Although alterations of these genes are responsible along with other genetic abnormalities for renal cyst formation [1,27,28], expression of both of these genes have been reported in various cell types involved in the extra-renal manifestations of ADPKD, including valvular heart disease, vascular aneurysm, gut diverticula, and hepatic cysts [1,28]. The presence of functional polycystin-1 in the motile cilia of human airway epithelial cells [8] and primary cilia of human airway smooth muscle cells [9] has also been demonstrated. These particular cells have been implicated in

airway ciliary function and injury repair with decreased function due to polycystin abnormality, perhaps an underlying mechanism by which ADPKD patients develop radiologic and clinical bronchiectasis. The negative impact of cigarette smoke may possibly hasten these effects. Although suggestive, more directed studies are needed to confirm this mechanism at a cellular level.

Strengths of our study include the review of ADPKD patients with both high resolution chest CT (as opposed to abdominal CT with lower lung cuts) and comprehensive PFT, allowing assessment and comparison of both radiologic and functional characteristics. While our cohort provided a more specific assessment of ADPKD-associated clinical and radiologic bronchiectasis, exclusion of ADPKD and control patients whom did not undergo CT and PFT may have underestimated the true prevalence of radiologic disease, explaining our lower prevalence of radiologic findings as compared to Driscoll and colleagues [8]. As well, such

Table 6. Location and distribution of ADPKD-associated radiologic bronchiectasis.

Lobe	Focal	Unilateral Multilobe	Diffuse (bilateral multilobe)	RUL*	RML	RLL	LUL	LML (lingula)	LLL
Group									
ADPKD (N)	7	2	10	1	6	13	0	2	13
Control (N)	6	1	2	2	3	3	1	1	4

*RUL = right upper lobe; RML = right middle lobe; RLL = right lower lobe; LUL = left upper lobe; LML = left middle lobe; LLL = left lower lobe.

selection may bias towards patients with other respiratory symptoms or pulmonary disease whose presentation may be difficult to differentiate from clinical bronchiectasis, and may not represent again a true estimate of less symptomatic bronchiectatic disease where chest CT and PFT would not have been obtained. However, our methodology was less likely to have missed ADPKD patients with more advanced or clinically relevant bronchiectasis, one of our study objectives. Another possible confounder is the inclusion of transplanted patients, whose immunosuppression may have led to increased risk of both radiologic and clinical bronchiectasis. While immunosuppression may be contributory, clinical bronchiectasis was infrequent and similar between the two groups with both groups having similar transplantation rates. As well, median time from date of transplantation to study CT was statistically similar making duration of transplantation over time less likely contributory to increased risk of infection or immuno-suppression related radiologic or clinical bronchiectasis. Finally, our study has all the limitations associated with retrospective data collection and reflects the patient population of a tertiary referral center. It did allow though for maximal accrual of selected patients

for a meaningful analysis using more strict radiologic and functional inclusion criteria.

In conclusion, we observed an increased prevalence of radiologic bronchiectasis among ADPKD patients who underwent high resolution chest CT. These changes most frequently involved mild-to-moderate cylindrical bronchiectasis with bilateral lower lung predominance. There were no differences in summary PFT abnormalities or frequency of clinical disease. A history of smoking in patients with APDKD may predispose to the development of radiologic and clinical bronchiectasis and smoking cessation should be generally encouraged. Radiologic bronchiectasis may be regarded as an extra-renal manifestation of ADPKD with further studies needed to explore this association.

Author Contributions

Conceived and designed the experiments: TM LZ DQ RH TH TP QQ. Performed the experiments: TM LZ RH TH. Analyzed the data: TM LZ QQ TP TH RH DQ. Wrote the paper: TM TP QQ.

References

1. Torres VE, Harris PC (2006) Mechanisms of Disease: autosomal dominant and recessive polycystic kidney diseases. Nature clinical practice Nephrology 2: 40–55; quiz 55.
2. Barua M, Pei Y (2010) Diagnosis of autosomal-dominant polycystic kidney disease: an integrated approach. Seminars in nephrology 30: 356–365.
3. Hopp K, Ward CJ, Hommerding CJ, Nasr SH, Tuan HF, et al. (2012) Functional polycystin-1 dosage governs autosomal dominant polycystic kidney disease severity. The Journal of clinical investigation 122: 4257–4273.
4. Gallagher AR, Germino GG, Somlo S (2010) Molecular advances in autosomal dominant polycystic kidney disease. Advances in chronic kidney disease 17: 118–130.
5. Qian Q, Hartman RP, King BF, Torres VE (2007) Increased occurrence of pericardial effusion in patients with autosomal dominant polycystic kidney disease. Clinical journal of the American Society of Nephrology: CJASN 2: 1223–1227.
6. Qian Q, Younge BR, Torres VE (2007) Retinal arterial and venous occlusions in patients with ADPKD. Nephrology, dialysis, transplantation : official publication of the European Dialysis and Transplant Association - European Renal Association 22: 1769–1771.
7. Kumar S, Adeva M, King BF, Kamath PS, Torres VE (2006) Duodenal diverticulosis in autosomal dominant polycystic kidney disease. Nephrology, dialysis, transplantation : official publication of the European Dialysis and Transplant Association - European Renal Association 21: 3576–3578.
8. Driscoll JA, Bhalla S, Liapis H, Ibricevic A, Brody SL (2008) Autosomal dominant polycystic kidney disease is associated with an increased prevalence of radiographic bronchiectasis. Chest 133: 1181–1188.
9. Wu J, Du H, Wang X, Mei C, Sieck GC, et al. (2009) Characterization of primary cilia in human airway smooth muscle cells. Chest 136: 561–570.
10. Naidich DP, McCauley DI, Khouri NF, Stitik FP, Siegelman SS (1982) Computed tomography of bronchiectasis. Journal of computer assisted tomography 6: 437–444.
11. Muller NL, Bergin CJ, Ostrow DN, Nichols DM (1984) Role of computed tomography in the recognition of bronchiectasis. AJR American journal of roentgenology 143: 971–976.
12. Kim JS, Muller NL, Park CS, Grenier P, Herold CJ (1997) Cylindrical bronchiectasis: diagnostic findings on thin-section CT. AJR American journal of roentgenology 168: 751–754.
13. Miller MR, Hankinson J, Brusasco V, Burgos F, Casaburi R, et al. (2005) Standardisation of spirometry. The European respiratory journal 26: 319–338.
14. Wanger J, Clausen JL, Coates A, Pedersen OF, Brusasco V, et al. (2005) Standardisation of the measurement of lung volumes. The European respiratory journal 26: 511–522.
15. Pellegrino R, Viegi G, Brusasco V, Crapo RO, Burgos F, et al. (2005) Interpretative strategies for lung function tests. The European respiratory journal 26: 948–968.
16. Jain R, Javidan-Nejad C, Alexander-Brett J, Horani A, Cabellon MC, et al. (2012) Sensory functions of motile cilia and implication for bronchiectasis. Frontiers in bioscience 4: 1088–1098.
17. Weycker D, Edelsberg J., Oster G., and Tino G. (2005) Prevalence and economic burden of bronchiectasis. Clinical Pulmonary Medicine 12: 205–209.
18. Seitz AE, Olivier KN, Adjemian J, Holland SM, Prevots R (2012) Trends in bronchiectasis among medicare beneficiaries in the United States, 2000 to 2007. Chest 142: 432–439.
19. Barker AF (2002) Bronchiectasis. The New England journal of medicine 346: 1383–1393.
20. O'Donnell AE (2008) Bronchiectasis. Chest 134: 815–823.
21. Kwak HJ, Moon JY, Choi YW, Kim TH, Sohn JW, et al. (2010) High prevalence of bronchiectasis in adults: analysis of CT findings in a health screening program. The Tohoku journal of experimental medicine 222: 237–242.
22. Tamashiro E, Xiong G, Anselmo-Lima WT, Kreindler JL, Palmer JN, et al. (2009) Cigarette smoke exposure impairs respiratory epithelial ciliogenesis. American journal of rhinology & allergy 23: 117–122.
23. Leopold PL, O'Mahony MJ, Lian XJ, Tilley AE, Harvey BG, et al. (2009) Smoking is associated with shortened airway cilia. PloS one 4: e8157.
24. Maestrelli P, Saetta M, Mapp CE, Fabbri LM (2001) Remodeling in response to infection and injury. Airway inflammation and hypersecretion of mucus in smoking subjects with chronic obstructive pulmonary disease. American journal of respiratory and critical care medicine 164: S76–80.
25. Simet SM, Sisson JH, Pavlik JA, Devasure JM, Boyer C, et al. (2010) Long-term cigarette smoke exposure in a mouse model of ciliated epithelial cell function. American journal of respiratory cell and molecular biology 43: 635–640.
26. Bhatta N, Dhakal SS, Rizal S, Kralingen KW, Niessen L (2008) Clinical spectrum of patients presenting with bronchiectasis in Nepal: evidence of linkage between tuberculosis, tobacco smoking and toxic exposure to biomass smoke. Kathmandu University medical journal 6: 195–203.
27. Chapin HC, Caplan MJ (2010) The cell biology of polycystic kidney disease. The Journal of cell biology 191: 701–710.
28. Al-Bhalal L, Akhtar M (2005) Molecular basis of autosomal dominant polycystic kidney disease. Advances in anatomic pathology 12: 126–133.

24

Analysis of a Urinary Biomarker Panel for Obstructive Nephropathy and Clinical Outcomes

Yuanyuan Xie[1], Wei Xue[2]*, Xinghua Shao[1], Xiajing Che[1], Weijia Xu[1], Zhaohui Ni[1], Shan Mou[1]*

1 Department of Nephrology, Molecular Cell Lab for Kidney Disease, Ren Ji Hospital, School of Medicine, Shanghai Jiao Tong University, Shanghai, P.R. China,
2 Department of Urology, Ren Ji Hospital, School of Medicine, Shanghai Jiao Tong University, Shanghai, P.R. China

Abstract

Objectives: To follow up renal function changes in patients with obstructive nephropathy and to evaluate the predictive value of biomarker panel in renal prognosis.

Methods: A total of 108 patients with obstructive nephropathy were enrolled in the study; 90 patients completed the follow-up. At multiple time points before and after obstruction resolution, urinary samples were prospectively collected in patients with obstructive nephropathy; the levels of urinary kidney injury molecule-1 (uKIM-1), liver-type fatty acid-binding protein (uL-FABP), and neutrophil gelatinase associated lipocalin (uNGAL) were determined by enzyme-linked immunosorbent assay (ELISA). After 1 year of follow-up, the predictive values of biomarker panel for determining the prognosis of obstructive nephropathy were evaluated.

Results: uKIM-1 ($r = 0.823$), uL-FABP ($r = 0.670$), and uNGAL ($r = 0.720$) levels were positively correlated with the serum creatinine level (all $P<0.01$). The levels of uKIM-1, uL-FABP, and uNGAL were higher in the renal function deterioration group than in the renal function stable group. Cox regression analysis revealed that the 72-h postoperative uKIM-1 level and the preoperative and 72-h postoperative uL-FABP levels were all risk factors for renal function deterioration (all $P<0.01$). The area under the curve of Receiver Operating Characteristic(ROC-AUCs) of 72-h postoperative uKIM-1, preoperative uL-FABP, and 72-h postoperative uL-FABP were 0.786, 0.911, and 0.875, respectively. When the combined preoperative uKIM-1, uL-FABP, and uNGAL levels or combined 72-h postoperative uKIM-1, uL-FABP, and uNGAL levels were considered, the accuracy of prediction for renal prognosis was markedly increased, with an ROC-AUC of 0.967 or 0.964, respectively. Kaplan-Meier survival curve analysis demonstrated that a 72-h postoperative uKIM-1>96.69 pg/mg creatinine (Cr), a preoperative uL-FABP>154.62 ng/mg Cr, and a 72-h postoperative uL-FABP>99.86 ng/mg Cr were all positively correlated with poor prognosis (all $P<0.01$).

Conclusion: Biomarker panel may be used as a marker for early screening of patients with obstructive nephropathy and for determining poor prognosis.

Editor: Jean-Claude Dussaule, INSERM, France

Funding: This study was supported in part by the National Basic Research Program of China 973 Program No. 2012CB517600 (No. 2012CB517602). The study was also sponsored by Hong Kong, Macao and Taiwan Science & Technology Cooperation Program of China (2014DFT30090), the National Natural Science Foundation of China (81102700, 81373865 and 81370794) and by grants 12401906400 and 14140903200 from the Science and Technology Commission of Shanghai Municipality, China, and ZYSNXD012-RC-ZXY017 from the Shanghai Health Bureau. Funding scheme for training young teachers in Colleges and universities in Shanghai was also included in the fund. The funders had no role in study design, data collection and analysis, decision to publish, or preparation of the manuscript.

Competing Interests: The authors have declared that no competing interests exist.

* Email: uroxuewei@163.com (WX); shan_mou@126.com (SM)

Introduction

Obstructive nephropathy is a common cause of acute kidney injury (AKI), chronic kidney disease (CKD) and end-stage renal disease (ESRD) [1–4]. Nephrolithiasis is an independent, albeit small, risk factor for CKD. The renal function of patients with obstructive nephropathy is initially slowly decreased, followed by rapid deterioration of renal function once AKI occurs. Even during the early stage of AKI, the occurrence of AKI may facilitate the progression of the disease as well as earlier progression into ESRD [5]. Ten years after discharge from the hospital, 24.0% to 61.6% of AKI patients have progressed into stage 3 and stage 5 CKD, respectively [6]. As a severe complication, AKI is now recognized as a short- and long-term risk factor for poor prognosis. Several biomarkers for the early diagnosis of AKI have been proposed, including kidney injury molecule-1 (KIM-1), liver-type fatty acid-binding protein (L-FABP), and neutrophil gelatinase-associated lipocalin (NGAL) [7]. However, the usefulness of these markers for evaluating renal disease progression remains unclear [8]. Studies of the application of urinary KIM-1 (uKIM-1) and urinary L-FABP (uL-FABP) in obstructive nephropathy have been limited, and further studies are needed to validate their use as predictive parameters for the prognosis of obstructive nephropathy progression. In this study, uKIM-1 and uL-FABP levels were measured at multiple time points during long-term follow-up of patients with obstructive nephropathy to investigate the potential predictive values of these biomarkers as renal prognostic parameters in patients with obstructive nephropathy.

Subjects and Methods

Subjects

The criteria for inclusion in the study were as follows: patients with obstructive nephropathy confirmed by surgery performed at our institute, age ≥18 years old, male or female, with complete clinical records and diagnosis using urinary system ultrasound, CT scan, or kidney radioisotope scanning. The etiology for obstructive nephropathy in all patients was lithiasis. There were unilateral incomplete obstructions, unilateral complete obstructions and bilateral incomplete obstructions. The exclusion criteria were as follows: patients <18 years old, ESRD with regular hemodialysis or peritoneal dialysis, AKI of other causation, prior history of kidney diseases, immune system diseases, solid tumors or other complications, or clinical presentation indicating acute or chronic infection.

Obstructive nephropathy refers to the renal disease resulting from impaired flow of urine or tubular fluid as a consequence of structural or functional abnormalities in the urinary tract [9].

Obstructive nephropathies in all subjects were confirmed by imaging results and surgery. Functional impairment referred to split renal function decline in radionuclide scan.

The study was approved by the Ethics Committee of Ren Ji Hospital, School of Medicine, Shanghai Jiao Tong University, Shanghai, 200127, P.R. China and all participants gave written informed consent.

Urine sample collection

A 10-mL sample of fresh urine was collected preoperatively and 4 h, 8 h, 12 h, 24 h, 48 h, and 72 h postoperatively, respectively, for each patient and centrifuged at 1,000×g for 15 min. The supernatant was transferred to an Eppendorf tube and stored at −80°C until use.

Determination of biological parameters

Serum creatinine (sCr) and urinary creatinine (uCr) were determined using an enzyme assay. uKIM-1 levels were determined by enzyme-linked immunosorbent assay (ELISA) (R&D Company, Minneapolis, USA). The corresponding concentrations in the samples were calculated based on the standard curve and expressed as pg/mg Cr after synchronous correction

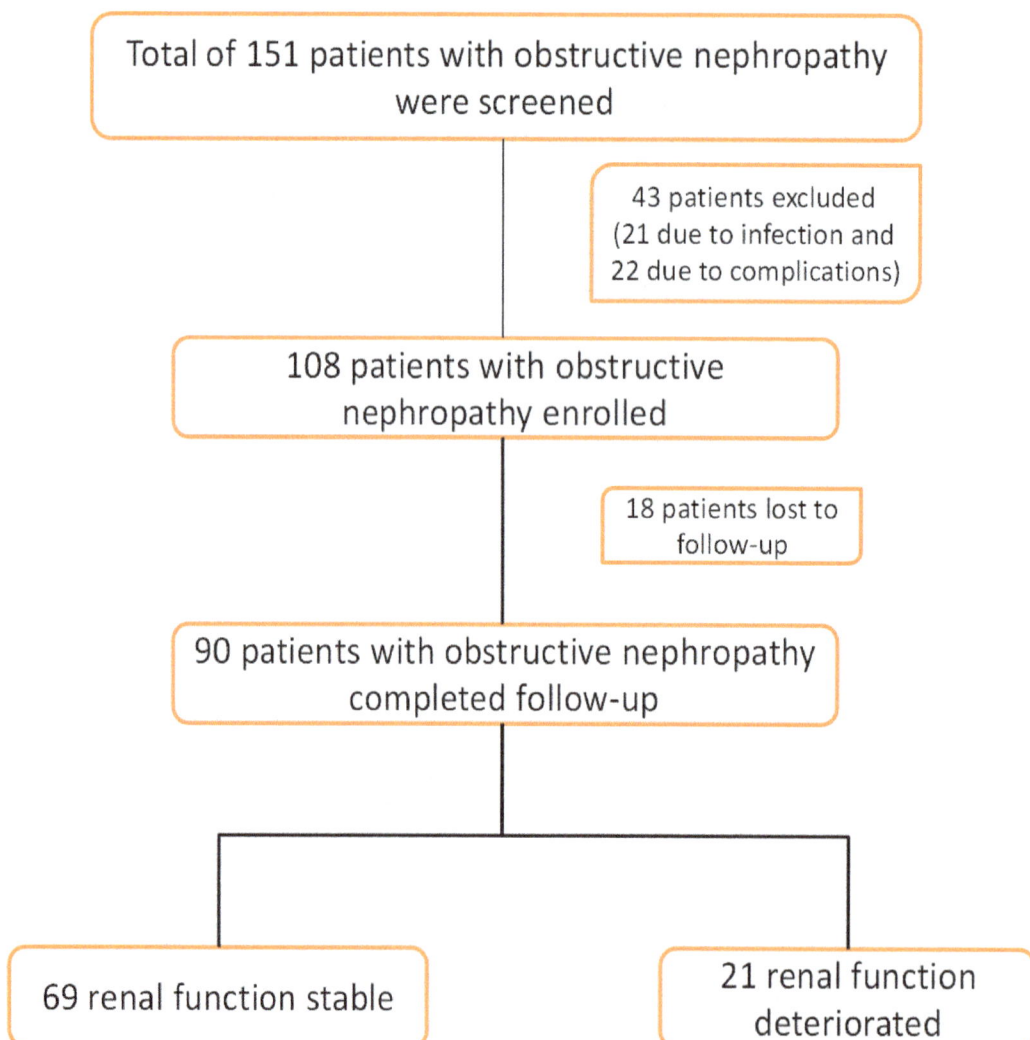

Figure 1. Study flow chart.

Table 1. Characteristics of the study group and healthy subjects.

Variable	ON patients	Healthy subjects	P
Sex (n; male/female)	90 (61/29)	28 (16/12)	NS
Age (years)	54.69±9.87	50.77±6.25	NS
Body weight (kg)	69.56±11.68	68.11±10.91	NS
RBC ($\times 10^{12}$/L)	4.15 (3.48–4.63)	5.10 (3.28–6.36)	NS
WBC ($\times 10^{9}$/L)	6.79 (5.63–8.84)	5.43 (4.85–8.66)	NS
Hemoglobin (g/dL)	129.45 (104.25–140.5)	130.69 (105.1–140.5)	NS
Serum albumin (g/L)	43.41 (39.5–46.81)	42.03 (37.41–45.65)	NS
ALT (IU/L)	20.34 (7.35–25.35)	21.2 (7.55–25.15)	NS
AST (U/L)	17.65 (14.25–25.35)	16.5 (12.35–23.8)	NS
Total cholesterol (mmol/L)	5.3 (3.96–6.52)	5.60 (3.66–7.56)	NS
Triglycerides (mmol/L)	1.55 (1.39–2.98)	1.77 (1.43–2.82)	NS
Renal function			
Serum creatinine (μmol/L)	454.64 (73.1–873.23)	71.96 (59.03–84.89)	0.001
GFR (ml/min/1.73 m^2)	9.7 (5.2–93)	96.18 (78.22–109.9)	0.000
Urinary NAG (U/mg)	20.53 (14.93–56.54)	2.1 (1.6–10.5)	0.001
Urinary L-FABP (ng/mg)	130.13 (36.67–755.07)	20.12 (16.43–93.69)	0.001
Urinary KIM-1 (pg/mg)	433.23 (160.43–628.12)	109.03 (54.21–266.36)	0.002
Urinary NGAL (ng/mg)	386.03 (103.25–1286.75)	65.61 (39.9–263.25)	0.000

GFR, glomerular filtration rate; AST, glutamate oxaloacetate transaminase; ALT, glutamate pyruvate transaminase; L-FABP, liver-type fatty acid-binding protein; NGAL, neutrophil gelatinase-associated lipocalin; KIM-1, kidney injury molecule-1; NAG, N-acetyl-β-D-glucosaminidase; RBC, red blood cells; WBC, white blood cells.

with uCr. The uL-FABP level was determined by ELISA (Hycult Biotech, Uden, The Netherlands). The corresponding concentrations in the samples were calculated based on the standard curve and expressed as ng/mg Cr after synchronous correction with uCr. The uNGAL level was determined by ELISA (Hycult Biotech, Uden, The Netherlands). The corresponding concentrations in the samples were calculated based on the standard curve and expressed as ng/mg Cr after synchronous correction with uCr. The glomerular filtration rate (GFR) was estimated using the simplified formulation of modified diet in renal disease (MDRD), i.e., eGFR = $186 \times (sCr/88.4)^{-1.154} \times age^{-0.203} \times (0.742, female)$ [10].

Grouping

After 1-year of follow-up, the patients were classified into two groups: the stable renal function group and the deteriorated renal function group. Stable renal function was defined as a sCr that decreased to the baseline level before obstruction, increased <50% versus the baseline level, or a stable sCr level within the normal range.

Statistical considerations

Statistical analysis was performed using SPSS13.0 software. Normally distributed data of normal were expressed as $mean \pm SD$, and the t test was used for inter-group comparisons; non-normally distributed data were expressed using the median (M) and interquartile range (P_{25}, P_{75}), and the rank sum test was used for inter-group comparison. Spearman correlation analysis was used to analyze correlations. The sensitivity and specificity of uKIM-1 and uL-FABP for renal prognosis were evaluated using the ROC curve and area under the curve. Relevant risk factors that might influence renal prognosis were analyzed using Cox multifactor regression analysis. The Kaplan-Meier survival curve was used to analyze the survival rate. Statistical significance was set at $P < 0.05$.

Results

General information

A total of 151 patients were screened, and 108 were enrolled in the study; 18 patients were lost to follow-up and excluded from the study. Ultimately, 90 patients with obstructive nephropathy were included in the study; of these, 54 patients progressed to AKI, and 36 did not progress to AKI. At 1-year follow-up, 69 patients were classified as renal function stable, and 21 were classified as renal function deteriorated (Figure 1).

The age of the 90 patients with obstructive nephropathy ranged from 37 to 76 years (average 54.69±9.87). The male/female ratio was 2.1:1. The level of serum creatinine (sCr) was 454.64 (73.1–873.23) μmol/L, eGFR was 9.7 (5.2–93) mL/min/1.73 m^2, uNAG was 20.53 (14.93–56.54) U/mg Cr, uKIM-1 was 433.23 (160.43–628.12) pg/mg Cr, uL-FABP was 130.13 (36.67–755.07) ng/mg Cr, and uNGAL was 386.03 (103.25–1286.75) ng/mg Cr. The uKIM-1, uNGAL, and uL-FABP levels were higher in patients with obstructive nephropathy than in the normal control group (Table 1).

uKIM-1, uL-FABP, and uNGAL levels and correlation with sCr and eGFR

The Spearman correlation analysis demonstrated that the uKIM-1 level was positively correlated with the serum creatinine level (r = 0.823; P = 0.000) and negatively correlated with eGFR (r = −0.869; P = 0.000). The uL-FABP level was positively correlated with the serum creatinine level (r = 0.670; P = 0.000) and negatively correlated with eGFR (r = −0.681; P = 0.000). The uNGAL level was positively correlated with the serum creatinine level (r = 0.720; P = 0.003) and negatively correlated with eGFR (r = −0.784; P = 0.001).

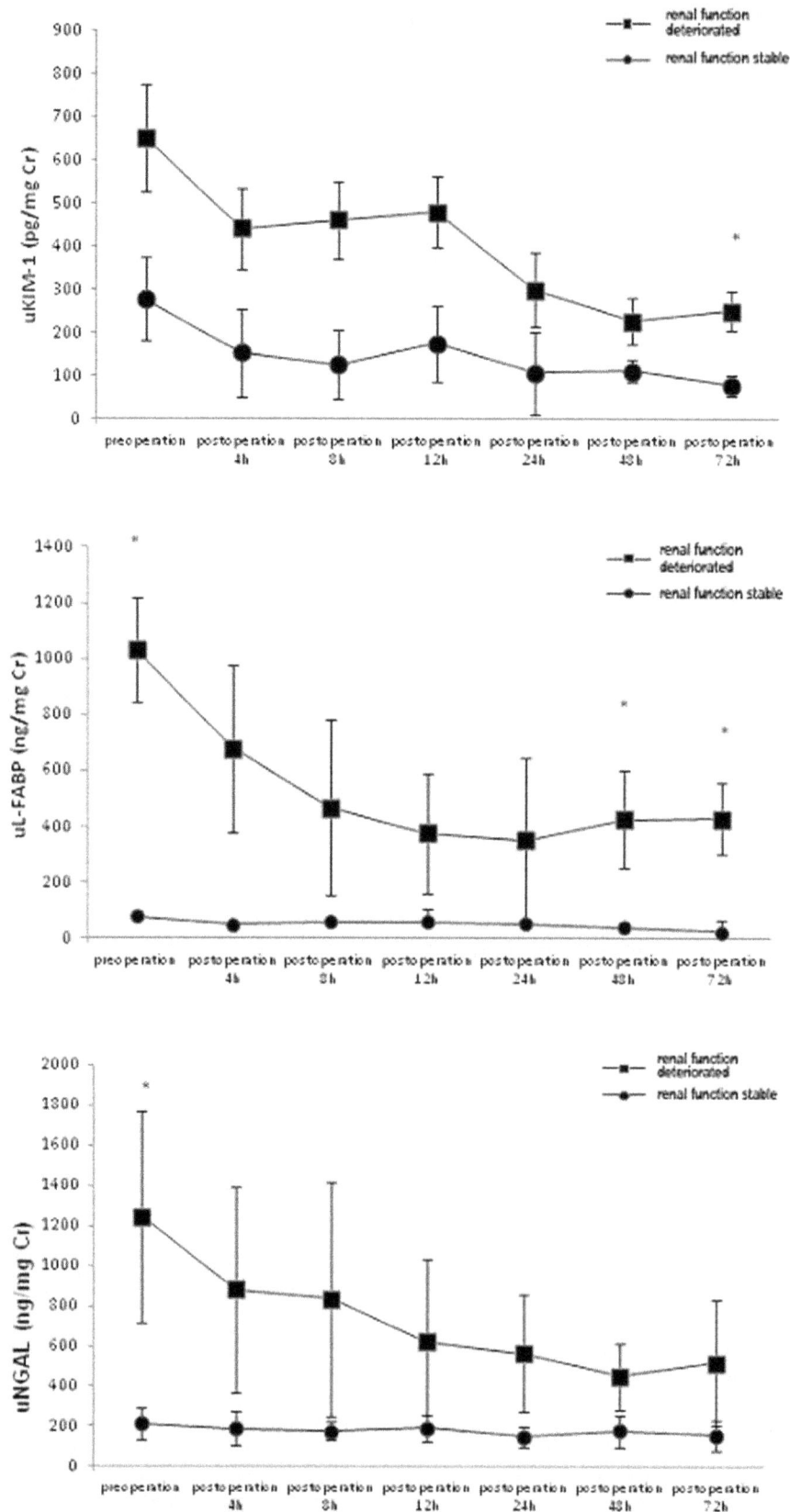

Figure 2. Comparison of the deteriorated renal function group and the stable group at 1-year follow-up. *The differences between the deteriorated renal function group and the stable group were statistically significant (P<0.05).

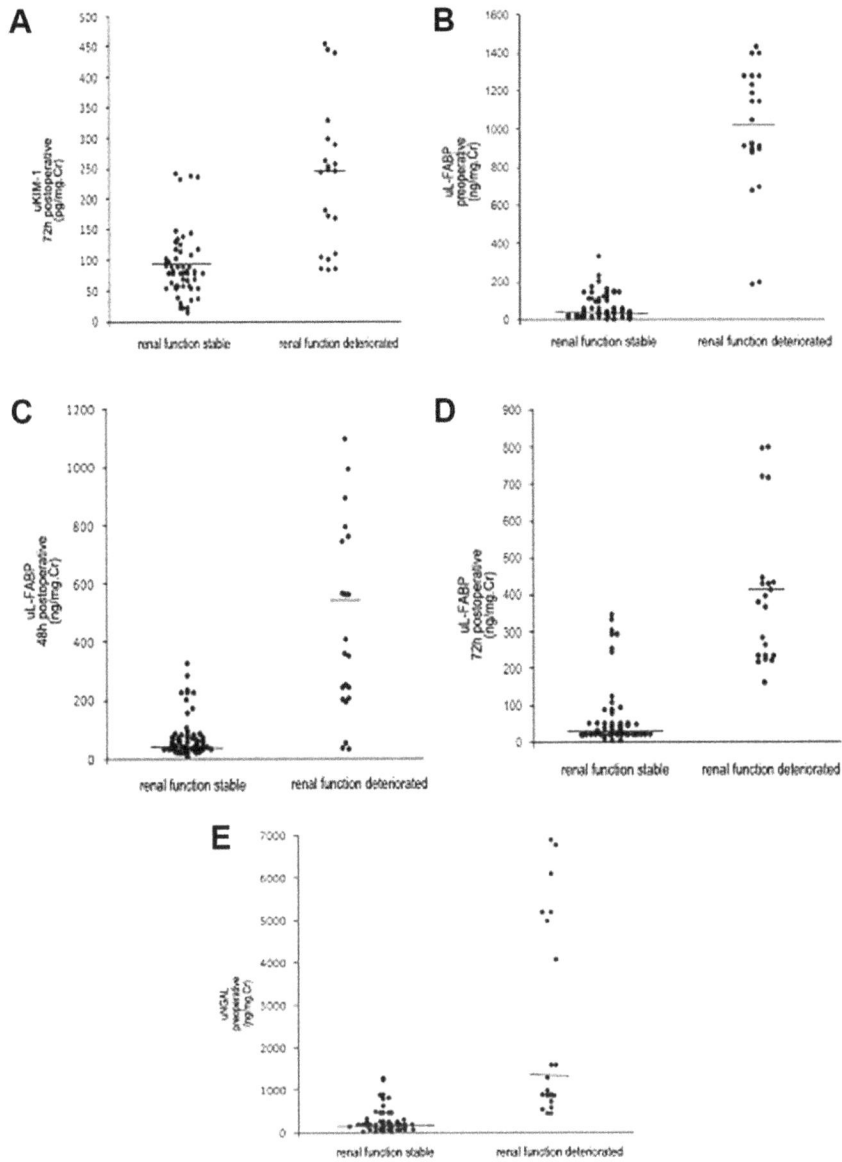

Figure 3. Distribution of biomarker levels in the deteriorated renal function group and the stable group at 1-year follow-up. A. Distribution of 72-h postoperative uKIM-1 levels in the deteriorated renal function group and the stable group at 1-year follow-up. B. Distribution of preoperative uL-FABP levels in the deteriorated renal function group and the stable group at 1-year follow-up. C. Distribution of 48-h postoperative uL-FABP levels in the deteriorated renal function group and the stable group at 1-year follow-up. D. Distribution of 72-h postoperative uL-FABP levels in the deteriorated renal function group and the stable group at 1-year follow-up. E. Distribution of preoperative uNGAL levels in the deteriorated renal function group and the stable group at 1-year follow-up.

Table 2. Relevant risk factors influencing the long-term renal prognosis of patients.

	Prognosis of patients		
	Mean ± standard deviation	HR (95% CI)	P
Preoperative uL-FABP (ng/mg Cr)	367.63±112.51	1.002 (1.001–1.004)	0.003
72 h postoperative uL-FABP (ng/mg Cr)	220.36±59.65	1.003 (1.001–1.007)	0.007
72 h postoperative uKIM-1 (pg/mg Cr)	132.68±29.34	1.008 (1.001–1.013)	0.009

Table 3. AUC for renal prognosis prediction.

	ROC-AUC	Cut-off	Sensitivity	Specificity
72-h postoperative uKIM-1 (pg/mg Cr)	0.786 (0.677–0.894)	96.69	85.7%	75%
preoperative uL-FABP (ng/mg Cr)	0.911 (0.851–0.971)	154.62	85.7%	87.5%
72-h postoperative uL-FABP (ng/mg Cr)	0.875 (0.781–0.969)	99.86	85.7%	75%
preoperative uL-FABP +72-h postoperative uL-FABP	0.857 (0.751–0.963)		85.7%	87.5%
72-h postoperative uKIM-1 +72-h postoperative uL-FABP	0.929 (0.879–0.978)		85.7%	87.5%
preoperative uL-FABP +preoperative uKIM-1	0.946 (0.902–0.991)		85.7%	100%
preoperative uL-FABP +preoperative uKIM-1 +preoperative uNGAL	0.967(0.919–1.000)		97.6%	97.9%
72-h postoperative uL-FABP +72-h postoperative uKIM-1 +72-h postoperative uNGAL	0.964 (0.932–0.997)		85.7%	100%

Comparison between the stable renal function group and the deteriorated renal function group

There were no significant differences in age, gender ratio, ALT, AST, total cholesterol (TC), triglycerides (TG), white blood cell count (WBC), red blood cell count (RBC), platelets (PLT), and uNAG levels between the stable renal function group and the deteriorated renal function group (all $P>0.05$). Hemoglobulin

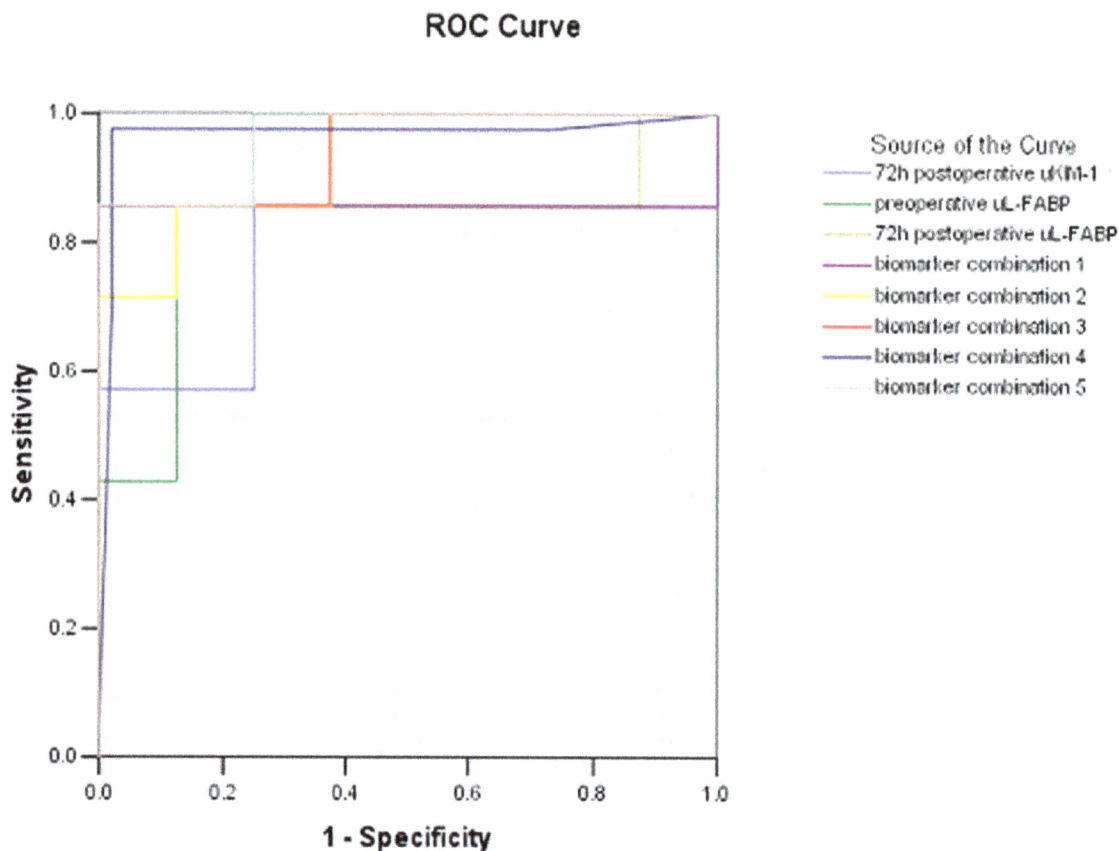

Figure 4. AUC for renal prognosis prediction. biomarker combination 1: combining preoperative uL-FABP and 72-h postoperative uL-FABP levels. biomarker combination 2: combining 72-h postoperative uL-FABP and uKIM-1 levels. biomarker combination 3: combining preoperative uL-FABP and uKIM-1 levels. biomarker combination 4: combining preoperative uL-FABP, uKIM-1, and uNGAL levels. biomarker combination 5: combining 72-h postoperative uL-FABP, uKIM-1, and uNGAL levels.

Survival Functions

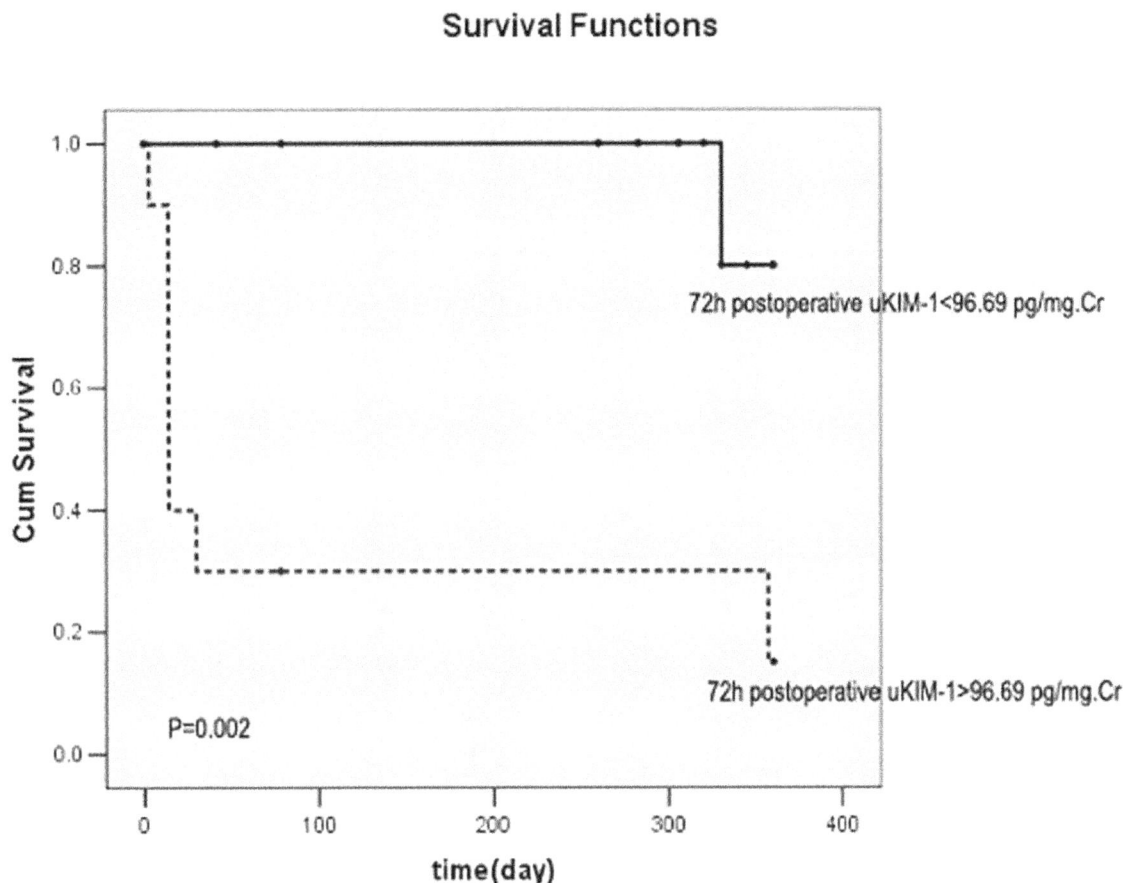

Figure 5. Relationship between the 72-h postoperative uKIM-1 level and renal prognosis. uKIM-1>96.69 pg/mg Cr was significantly correlated with poor prognosis.

(Hb) and albumin (Alb) levels were higher in the deteriorated renal function group than the stable renal function group (all $P<0.05$).

uL-FABP, uKIM-1, uNGAL, and sCr levels were evaluated at various time points and compared between the stable renal function group and the deteriorated renal function group. The 48-h and 72-h postoperative uL-FABP levels were significantly higher in the deteriorated group than in the stable group. The 72-h postoperative uKIM-1 level was significantly higher in the stable group than in the deteriorated group. The preoperative uNGAL level was significantly higher in the deteriorated group than in the stable group. These differences were significant (all $P<0.05$) (Figure 2,3), whereas the sCr level was not statistically different between the two groups.

Risk factor analysis of renal prognosis

Stepwise Cox regression analysis revealed that a 72-h postoperative uKIM-1 of 132.68 ± 29.34 pg/mg Cr ($HR=1.008$; 95% CI, 1.001–1.013); preoperative uL-FABP of 367.63 ± 112.51 ng/mg Cr ($HR=1.002$; 95% CI, 1.001–1.004); and 72-h postoperative uL-FABP of 220.36 ± 59.65 ng/mg Cr ($HR=1.003$; 95% CI, 1.001–1.007) were all risk factors for poor kidney prognosis (all $P<0.01$), whereas gender, age, and uNGAL level were not significantly correlated with prognosis (Table 2). Each 1 pg/mg drop in the 72-h postoperative uKIM-1,1 ng/mg drop in the preoperative uL-FABP and 1 ng/mg drop in the 72-h postoperative uL-FABP was associated with a 0.8%, 0.2% and 0.3% increase in the risk of renal progression relatively.

ROC curve analysis

The area under the curve (AUC) of 72-h postoperative uKIM-1 was 0.786 (95% CI, 0.677–0.894; $P=0.008$); when the intercept of detection was 96.69 pg/mg Cr, the sensitivity and specificity were 85.7% and 75%, respectively. The AUC of preoperative uL-FABP was 0.911 (95% CI, 0.851–0.971; $P=0.000$); when the intercept of detection was 154.62 ng/mg Cr, the sensitivity and specificity were 85.7% and 87.5%, respectively. The AUC of 72-h postoperative uL-FABP was 0.875 (95% CI, 0.781–0.969, $P=0.000$); when the intercept of detection was 99.86 ng/mg Cr, the sensitivity and specificity were 85.7% and 75%, respectively. When the preoperative uL-FABP and 72-h postoperative uL-FABP levels were substituted in the multifactor logistic regression model, the AUC of the combined biomarker was 0.857 (95% CI, 0.751–0.963, $P=0.001$), with a sensitivity of 85.7% and a specificity of 87.5%. When the 72-h postoperative uL-FABP and uKIM-1 levels were substituted in the multifactor logistic regression model, the AUC of the combined biomarker was 0.929 (95% CI, 0.879–0.978; $P=0.000$), with a sensitivity of 85.7% and a specificity of 87.5%. When the preoperative uL-FABP and uKIM-1 levels were substituted in the multifactor logistic regression model, the AUC of the combined biomarker was 0.946 (95% CI, 0.902–0.991; $P=0.000$), with a sensitivity of 85.7% and a specificity of 100%. When the preoperative uL-FABP, uKIM-1, and uNGAL levels were substituted in the multifactor logistic regression model, the AUC of the combined biomarker was 0.967 (95%CI, 0.919–1.000; $P=0.000$), with a

Survival Functions

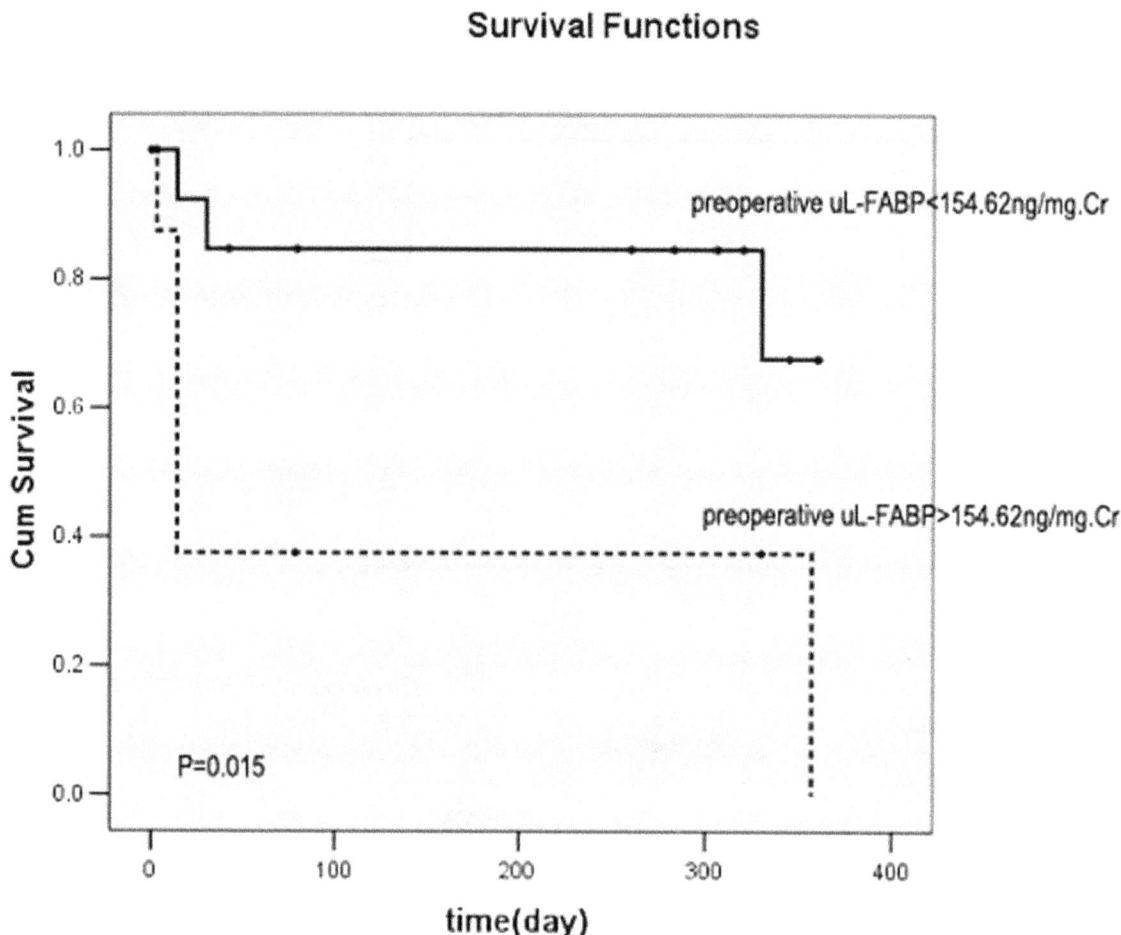

Figure 6. Relationship between the preoperative uL-FABP level and renal prognosis. uL-FABP>154.62 ng/mg Cr was significantly correlated with poor prognosis.

sensitivity of 97.6% and a specificity of 97.9%. When the 72-h postoperative uL-FABP, uKIM-1, and uNGAL levels were substituted in the multifactor logistic regression model, the AUC of the combined biomarker was 0.964 (CI, 0.932–0.997; $P = 0.000$), with a sensitivity of 85.7% and a specificity of 100% (Figure 4, Table 3).

Relationship between uKIM-1/uL-FABP and renal prognosis

A 72-h postoperative uKIM-1>96.69 pg/mg Cr, preoperative uL-FABP>154.62 ng/mg Cr, and uL-FABP>99.86 ng/mg Cr were all positively correlated with poor kidney prognosis (all $P < 0.01$) (Figures 5–7).

Discussion

Obstructive nephropathy is a disease of renal functional and organic impairment that is caused by urine flow occlusion. Renal interstitial fibrosis is the characteristic pathological manifestation of obstructive nephropathy. Progressive renal interstitial fibrosis is directly related to renal function impairment and causes progressive renal function deterioration. Researchers and nephrologists aim to delay or block the deterioration of renal function and to establish parameters for prognosis prediction and early interven-

tion to delay the progression of renal function deterioration [11–13].

KIM-1 is a transmembrane protein that is not expressed in normal kidneys but is secreted in large amounts by the renal proximal tubule cells in patients with renal diseases, renal ischemia, and renal toxic injury [14]. Pre-clinical experiments [15] have demonstrated that KIM-1 is an excellent marker for renal toxic injury. The uKIM-1 level has been correlated to various extents with tubular injury in 13 different AKI models, particularly mild tubular injury, in which uKIM-1 was more sensitive than sCr, blood urine nitrogen (BUN), and NAG. Chaturvedi et al [16] demonstrated that KIM-1 persists until the tubular cell injury is completely repaired. A large-scale clinical study [17] that examined renal needle biopsy samples from nephropathy patients with various etiologies demonstrated that proximal tubular cells from all patients secreted KIM-1 and that tissue KIM-1 expression was correlated with inflammation. uKIM-1 could reflect the KIM-1 level in tissues and correlate with renal interstitial inflammation and renal function. These factors indicated that KIM-1 is a biomarker for not only acute renal proximal tubular injury but also chronic renal interstitial inflammation and fibrosis. Our previous study [18] of AKI patients with obstructive nephropathy in our center showed that uKIM-1 could predict the renal outcome of AKI caused by obstructive nephropathy. In this study we found that uKIM-1

Survival Functions

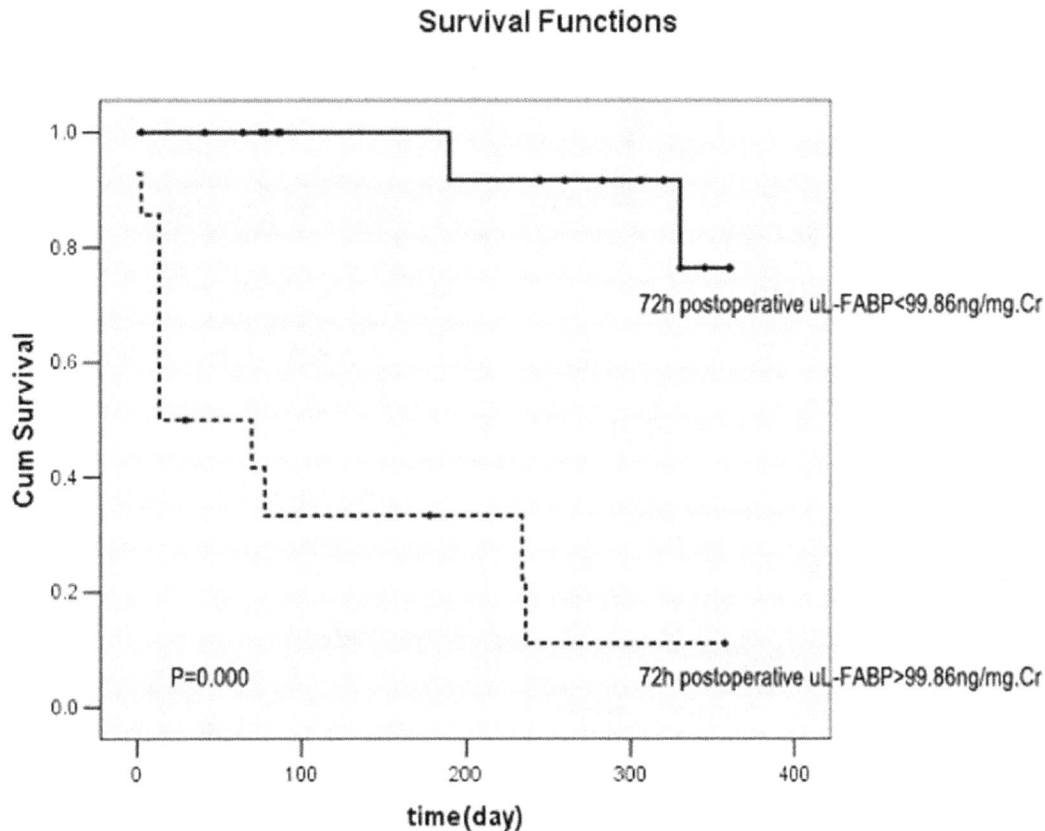

Figure 7. Relationship between the 72-h postoperative uL-FABP level and renal prognosis. uL-FABP>99.86 ng/mg Cr was significantly correlated with poor prognosis.

levels in patients with obstructive nephropathy were higher than healthy people. The results of this study demonstrated that uKIM-1 levels in patients with obstructive nephropathy were significantly different between the deteriorated renal function group and the stable renal function group; Cox regression analysis revealed that the 72-h postoperative uKIM-1 level after obstruction resolution was a risk factor for renal prognosis, with an AUC of 0.786; i.e., it could accurately predict renal function prognosis.

L-FABP is a small molecular protein that is secreted in large amounts at the site of active fatty acid metabolism and participates in and promotes the β-oxidation of fatty acids in the mitochondria or peroxisomes [19]. Under normal conditions, L-FABP exits the renal proximal tubular cells and participates in the metabolism of free fatty acids (FFAs) in renal tubules. By contrast, under various stress situations, the FFAs over-aggregate in the renal proximal tubules; the oxidated and peroxidated products may increase renal tubular injury, and L-FABP is expressed in the epithelial cells in large amounts [20]. In a clinical trial [21], uL-FABP levels were increased before angiography in 13 (high uL-FABP group) of 66 patients who underwent non-emergency angiography; during the follow-up period, these 13 patients were all diagnosed with contrast-associated nephropathy (CAN), whereas none of the patients with low uL-FABP levels (low uL-FABP group) were diagnosed with CAN. The pre-angiography sCr level was not significantly different between the two groups ($P>0.05$). These findings indicated that uL-FABP is a more sensitive biomarker than sCr for AKI prediction and may be used as a clinical parameter for the prediction of CAN. In a multicenter trial [22], 48 patients with non-diabetic nephropathy were retrospectively

classified into a progression group and non-progression group and monitored for 7 to 13 months. The creatinine clearance rates (CCr) of the two groups were similar, whereas the uL-FABP level was significantly higher in the progression group than in the non-progression group ($P<0.05$). This finding indicated that L-FABP might predict the progression of chronic nephropathy. A study of chronic glomerulonephritis (CGN) conducted by our study group [23] demonstrated that uL-FABP levels were significantly higher in CGN patients than in the normal population. After 5 years of follow-up, uL-FABP levels were shown to be an important indicator of CGN progression; uL-FABP levels were significantly higher in the progression group than in the non-progression group. These findings indicated that uL-FABP is valuable for predicting CGN progression. Our previous study [24] of AKI caused by obstructive nephropathy had shown that uL-FABP was an early screening parameter for the poor prognosis of AKI patients with obstructive nephropathy. The uL-FABP levels were significantly higher in patients with obstructive nephropathy than in healthy people. All obstructive nephropathy patients had renal impairment, including the patients who did not develop AKI at the onset. The results of the present study demonstrated that there was a significant difference in uL-FABP levels between the deteriorated renal function group and the stable group and that the preoperative and 72-h postoperative uL-FABP levels are risk factors for renal prognosis that are positively correlated with poor prognosis. The AUC of preoperative uL-FABP was 0.911, and the sensitivity and specificity were 85.7% and 87.5%, respectively, when the detection intercept was 154.62 ng/mg Cr. The AUC of 72-h postoperative uL-FABP was 0.875, and the sensitivity and specificity were 85.7% and 75%, respectively, when the detection intercept was 99.86 ng/mg Cr. These findings all indicated that uL-FABP is an important marker of renal function deterioration in patients with obstructive nephropathy.

NGAL is a 25-kDa protein that is primarily secreted by neutrophils and various epithelial cells, including proximal tubular cells [25]. A meta-analysis [26] demonstrated that uNGAL was not only helpful for the early diagnosis of AKI but was also useful for predicting whether patients need RRT therapy and determining their short-term prognosis. In a large-scale community study of atherosclerosis risks [27], the uNGAL level was correlated with CKD stage 3 prediction and was a potential risk factor for predicting CKD. The predictive value of uNGAL for kidney function was not as high in our study of obstructive nephropathy.

Combining multiple biomarkers has recently been proposed to increase the accuracy of AKI prediction. Studies have demonstrated that combining markers with different sensitivities and specificities as well as combining different markers at various time points could increase the accuracy of the effective prediction of AKI [28,29]. A prospective, multicenter cohort study that enrolled 1219 adults and 311 children demonstrated that there were several correlations between these biomarkers and that combining the uIL-18 and uL-FABP levels at various time points or combining the uIL-18, uNGAL. and uL-FABP levels at various time points increased the ROC-AUC of AKI prediction to 0.78. Because the etiology of AKI varies, combining different biomarkers was more beneficial for determining renal prognosis. A study [30] in 76 AKI patients receiving renal support therapy (RST) demonstrated that the maximal ROC-AUC of renal prognosis prediction was 0.94 when combining various biomarkers (uHGF, uNGAL, uCystatin C, uNGAL/MMP-9, and uIL-18) at multiple time points. The subjects in our study were patients with obstructive nephropathy, and when the various biomarker levels at different time points were substituted in the multifactor logistic regression model [31], the AUCs for determining obstructive nephropathy prognosis were 0.929 and 0.946, respectively, when combining biomarkers 72 h postoperative uKIM-1 and uL-FABP, preoperative uL-FABP and uKIM-1. The AUCs were 0.964 (sensitivity 85.7%, specificity

100%) and 0.967 (sensitivity 97.6%, specificity 97.9%), respectively, when combining biomarkers 72 h postoperative uKIM-1, uL-FABP and uNGAL, preoperative uKIM-1, uL-FABP and uNGAL. These results indicate that combining multiple biomarkers could markedly increase the accuracy of renal prognosis in patients with obstructive nephropathy.

This study is limited because it was a single-centered, small-sample clinical trial that followed renal function changes for 1 year without additional follow-up of biomarker level changes. Therefore, a large-scale, multicenter study is necessary to follow up the biomarker level changes during the progress of nephropathy and confirm the value of these markers in renal prognosis monitoring.

uKIM-1 and uL-FABP levels may accurately predict the renal prognosis of patients with obstructive nephropathy. The sensitivity and specificity of uL-FABP were superior to those of uKIM-1, which may be used as an early screening parameter for determining poor prognosis in patients with obstructive nephropathy. Combining various biomarkers may further increase the accuracy of renal prognosis in patients with obstructive nephropathy and thus help physicians give their patients timely intervention to prevent disease progression.

Acknowledgments

This study was supported in part by the National Basic Research Program of China 973 Program No. 2012CB517600 (No. 2012CB517602). The study was also sponsored by HongKong, Macao and Taiwan Science & Technology Cooperation Program of China (2014DFT30090), the National Natural Science Foundation of China (81102700, 81373865 and 81370794) and by grants 12401906400 and 14140903200 from the Science and Technology Commission of Shanghai Municipality, China, and ZYSNXD012-RC-ZXY017 from the Shanghai Health Bureau. Funding scheme for training young teachers in Colleges and universities in Shanghai was also included in the fund.

Author Contributions

Conceived and designed the experiments: SM W. Xue. Performed the experiments: YX. Analyzed the data: XS XC W. Xu. Contributed reagents/materials/analysis tools: ZN. Wrote the paper: YX.

References

1. Smith JM, Stablein DM, Munoz R, Hebert D, McDonald RA (2007) Contributions of the transplant registry: The 2006 Annual Report of the North American Pediatric Renal Trials and Collaborative Studies (NAPRTCS). Pediatr Transplant 11: 366–373.

2. Klahr S, Morrissey J (2002) Obstructive nephropathy and renal fibrosis. Am J Physiol Renal Physiol 283: F861–F875.

3. Chevalier RL, Thornhill BA, Forbes MS, Kiley SC (2010) Mechanisms of renal injury and progression of renal disease in congenital obstructive nephropathy. Pediatr Nephrol 25: 687–697.

4. Tang X, Lieske JC (2014) Acute and chronic kidney injury in nephrolithiasis. Curr Opin Nephrol Hypertens. 23: 385–390.

5. Dear JW, Yuen PST (2008) Setting the stage for acute-on-chronic kidney injury. Kidney Int 74: 7–9.

6. Ponte B, Felipe C, Muriel A, Tenorio MT, Liaño F (2008) Long-term functional evolution after an acute kidney injury: a 10-year study. Nephrol Dial Transplant 23: 3859–3866.

7. Siew ED, Ware LB, Ikizler TA (2011) Biological markers of acute kidney injury. J Am Soc Nephrol 22: 810–820.

8. Bonventre JV (2009) Kidney injury molecule-1 (KIM-1): a urinary biomarker and much more. Nephrol Dial Transplant 24: 3265–3268.

9. Klahr S (1991) New Insights Into the Consequences and Mechanisms of Renal Impairment in Obstructive Nephropathy. Am J Kidney Dis.18: 689.

10. Levey AS, Coresh J, Greene T, Marsh J, Stevens LA, et al. (2007) Expressing the Modification of Diet in Renal Disease Study Equation for Estimating Glomerular Filtration Rate with Standardized Serum Creatinine Values. Clin. Chem 53: 766–772.

11. Trnka P, Ivanova L, Hiatt MJ, Matsell DG (2012) Urinary Biomarkers in Obstructive Nephropathy. Clin J Am Soc Nephrol 7: 1567–1575.

12. Butt MJ, Tarantal AF, Jimenez DF, Matsell DG (2007) Collecting duct epithelial-mesenchymal transition in fetal urinary tract obstruction. Kidney Int. 72: 936–944.

13. Fu P, Huang XQ, Yuan AH, Yu G, Mei XB, et al. (2012) Effects of salvianolate combined with alprostadil and reduced glutathione on progression of chronic renal failure in patients with chronic kidney diseases: a long-term randomized controlled trial. Journal of Integrative Medicine 10: 641–646.

14. Wasilewska A, Taranta-Janusz K, Dębek W, Zoch-Zwierz W, Kuroczycka-Saniutycz E (2011) KIM-1 and NGAL: new markers of obstructive nephropathy. Pediatr Nephrol 26: 579–586.

15. Vaidya VS, Ozer JS, Dieterle F, Collings FB, Ramirez V, et al. (2010) Kidney injury molecule-1 outperforms traditional biomarkers of kidney injury in preclinical biomarker qualification studies. Nat Biotechnol. 28: 478–485.

16. Chaturvedi S, Farmer T, Kapke GF (2009) Assay validation for KIM-1: human urinary renal dysfunction biomarker. Int J Biol Sci 5: 128–134.

17. van Timmeren MM, van den Heuvel MC, Bailly V, Bakker SJ, van Goor H, et al. (2007) Tubular kidney injury molecule-1 (KIM-1) in human renal disease. J Pathol 212: 209–217.

18. Xue W, Xie Y, Wang Q, Xu W, Mou S, et al. (2014) Diagnostic performance of urinary kidney injury molecule-1 and neutrophil gelatinase-associated lipocalin for acute kidney injury in an obstructive nephropathy patient. Nephrology 19: 186–194.

19. Portilla D, Dent C, Sugaya T, Nagothu KK, Kundi I, et al. (2008) Liver-type fatty acid-binding protein as a biomarker of acute kidney injury after cardiac surgery. Kidney Int 73: 465–472.

20. Kamijo A, Sugaya T, Hikawa A, Okada M, Okumura F, et al. (2004) Urinary excretion of fatty acid-binding protein reflects stress overload on the proximal tubules. Am J Pathol 165: 1243–1255.

21. Nakamura T, Sugaya T, Node K, Ueda Y, Koide H (2006) Urinary excretion of liver-type fatty acid-binding protein in contrast mediun-induced nephropathy. Am J Kidney Dis 47: 439–444.

22. Kamijo A, Sugaya T, Hikawa A, Yamanouchi M, Hirata Y, et al. (2005) Clinical evaluation of urinary excretion of liver-type fatty acid-binding protein as a

marker for the monitoring of chronic kidney disease: a multicenter trial. J Lab Clin Med 145: 125–133.

23. Mou S, Wang Q, Li J, Shi B, Ni Z (2012) Urinary excretion of liver-type fatty acid-binding protein as a marker of progressive kidney function deterioration in patients with chronic glomerulonephritis. Clin Chim Acta. 413: 187–191.

24. Xie Y, Xu W, Wang Q, Shao X, Mou S, et al. (2014) Urinary excretion of liver-type FABP as a new clinical marker for the progression of obstructive nephropathy. Biomark Med. 8: 543–556.

25. Soni SS, Ronco C, Katz N, Cruz DN (2009) Early diagnosis of acute kidney injury: the promise of novel biomarkers. Blood Purif 28: 165–174.

26. Haase M, Bellomo R, Devarajan P, Schlattmann P, Haase-Fielitz A, et al. (2009) Accuracy of neutrophil gelatinase-associated lipocalin (NGAL) in diagnosis and prognosis in acute kidney injury: a systematic review and meta-analysis. Am J Kidney Dis. 54: 1012–1024.

27. Bhavsar NA, Köttgen A, Coresh J, Astor BC (2012) Neutrophil Gelatinase-Associated Lipocalin (NGAL) and Kidney Injury Molecule 1 (KIM-1) as

Predictors of Incident CKD Stage 3: The Atherosclerosis Risk in Communities (ARIC) Study. Am J Kidney Dis. 60: 233–240.

28. Parikh CR, Thiessen-Philbrook H, Garg AX, Kadiyala D, Shlipak MG, et al. (2013) Performance of kidney injury molecule-1 and liver-type fatty acid-binding protein and combined biomarkers of AKI after cardiac surgery. Clin J Am Soc Nephrol. 8: 1079–1088.

29. Shao X, Tian L, Xu W, Zhang Z, Mou S., et al. (2014) Diagnostic Value of Urinary Kidney Injury Molecule 1 for Acute Kidney Injury: A Meta-analysis. PLOS ONE. 9: e84131.

30. Srisawat N, Wen X, Lee M, Kong L, Elder M, et al. (2011) Urinary biomarkers and renal recovery in critically ill patients with renal support. Clin J Am Soc Nephrol. 6: 1815–1823.

31. Han WK, Wagener G, Zhu Y, Wang S, Lee HT (2009) Urinary biomarkers in the early detection of acute kidney injury after cardiac surgery. Clin J Am Soc Nephml 4: 873–882.

25

Hemodynamics and Function of Resistance Arteries in Healthy Persons and End Stage Renal Disease Patients

Morten K. Borg[1], Per Ivarsen[2], Emil Brøndum[1], Johan V. Povlsen[2], Christian Aalkjær[1]*

1 Department of Biomedicine, Aarhus University, Aarhus, Denmark, **2** Department of Renal Medicine, Aarhus University Hospital and Department of Clinical Medicine, Faculty of Health, Aarhus University, Aarhus, Denmark

Abstract

Introduction: Cardiovascular disease is the leading cause of death in patients with end stage renal disease (ESRD). The vasodilator mechanisms in small resistance arteries are in earlier studies shown to be reduced in patients with end stage renal disease. We studied whether endothelium dependent vasodilatation were diminished in ESRD patients and the interaction between the macro- and microcirculation.

Methods: Eleven patients with ESRD had prior to renal transplant or insertion of peritoneal dialysis catheter measured pulse wave velocity. During surgery, a subcutaneous fat biopsy was extracted. Resistance arteries were then dissected and mounted on a wire myograph for measurements of dilator response to increasing concentrations of acetylcholine after preconstriction with noradrenaline. Twelve healthy kidney donors served as controls.

Results: Systolic blood pressure was elevated in patients compared to the healthy controls; no difference in the concentration of asymmetric dimethyl arginine was seen. No significant difference in the endothelium dependent vasodilatation between patients and controls was found. Correlation of small artery properties showed an inverse relationship between diastolic blood pressure and nitric oxide dependent vasodilatation in controls. Pulse pressure was positively correlated to the total endothelial vasodilatation in patients. A negative association between S-phosphate and endothelial derived hyperpolarisation-like vasodilatation was seen in resistance arteries from controls.

Conclusion: This study finds similar vasodilator properties in kidney patients and controls. However, correlations of pulse pressure and diastolic blood pressure with resistance artery function indicate compensating measures in the microcirculation during end stage renal disease.

Editor: Emmanuel A Burdmann, University of Sao Paulo Medical School, Brazil

Funding: The study was funded by the P Carl Petersen Foundation and the Danish Kidney Association. The funders had no role in study design, data collection and analysis, decision to publish, or preparation of the manuscript.

Competing Interests: The authors have declared that no competing interests exist.

* E-mail: ca@fi.au.dk

Introduction

Cardiovascular disease (CVD) is overrepresented in patients with reduced kidney function, and the risk increases with declining kidney function, why CVD is the major cause of death in patients with end stage renal disease (ESRD) [1]. Both arterial stiffness and small artery structural and functional alterations are involved in the pathophysiology leading to changes in the cardiovascular system, but the mechanisms responsible are not fully elucidated.

Arterial stiffness, defined as decreased ability and degree of the conductive arteries to absorb the pulse pressure is related to mortality in dialysis and non-dialysis patients [2,3]. The degree of arterial stiffness can be estimated by measuring pulse pressure, pulse wave velocity (PWV) or augmentation index (AI). The mechanisms inducing stiffening of the conductive arteries are complex and include both non-renal risk factors e.g. smoking, diabetes, hypertension and renal risk factors such as calcification, increased plasma concentration of asymmetric dimethylarginine (ADMA), inflammation and oxidative stress [4,5].

The function of the large arteries' viscoelasticity reduces the pulsative pressure and flow that results from the intermittent ventricular ejection, securing a stabile pressure and flow at the level of small arteries. When stiffness increases, an augmentation of the pulse wave is present because of changes in the timing and size of reflection. This might induce damage and change the functionality of the vascular microcirculation as it is exposed to a higher pulsative pressure and flow.

Endothelium-dependent vasodilatation occurs via three main pathways; cyclooxygenase (COX) products, nitric oxide (NO) and endothelium-derived hyperpolarisation (EDH) [6]. Endothelium-dependent vasodilatation in the large arteries from ESRD patients has been examined with forearm blood flow measurements and shown to be associated with an impairment of the vasodilator properties due to a defect in the NO-pathway [7]. Similar results have been obtained in brachial artery, where shear stress induced vasodilatation in ESRD patients was found attenuated at maximal shear stress [8]. The diminished vasodilator function in the macro circulation of ESRD patients, measured as post-ischemic reactive hyperemia, is associated with increased all-cause mortality [9].

Investigations of the micro circulation (the resistance arteries) of ESRD patients show no difference from similar arteries from healthy controls when comparing morphology and sensitivity to vasoconstrictors [10]. Endothelium independent vasodilatation is also found unchanged, whereas studies examining the endothelium dependent vasodilatation have yielded different results, as resistance arteries from ESRD patients have shown to have a reduced relaxation to acetylcholine (ACh) [11]. This appears to be due to a defect in the NO-pathway [12], while another study shows that the EDHF-response is attenuated, but only when using bradykinin as the agonist and not ACh [13].

In this study we wanted to evaluate differences in vascular function in arteries from patients with ESRD and normal controls and to study the interaction between the macro- and microcirculation. Especially we wanted to test whether endothelium dependent vasodilatation was diminished in ESRD patients with well controlled blood pressure.

Materials and Methods

Study population

Eleven patients with ESRD were enrolled in the study. Nine had living related donor renal transplant and two insertion of peritoneal dialysis catheter. Patients included were above 18 years of age. Exclusion criteria were persisting cardiac arrhythmias, severe congestive heart failure, reduced pulmonary function, severe psychiatric disease, acute infection and leg-amputation. Five patients were treated with peritoneal dialysis (vintage 252 days (101-568) median (range)); four with hemodialysis (vintage 769 days (14-1201)) and two were not on dialysis. Patient's kidney diseases were glomerulonephritis (n = 5), adult polycystic kidney disease (n = 2), obstructive nephropathy (n = 2), type 1 diabetes mellitus (n = 1) and vasculitis (n = 1). No patient had diabetes mellitus as comorbidity. Nine out of eleven were treated with antihypertensive medication. Two were treated with angiotensin converting enzyme inhibitors, four with angiotensin receptor blockade, six with calcium antagonists, four with beta-blockers, six with diuretics, ten with erythropoietin analogs and one with statins.

The majority of patients were cardiovascular assessed as part of the pre-transplantation assessment or ESRD regular control with echocardiography, coronary angiogram and CT scans of the iliac arteries. All investigation was performed in the year before the study and none had any cardiovascular event between the cardiovascular assessment and transplantation. All patients had an echocardiography; ten had normal ejection fraction (EF) while one patient had an EF of 40%. One of the patients had indication of a light aortastenosis and five patients had light left ventricular hypertrophy. Nine patients had a coronary angiogram; seven patients had normal coronary arteries, one had earlier coronary by-pass and one had some calcification but no stenosis. Seven had a CT scan of the iliac arteries; five had no calcification, 2 had mild to moderate calcification. Cholesterol was measured in six patients, with a mean value of 4.9 mmol/l. Inflammatory profile were assessed with c-reactive protein in ten of eleven patients prior to surgery; all values were less than 10 mg/l.

Twelve kidney donors with no preexisting medical conditions or drug intake served as healthy controls. Before surgery the kidney recipients received 2 days of immunosuppressive therapy consisting of 0.2 mg/kg tacrolimus, 1.5 g mycophenolat mofetil acid and 20 mg prednisolone. The study was performed in accordance with the Declaration of Helsinki. Protocol and consent forms were approved by the local research Ethics Committee (Central Denmark Region), and all participants gave written informed consent before inclusion.

Protocol

Participant's body weight, height and blood pressure were measured and hemodynamic data were calculated the day before surgery. Patient's type of dialysis, vintage, underlying condition and drug intake were obtained from medical records. Blood samples were taken on the day of surgery. During surgery a 2×3 cm biopsy containing skin and subcutaneous fat was removed from the abdominal wall with scalpel without the use of diathermy.

Microvascular function

Subcutaneous fat biopsies were immediately after extraction placed in $5\,°C$ physiological salt solution (PSS), transported to the lab where 2 mm long segments of arteries were isolated and mounted on two stainless steel wires (40 µm diameter) in the organ baths of a 4-channel wire myograph (model 610M, Danish Myo Technology (DMT), Aarhus, Denmark) or in a double channel myograph (model 410A, DMT) for isometric force measurement. The myograph contained PSS at $37\,°C$, continuously bubbled with a gas mixture containing 5% CO_2 and 21% O_2 in a nitrogen based gas to keep pH at 7.4 at all times. Upon mounting, the arteries were left 20 min to equilibrate before stepwise stretching, characterizing the elastic properties as described by Mulvany and Halpern [14]. Experiments were conducted at 90% of L_{100} (defined as the circumference of the relaxed artery exposed to a transmural pressure of 100 mmHg). Viability of the arteries was tested using 10 µM noradrenaline (NA) twice before beginning the experiments. The arteries were preconstricted with 3 µM NA and subsequent relaxation using increasing concentrations of the endothelium-dependent vasodilator ACh. The experiment were repeated after incubation (20 min) with first the COX-inhibitor indomethacin (3 µM) and then the combination of the NOS inhibitor L-NAME (100 µM) and indomethacin.

To ensure that the endothelium was viable no artery was submitted to more than 3 endothelium-dependent relaxation curves and were left resting for 20 minutes between curves during incubation.

The composition of PSS was (mM): NaCl 119, KCl 4.7, KH_2PO_4 1.18, $MgSO_4$ 1.17, $NaHCO_3$ 25, $CaCl_2$ 1.6, EDTA 0.026, and glucose 5.5. The chemicals were obtained from Sigma (St.Louis, MO, USA). Indomethacin was dissolved in ethanol, the other chemicals in distilled water.

Hemodynamics

Cardiac output (CO) was measured by rebreathing technique in a closed system containing a gas mixture of sulfahexafloride and nitrous oxide in a mixture of oxygen and nitrogen (Innocor, Denmark). Rebreathing was performed in the sitting position during 15 s with a breathing rate of 14–16 min^{-1} and a volume of 1.8 l after a rest of at least 10 min [15]. Gas was sampled continuously from the mouthpiece and analyzed online on an infrared gas analyzer. Pulmonary blood flow (PBF) was calculated from uptake rate of nitrous oxide into the blood. The first two or three breaths were excluded from analysis if the total lung volume measured by sulfahexafloride indicated incomplete gas mixture. In the majority of patients without pulmonary arterio-venous shunt PBF equals CO [16,17]. In contrast in patients with pulmonary shunt, the shunt fraction is calculated and added to PBF to get CO. The shunt fraction is calculated from the oxygen concentration [18]. The calculations were performed assuming that the gasses were mixed completely and that the equilibration of gasses between alveoli and capillary was rapid and that lung flow was constant. Systolic blood pressure (SBP) and diastolic blood pressure (DBP) were measured by an automatic device connected to the Innocor. Systemic vascular resistance index (SVRi) was calculated as: (Mean arterial blood pressure − central venous pressure)/Cardiac output and indexed to body surface by Innocor. The measurement was performed twice, and the mean values were used in data analysis.

PWV and AI were measured in the supine position after 10 min of rest. Carotid –femoral PWV was measured with SphygmoCor, AtCor Medical, Texas, US, using the integral software.

Augmentation pressure was calculated as the difference between the second and first systolic peaks, and AI was calculated as the augmentation pressure expressed as percentage of pulse pressure. AI was measured for aorta. All of the measurements were made in duplicate by one trained study nurse, and the mean values were used in the subsequent analysis.

Biochemistry

Asymmetric dimethyl arginine (ADMA) was measured using ELISA (DLD Diagnostika GmbH, Germany). All other biochemistry was analysed at the Department of Clinical Biochemistry, Aarhus University Hospital. EGFR was calculated from the 4 point MDRD formula.

Statistics

Data in figures are presented as mean ± SEM, in tables as mean ± SEM or median (range). Concentration-response curves to ACh are given as percentage relaxation of the pre-constriction to NA. EC_{50} values are calculated by non-linear regression for variable slope for each vessel and presented as the negative logarithmic value in mol/L (pEC50). NO dependent response was calculated as the difference between EC_{50} values of indomethacin and indomethacin/L-NAME curves respectively (ΔpEC_{50}). Mean pEC_{50}, ΔpEC_{50} and baseline characteristics on patients were compared using unpaired student's t-test. Associations between variables were calculated using Pearson's correlation. P<0.05 were considered significant. All statistical analyses were performed with GraphPad Prism (v. 4.03 GraphPad Software Inc., CA, US)

Results

Study population

Kidney function was significant lower in ESRD patient, as expected. Age, weight and BMI were similar, whereas systolic, but not diastolic, blood pressure was significantly elevated in ESRD patients (Table 1), despite antihypertensive treatment. Blood hemoglobin concentration was decreased in ESRD patients, whereas no significant difference in ADMA concentration was found.

Microvascular function

Relaxation of subcutaneous resistance arteries with ACh was not significantly different between ESRD patients and controls (Figure 1A). Both maximal relaxation and pEC50 were comparable (maximal relaxation: 84±4% vs. 90±2%, p = 0.22; pEC50: 7.06±0.12 vs. 6.97±0.06, p = 0.52).

The EDH-like relaxation was recorded after blockade of eNOS and COX (Figure 1B). The maximal relaxation and sensitivity to ACh was similar between the two groups (maximal relaxation: 68±5% vs. 66±5%, p = 0.82; pEC50: 6.39±0.17 vs. 6.15±0.21, p = 0.38).

The NO-dependent vasodilatation was calculated as ΔpEC_{50} for concentration response curves incubated with indomethacin and indomethacin + L-NAME respectively (figure 2). No

Table 1. Baseline characteristics for end stage renal disease (ESRD) patients and healthy controls.

Variable	ESRD (n = 11)	Controls (n = 12)
Sex (male/female)	6/5	4/8
Age (years)	51(19–85)	54(36–70)
S-Creatinine (µmol/mL)	806±82*	68±3
eGFR (mL/min/1,73 m²)	6.7±0.7*	87.5±4.2
Systolic blood pressure (mmHg)	130±2*§	119±4#
Diastolic blood pressure (mmHg)	78±3§	76±2#
Pulse pressure (mmHg)	52±3§	43±4#
Weight (kg)	73.2±3.2§	75.9±3.8#
BMI (kg/m²)	24.6±1.2§	26.2±0.9#
Hemoglobin (mmol/L)	7.2±0.3*	8.2±0.2
S-Calcium-ion (mmol/L)	1.18±0.03	1.22±0.02
S-Phosphate (mmol/l)	1.87±0.10*	1.14±0.03
S-PTH (pmol/l)	24.9±5.1	NA
Albuminuria (g/day)	3.38±1.30*§	0±0
ADMA (µmol/L)	0.78±0.04§	0.72±0.02

Data are mean±SEM, except for age which is median (range); * p<0.05, § n = 10, # n = 11.

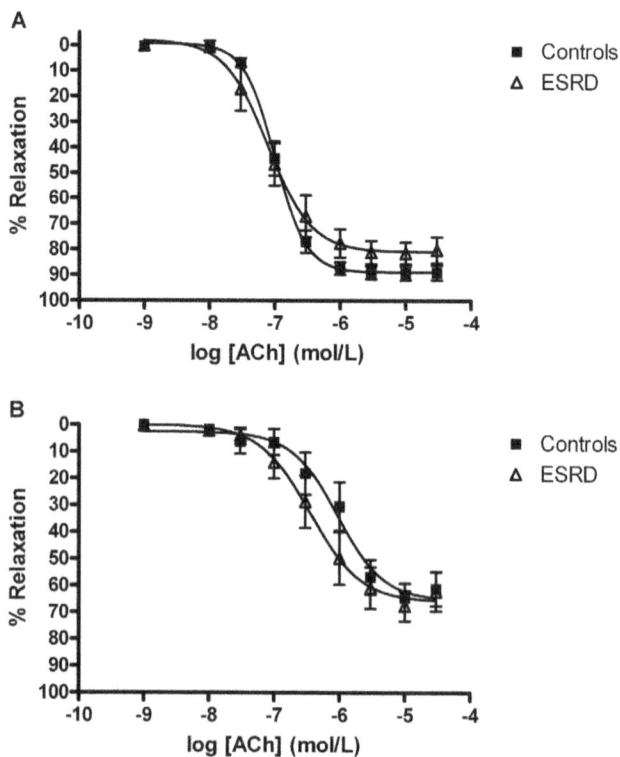

Figure 1. Concentration-response relaxation curves to acetylcholine in arteries from healthy controls and patients with end stage renal disease. A: Endothelium dependent vasodilatation; p = ns. B: Endothelium-derived hyperpolarisation-like relaxation in the presence of indomethacin and L-NAME; p = ns.

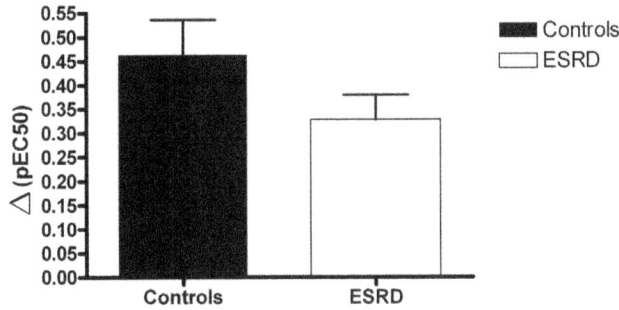

Figure 2. Nitric oxide dependent-response, calculated as the difference between pEC_{50}-values of concentration response curves incubated with indomethacin and indomethacin/L-NAME respectively – ΔpEC_{50}; controls (n = 10), ESRD (n = 11); p = 0.15.

Table 2. Hemodynamics in patients with end stage renal disease (ESRD) and healthy controls.

Variable	ESRD (n = 5)	Controls (n = 12)
Pulse wave velocity (m/s)	11.38±3.33[§]	7.11±0.39[#]
Augmentation index (%)	122±7*	154±9[#]
Cardiac output index (L/min/m²)	3.58±0.42*	2.79±0.14
SVR index (mmHg/(L/min)/m²)	28.05±2.99	32.58±1.40

Systemic vascular resistance (SVR).
Data are mean±SEM; * p<0.05; [§] n = 4; [#] n = 10.

significant difference between ESRD and controls was found (ΔpEC_{50} was 0.33±0.05 vs. 0.46±0.07, ESRD and controls, respectively, p = 0.15).

To assess whether three concentration response curves to acetylcholine can be obtained, time control experiments were performed. Three concentration response curves, with 20 minutes of rest in between, were conducted; without use of any blocking agent (figure 3). As seen there was no deterioration in the response to acetylcholine with time.

Hemodynamics

PWV and SVRi were not significantly different in the two groups, while AI was lower in the ESRD group (table 2), which was not expected. This was probably because of small sample size.

Associations between micro- and macrovascular functions

DBP was inversely related to the NO-dependent vasorelaxation in controls (r = −0.59; p<0.05) (figure 4). The inverse relation was not significant in ESRD (r = −0.44; p = 0.10).

Pulse pressure was positively correlated to ACh induced vasodilatation in ESRD (r = 0.81; p<0.01), this was not the case in control subjects (r = −0.17; p = 0.31) (figure 5).

Correlation of ADMA and NO-response showed a trend in controls (figure 6), although not statistically significant (r = 0.49; p = 0.07), whereas no trend was seen in ESRD (r = 0.01; p = 0.97).

As expected S-phosphate levels were different in the two groups. A negative association was found between S-phosphate and EDH-like response in controls(r = −0.66; p<0.05), but not in ESRD (r = −0.30; p = 0.18) (figure 7).

Cardiac output and vasodilatation were inversely related in controls (figure 8), higher cardiac output resulted in a diminished vasorelaxation (r = −0.50; p = 0.05). While no relation was present in ESRD (r = 0.76; p = 0.12).

Discussion

In the present study, we evaluated micro- and macrovascular differences in ESRD patients and healthy controls and for the first time correlated these findings. The ESRD patients had little comorbidity and well controlled blood pressure. In the microvascular function no significant different response to endothelium dependent vasodilatation was seen between ESRD and healthy controls. In the macrovascular arteries a significant higher SBP was present in the ESRD patients. Micro- and macrovascular function was correlated, DBP and the NO-dependent vasorelaxation was inversely related in controls. Pulse pressure was positively correlated to endothelial vasodilatation in ESRD and interestingly a negative correlation between S-phosphate and EDH-like response was found in controls.

The microvascular endothelial dependent vasodilator response to ACh has earlier been shown to be diminished in ESRD, while attempts to determine the affected pathway, has yielded diverging

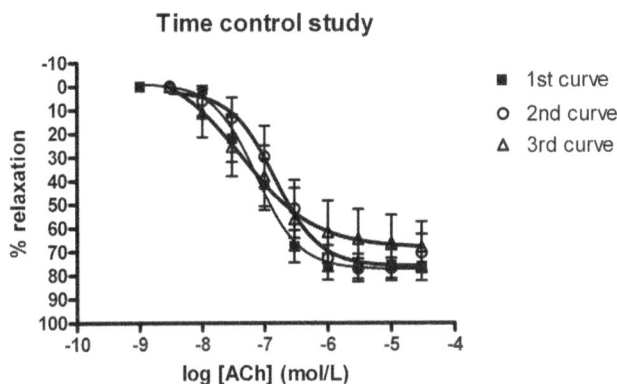

Figure 3. Time control experiments; three consecutive concentration response curves, with 20 minutes of rest in between, without use of blocker.

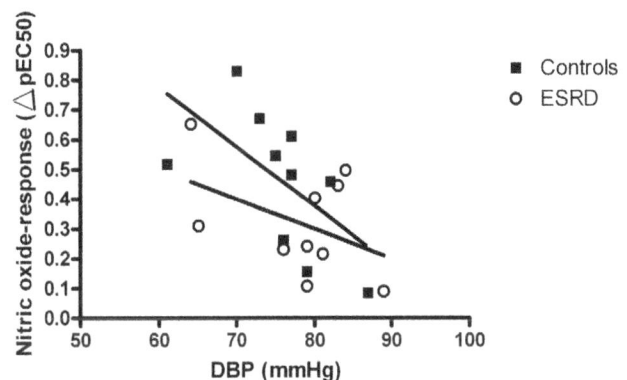

Figure 4. Association between diastolic blood pressure and nitric oxide-response (ΔpEC_{50}) in controls (r = −0.59; p<0.05) and ESRD (r = −0.44; p = 0.10), Pearson one-tailed correlation.

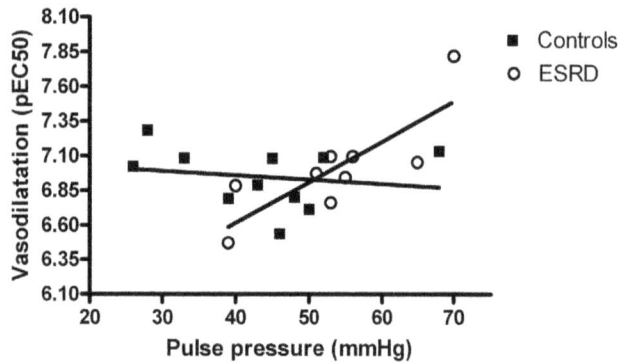

Figure 5. Association between pulse pressure and vasodilatation (pEC$_{50}$) in controls (r = −0.17; p = 0.31) and ESRD (r = 0.81; p<0.01), Pearson one-tailed correlation.

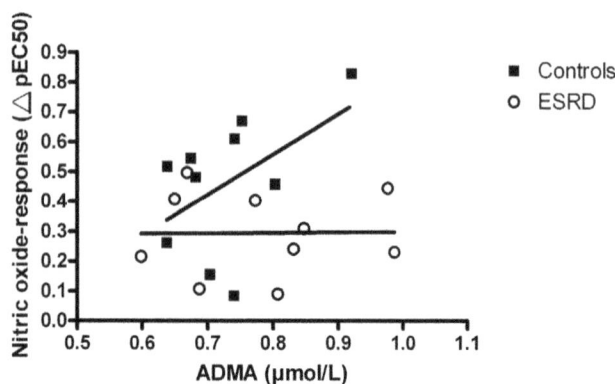

Figure 7. Association between S-Phosphate and EDH-like relaxation (pEC$_{50}$) in controls (r = −0.66; p<0.05) and ESRD (r = −0.30; p = 0.18), Pearson one-tailed correlation.

results [11–13]. In our study a similar vasodilator response to ACh was found, both under control conditions and after inhibition of NOS and COX dependent pathways. The earlier studies suggested that the ACh induced vasodilatation is diminished in ESRD patients [11]; others have confirmed this and suggested that the affected pathway is NOS dependent [12] or involves EDH-like relaxation [13]. Luksha et al. [13] found that only bradykinin-induced EDH-like relaxation was reduced, while ACh-induced EDH-like relaxation was similar in the two groups. Hence parts of our results differ from earlier studies. The diverging results must rely on a complex mixture of a different period of exposure to the uremic milieu, patients' age, physical form, pharmacological treatment, dialysis and blood pressure levels while the experimental setup seems comparable. The lack of a significant difference in resistance artery function in the two groups is consistent with the similar SVRi in the two groups.

Our patients have substantial lower blood pressure than the patients in the aforementioned papers. Since diastolic hypertension is known to cause an attenuated ACh induced vasorelaxation in the resistance arteries [19], the possibility of normal endothelial function in resistance arteries of ESRD patients with well controlled blood pressures seems feasible. We found a negative association between diastolic blood pressure and NO-response in controls (figure 4), while this was not statistically significant in ESRD. This further suggests a greater role of high blood pressure in the attenuation of endothelial function in resistance arteries

than the uremia per se. The similar ADMA levels in patients and controls additionally suggest a relative low exposure to the uremic toxicity indicating well treated dialysis patients. This contrasts with the patients used in the previous studies [12,13] where ADMA levels were significantly increased.

Interestingly we found a positive correlation between pulse pressure and micro-vascular vasodilatation in ESRD patients, which was not present in control subjects. This indicates that higher pulse pressure, which could translate into arterial stiffness, generates a process in the microcirculation that increases the vasodilator properties. Knowing that our patients are well treated in terms of blood pressure and with exposure to uremic toxins, we can speculate, that with longer exposure to renal deficiency, this compensation reaches its maximum and instead diminishing of the vasodilatation starts, as shown in other studies [11–13].

As expected the pulse wave velocity was increased in the ESRD population [20] – although in our study not statistically significant. At the same time cardiac output was higher possibly as a consequence of a reduced hemoglobin level.

Interestingly, we showed that the EDH-like response in healthy controls is dependent on the S-phosphate level, with a decreased vasodilator response with higher S-phosphate, even within the normal range of S-phosphate. We believe that further studies in this field are required to finally establish this correlation. Interestingly is has recently been shown that incubating resistance vessels from both healthy controls and patients with chronic kidney disease with a higher concentration of phosphate decrease the endothelium dependent vasodilatation [21]. The same group

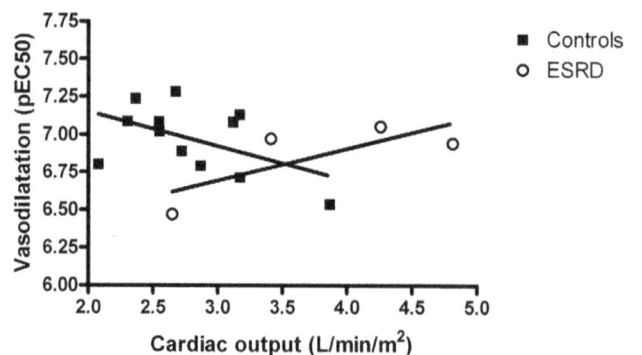

Figure 6. Association between ADMA and NOS dependent relaxation (ΔpEC$_{50}$) in controls (r = 0.49<; p = 0.07) and ESRD (r = 0.01; p = 0.97), Pearson one-tailed correlation.

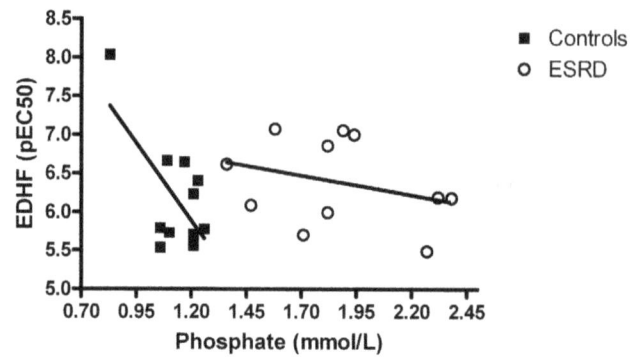

Figure 8. Association between cardiac output and vasodilatation (pEC$_{50}$) in controls (r = −0.50; p = 0.05) and ESRD (r = 0.76; p = 0.12), Pearson one-tailed correlation.

has shown that loading healthy people with phosphate reduces flow-mediated dilatation, indicating impaired endothelial function. After loading, S-phosphate was still within normal range [21]. Other studies have shown that FGF23, which might be an indicator of dietary phosphate load [22] is related to a reduced flow-mediated dilatation [23]. Our data indicates that the level of S-phosphate might affect the vasorelaxation.

When assessing cardiac output and sensitivity of resistance arteries to ACh, opposing associations were seen in controls and ESRD (figure 8). This could suggest that in healthy subjects, better vasodilator capacity in the resistance arteries is associated with a lower cardiac output, which could translate into diminished workload on the heart in the long term, and subsequent a lower risk of cardiac failure.

Study limitation

The sample size of study groups was relatively small which possess a risk of committing type II errors and overinterpretation of the correlations. The majority of patients was receiving kidney transplants, and was therefore with less comorbidity than most patients in dialysis. This could explain why we see little difference between healthy controls and kidney patients in some of our assays.

Conclusions

In conclusion this study finds similar vasodilator properties in small resistance arteries of ESRD and control subjects. ESRD patients were well controlled in terms of blood pressure and uremic exposure. However correlations of pulse pressure, diastolic blood pressure and cardiac output with micro-vascular functions, indicate compensating measures in the microcirculation of ESRD patients.

Acknowledgments

The authors wish to thank the included patients and staff at Aarhus University Hospital involved in sample collection. Special thanks to laboratory technician Jørgen Andresen and project nurse Karin Hansen for excellent technical assistance.

Author Contributions

Conceived and designed the experiments: MB PI CA EB JP. Performed the experiments: MB PI CA. Analyzed the data: MB PI CA. Contributed reagents/materials/analysis tools: MB PI CA JP. Wrote the paper: MB PI CA.

References

1. Foley RN, Parfrey PS (1998) Cardiovascular disease and mortality in ESRD. J Nephrol 11: 239–245.
2. Pannier B, Guerin AP, Marchais SJ, Safar ME, London GM (2005) Stiffness of capacitive and conduit arteries: prognostic significance for end-stage renal disease patients. Hypertension 45: 592–596.
3. Blacher J, Guerin AP, Pannier B, Marchais SJ, Safar ME, et al. (1999) Impact of aortic stiffness on survival in end-stage renal disease. Circulation 99: 2434–2439.
4. Mallamaci F, Tripepi G, Cutrupi S, Malatino LS, Zoccali C (2005) Prognostic value of combined use of biomarkers of inflammation, endothelial dysfunction, and myocardiopathy in patients with ESRD. Kidney Int 67: 2330–2337.
5. Tripepi G, Mattace RF, Sijbrands E, Seck MS, Maas R, et al. (2011) Inflammation and asymmetric dimethylarginine for predicting death and cardiovascular events in ESRD patients. Clin J Am Soc Nephrol 6: 1714–1721.
6. Triggle CR, Samuel SM, Ravishankar S, Marei I, Arunachalam G, et al. (2012) The endothelium: influencing vascular smooth muscle in many ways. Can J Physiol Pharmacol 90: 713–738.
7. Passauer J, Pistrosch F, Bussemaker E, Lassig G, Herbrig K, et al. (2005) Reduced agonist-induced endothelium-dependent vasodilation in uremia is attributable to an impairment of vascular nitric oxide. J Am Soc Nephrol 16: 959–965.
8. Verbeke FH, Pannier B, Guerin AP, Boutouyrie P, Laurent S, et al. (2011) Flow-mediated vasodilation in end-stage renal disease. Clin J Am Soc Nephrol 6: 2009–2015.
9. London GM, Pannier B, Agharazii M, Guerin AP, Verbeke FH, et al. (2004) Forearm reactive hyperemia and mortality in end-stage renal disease. Kidney Int 65: 700–704.
10. Aalkjaer C, Pedersen EB, Danielsen H, Fjeldborg O, Jespersen B, et al. (1986) Morphological and functional characteristics of isolated resistance vessels in advanced uraemia. Clin Sci (Lond) 71: 657–663.
11. Morris ST, McMurray JJ, Spiers A, Jardine AG (2001) Impaired endothelial function in isolated human uremic resistance arteries. Kidney Int 60: 1077–1082.
12. Luksha N, Luksha L, Carrero JJ, Hammarqvist F, Stenvinkel P, et al. (2011) Impaired resistance artery function in patients with end-stage renal disease. Clin Sci (Lond) 120: 525–536.
13. Luksha L, Stenvinkel P, Hammarqvist F, Carrero JJ, Davidge ST, et al. (2012) Mechanisms of endothelial dysfunction in resistance arteries from patients with end-stage renal disease. PLoS One 7: e36056.
14. Halpern W, Mulvany MJ (1977) Tension responses to small length changes of vascular smooth muscle cells [proceedings]. J Physiol 265: 21P–23P.
15. Damgaard M, Norsk P (2005) Effects of ventilation on cardiac output determined by inert gas rebreathing. Clin Physiol Funct Imaging 25: 142–147.
16. Friedman M, Wilkins SA Jr, Rothfeld AF, Bromberg PA (1984) Effect of ventilation and perfusion imbalance on inert gas rebreathing variables. J Appl Physiol 56: 364–369.
17. Petrini MF, Peterson BT, Hyde RW (1978) Lung tissue volume and blood flow by rebreathing theory. J Appl Physiol 44: 795–802.
18. Clemensen P, Christensen P, Norsk P, Gronlund J (1994) A modified photo- and magnetoacoustic multigas analyzer applied in gas exchange measurements. J Appl Physiol 76: 2832–2839.
19. Olsen MH, Wachtell K, Aalkjaer C, Devereux RB, Dige-Petersen H, et al. (2001) Endothelial dysfunction in resistance arteries is related to high blood pressure and circulating low density lipoproteins in previously treated hypertension. Am J Hypertens 14: 861–867.
20. Townsend RR, Wimmer NJ, Chirinos JA, Parsa A, Weir M, et al. (2010) Aortic PWV in chronic kidney disease: a CRIC ancillary study. Am J Hypertens 23: 282–289.
21. Abstracts of the 50th ERA-EDTA (European Renal Association-European Dialysis and Transplant Association) Congress. May 18-21, 2013. Istanbul, Turkey. Nephrol Dial Transplant 28 Suppl 1: i1–553.
22. Isakova T, Gutierrez OM, Wolf M (2009) A blueprint for randomized trials targeting phosphorus metabolism in chronic kidney disease. Kidney Int 76: 705–716.
23. Yilmaz MI, Sonmez A, Saglam M, Yaman H, Kilic S, et al. (2013) Longitudinal analysis of vascular function and biomarkers of metabolic bone disorders before and after renal transplantation. Am J Nephrol 37: 126–134.

26

Metabolic Syndrome and Chronic Kidney Disease in an Adult Korean Population: Results from the Korean National Health Screening

Yong Un Kang, Ha Yeon Kim, Joon Seok Choi, Chang Seong Kim, Eun Hui Bae, Seong Kwon Ma, Soo Wan Kim*

Department of Internal Medicine, Chonnam National University Medical School, Gwangju, Korea

Abstract

Background: This study was aimed to examine the prevalence of metabolic syndrome (MS) and chronic kidney disease (CKD), and the association between MS and its components with CKD in Korea.

Methods: We excluded diabetes to appreciate the real impact of MS and performed a cross-sectional study using the general health screening data of 10,253,085 (48.86±13.83 years, men 56.18%) participants (age, ≥20 years) from the Korean National Health Screening 2011. CKD was defined as dipstick proteinuria ≥1 or an estimated glomerular filtration rate (eGFR) <60 ml/min/1.73 m^2.

Results: The prevalence of CKD was 6.15% (men, 5.37%; women, 7.15%). Further, 22.25% study population had MS (abdominal obesity, 27.98%; hypertriglyceridemia, 30.09%; low high-density cholesterol levels, 19.74%; high blood pressure, 43.45%; and high fasting glucose levels, 30.44%). Multivariate-adjusted analysis indicated that proteinuria risk increased in participants with MS (odds ratio [OR] 1.884, 95% confidence interval [CI] 1.867–1.902, $P<0.001$). The presence of MS was associated with eGFR<60 mL/min/1.73 m^2 (OR 1.364, 95% CI 1.355–1.373, $P<0.001$). MS individual components were also associated with an increased CKD risk. The strength of association between MS and the development of CKD increase as the number of components increased from 1 to 5. In sub-analysis by men and women, MS and its each components were a significant determinant for CKD.

Conclusions: MS and its individual components can predict the risk of prevalent CKD for men and women.

Editor: Giovanni Targher, University of Verona, Ospedale Civile Maggiore, Italy

Funding: This research was supported by a fund under the Korea Centers for Disease Control and Prevention (2012-E33024-00), by the National Research Foundation of Korea (NRF) grant (MRC for Gene Regulation, 2011-0030132) funded by the Korea government (MSIP), and by Basic Science Research Program through the National Research Foundation of Korea (NRF) funded by the Ministry of Science, ICT and future Planning (2013R1A2A2A01067611). The funders had no role in study design, data collection and analysis, decision to publish, or preparation of the manuscript.

Competing Interests: The authors have declared that no competing interests exist.

* E-mail: skimw@chonnam.ac.kr

Introduction

Metabolic syndrome (MS) includes various metabolic abnormalities that have been associated with cardiovascular disease, stroke, and all-cause mortality in the general population [1]. The components of MS include central obesity, elevated blood pressure, and impaired fasting glucose and high triglyceride (TG) and low high-density lipoprotein (HDL) cholesterol levels, and these components are present in approximately 20% adults in USA [2]. In Korea, recent changes in lifestyle and diet have resulted in an increased prevalence of MS, becoming an important public health concern. The prevalence of MS has been reported to be about 14.2% in men and 17.7% in women in the general population [3]. Another study suggested that the prevalence of MS has increased to approximately 19.0% [4].

The burden of chronic kidney disease (CKD) has also been increasing worldwide over the last decade and is expected to increase further [5]. The increased incidence of CKD in recent years paralleled with an increasing prevalence of MS [6,7]. Previous observational studies have reported an independent association between MS and microalbuminuria or proteinuria and CKD [8,9]. In a large cohort survey, both MS and microalbuminuria had strong adverse effects on the estimated glomerular filtration rate (eGFR), and this relationship was even more pronounced in the presence of both factors [10]. However, a few studies have shown statistically insignificant association between MS and low eGFR after adjustment for albuminuria [11].

Additionally, the reported studies used varying definitions for MS and studied different populations. Thus, the data on MS or its relationship with CKD in large population-based studies are limited. Therefore, we aimed to assess the prevalence of MS and CKD, and the association between MS and its components with CKD in an adult Korean population.

Materials and Methods

Study Population

Korean National Health Screening is an annual health examination to improve the health of people and reduce healthcare costs by preventing cardiocerebrovascular diseases affected by lifestyle habits, such as hypertension, diabetes, dyslipidemia, and by detecting five major forms of cancer at an early stage. General Health Screening was the first-step screening test for an early detection. We performed a cross-sectional study using the general health screening data of 11,828,803 participants (age$\geq$20 years) from the 2011 Korean National Health Screening database. Of these, 10,549,230 subjects with information on renal function, such as serum creatinine and urine analysis, and all parameters related to MS were included in this analysis. 296,145 subjects with diabetes were excluded to appreciate the real impact of MS. Finally, 10,253,085 subjects were recruited in our study to assess the prevalence and association between MS and CKD.

This study was approved by the institutional review board of Chonnam National University Hospital, Gwangju, Republic of Korea. This institutional review board waived the need for consent given the retrospective design of the project. The study was performed in accordance with the Helsinki Declaration of 1975, as revised in 2000.

Data Collection

Health examination included data for anthropometric measurement, blood pressure, and blood chemistry tests. Information on sex, age, and other pertinent medical data were obtained. Anthropometric measurements, including height, weight, and waist circumference, were determined, and the body mass index (BMI) was calculated by dividing the weight in kilograms by height in meters squared. Trained nurses measured blood pressure at the health screening facilities using a standard protocol. Blood samples were collected in the morning after an overnight fast of at least 8 h. Plasma glucose levels were measured using a hexokinase enzyme reference method. At the health screening facilities, serum HDL cholesterol and TG levels were measured enzymatically by using a commercially available reagent mixture, and serum creatinine was measured using the modified Jaffe kinetic reaction.

Definitions

MS was defined using the current criteria in the National Cholesterol Education Program Adult Treatment Panel III (ATP III) (NCEP) guidelines with a modification for waist circumference. Specifically, elevated blood pressure was defined as systolic or diastolic blood pressure of 130/85 mmHg or higher and the current use of antihypertensive medication. Elevated blood glucose level was defined as a fasting blood glucose level of $\geq$100 mg/dL or use of glucose level-lowering medicine. Low HDL cholesterol level was defined as that <40 mg/dL in men and <50 mg/dL in women. Hypertriglyceridemia was defined as a serum TG level of $\geq$150 mg/dL. Abdominal obesity was defined as a waist circumference >90 cm in men and >80 cm in women according to the Asia-Pacific criteria. MS was defined as the presence of three or more of these five components [12].

Diabetes mellitus (DM) was defined as a self-reported history of a previous diagnosis of diabetes or a fasting plasma glucose level of $\geq$126 mg/dL. Hypertension (HT) was defined as self-reported history of a previous diagnosis of HT or systolic blood pressure $\geq$ 140 mmHg or diastolic blood pressure $\geq$90 mmHg. eGFR was calculated using The Chronic Kidney Disease Epidemiology Collaboration (CKD-EPI) equation [13]. The definition of proteinuria was based on a dipstick urinalysis score of 1+ or more. CKD was defined as an eGFR<60 mL/min/1.73 m^2 or dipstick proteinuria ($\geq$1+) [14].

Statistical Analysis

The prevalence of CKD, MS, and its individual components (abdominal obesity, high blood pressure, and high TG, low HDL cholesterol, and high fasting glucose levels) was determined for the overall population. Data were presented as the mean $\pm$ SD for continuous variables and as proportions for categorical variables. The characteristics of the subjects were compared using the chi-squared test for categorical variables. Student's t-test was used for continuous variables. Multivariate logistic regression was used to estimate odds ratio (OR), and 95% confidence interval (CI) was used for determining the relationship between MS and proteinuria or eGFR<60 mL/min/1.73 m^2. Covariates considered as potential confounders (age and sex) were included in multivariable models. Model 1 was unadjusted, model 2 included age and sex. For the eGFR analysis, model 3 included age, sex, and proteinuria. The associations between MS components and CKD were analysed using multivariate logistic regression models after adjustments for age and sex. Statistical analysis was performed with the SAS (Version 8.2, SAS Institute Inc., Cary, NC, USA). A P-value of <0.05 was considered statistically significant.

Results

Clinical Characteristics

We studied 10,253,085 (56.18% men) participants (mean age, 48.86$\pm$13.83 years). Women had significantly older age, higher proportion of hypertension, total cholesterol levels, low-density lipoprotein cholesterol levels, HDL cholesterol levels, and proportion of eGFR<60 mL/min/1.73 m^2 but lower BMI, waist circumference, TG levels, systolic blood pressure, diastolic blood pressure, fasting glucose levels, eGFR, and serum creatinine levels than men. However, proportion of proteinuria was not different between men and women (Table 1).

Prevalence of MS and CKD

The overall prevalence of CKD was 6.15% (men, 5.37%; women, 7.15%). The prevalence of CKD according to the stage was 0.81% in stage 1, 0.86% in stage 2, 3.52% in stage 3, and 0.96% in stage 4 or 5 (Table 2). We identified 2,281,675 (22.25%) subjects who met the current ATP III criteria. Among all subjects, 27.98% had abdominal obesity, 30.09% had hypertriglyceridemia, 19.74% had low HDL cholesterol levels, 43.45% had high blood pressure, and 30.44% had high fasting glucose levels. Women had significantly higher proportion of abdominal obesity and low HDL cholesterol but lower that of hypertriglyceridemia, high blood pressure, and high fasting glucose than men (Table 1).

Subjects with MS had a higher prevalence of CKD than those without MS (10.48% vs. 4.91%, P<0.001). 37.93% of the participants with total CKD (n = 239,137) had MS (40.04% for abdominal obesity; 34.46% for hypertriglyceridemia; 27.1% for low HDL cholesterol; 62.74% for high blood pressure; and 43.61% for high fasting glucose). The prevalence of MS increased with an increase in CKD stage. On the other hand, that of MS in CKD stage 4 or 5 was the lowest compared to those with other CKD stages. High blood pressure was the most common MS component in each CKD stage (Figure 1).

Association between MS and CKD

In multivariate logistic regression models, the participants with MS had a 1.884-fold increased OR (95% CI 1.867–1.902, P<

Table 1. Clinical characteristics.

	Overall	Men	Women	P
Number of subjects	10,253,085	5,760,643 (56.18)	4,492,442 (43.82)	<0.001
Age (years)	46.86±13.83	45.12±13.40	49.10±14.05	<0.001
Hypertension (%)	238,989 (2.33)	123,447 (2.14)	115,542 (2.57)	<0.001
Body mass index (kg/m²)	23.88±3.23	24.28±3.07	23.46±3.36	<0.001
Waist circumference (cm)	80.67±9.02	83.80±7.83	76.66±8.84	<0.001
TC (mg/dL)	195.84±35.82	194.43±35.08	197.52±36.67	<0.001
LDL cholesterol (mg/dL)	114.74±33.02	113.41±32.48	116.45±33.62	<0.001
Triglyceride (mg/dL)	132.71±72.26	146.52±77.92	115.01±59.78	<0.001
HDL cholesterol (mg/dL)	54.66±13.45	51.99±12.62	58.07±13.70	<0.001
Systolic blood pressure (mmHg)	122.65±14.71	124.50±13.76	120.08±15.49	<0.001
Diastolic blood pressure (mmHg)	76.44±9.89	77.97±9.58	74.48±9.93	<0.001
Fasting glucose (mg/dL)	95.81±18.40	97.27±19.92	93.92±16.04	<0.001
eGFR (mL/min/1.73 m²)	90.02±19.64	91.19±19.24	90.81±20.14	<0.001
Serum creatinine (mg/dL)	0.96±0.71	1.06±0.75	0.82±0.62	<0.001
Proteinuria (%)	202,928 (1.98)	113,838 (1.98)	89,090 (1.98)	0.426
eGFR<60 mL/min/1.73 m² (%)	459,032 (4.48)	213,207 (3.70)	245,825 (5.47)	<0.001
Chronic kidney disease (%)	630,420 (6.15)	309,360 (5.37)	321,060 (7.15)	<0.001
Metabolic syndrome (%)	2,281,675 (22.25)	1,270,105 (22.05)	1,011,570 (22.52)	<0.001
Individual component (%)				
Abdominal obesity	2,868,480 (27.98)	1,266,208 (21.98)	1,602,272 (35.67)	<0.001
Hypertriglyceridemia	3,085,216 (30.09)	2,163,829 (37.56)	921,387 (20.51)	<0.001
Low HDL cholesterol	2,023,489 (19.74)	786,802 (13.66)	1,236,687 (27.53)	<0.001
High blood pressure	4,454,799 (43.45)	2,757,750 (47.87)	1,697,049 (37.78)	<0.001
High fasting glucose	3,120,707 (30.44)	1,963,828 (34.09)	1,156,879 (25.75)	<0.001

Abbreviations: TC, total cholesterol; LDL, low-density lipoprotein; HDL, high-density lipoprotein; eGFR, estimated glomerular filtration rate.

0.001) for proteinuria compared with those without MS. In addition, the presence of MS was a significant determinant of eGFR<60 mL/min/1.73 m² (OR 1.364, 95% CI 1.355–1.373, P<0.001) and CKD (OR 1.526, 95% CI 1.518–1.535, P<0.001) compared with those without MS. In sub-analysis by men and women, the presence of MS was also a significant determinant for proteinuria, eGFR<60 mL/min/1.73 m², and CKD compared with those without MS (Table 3).

Association between MS Components and their Risk for Development of CKD

In models adjusted for age and sex, we further examined the associations of individual components of MS and the risk of CKD by dividing each components of MS, in quartiles and making the groups accordingly. Increasing component levels of MS showed a positive association with the development of CKD compared with the lowest quartile for men and women, respectively. On the other hand, decreasing HDL cholesterol levels was linked clearly to CKD compared with the lowest quartile for men and women, respectively. The OR for CKD for high fasting glucose as an MS component was higher than that for other MS components (Table 4). The prevalence of markers of CKD was higher with increasing number of MS components (Figure 2). The participants with 1–5 component of MS had an increased OR for CKD: 1.062 (95% CI 1.053–1.071), 1.281 (95% CI 1.270–1.292), 1.575 (95% CI 1.561–1.590), 1.942 (95% CI 1.921–1.962), and 2.367 (95% CI 2.329–2.406) compared with those with no MS components (P<

0.001). In sub-analysis for men and women, the strength of association between MS and the development of CKD also appeared to increase as the number of components increased from 1 to 5 (Table 4).

Discussion

The results of our study identified a strong, positive relationship between MS and the prevalence of CKD. A rise in the incidence of CKD in recent years has been associated with an increasing prevalence of MS [6,7]. The prevalence of MS is about 24.7% of adults in USA [8]. A recent study demonstrated that the prevalence of MS has increased to approximately 19.0% in Korea [4]. Although we excluded subjects with diabetes to appreciate the real impact of MS, the present study reported an even higher prevalence of MS (22.25%), reflecting a rapidly increasing prevalence in Korea. The identification of MS is important in patients with a high risk of developing end-stage renal disease (ESRD).

Chen et al. [8] demonstrated a significant correlation between the number of MS traits and both albuminuria and eGFR< 60 mL/min/1.73 m². In a prospective cohort survey, Luk et al. [10] reported that the presence of MS independently predicted the development of CKD in subjects with type 2 diabetes. According to the National Health and Nutrition Examination survey, MS is independently associated with CKD in the general population and in non-diabetic adults [4,15]. Palaniappan et al. [16] showed a higher risk for microalbuminuria in men and women with MS.

Table 2. The prevalence of kidney function and chronic kidney disease stage.

Kidney function				Chronic kidney disease			
eGFR[a]	Overall[b]	Men[b]	Women[b]	Stage	Overall[b]	Men[b]	Women[b]
≥90	5,492,524 (53.57)	3,096,868 (53.76)	2,393,565 (53.33)	1	82,770 (0.81)	44,763 (0.78)	38,007 (0.85)
60–89	4,301,529 (41.95)	2,450,568 (42.54)	1,850,961 (41.20)	2	88,618 (0.86)	51,390 (0.89)	37,228 (0.83)
30–59	360,641 (3.52)	156,994 (2.73)	203,647 (4.53)	3	360,641 (3.52)	156,994 (2.73)	203,647 (4.53)
<30	98,391 (0.96)	56,213 (0.97)	42,178 (0.94)	4 or 5	98,391 (0.96)	56,213 (0.97)	42,178 (0.94)
Total	10,253,085 (100)	5,760,643 (100)	4,492,442 (100)	All	630,420 (6.15)	309,360 (5.37)	321,060 (7.15)

Abbreviations: eGFR, estimated glomerular filtration rate.
[a] eGFR, mL/min/1.73 m² by CKD-PEI equation.
[b] All P value for trend<0.001.

These data support the importance of MS in the development of CKD. In a recent meta-analysis, although the results for proteinuria outcomes were debated because of the small number of prospective cohort studies, MS and its components were associated with the development of eGFR<60 mL/min/1.73 m² and microalbuminuria or overt proteinuria [17]. All of these studies confirmed a relationship between MS and CKD. Also, our study results showed a strong relationship between MS and CKD in non-diabetic adult Korean population. In sub-analysis by men and women, MS was a significant determinant for CKD. These findings have important clinical and public health implications because the prevalence of the MS is rapidly increasing in Korea.

Our findings revealed each component of MS was an independent predictor of CKD. We analysed individual components to explore their differential effect in the presence of MS, and thus, the risk estimates were interpreted in the context of MS. In addition, the number of MS components and the risk for CKD showed a graded association. Moreover, the prevalence of markers of CKD increased with an increasing number of MS components. Therefore, therapeutic strategies that targeted individual MS components seem highly reasonable for preventing CKD.

Obesity is a significant risk factor for CKD. Visceral obesity is highly correlated with insulin resistance, and indices of visceral obesity may be more sensitive predictors of kidney disease than BMI [18]. Adipose tissue is a significant source of inflammatory and immunomodulatory factors; the interaction between adipocytes and macrophages may contribute to insulin resistance and many of the features that characterise MS [19–21]. Obesity occurs probably via the mechanisms associated with renal hyperfiltration and hyperperfusion as focal glomerulosclerosis and other histological changes have been observed in kidneys of obese patients [22,23]. Previous studies reporting obesity as a significant risk factor for eGFR<60 ml/min/1.73 m² used waist circumference criteria (a better measure of central adiposity) rather than BMI [24,25]. Our study results indicated a 69.1% and 37.6% higher risk of developing CKD with abdominal obesity compared with the lowest quartile for men and women, respectively.

Dyslipidemia is also an important risk factor for proteinuria and decline of renal function [26]. In a prospective study of 12,728 subjects, high TG and low HDL cholesterol levels predicted an increased risk of renal dysfunction [27]. According to Ryu et al. [28] both high TG and low HDL cholesterol levels were associated with a significantly increased risk of CKD. These results remained unchanged, even after additional adjustment for incident HT and DM. The mechanisms underlying the contribution of lipids to renal injury are not completely understood. Dyslipidemia is associated with glomerular capillary endothelial and mesangial cell as well as podocyte injury, which further leads to mesangial sclerosis [29,30]. The accumulation of lipoproteins in the glomerular mesangium can stimulate matrix production and glomerulosclerosis [31]. Although hypertriglyceridemia and low HDL cholesterol levels have been previously associated with an increased risk for CKD [26–28], these factors are often overlooked in clinical practice. Our results suggest that these could be potential targets for reducing the risk of CKD.

DM and HT are the most common risk factors for ESRD [14], and MS is frequently associated with these factors. The PAMELA (Pressioni Arteriose Monitorate E Loro Associazioni) population study revealed high normal blood pressure values and HT in 80% individuals with MS [32,33]. According to the results of a previous study, insulin resistance and central obesity have been considered the main factors involved in hypertension pathophysiology associated with MS [34]. Recent community-based prospective observational cohort studies reported a significant risk for impaired

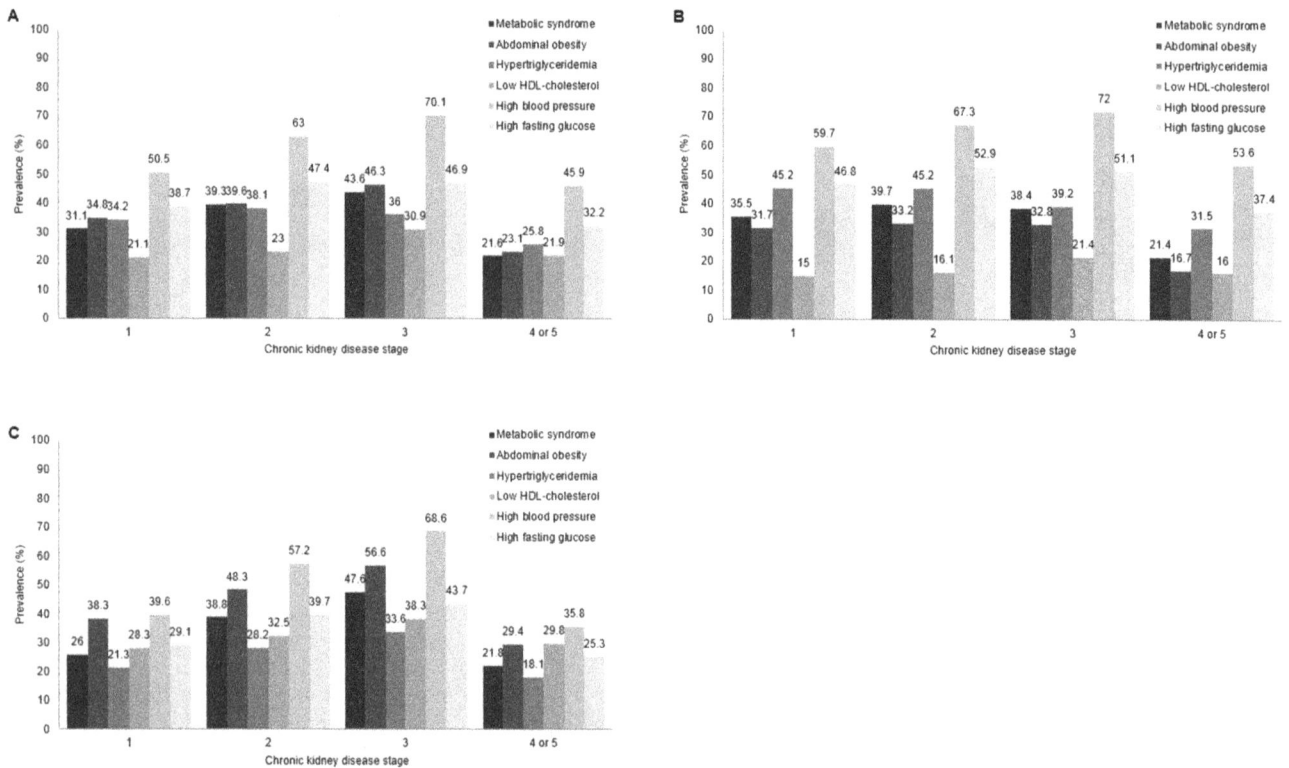

Figure 1. The prevalence of metabolic syndrome and its components according to chronic kidney disease stages. (A) Overall. (B) Men. (C) Women.

fasting glucose and development of eGFR<60 mL/min/1.73 m^2 in Asia [35,36]. Evidence has shown that hyperinsulinemia occurs well before the onset of glucose intolerance, and this evidence suggests insulin resistance at levels of the muscle and liver, which is not directly indicated in the NCEP-ATP III criteria for MS. Thus, insulin resistance and subsequent hyperinsulinemia in addition to mild hyperglycemia may be accountable for the association between impaired fasting glucose level and CKD [37,38]. In our analysis, we excluded subjects with diabetes to appreciate the real

impact of MS. both high blood pressure and high fasting glucose levels were associated with significantly increased risk of CKD for men and women.

The present study has several limitations. First, the cross-sectional study design makes it difficult to infer causality between MS and the risk of developing CKD. Second, laboratory tests, specifically estimation of serum creatinine levels were performed in each hospital. Therefore, inter-laboratory variability may be present. A systematic difference in creatinine measurements

Table 3. Odds ratios for the association between metabolic syndrome and chronic kidney disease.

Description of model covariates	Odds ratio (95% CI)		
	Overall[a]	Men[a]	Women[a]
Proteinuria			
Model 1: unadjusted	2.148 (2.128–2.167)	2.317 (2.290–2.346)	1.947 (1.920–1.974)
Model 2: adjusted for age, sex	1.884 (1.867–1.902)	2.071 (2.046–2.096)	1.815 (1.788–1.843)
eGFR<60 mL/min/1.73 m^2			
Model 1: unadjusted	2.328 (2.314–2.342)	1.866 (1.849–1.884)	2.806 (2.783–2.829)
Model 2: adjusted for age, sex	1.400 (1.391–1.409)	1.450 (1.437–1.464)	1.366 (1.353–1.378)
Model 3: adjust for age, sex, proteinuria	1.364 (1.355–1.373)	1.394 (1.381–1.407)	1.341 (1.329–1.353)
Chronic kidney disease			
Model 1: unadjusted	2.268 (2.256–2.280)	2.000 (1.984–2.015)	2.557 (2.538–2.576)
Model 2: adjusted for age, sex	1.526 (1.518–1.535)	1.626 (1.613–1.639)	1.452 (1.440–1.463)

Abbreviations: eGFR; estimated glomerular filtration rate; CI, confidence interval.
[a]All P value for trend<0.001.

Table 4. Association between metabolic syndrome components and the risk of development of chronic kidney disease.

Variables	Odds ratio (95% CI)		
	Overall	Men	Women
Abdominal obesity[a]			
Q2	1.132 (1.121–1.142)[e]	1.261 (1.243–1.279)[e]	1.048 (1.036–1.061)[e]
Q3	1.228 (1.217–1.238)[e]	1.320 (1.303–1.338)[e]	1.153 (1.139–1.166)[e]
Q4	1.487 (1.475–1.500)[e]	1.691 (1.669–1.714)[e]	1.376 (1.361–1.391)[e]
Hypertriglyceridemia[a]			
Q2	1.140 (1.129–1.151)[e]	1.132 (1.118–1.146)[e]	1.159 (1.142–1.176)[c]
Q3	1.199 (1.188–1.210)[e]	1.204 (1.189–1.220)[e]	1.200 (1.183–1.217)[e]
Q4	1.308 (1.296–1.320)[e]	1.321 (1.305–1.338)[e]	1.302 (1.284–1.321)[e]
Low HDL cholesterol[a]			
Q2	0.878 (0.866–0.891)[e]	0.864 (0.843–0.886)[e]	0.879 (0.864–0.895)[d]
Q3	0.828 (0.816–0.840)[e]	0.799 (0.779–0.819)[e]	0.837 (0.822–0.852)[e]
Q4	0.734 (0.726–0.742)[e]	0.654 (0.642–0.665)[e]	0.778 (0.769–0.788)[e]
Systolic blood pressure[a]			
Q2	1.154 (1.144–1.163)[e]	1.233 (1.220–1.245)[e]	1.032 (1.017–1.047)[e]
Q3	1.201 (1.191–1.212)[e]	1.297 (1.280–1.313)[e]	1.119 (1.105–1.133)[d]
Q4	1.402 (1.390–1.414)[e]	1.555 (1.535–1.575)[e]	1.292 (1.278–1.307)[e]
Diastolic blood pressure[a]			
Q2	1.069 (1.056–1.082)[e]	1.111 (1.095–1.128)[e]	1.000 (0.981–1.021)[e]
Q3	1.163 (1.151–1.175)[e]	1.166 (1.150–1.183)[c]	1.162 (1.145–1.179)[e]
Q4	1.344 (1.330–1.358)[e]	1.388 (1.369–1.407)[e]	1.290 (1.270–1.311)[e]
High fasting glucose[a]			
Q2	1.137 (1.127–1.148)[e]	1.141 (1.127–1.156)[e]	1.133 (1.119–1.148)[e]
Q3	1.266 (1.255–1.277)[e]	1.256 (1.241–1.271)[e]	1.279 (1.263–1.296)[e]
Q4	1.568 (1.556–1.581)[e]	1.585 (1.568–1.602)[e]	1.549 (1.531–1.568)[e]
Number of components model[b]			
1 component	1.062 (1.053–1.071)[e]	1.198 (1.183–1.214)[e]	0.967 (0.955–0.979)[e]
2 components	1.281 (1.270–1.292)[e]	1.493 (1.474–1.512)[e]	1.125 (1.111–1.139)[e]
3 components	1.575 (1.561–1.590)[e]	1.875 (1.850–1.900)[e]	1.364 (1.346–1.382)[e]
4 components	1.942 (1.921–1.962)[e]	2.398 (2.360–2.436)[e]	1.653 (1.629–1.678)[e]
5 components	2.367 (2.329–2.406)[e]	2.911 (2.830–2.995)[e]	2.070 (2.027–2.112)[e]

Note: Adjusted for factors included in age and sex.
Abbreviations: CI, confidence interval; HDL, high-density lipoprotein.
[a]Reference group is lowest quartile (Q1) for each set of quartiles of factors.
[b]Reference group is 0 component for number of compomants model.
[c]P value for trend>0.05.
[d]P value for trend<0.05.
[e]P value for trend<0.001.

between laboratories could have affected the association between MS and CKD. Third, CKD was defined as an eGFR<60 mL/min/1.73 m^2 or dipstick proteinuria (≥1+). This definition didn't include another kidney damages (e.g. abnormal urine sediment, abnormal blood and urine chemistry, abnormal imaging studies) and repeated measurements of creatinine levels and proteinuria were not performed. These factors could have led to underestimation or overestimation of the prevalence of CKD. Finally, other parameters associated with obesity and glucose metabolism, such as physical activity and alcohol consumption, were not evaluated in the present study. However, we believe most of these potential limitations should be consistently attenuated by the large sample size of the study.

In conclusion, our study confirmed MS and its individual components as a strong and independent risk factor for men and women with CKD. In addition, we found a graded relationship between the number of MS components and the risk for CKD. Our results emphasise that individuals with metabolic risk factors should be identified that an early stage and should undergo multidisciplinary interventions, particularly lifestyle modifications, to impede the development of CKD.

Author Contributions

Conceived and designed the experiments: YUK SWK. Performed the experiments: YUK HYK JSC CSK. Analyzed the data: YUK EHB SKM SWK. Contributed reagents/materials/analysis tools: YUK HYK JSC CSK. Wrote the paper: YUK SWK.

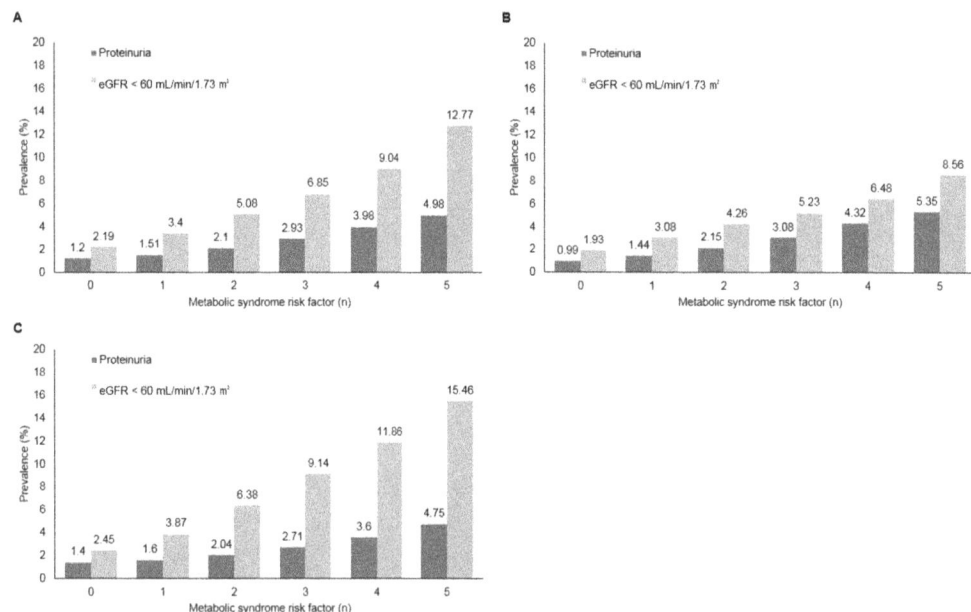

Figure 2. The prevalence of markers of chronic kidney disease according to number of metabolic syndrome components. (A) Overall. (B) Men. (C) Women.

References

1. Alberti KG, Eckel RH, Grundy SM, Zimmet PZ, Cleeman JI, et al. (2009) Harmonizing the metabolic syndrome: a joint interim statement of the International Diabetes Federation Task Force on Epidemiology and Prevention; National Heart, Lung, and Blood Institute; American Heart Association; World Heart Federation; International Atherosclerosis Society; and International Association for the Study of Obesity. Circulation 120: 1640–1645.

2. Ford ES, Giles WH, Dietz WH (2002) Prevalence of the metabolic syndrome among US adults: Findings from the third National Health and Nutrition Examination survey. JAMA 287: 356–359.

3. Park HS, Oh SW, Cho SI, Choi WH, Kim YS (2004) The metabolic syndrome and associated lifestyle factors among South Korean adults. Int J Epidemiol 33: 328–336.

4. Chang IH, Han JH, Myung SC, Kwak KW, Kim TH, et al. (2009) Association between metabolic syndrome and chronic kidney disease in the Korean population. Nephrology 14: 321–326.

5. Levey AS, Atkins R, Coresh J, Cohen EP, Collins AJ, et al. (2007) Chronic kidney disease as a global public health problem: approaches and initiatives–a position statement from kidney disease improving global outcomes. Kidney Int 72: 247–259.

6. Ford ES, Giles WH, Mokdad AH (2004) Increasing prevalence of the metabolic syndrome among U.S. adults. Diabetes Care 27: 2444–2449.

7. Nestel P, Lyu R, Low LP, Sheu WH, Nitiyanant W, et al. (2007) Metabolic syndrome: recent prevalence in East and Southeast Asian populations. Asia Pac J Clin Nutr 16: 362–367.

8. Chen J, Muntner P, Hamm LL, Jones DW, Batuman V, et al. (2004) The metabolic syndrome and chronic kidney disease in U.S. adults. Ann Intern Med 140: 167–174.

9. Lucove J, Vupputuri S, Heiss G, North K, Russell M (2008) Metabolic syndrome and the development of CKD in American Indians: The Strong Heart Study. Am J Kidney Dis 51: 21–28.

10. Luk AO, So WY, Ma RC, Kong AP, Ozaki R, et al; Hong Kong Diabetes Registry. (2008) Metabolic syndrome predicts new onset of chronic kidney disease in 5829 patients with type 2 diabetes. Diabetes Care 31: 2357–2361.

11. Athyros VG, Karagiannis A, Ganotakis ES, Paletas K, Nicolaou V, et al; Assessing The Treatment Effect in Metabolic syndrome without Perceptible diabeTes (ATTEMPT) Collaborative Group. (2011) Association between changes in renal function and serum uric acid levels during multifactorial intervention and clinical outcome in patients with metabolic syndrome. A post hoc analysis of the ATTEMPT study. Curr Med Res Opin 27: 1659–1668.

12. Grundy SM, Cleeman JI, Daniels SR, Donato KA, Eckel RH, et al; American Heart Association, National Heart, Lung, and Blood Institute (2005) Diagnosis and management of the metabolic syndrome: an American Heart Association/National Heart, Lung, and Blood Institute Scientific Statement. Circulation 112: 2735.

13. Levey AS, Stevens LA, Schmid CH, Zhang YL, Castro AF 3rd, et al; CKD-EPI (Chronic Kidney Disease Epidemiology Collaboration) (2009) A new equation to estimate glomerular filtration rate. Ann Intern Med 150: 604–612.

14. National Kidney Foundation (2002) K/DOQI Clinical practice guidelines for chronic kidney disease: evaluation, classification and stratification. Am J Kidney Dis 39 (Suppl 1): S1–S266.

15. Kurella M, Lo JC, Chertow GM (2005) Metabolic syndrome and the risk for chronic kidney disease among nondiabetic adults. J Am Soc Nephrol 16: 2134–2140.

16. Palaniappan L, Carnethon M, Fortmann SP (2003) Association between microalbuminuria and the metabolic syndrome: NHANES III. Am J Hypertens 16: 952–958.

17. Thomas G, Sehgal AR, Kashyap SR, Srinivas TR, Kirwan JP, et al. (2011) Metabolic syndrome and kidney disease: a systematic review and meta-analysis. Clin J Am Soc Nephrol 6: 2364–2373.

18. Pinto-Sietsma SJ, Navis G, Janssen WM, de Zeeuw D, Gans RO, et al. (2003) A central body fat distribution is related to renal function impairment, even in lean subjects. Am J Kidney Dis 41: 733–741.

19. Bagby SP (2004) Obesity-initiated metabolic syndrome and the kidney: A recipe for chronic kidney disease? J Am Soc Nephrol 15: 2775–2791.

20. Schelling JR, Sedor JR (2004) The metabolic syndrome as a risk factor for chronic kidney disease: More than a fat chance? J Am Soc Nephrol 15: 2773–2774.

21. Wisse BE (2004) The inflammatory syndrome: The role of adipose tissue cytokines in metabolic disorders linked to obesity. J Am Soc Nephrol 15: 2792–2800.

22. Kopple JD, Feroze U (2011) The effect of obesity on chronic kidney disease. J Ren Nutr 21: 66–71.

23. Tomaszewski M, Charchar FJ, Maric C, McClure J, Crawford L, et al. (2007) Glomerular hyperfiltration: a new marker of metabolic risk. Kidney Int 71: 816–821.

24. Rashidi A, Ghanbarian A, Azizi F (2007) Are patients who have metabolic syndrome without diabetes at risk for developing chronic kidney disease? Evidence based on data from a large cohort screening population. Clin J Am Soc Nephrol 2: 976–983.

25. Sun F, Tao Q, Zhan S (2010) Metabolic syndrome and the development of chronic kidney disease among 118,924 non-diabetic Taiwanese in a retrospective cohort. Nephrology 15: 84–92.

26. Tozawa M, Iseki K, Iseki C, Oshiro S, Ikemiya Y, et al. (2002) Triglyceride, but not total cholesterol or low-density lipoprotein cholesterol levels, predict development of proteinuria. Kidney Int 62: 1743–1749.

27. Muntner P, Coresh J, Smith JC, Eckfeldt J, Klag MJ (2000) Plasma lipids and risk of developing renal dysfunction: The atherosclerosis risk in communities study. Kidney Int 58: 293–301.

28. Ryu S, Chang Y, Woo HY, Lee KB, Kim SG, et al. (2009) Time-dependent association between metabolic syndrome and risk of CKD in Korean men without hypertension or diabetes. Am J Kidney Dis 53: 59–69.

29. Cases A, Coll E (2005) Dyslipidemia and the progression of renal disease in chronic renal failure patients. Kidney Int 68: S87–93.

30. Joles JA, Kunter U, Janssen U, Kriz W, Rabelink TJ, et al. (2000) Early mechanisms of renal injury in hypercholesterolemic or hypertriglyceridemic rats. J Am Soc Nephrol 11: 669–683.

31. Gluba A, Rysz J, Banach M (2010) Statins in patients with chronic kidney disease: why, who and when? Expert Opin Pharmacother 11: 2665–2674.

32. Mancia G, Bombelli M, Corrao G, Facchetti R, Madotto F, et al. (2007) Metabolic syndrome in the Pressioni Arteriose Monitorate E Loro Associazioni (PAMELA) study: daily life blood pressure, cardiac damage, and prognosis. Hypertension 49: 40–74.

33. Deedwania P (2011) Hypertension, dyslipidemia, and insulin resistance in patients with diabetes mellitus or the cardiometabolic syndrome: benefits of vasodilating β-blockers. J Clin Hypertens (Greenwich) 13: 52–59.

34. Banach M, Rysz J (2010) Current problems in hypertension and nephrology. Expert Opin Pharmacother 11: 2575–2578.

35. Kitiyakara C, Yamwong S, Cheepudomwit S, Domrongkitchaiporn S, Unkurapinun N, et al. (2007) The metabolic syndrome and chronic kidney disease in a southeast Asian cohort. Kidney Int 71: 693–700.

36. Watanabe H, Obata H, Watanabe T, Sasaki S, Nagai K, et al. (2010) Metabolic syndrome and risk of development of chronic kidney disease: The Niigata Preventive Medicine Study. Diabetes Metab Res Rev 26: 26–32.

37. Eckel RH, Alberti KG, Grundy SM, Zimmet PZ (2010) The metabolic syndrome. Lancet 375: 181–183.

38. Tabak AG, Jokela M, Akbaraly TN, Brunner EJ, Kivimaki M, et al. (2009) Trajectories of glycaemia, insulin sensitivity, and insulin secretion before diagnosis of type 2 diabetes: An analysis from the Whitehall II Study. Lancet 373: 2215–2221.

27

One-Year Mortality Associations in Hemodialysis Patients after Traumatic Brain Injury

Jen-Chieh Liao[1]◗, Chung-Han Ho[2,5]◗, Fu-Wen Liang[3], Jhi-Joung Wang[2], Kao-Chang Lin[2,4], Chung-Ching Chio[1], Jinn-Rung Kuo[1,2,4]*

1 Department of Neurosurgery, Chi-Mei Medical Center, Tainan, Taiwan, 2 Department of Medical Research, Chi-Mei Medical Center, Tainan, Taiwan, 3 Institute of Public Health, College of Medicine, National Cheng Kung University, Tainan, Taiwan, 4 Department of Biotechnology, Southern Taiwan University of Science and Technology, Tainan, Taiwan, 5 Department of Hospital and Health Care Administration, Chia Nan University of Pharmacy and Science, Tainan, Taiwan

Abstract

Purpose: This study aimed to investigate the one-year mortality associations in hemodialysis patients who underwent neurosurgical intervention after traumatic brain injury (TBI) using a nationwide database in Taiwan.

Materials and Methods: An age- and gender-matched longitudinal cohort study of 4416 subjects, 1104 TBI patients with end-stage renal disease (ESRD) and 3312 TBI patients without ESRD, was conducted using the National Health Insurance Research Database in Taiwan between January 2000 and December 2007. The demographic characteristics, length of stay (LOS), length of ICU stay, length of ventilation (LOV), and tracheostomy were collected and analyzed. The co-morbidities of hypertension (HTN), diabetes mellitus (DM), myocardial infarction (MI), stroke, and heart failure (HF) were also evaluated.

Results: TBI patients with ESRD presented a shorter LOS, a longer length of ICU stay and LOV, and a higher percentage of comorbidities compared with those without ESRD. TBI patients with ESRD displayed a stable trend of one-year mortality rate, 75.82% to 76.79%, from 2000–2007. For TBI patients with ESRD, the median survival time was 0.86 months, and pre-existing stroke was a significant risk factor of mortality (HR: 1.29, 95% C.I.: 1.08–1.55). Pre-existing DM (HR: 1.35, 95% C.I.: 1.12–1.63) and MI (HR: 1.61, 95% C.I.: 1.07–2.42) effect on the mortality in ESRD patients who underwent TBI surgical intervention in the younger (age<65) and older (age≥65) population, respectively. In addition, the length of ICU stay and tracheostomy may provide important information to predict the mortality risk.

Conclusions: This is the first report indicating an increased risk of one-year mortality among TBI patients with a pre-existing ERSD insult. Comorbidities were more common in TBI patients with ESRD. Physicians should pay more attention to TBI patients with ESRD based on the status of age, comorbidities, length of ICU stay, and tracheostomy to improve their survival.

Editor: Daqing Ma, Imperial College London, Chelsea & Westminster Hospital, United Kingdom

Funding: The authors have no support or funding to report.

Competing Interests: The authors have declared that no competing interests exist.

* E-mail: kuojinnrung@gmail.com

◗ These authors contributed equally to this work.

Introduction

The population of patients with end-stage renal disease (ESRD) requiring dialysis is progressively growing, and the mortality rate of this group is much higher than that of the general population in the USA in recent decades[1]. In Taiwan, cases of ESRD requiring hemodialysis also have increased considerably over the past few decades [2,3]. The country has had the greatest incidence and the second greatest prevalence of ESRD since 2000, according to an international comparison based on data from the US Renal Data System [4,5].

Patients who have pre-existing ESRD and are admitted to the intensive care unit (ICU) with different etiologies, such as medical [6,7] or surgical problems [8,9], have a higher mortality than patients without ESRD. The data also indicate that ESRD patients have a greater number of comorbidities, such as diabetes, stroke, hypertension, and heart disease, than non-ESRD patients admitted to the ICU [10]. Thus, these comorbidities are often one of the risk factors for mortality [11].

According to the Centers for Disease Control and Prevention, the annual incidence of traumatic brain injury (TBI) in the United States is ∼1.7 million [12]. Incidence rates of 103 and 344 per 100 000 people have been reported in the United States [13] and Taiwan [14], respectively. At present, TBI is a major cause of death and disability in humans and remains a critical public health challenge. Cases of ESRD requiring hemodialysis have increased in Taiwan. Therefore, neurosurgeons can expect to see more dialysis patients presenting with TBI in daily practice.

Table 1. Demographic characteristics and clinical information of TBI surgery patients with and without pre-existing E SRD from 2000 to 2007 in Taiwan.

	With ESRD (N = 1104)	Without ESRD (N = 3312)	*p*-value*
Age (mean±SD)	60.05±12.29	60.05±12.29	0.9995
Age (%)			
<65	708(64.13)	2124(64.13)	1.0000
>=65	396(35.87)	1188(35.87)	
Gender (%)			
Male	588(53.26)	1764(53.26)	1.0000
Female	516(46.74)	1548(46.74)	
Level of Urbanization (%)			
1	418(37.86)	1274(38.47)	0.8445
2	488(44.20)	1431(43.21)	
>=3	198(17.93)	607(18.33)	
Time to death, months			
Median(IQR)	0.86(0.26–8.91)	29.36(4.18–59.57)	<.0001
Death (%)			
Yes	959(86.87)	1332(40.22)	<.0001
No	145(13.13)	1980(59.78)	
Time to death at one year, month			
Median (IQR)	0.86(0.26–8.91)	12(4.18–12.00)	<.0001
Death at one year(%)			
Yes	847(76.72)	986(29.77)	<.0001
No	257(23.28)	2326(70.23)	
Hospitalization Death (%)			
Yes	219(19.84)	227(6.85)	<.0001
No	885(80.16)	3085(93.15)	
Length of Stay, days			
Median (IQR)	14(6–28)	21(11–30)	<.0001
Length of ICU, days			
Median (IQR)	10(5–19)	8(4–16)	<.0001
Length of ventilation, days			
Median (IQR)	9(5–17)	6(3–14)	<.0001
Tracheostomy (%)			
Yes	213(19.29)	614(18.54)	0.5777
No	891(80.71)	2698(81.46)	
Comorbidity			
Hypertension (%)			
Yes	965(87.41)	1861(56.19)	<.0001
No	139(12.59)	1451(43.81)	
Diabetes mellitus (%)			
Yes	589(53.35)	895(27.02)	<.0001
No	515(46.65)	2417(72.98)	
Myocardial infarction (%)			
Yes	68(6.16)	91(2.75)	<.0001
No	1036(93.84)	3221(97.25)	
Stroke (%)			
Yes	889(80.53)	2168(65.46)	<.0001
No	215(19.47)	1144(34.54)	
Heart failure (%)			
Yes	196(17.75)	168(5.07)	<.0001
No	908(82.25)	3144(94.93)	

*p-values were derived from the Student t test for continuous variables and chi-square test for categorical variables.
ESRD: end-stage renal disease; SD: standard deviation; IQR: interquartile range; ICU: Intensive Care Unit.

In central nervous system insults, several studies have demonstrated that the mortality rate after stroke is higher in ESRD patients than in the general population [15–18]. However, the long-term prognosis, the mortality rate, and possible risk factors in TBI patients with ESRD remain unclear. Therefore, the aim of this study was to evaluate the one-year mortality risk factors for TBI patients with ESRD using data from the nationwide database of the National Health Insurance (NHI) Program in Taiwan (2000–2007). We believe that awareness of the possibility of developing mortality post-TBI can improve not only one's understanding of the sequelae of brain injury but also the patient treatment and prevention protocol.

Materials and Methods

Data source

In this study, the inpatient medical claims data between January 1997 and December 2008 were retrieved from the Taiwan's National Health Insurance Research Database (NHIRD). NHIRD was established by the Taiwan's National Health Research Institute to enhance medical research. The NHIRD have has been used extensively in various published studies[19]. The database comprises detailed information about clinical visits for each insured subject, including diagnostic codes according to the clinical modification of the International Classification of Diseases, Ninth Revision, Clinical Modification (ICD-9CM) code. The confidentiality of individuals was protected using encrypted personal identification to avoid the possibility of the ethical violations related to the data. Exemption was obtained from the institutional review board of Chi Mei Medical Center.

Patient selection and definition

The inpatient medical claims data during 2000–2007 was analyzed in this study. TBI patients were defined as those claiming medical expenditure applications for TBI surgery. The patients with ESRD were identified using the catastrophic illness certification records, as patients who underwent hemodialysis for more than three months could apply for a catastrophic illness card. A total of 74226 TBI patients received surgery, and of those, 1104 patients with ESRD were selected as the study sample. We then randomly selected 3312 TBI patients without ESRD (three for every patient with TBI) who were matched with the study cohort in terms of age and gender. The disease records for these patients were consistent with the format of ICD-9CM code. The co-morbidities of hypertension (HTN), diabetes mellitus (DM), myocardial infarction (MI), stroke, and heart failure (HF) were based on the records from one year before the date of TBI diagnosis. HTN was coded by hypertensive disease (ICD-9CM: 401-405), hypertensive encephalopathy (ICD-9CM: 437.2), and hypertensive retinopathy (ICD-9CM: 362.11). The DM was coded as follows: diabetes mellitus (ICD-9CM: 250), polyneuropathy in diabetes (ICD-9CM: 357.2), diabetic retinopathy (ICD-9CM: 362.0), and diabetic cataract (ICD-9CM: 366.41). MI was coded by acute myocardial infarction (ICD-9CM: 410) and old myocardial infarction (ICD-9CM: 412). Stroke was coded by cerebrovascular disease (ICD-9CM: 430-438). HF was coded by heart failure (ICD-9CM: 428), rheumatic heart failure (ICD-9CM: 398.91), acute myocarditis (ICD-9CM: 422), cardiomyopathy (ICD-9CM: 425), hypertensive heart disease with heart failure (ICD-9CM: 402.01, 402.11, and 402.91), and hypertensive heart and chronic kidney disease with heart failure (ICD-9CM: 404.01, 404.03, 404.11, 404.13, 404.91, and 404.93).

Measurements

The main event in this study was one-year mortality as TBI patients with ESRD had short survival after surgery. Survival time was calculated from the date of TBI surgery to the date of death or to one year after admission. Demographic and clinical characteristics, including age, gender, level of urbanization[20], DM, HTN, MI, stroke, heart failure, length of stay (LOS), length of ICU stay,

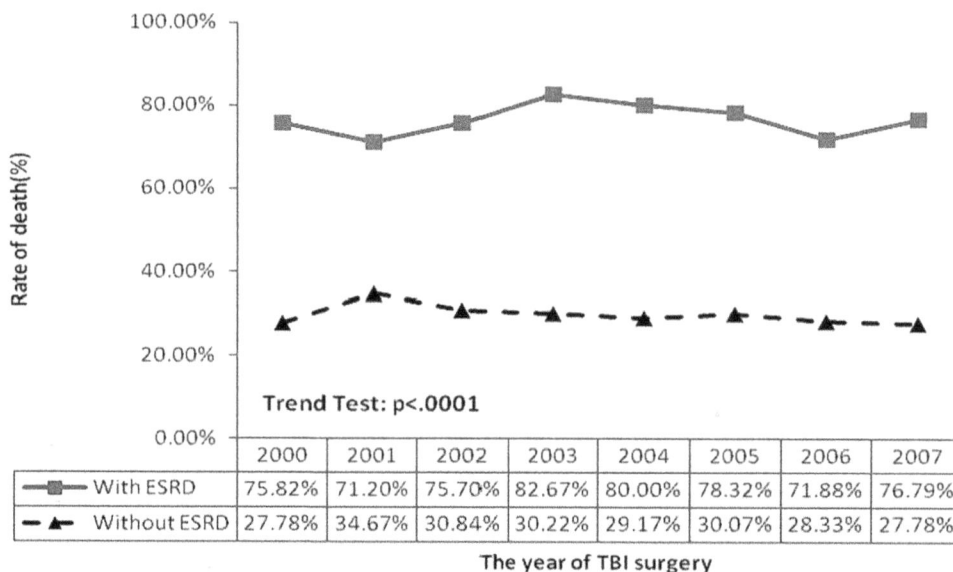

	2000	2001	2002	2003	2004	2005	2006	2007
With ESRD	75.82%	71.20%	75.70%	82.67%	80.00%	78.32%	71.88%	76.79%
Without ESRD	27.78%	34.67%	30.84%	30.22%	29.17%	30.07%	28.33%	27.78%

The year of TBI surgery

Trend Test: p<.0001

Figure 1. Trend of one-year mortality rate for TBI patients receiving surgery with and without pre-existing ESRD.

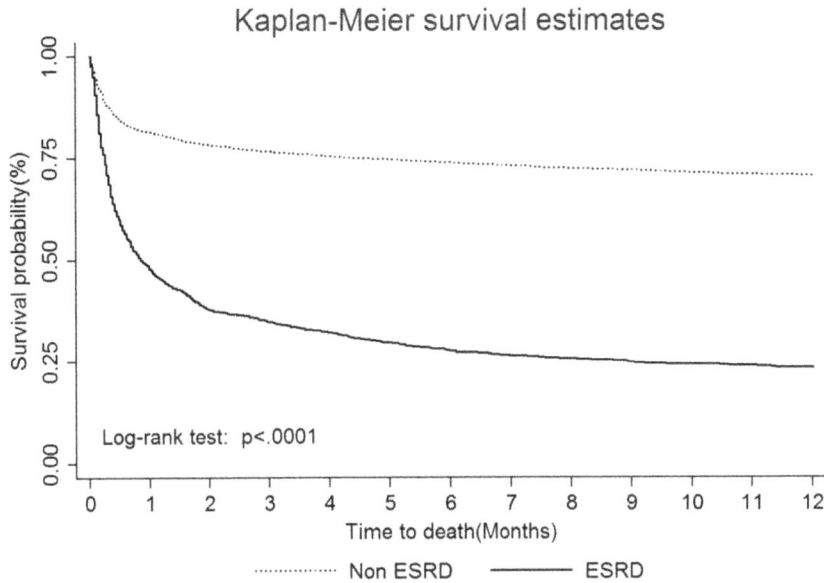

Figure 2. Kaplan-Meier survival curves for mortality of TBI surgery patients with and without pre-existing ESRD.

length of ventilation (LOV), and tracheostomy, were also used to estimate the risk of one-year mortality. For stratified analysis, patients were further classified into three groups according to their length of ICU stay: shorter group (first quartile), in-between group (first quartile to third quartile), and prolonged group (third quartile). This approach has been used on some previous studies for the distribution of ICU length of stay [21,22].

Statistical analysis

Comparisons between TBI patients with/without ESRD were performed using Pearson's chi-square test or Fisher's exact test for categorical variables and the Student's t test or Wilcoxon rank-sum test for continuous variables. The Kaplan-Meier plot was constructed to describe the proportion of patients who were still alive after one year, and the log-rank test was used to compare the mortality risk difference between two subgroups. The Cox proportional regression model was applied to estimate the hazards of mortality adjusted by potential confounding factors. To test the hypothesis that for TBI patients, the effect of pre-existing ESRD on mortality varied by age and the length of ICU stay, the model was also stratified by age and the length of ICU stay group to evaluate the potential risk factors. A p-value <0.05 was considered significant. All analyses were performed using Statistical Analysis System (SAS) statistical software (version 9.3; SAS Institute, Inc., Cary, NC). The Kaplan-Meier curves were plotted using STATA (version 12; Stata Corp., College Station, TX).

Results

Table 1 shows the distribution of demographical and clinical variables for TBI patients with and without ESRD. A total of 4416 subjects (1104 TBI patients with ESRD and 3312 TBI patients without ESRD) were enrolled in this study. Of the TBI patients, most (64.13%) were younger than 65 years of age, and there were more males than females. The distribution of overall mortality indicated a significant difference between TBI patients with ESRD and those without ESRD. The median survival time was 0.86 (0.26–8.91) months for TBI patients with ESRD and 29.36 (4.18–59.57) months for those without ESRD. TBI patients with ESRD

have a higher percentage of hospitalization deaths than do patients without ESRD. As most TBI patients with ESRD did not survive more than one year, the one-year mortality was used in this study to understand the potential risk factors. In addition, TBI patients with ESRD also presented a shorter LOS, a longer length of ICU days and LOV, and a higher percentage of comorbidities (HTN, DM, MI, stroke, and heart failure) compared with patients without ESRD.

Figure 1 shows that both TBI patients with ESRD and without ESRD had a stable trend in one-year mortality rate during the follow-up period. The result of a trend test indicated there was a significant trend difference between TBI with ESRD patients and patients without ESRD ($p<.0001$).

The Kaplan-Meier survival curves for TBI patients with and without ESRD are presented in Figure 2. There was a significant difference in survival between the two groups ($p<.0001$). In addition, after controlling for age, gender, and clinical characteristics, TBI patients with ESRD were more likely to die within one year (HR: 2.85, 95%C.I.: 2.56–3.17) compared with TBI patients without ESRD. Kaplan-Meier plots indicated a mortality rate of 52.36% at 1 month, 65.40% threat 3 months, 72.46% at 6 months, and 76.63% for one year.

Table 2 shows the hazard ratios of one-year mortality for TBI patients with ESRD. The hazard ratio (HR) for TBI patients indicates that an age ≥65 years (HR: 1.21, 95% C.I.: 1.05–1.39), stroke (HR: 1.29, 95% C.I.: 1.08–1.55), and prolonged use of a ventilator (HR: 1.06, 95% C.I.: 1.05–1.08) were associated with a significantly higher risk of mortality. However, a longer LOS (HR: 0.93, 95% C.I.: 0.92–0.94), longer ICU stays, and tracheostomy use were associated with a significantly lower risk of mortality.

In Figure 3, the Kaplan-Meier plots show that the risk of mortality for TBI patients with ESRD is significantly different between the <65 y/o and ≥65 y/o patients ($p=0.0026$). However, at the beginning of the study period, the survival probability was similar between these two groups. About one month after surgery, TBI patients with ESRD who were ≥65 years old presented a higher risk of mortality than did the younger patients.

When stratified by age, DM (HR: 1.35, 95% C.I.: 1.12–1.63) and LOV (HR: 1.07, 95% C.I.: 1.05–1.09) were significant risk

Table 2. Univariate and multivariable Cox proportional hazards regression analysis for the mortality rate ratios of composite outcome among TBI patients with pre-existing ESRD.

	Crude Hazards (95% C.I.)	*p*-value	Adjusted Hazards* (95% C.I.)	*p*-value
Age				
<65	1.00(Ref.)		1.00(Ref.)	
>=65	1.23(1.07–1.42)	0.0030	1.21(1.05–1.39)	0.0081
Gender				
Female	1.00(Ref.)		1.00(Ref.)	
Male	0.98(0.86–1.12)	0.7633	0.96(0.83–1.10)	0.5151
Level of Urbanization				
>=3	1.00(Ref.)		1.00(Ref.)	
1	0.93(0.77–1.12)	0.4324	0.94(0.77–1.13)	0.4951
2	0.85(0.70–1.03)	0.0896	0.94(0.77–1.13)	0.4891
Hypertension				
No	1.00(Ref.)		1.00(Ref.)	
Yes	0.83(0.69–1.02)	0.0720	0.88(0.71–1.08)	0.2252
Diabetes mellitus				
No	1.00(Ref.)		1.00(Ref.)	
Yes	1.10(0.96–1.26)	0.1766	1.14(0.98–1.31)	0.0810
Myocardial infarction				
No	1.00(Ref.)		1.00(Ref.)	
Yes	1.02(0.77–1.35)	0.8970	1.04(0.78–1.39)	0.7708
Stroke				
No	1.00(Ref.)		1.00(Ref.)	
Yes	1.21(1.02–1.44)	0.0339	1.29(1.08–1.55)	0.0052
Heart failure				
No	1.00(Ref.)		1.00(Ref.)	
Yes	1.08(0.91–1.29)	0.3754	0.96(0.80–1.15)	0.6321
Length of Stay, days	0.95(0.94–0.96)	<.0001	0.93(0.92–0.94)	<.0001
Length of ICU stay, days				
<=5	1.00(Ref.)		1.00(Ref.)	
6~19	0.59(0.50–0.69)	<.0001	0.61(0.51–0.73)	<.0001
>19	0.40(0.33–0.48)	<.0001	0.52(0.38–0.72)	<.0001
Length of ventilation, days	0.99(0.98–0.99)	<.0001	1.06(1.05–1.08)	<.0001
Tracheostomy				
No	1.00(Ref.)		1.00(Ref.)	
Yes	0.61(0.51–0.72)	<.0001	0.73(0.59–0.90)	0.0034

*The model was adjusted by the variables which were listed above.
C.I.: confidence interval; Ref.: reference; ICU: Intensive Care Unit.

factors for TBI patients with ESRD who were younger than 65 y/o (Table 3). For older patients (age ≥65 y/o), MI (HR: 1.61, 95% C.I.: 1.07–2.42) and LOV (HR: 1.05, 95% C.I.: 1.03–1.07) were significant risk factors. LOS and length of ICU stay were the protective factors of mortality regardless of age. Although tracheostomy was a protective factor, it was significant for young patients and borderline significant for older patients.

In addition, stratified analysis by the length of ICU stay was presented in the Table 4. LOS is a significant protective factor for all subgroups. For shorter length of ICU stay, older TBI patients with ESRD had a 30% increased risk of one-year mortality compared to younger TBI patients. For patients with prolonged length of ICU stays, LOV days (HR: 1.03, 95% C.I.: 1.02–1.04) was the significant risk factor, but the comorbidity of HTN and

LOS were the protective factors of one-year mortality. For the in-between group, stroke (HR: 1.35, 95% C.I.: 1.03–1.77) and LOV days (HR: 1.04, 95% C.I.: 1.02–1.07) were associated with increased risk of mortality whereas tracheostomy was associated with lower risk (HR: 0.68, 95% C.I.: 0.49–0.93).

Discussion

To the best of our knowledge, this is the first study to report one-year mortality associations in ESRD patients after TBI using population-based administrative data. The main findings of our study were that (1) TBI patients with ESRD had more comorbidity, higher one-year mortality, and longer length of ventilator use compared with non-ESRD TBI patients; (2) age,

Kaplan-Meier survival estimates

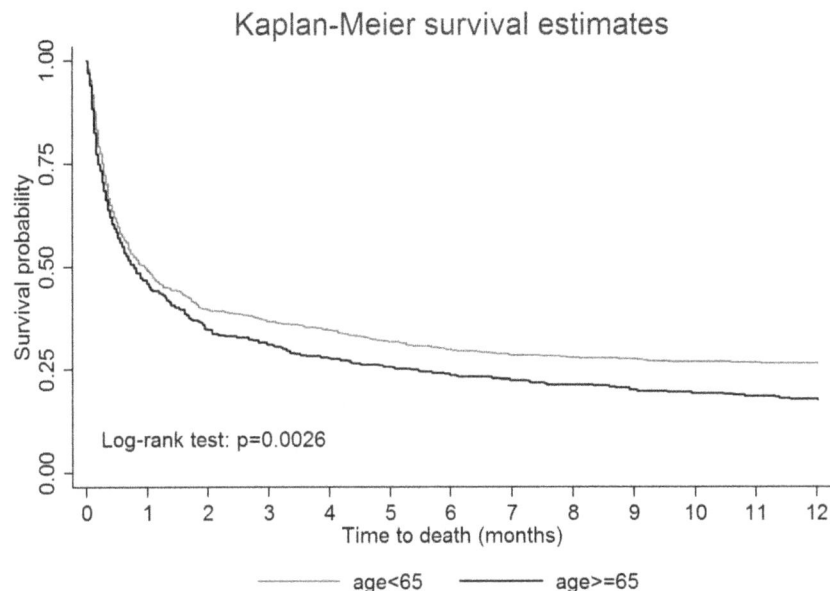

Figure 3. Kaplan-Meier survival curves for mortality of TBI patients with pre-existing ESRD, stratified by age.

comorbidity of stroke, and LOV were the risk factors of mortality for TBI patients with ESRD. However, LOS, length of ICU stay, and tracheostomy were protective factors for the same patients; (3) DM was a mortality predictor for ESRD patients whose age < 65 y/o, and MI was a mortality predictor for those patients ≥65 years of age; and (4) the risk factors for mortality among TBI patients with ESRD varied by length of ICU stays. Given that the NHIRD covers nearly 99% of inpatient and outpatient medical benefit claims for the 23 million residents in Taiwan, the data here closely approximate the true distribution of ESRD in TBI patients. For patients belonging to one of the high-risk groups, this information is critical to clinicians when they perform the TBI surgery and when they explain the prognosis to the patient's family.

High mortality rate was observed in TBI patients with ESRD who underwent surgical intervention compared with patients without ESRD

Several studies have reported that acute kidney injury may develop due to renal ischemia following hypoperfusion as a complication of traumatic brain injury [23,24]. However, pre-existing ESRD effects on TBI patients were not evaluated. Our finding indicated that TBI patients with ESRD had a higher percentage of hospitalization and one-year mortality, ICU days, length of ventilation, and comorbidities than patients without ESRD. The hazard ratio of one-year mortality, which was adjusted by age, gender, and clinical variables for TBI patients between those with ESRD and those without ESRD, is 2.85 (95% C.I.: 2.56–3.17). The results provide evidence supporting a new concept that pre-existing ESRD is a risk factor of mortality after TBI surgery. In addition, ESRD is associated with increased mortality among patients who are admitted to the ICU, and this effect is mostly a result of comorbidity [10,25]. Our results are also consistent with previous reports that ESRD patients have a greater incidence of comorbidities such as diabetes, stroke, hypertension, heart disease than patients without ESRD. This may support that the conclusion that ESRD patients use a significantly greater

amount of resources than do non-ESRD patients [26,27]. Therefore, the investigation of the impact of neurosurgical interventions on healthcare costs and economic burden in dialysis patients, who are a growing population with high co-morbidity, is a very important issue for the future.

In addition, our results are consistent with those of Chapman et al. [28], who reported that the majority of deaths occurred within the first month of ICU admission, depending on the medical etiology. In the current study, we found that the majority of deaths occurred at 0.86 months (IQR: 0.26–8.91), with a one-month post-ICU admission mortality rate of 52.36% (49.44%–55.33%). In our study, the one-year mortality rate of 76.63% (74.10%–79.08%) was higher than the previously reported 40% to 65% for critically ill ESRD patients [7,29,30]. Our results are also consistent with those of Rhodes et al. and Dhanani et al. who indicated that patients who had pre-existing ESRD after major surgery had a higher mortality than patients without ESRD [8,31]. Furthermore, in the current study, the one-year mortality trend test from 2000 to 2007 between TBI patients with ESRD and TBI patients without ESRD revealed significant differences (76.63% vs. 29.77%). These results imply that despite aggressive surgical intervention, the one-year mortality remained high and stable (76.63%). Thus, patients with pre-existing ERSD who suffer TBI and require neurosurgical intervention should be considered to have a serious and critical condition. This important information can be useful to surgeons, families, intensivists and nephrologists when considering surgical intervention and defining goals for treatment.

Studies have shown that hypertension, DM, MI, stroke, and heart failure are associated with higher mortality in TBI patients [32,33]. However, how these comorbidities affect the prognosis in TBI patients with ESRD is still unknown. This is the first study to examine the effect of comorbidities on mortality among TBI with ESRD after controlling for potential risk factors. With the insult of ESRD, hypertension, DM, MI, and heart failure are not significantly associated with higher mortality for TBI patients.

Table 3. Mortality rate ratios of composite outcome among TBI patients with pre-existing ESRD, stratified by age.

	Age<65	*p*-value	Age> = 65	*p*-value
	Adjusted Hazards* (95% C.I.)		Adjusted Hazards* (95% C.I.)	
Gender				
Female	1.00(Ref.)		1.00(Ref.)	
Male	0.98(0.83–1.17)	0.8487	0.89(0.72–1.11)	0.3173
Level of Urbanization (%)				
>=3	1.00(Ref.)		1.00(Ref.)	
1	1.00(0.78–1.29)	0.9839	0.94(0.69–1.29)	0.7139
2	0.90(0.71–1.16)	0.4261	1.04(0.77–1.42)	0.7887
Hypertension				
No	1.00(Ref.)		1.00(Ref.)	
Yes	0.93(0.72–1.20)	0.5688	0.86(0.60–1.23)	0.3993
Diabetes mellitus				
No	1.00(Ref.)		1.00(Ref.)	
Yes	1.35(1.12–1.63)	0.0016	0.85(0.67–1.07)	0.1646
Myocardial infarction				
No	1.00(Ref.)		1.00(Ref.)	
Yes	0.74(0.48–1.13)	0.1591	1.61(1.07–2.42)	0.0211
Stroke				
No	1.00(Ref.)		1.00(Ref.)	
Yes	1.22(0.95–1.57)	0.1118	1.27(0.98–1.66)	0.0741
Heart failure				
No	1.00(Ref.)		1.00(Ref.)	
Yes	1.03(0.80–1.31)	0.8456	0.88(0.67–1.17)	0.3839
Length of Stay, days	0.92(0.91–0.93)	<.0001	0.95(0.93–0.96)	<.0001
Length of ICU group				
<=5	1.00(Ref.)		1.00(Ref.)	
6~19	0.69(0.54–0.88)	0.0029	0.53(0.40–0.71)	<.0001
>19	0.61(0.40–0.93)	0.0203	0.43(0.27–0.71)	0.0008
Length of ventilation, days	1.07(1.05–1.09)	<.0001	1.05(1.03–1.07)	<.0001
Tracheostomy				
No	1.00(Ref.)		1.00(Ref.)	
Yes	0.73(0.56–0.96)	0.0230	0.72(0.51–1.01)	0.0600

*The model was adjusted by the variables which were listed above.
C.I.: confidence interval; Ref.: reference; ICU: Intensive Care Unit.

Pre-existing stroke is a risk factor of mortality for ESRD patients with TBI who underwent surgical intervention

The overall mortality of spontaneous intracerebral hemorrhage in ESRD patients was 61% to 71.4%, and the mortality rate after stroke was 46.6% at one month and 64.3% at one year [17,18]. Thus, stroke is an important risk factor of mortality for ESRD patients. In addition, the study by Thompson and colleagues demonstrated that the cerebrovascular disease had high association with mortality [32]. Our findings also indicate that pre-existing stroke is a significant risk factor for ESRD patients with TBI who underwent surgical intervention. Among these patients, those with preexisting stroke displayed a 29% increase in mortality risk compared with those without preexisting stroke (HR: 1.29, 95% C.I.: 1.08–1.55).

However, we believe that the effects of different types of intracranial hemorrhage, such as epidural hemorrhage, subdural hemorrhage, and intracerebral hemorrhage, on TBI mortality rate deserve to be investigated in the future. Therefore, we recommend the link between pre-existing stroke and TBI, effects of severity, subtypes, and external causes of TBI should be examined in future studies.

Pre-existing DM and MI effects on the mortality in ESRD patients who underwent TBI surgical intervention in the younger (age<65) and older (age≥65) population, respectively

Age has long been recognized as an independent adverse outcome predictor following TBI in various studies. Older age is associated with poorer outcome in patients with TBI [34–36]. Consistent with previous studies, we found the long-term mortality rate starting from one month (60.45% vs. 65.66%) to one year (73.45% vs 82.32%) after TBI in ESRD patients was significantly

Table 4. Mortality rate ratios of composite outcome among TBI patients with pre-existing ESRD, stratified by the length of ICU stay.

Adjusted Hazards* (95% C.I.)	Length of ICU stay, <=5 days (N=337)	p-value	Length of ICU stay, 6~19 days (N=501)	p-value	Length of ICU stay, >19 days (N=266)	p-value
Age						
<65	1.00(Ref.)		1.00(Ref.)		1.00(Ref.)	
>=65	1.30(1.01–1.67)	0.0409	1.07(0.86–1.33)	0.5660	1.20(0.89–1.62)	0.2260
Gender						
Female	1.00(Ref.)		1.00(Ref.)		1.00(Ref.)	
Male	1.09(0.85–1.39)	0.5156	0.97(0.79–1.18)	0.7306	0.79(0.58–1.06)	0.1142
Level of urbanization						
>=3	1.00(Ref.)		1.00(Ref.)		1.00(Ref.)	
1	0.86(0.62–1.21)	0.3940	0.98(0.74–1.30)	0.8653	1.06(0.67–1.68)	0.7967
2	0.97(0.69–1.35)	0.8420	0.88(0.66–1.16)	0.3610	1.07(0.68–1.68)	0.7743
Hypertension						
No	1.00(Ref.)		1.00(Ref.)		1.00(Ref.)	
Yes	0.98(0.69–1.39)	0.9229	0.79(0.58–1.09)	0.1482	0.53(0.33–0.84)	0.0077
Diabetes mellitus						
No	1.00(Ref.)		1.00(Ref.)		1.00(Ref.)	
Yes	1.20(0.94–1.53)	0.1523	1.23(0.98–1.53)	0.0709	1.09(0.80–1.47)	0.5964
Myocardial infarction						
No	1.00(Ref.)		1.00(Ref.)		1.00(Ref.)	
Yes	1.18(0.74–1.89)	0.4777	0.77(0.45–1.30)	0.3224	1.17(0.67–2.04)	0.5765
Stroke						
No	1.00(Ref.)		1.00(Ref.)		1.00(Ref.)	
Yes	1.11(0.81–1.52)	0.5218	1.35(1.03–1.77)	0.0322	1.05(0.71–1.55)	0.8044
Heart failure						
No	1.00(Ref.)		1.00(Ref.)		1.00(Ref.)	
Yes	0.91(0.66–1.25)	0.5508	0.91(0.67–1.22)	0.5156	1.34(0.91–1.98)	0.1339
Length of Stay, days	0.84(0.81–0.88)	<.0001	0.92(0.91–0.94)	<.0001	0.97(0.95–0.98)	<.0001
Length of ventilation, days	1.06(0.99–1.13)	0.0880	1.04(1.02–1.07)	<.0001	1.03(1.02–1.04)	<.0001
Tracheostomy						
No	1.00(Ref.)		1.00(Ref.)		1.00(Ref.)	
Yes	0.30(0.04–2.15)	0.2282	0.68(0.49–0.93)	0.0169	0.82(0.61–1.12)	0.2207

*The model was adjusted by the variables which were listed above.
C.I.: confidence interval; Ref.: reference; ICU: Intensive Care Unit.

different between patients <65 y/o and patients ≥65 y/o. We also found significantly elevated one-year mortality rates in the older dialysis patients compared with the younger patients after TBI surgery (HR: 1.21, 95% C.I.: 1.05–1.39). These findings are consistent with the US Renal Data Service annual report that indicates that among dialysis patients age 65 and older, the mortality is twice as high as that in the general population [37]. Given that societal aging may increase the number of surgical cases of ESRD with TBI and that the older population presents a high mortality risk, neurosurgeons should be more cautious when performing surgical intervention in older ESRD patients if TBI has occurred.

Currently, diabetic nephropathy is the leading cause of ESRD in Germany and Taiwan [27,38]. Many studies have reported an association between pre-existing DM at the initiation of dialysis and a poor outcome in ESRD patients undergoing dialysis [38,39]. We further elucidated that for TBI patients with ESRD, pre-existing DM is a risk factor of one-year mortality (HR: 1.35, 95%

C.I.: 1.12–1.63) for patients <65 years of age. One possible hypothesis is that younger ESRD patients have a longer follow-up related to DM, so a poorer health condition leads to a higher mortality risk for those who undergo surgical intervention. We believe that the management of TBI patients with ESRD derived from DM will represent a serious problem in the future.

In addition, pre-existing MI was associated with a significantly increased risk of mortality (HR: 1.61, 95% CI: 1.07–2.42) in the older population (age≥65). The reason for this result might be that pre-existing MI in older patients is a key factor to determine mortality compared with other comorbidities. Because we evaluated neither the time interval since MI nor the severity of MI, which would influence cardiac function and mortality, we believe this information encourages us to pay more attention to these new high-risk groups during the decision-making process for surgical intervention.

Length of ICU stay could be a mortality predicator and a surrogate of disease severity for ESRD patients who underwent TBI surgery

Previous studies found that the TBI patients with prolonged ICU stays have greater disease severity or poor functional outcome according to the different scores [40–44]. Since the TBI patients were unstable after TBI surgery at the beginning of ICU stay, and longer ICU lengths of stay might be associated with greater disease severity, examining the risk factors for mortality by different lengths of ICU stay among TBI patients is meaningful. Results of stratified analysis indicated that patients with different lengths of ICU stays have different risk factors for mortality: for patients with short ICU stays, age was an independent risk factor for mortality, and it was similar as former studies that age is the most frequently documented risk factor [45,46]; for those with prolonged ICU stays, HTN was a protective factor, and this " reverse epidemiology" had also been reported on the some studies for ESRD patients [47,48]; for in-between groups, stroke and LOV were associated with increased risk of death, but tracheostomy was associated with lower risk.

One reason for tracheostomy need may be related to general clinical practices and the general consensus of neurosurgeons that tracheostomy is not required for patients who have a critical condition and less opportunity to survive. The previous studies indicated that the benefits of tracheostomy have been demonstrated for critically ill patients, especially for patients with limited neurological recovery, without spontaneous ventilation, excessive secretion, and long-term functional outcome [49–51]. However, the association between the tracheostomy and mortality is still unclear. A meta-analysis review indicated that the tracheostomy could reduce the risk of mortality, but it is no significant [21]. Only one study demonstrated that tracheostomy could significantly reduce mortality [52]. In our study, the effect of tracheostomy on mortality presented the protective information in the different ICU stays, only the in-between ICU stays group of TBI patients with ESRD who received tracheostomy displayed a 32% reduction in the one-year mortality rate compared with those who did not receive tracheostomy (HR: 0.68, 95% C.I.: 0.49–0.93). Since trauma patients are unstable at short length of ICU stay, tracheostomy may not be applied according the guideline

[49–51]. Thus, it could not be significant for protecting the mortality. Considering of the severity of TBI, TBI patients with ESRD within prolonged ICU days may have the poor functional outcomes. The non-significant protective effect on mortality is consistency as previous studies [21,22,41]. Therefore, the tracheostomy may still have some benefit for some restricted patients. This information can be provided to the families of patients if they have doubts about the tracheotomy procedure in ESRD patients who underwent TBI surgery.

Limitations

There are several limitations in our study. First, the diagnoses, including comorbidities, all relied on the claims data and ICD-9-CM diagnosis codes; thus, there may be some disease misclassification. Second, we were unable to take into account the illness severity scores of TBI and ESRD because the data were unavailable. Third, the data concerning the onset, duration of tracheostomy, and severity of DM, MI, and stroke were also unavailable for evaluation.

Conclusions

TBI patients with ESRD have more co-morbidity and higher one-year mortality than with non-ESRD TBI patients. Age, history of comorbidities, length of ICU stay, and tracheostomy are associated with higher mortality in TBI patients with ESRD. When performing TBI surgery or explaining the prognosis to the families of patients, physicians should keep these factors in mind to the aforementioned high-risk groups.

Acknowledgments

The authors thank Dr. Chih-Chiang Chien for his critical advice during the preparation of this article.

Author Contributions

Conceived and designed the experiments: JCL JRK JJW CHH. Performed the experiments: JCL JRK CCC. Analyzed the data: CHH FWL JRK KCL. Contributed reagents/materials/analysis tools: JJW CCC. Wrote the paper: CHH JRK FWL KCL CCC.

References

1. Collins AJ, Foley RN, Chavers B, Gilbertson D, Herzog C, et al. (2012) 'United States Renal Data System 2011 Annual Data Report: Atlas of chronic kidney disease & end-stage renal disease in the United States. Am J Kidney Dis 59: A7, e1–420.
2. Hwang SJ, Yang WC (2000) National dialysis surveillance in Taiwan-1999. Acta Nephrol (Taiwan SocNephrol) 14: 139–169.
3. Kuo HW, Tsai SS, Tiao MM, Yang CY (2007) Epidemiological features of CKD in Taiwan. Am J Kidney Dis 49: 46–55.
4. Insurance BoNH (2002) National Health Insurance Annual Statistical Report, 2000. Executive Yuan.
5. System USRD (2005) USRDS 2005 Annual Data Report: Atlas of End-Stage Renal Disease in the United States. Bethesda, MD.
6. Chan M, Ostermann M (2013) Outcomes of chronic hemodialysis patients in the intensive care unit. Crit Care Res Pract 2013: 715807.
7. Sood MM, Miller L, Komenda P, Reslerova M, Bueti J, et al. (2011) Long-term outcomes of end-stage renal disease patients admitted to the ICU. Nephrol Dial Transplant 26: 2965–2970.
8. Rhodes A, Moreno RP, Metnitz B, Hochrieser H, Bauer P, et al. (2011) Epidemiology and outcome following post-surgical admission to critical care. Intensive Care Med 37: 1466–1472.
9. Gogbashian A, Sedrakyan A, Treasure T (2004) EuroSCORE: a systematic review of international performance. Eur J Cardiothorac Surg 25: 695–700.
10. Strijack B, Mojica J, Sood M, Komenda P, Bueti J, et al. (2009) Outcomes of chronic dialysis patients admitted to the intensive care unit. J Am Soc Nephrol 20: 2441–2447.
11. Chae JW, Song CS, Kim H, Lee KB, Seo BS, et al. (2011) Prediction of mortality in patients undergoing maintenance hemodialysis by Charlson Comorbidity Index using ICD-10 database. Nephron Clin Pract 117: c379–384.
12. Prevention CfDCa (2010) Get the Stats on Traumatic Brain Injury in the United States. Centers for Disease Control and Prevention, Atlanta, Georgia, USA 2010.
13. Langlois JA, Rutland-Brown W, Thomas KE (2005) The incidence of traumatic brain injury among children in the United States: differences by race. J Head Trauma Rehabil 20: 229–238.
14. Chiu WT, Yeh KH, Li YC, Gan YH, Chen HY, et al. (1997) Traumatic brain injury registry in Taiwan. Neurol Res 19: 261–264.
15. Iseki K, Fukiyama K (1996) Predictors of stroke in patients receiving chronic hemodialysis. Kidney Int 50: 1672–1675.
16. Iseki K, Fukiyama K, Okawa Dialysis Study G (2000) Clinical demographics and long-term prognosis after stroke in patients on chronic haemodialysis. The Okinawa Dialysis Study (OKIDS) Group. Nephrol Dial Transplant 15: 1808–1813.
17. Kawamura M, Fijimoto S, Hisanaga S, Yamamoto Y, Eto T (1998) Incidence, outcome, and risk factors of cerebrovascular events in patients undergoing maintenance hemodialysis. Am J Kidney Dis 31: 991–996.
18. Murakami M, Hamasaki T, Kimura S, Maruyama D, Kakita K (2004) Clinical features and management of intracranial hemorrhage in patients undergoing maintenance dialysis therapy. Neurol Med Chir (Tokyo) 44: 225–232; discussion 233.
19. Chen Y-C, Yeh H-Y, Wu J-C, Haschler I, Chen T-J, et al. (2011) Taiwan's National Health Insurance Research Database: administrative health care database as study object in bibliometrics. Scientometrics 86: 365–380.
20. Liu CY, Hung YT, Chuang YL, Chen YJ, Weng WS, et al. (2006) Incorporating development stratification of Taiwan townships into sampling design of large scale health interview survey. Journal of Health Management 4: 1–22.

21. Weissman C (1997) Analyzing intensive care unit length of stay data: problems and possible solutions. Crit Care Med 25: 1594–1600.

22. Weissman C (2000) Analyzing the impact of long-term patients on ICU bed utilization. Intensive care medicine 26: 1319–1325.

23. Davenport A (2001) Renal replacement therapy in the patient with acute brain injury. Am J Kidney Dis 37: 457–466.

24. Schirmer-Mikalsen K, Moen KG, Skandsen T, Vik A, Klepstad P (2013) Intensive care and traumatic brain injury after the introduction of a treatment protocol: a prospective study. Acta Anaesthesiol Scand 57: 46–55.

25. System URD (1998) USRDS 1998 Annual data report: atlas of chronic kidney disease and end-stage renal disease in the United States. National Institutes of Health.

26. Hamilton MA, Cecconi M, Rhodes A (2011) A systematic review and meta-analysis on the use of preemptive hemodynamic intervention to improve postoperative outcomes in moderate and high-risk surgical patients. Anesth Analg 112: 1392–1402.

27. Yang WC, Hwang SJ, Taiwan Society of N (2008) Incidence, prevalence and mortality trends of dialysis end-stage renal disease in Taiwan from 1990 to 2001: the impact of national health insurance. Nephrol Dial Transplant 23: 3977–3982.

28. Chapman RJ, Templeton M, Ashworth S, Broomhead R, McLean A, et al. (2009) Long-term survival of chronic dialysis patients following survival from an episode of multiple-organ failure. Crit Care 13: R65.

29. Bagshaw SM, Mortis G, Doig CJ, Godinez-Luna T, Fick GH, et al. (2006) One-year mortality in critically ill patients by severity of kidney dysfunction: a population-based assessment. Am J Kidney Dis 48: 402–409.

30. Bell M, Granath F, Schon S, Lofberg E, Swing, et al. (2008) End-stage renal disease patients on renal replacement therapy in the intensive care unit: short- and long-term outcome. Crit Care Med 36: 2773–2778.

31. Dhanani J, Mullany DV, Fraser JF (2013) Effect of preoperative renal function on long-term survival after cardiac surgery. J Thorac Cardiovasc Surg 146: 90–95.

32. Thompson HJ, Rivara FP, Nathens A, Wang J, Jurkovich GJ, et al. (2010) Development and validation of the mortality risk for trauma comorbidity index. Annals of surgery 252: 370.

33. Gale SC, Sicoutris C, Reilly PM, Schwab CW, Gracias VH (2007) Poor glycemic control is associated with increased mortality in critically ill trauma patients. The American Surgeon 73: 454–460.

34. Coronado VG, Thomas KE, Sattin RW, Johnson RL (2005) The CDC traumatic brain injury surveillance system: characteristics of persons aged 65 years and older hospitalized with a TBI. J Head Trauma Rehabil 20: 215–228.

35. Hukkelhoven CW, Steyerberg EW, Rampen AJ, Farace E, Habbema JD, et al. (2003) Patient age and outcome following severe traumatic brain injury: an analysis of 5600 patients. J Neurosurg 99: 666–673.

36. McIntyre A, Mehta S, Aubut J, Dijkers M, Teasell RW (2013) Mortality among older adults after a traumatic brain injury: a meta-analysis. Brain Inj 27: 31–40.

37. System USRD (2012) USRDS 2012 Annual Data Report: Atlas of Chronic Kidney Disease and End-Stage Renal Disease in the United States. National Institutes of Health, Bethesda, MD.

38. Hoffmann F, Haastert B, Koch M, Giani G, Glaeske G, et al. (2011) The effect of diabetes on incidence and mortality in end-stage renal disease in Germany. Nephrol Dial Transplant 26: 1634–1640.

39. Lok CE, Oliver MJ, Rothwell DM, Hux JE (2004) The growing volume of diabetes-related dialysis: a population based study. Nephrol Dial Transplant 19: 3098–3103.

40. Heyland DK, Konopad E, Noseworthy TW, Johnston R, Gafni A (1998) Is itworthwhile'to continue treating patients with a prolonged stay (>14 days) in the ICU? An economic evaluation. CHEST Journal 114: 192–198.

41. Higgins TL, McGee WT, Steingrub JS, Rapoport J, Lemeshow S, et al. (2003) Early indicators of prolonged intensive care unit stay: impact of illness severity, physician staffing, and pre-intensive care unit length of stay. critical care medicine 31: 45–51.

42. Rothen HU, Stricker K, Einfalt J, Bauer P, Metnitz PG, et al. (2007) Variability in outcome and resource use in intensive care units. Intensive care medicine 33: 1329–1336.

43. Arabi Y, Venkatesh S, Haddad S, Al Shimemeri A, Al Malik S (2002) A prospective study of prolonged stay in the intensive care unit: predictors and impact on resource utilization. International Journal for Quality in Health Care 14: 403–410.

44. Laupland KB, Kirkpatrick AW, Kortbeek JB, Zuege DJ (2006) Long-term mortality outcome associated with prolonged admission to the ICU. CHEST Journal 129: 954–959.

45. Miller RS, Patton M, Graham RM, Hollins D (2000) Outcomes of trauma patients who survive prolonged lengths of stay in the intensive care unit. The Journal of Trauma and Acute Care Surgery 48: 229–234.

46. Taylor MD, Tracy JK, Meyer W, Pasquale M, Napolitano LM (2002) Trauma in the elderly: intensive care unit resource use and outcome. The Journal of Trauma and Acute Care Surgery 53: 407–414.

47. Chien C-C, Yen C-S, Wang J-J, Chen H-A, Chou M-T, et al. (2012) Reverse epidemiology of hypertension-mortality associations in hemodialysis patients: a long-term population-based study. American journal of hypertension 25: 900–906.

48. Tomita J, Kimura G, Inoue T, Inenaga T, Sanai T, et al. (1995) Role of systolic blood pressure in determining prognosis of hemodialyzed patients. American journal of kidney diseases 25: 405–412.

49. Freeman BD, Borecki IB, Coopersmith CM, Buchman TG (2005) Relationship between tracheostomy timing and duration of mechanical ventilation in critically ill patients. Crit Care Med 33: 2513–2520.

50. Plummer AL, Gracey DR (1989) Consensus conference on artificial airways in patients receiving mechanical ventilation. Chest 96: 178–180.

51. Wang HK, Lu K, Liliang PC, Wang KW, Chen HJ, et al. (2012) The impact of tracheostomy timing in patients with severe head injury: an observational cohort study. Injury 43: 1432–1436.

52. Rumbak MJ, Newton M, Truncale T, Schwartz SW, Adams JW, et al. (2004) A prospective, randomized, study comparing early percutaneous dilational tracheotomy to prolonged translaryngeal intubation (delayed tracheotomy) in critically ill medical patients. Critical care medicine 32: 1689–1694.

28

Prognosis in IgA Nephropathy: 30-Year Analysis of 1,012 Patients at a Single Center

Takahito Moriyama*, Kayu Tanaka, Chihiro Iwasaki, Yasuko Oshima, Ayami Ochi, Hiroshi Kataoka, Mitsuyo Itabashi, Takashi Takei, Keiko Uchida, Kosaku Nitta

Department of Medicine, Kidney Center, Tokyo Women's Medical University, Tokyo, Japan

Abstract

Background: Little is known about the long-term prognosis of patients with IgA nephropathy (IgAN).

Methods: This retrospective cohort analysis evaluated clinical and histological findings at the time of renal biopsy, initial treatment, patient outcomes over 30 years, and risk factors associated with progression in 1,012 patients diagnosed with IgAN at our center since 1974.

Results: Of the 1,012 patients, 40.5% were male. Mean patient age was 33 ± 12 years and mean blood pressure was $122\pm17/75\pm13$ mmHg. Mean serum creatinine concentration was 0.89 ± 0.42 mg/dL, and mean estimated glomerular filtration rate (eGFR) was 78.5 ± 26.2 ml/min/1.73 m^2. Mean proteinuria was 1.19 ± 1.61 g/day, and mean urinary red blood cells were 36.6 ± 35.3/high-powered field. Histologically, mesangial hypercellularity was present in 47.6% of patients, endothelial hypercellularity in 44.3%, segmental sclerosis in 74.6%, and tubular atrophy/interstitial fibrosis in 28.8% by Oxford classification. Initial treatment consisted of corticosteroids in 26.9% of patients, renin-angiotensin-aldosterone system inhibitor in 28.9%, and tonsillectomy plus steroids in 11.7%. The 10-, 20-, and 30-year renal survival rates were 84.3, 66.6, and 50.3%, respectively. Tonsillectomy plus steroids dramatically improved renal outcome. Cox multivariate regression analysis showed that higher proteinuria, lower eGFR, and higher uric acid at the time of renal biopsy were independent risk factors for the development of end stage renal disease (ESRD).

Conclusions: IgAN is not a benign disease, with about 50% of patients progressing to ESRD within 30 years despite treatment.

Editor: Ivan Cruz Moura, Institut national de la santé et de la recherche médicale (INSERM), France

Funding: The authors have no support or funding to report.

Competing Interests: The authors have declared that no competing interests exist.

* E-mail: takamori@kc.twmu.ac.jp

Introduction

Mesangial proliferative glomerulonephritis with mesangial deposition of immunoglobulin A (IgA) and IgG, now recognized as IgA nephropathy (IgAN) was first described in 1968 [1]. Since then, the mechanism of onset and progression of this disease have been described, along with treatment modalities, patient prognosis, and risk factors. Although IgAN was initially regarded as a benign disease, a study in the 1990s reported that about 40% of patients with IgAN progressed to end stage renal disease (ESRD) within 20 years [2,3]. Since the first report, in 1986, showing that steroid therapy had a beneficial effect in patients with IgAN [4], steroids have been frequently used to treat IgAN patients with massive proteinuria (>1 g/day), active histological findings such as crescent formation, and normal renal function. A randomized controlled trial in 1999 found that steroid pulse therapy could decrease amount of proteinuria and improve patient prognosis [5]. Moreover, steroid pulse therapy was found to have long term efficacy in these patients [6] and has been widely recognized as the most effective treatment for IgAN. Since a retrospective analysis in 2001 found that the combination of tonsillectomy plus steroid

pulse therapy induced complete remission of proteinuria and hematuria and prevented deterioration of renal function [7], the number of institutions in Japan performing tonsillectomy plus steroid pulse therapy in patients with IgAN has dramatically increased [8,9]. Although these intensive therapies may improve the prognosis of patients with IgAN, the mechanisms underlying the onset and progression of IgAN, the risk factors for progression and the long term prognosis of these patients have not been determined. Indeed, despite intensive treatment, many patients with IgAN progress to ESRD.

This retrospective cohort study was performed to analyze the long term outcomes in patients with IgAN and their prognosis over 30 years. We therefore analyzed clinical and histological findings at renal biopsy and risk factors for progression in 1,012 IgAN patients diagnosed at our institution.

Materials and Methods

Ethics statement

This cohort study was conducted in accordance with the Declaration of Helsinki, and approved by the Medical Ethics

Table 1. Clinical and laboratory findings at renal biopsy.

Variables	Values
Clinical Findings	
Sex	410/602 (Male/Female)
Age	32.9±12.0 years
Body Mass Index	21.6±3.1 kg/m^2
Systolic Blood Pressure	121.7±17.1 mmHg
Diastolic Blood Pressure	74.6±12.8 mmHg
Mean arterial Pressure	90.4±12.8 mmHg
Interval from onset	5.8±6.6 years
Observation period	7.9±7.1 years
Laboratory Findings	
Total Protein	6.69±0.73 g/dl
Serum Albumin	3.92±0.53 g/dl
Blood Urea Nitrogen	15.8±5.7 mg/dl
Serum Creatinine	0.89±0.42 mg/dl
eGFR	78.5±26.2 ml/min/1.73m^2
Uric Acid	5.71±1.62 mg/dl
Total Cholesterol	197.3±48.5 mg/dl
HDL Cholesterol	56.4±16.7 mg/dl
Triglyceride	123.7±82.2 mg/dl
IgG	1158.1±341.2 mg/dl
IgA	325.1±126.6 mg/dl
IgM	144.7±75.7 mg/dl
CH50	40.6±8.4 mg/dl
C3	87.5±35.2 mg/dl
C4	29.0±15.5 mg/dl
Urinary protein excretion	1.19±1.61 g/day
U-RBC	36.6±35.3 counts/HF

Table 2. Histological findings (glomerular lesions and Oxford classification).

Glomerular lesions	Values
Number of glomeruli	16.1±10.4 (number)
Global Sclerosis	15.5±16.6 %
Segmental Sclerosis or Adhesion	13.6±13.7 %
Crescent	9.12±12.3 %
Cellular or Fibro-Cellular	6.72±10.5 %
Fibrous	2.25±5.76 %
Oxford Classification [number/(%)]	**Values [number(%)]**
Mesangial hypercellularity: M0/M1	449/408 (52.4/47.6%)
Endocapillary hypercellularity: E0/E1	477/380 (55.7/44.3%)
Segmental glomerulosclerosis: S0/S1	218/639 (25.4/74.6%)
Tubular atrophy/Interstitial fibrosis: T0/T1/T2	610/197/50 (71.2/23.0/5.8%)
Not evaluated	155 (15.3%)

Committee of Tokyo Women's Medical University (#2962). Written informed consent for renal biopsy was obtained from all patients and for use of clinical data at the time of renal biopsy and subsequent histological data was obtained from all recent patients.

Patients

Between 1974 and 2011, 1,012 patients at Tokyo Women's Medical University were diagnosed with primary IgAN by renal biopsy. IgAN was diagnosed based on light microscopic findings of mesangial proliferative changes, immunofluorescence findings of mesangial IgA and C3 deposition, and electron microscopic findings of electron-dense deposits in the mesangial area. Patients were observed for a mean 7.9 ± 7.1 years (maximum 36 years); 4 patients died during the observation period.

Histological evaluation of renal biopsy specimens

All renal biopsy specimens were obtained by percutaneous needle biopsy. The specimens were fixed in 10% phosphate-buffered formalin (pH 7.2), embedded in paraffin, and cut into 4-μm-thick sections. The sections were stained with hematoxylin and eosin, periodic acid–Schiff, silver methenamine, and Masson trichrome and examined by light microscopy. The percentage of glomerular lesions, such as global sclerosis, segmental sclerosis or adhesion, cellular or fibrocellular crescents, and fibrous crescents, were evaluated. The histological findings were also graded according to the Oxford classification [11,12], which scored four key pathological features in each specimen. (i) Mesangial hypercellularity was scored as M0 if >50% of glomeruli had fewer than three cells per mesangial area or M1 if >50% of glomeruli had more than three cells per mesangial area. (ii) Segmental glomerulosclerosis was scored as absent (S0) or present (S1). (iii) Endocapillary hypercellularity was scored as absent (E0) or present (E1). (iv) Tubular atrophy/interstitial fibrosis score was based on the ratio of tubular atrophy/interstitial fibrosis in the total interstitium and scored as T0 (0–25%), T1 (26–50%), or T2 (>51%). Biopsies containing fewer than 8 glomeruli were excluded from analysis.

Demographic and clinical data

Patient sex, age, body mass index (BMI), systolic blood pressure (S-BP), diastolic blood pressure (D-BP), mean arterial pressure (MAP), and time from onset of IgAN were recorded. In Japan, a large proportion of the population can receive free annual medical

examinations, including annual urinary screening. These screenings are regularly performed in school, the workplace, and in municipal facilities. These screenings enable recognition of the onset of IgAN as the first manifestation of a urinary abnormality or a finding of macrohematuria. Laboratory data included serum total protein, albumin, creatinine, uric acid, total cholesterol, HDL-cholesterol, triglyceride, IgG, IgA, IgM, C3, and C4 concentrations; blood urea nitrogen concentration; estimated glomerular filtration rate (eGFR), CH50 activity; urinary protein excretion (U-Prot), and urinary red blood cells (U-RBC). These clinical and laboratory findings were measured at the time of renal biopsy. Time to progression to ESRD, defined as requiring dialysis or renal transplantation, and the risk factors associated with progression to ESRD were also evaluated. Initial treatment, defined as treatment performed during the first year after renal biopsy, and renal survival rate relative to treatment were evaluated. The eGFR was calculated by the modified isotope dilution mass spectorometry – modification of diet in renal disease (IDMS-MDRD) study for Japanese [eGFR = $194 \times$ S-Cre$^{-1.094} \times$ age$^{-0.287} \times 0.739$ (if female)] [10].

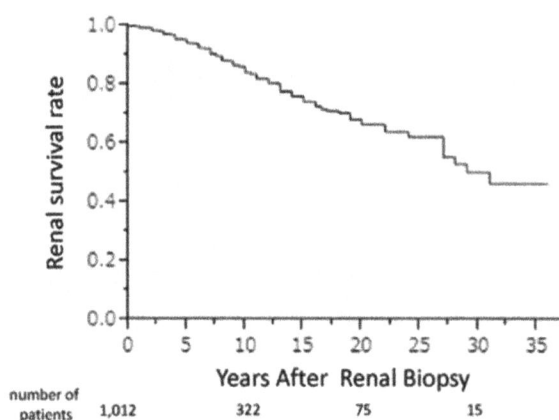

Figure 1. Cumulative renal survival rate from renal biopsy until ESRD in all 1,012 patients with IgAN.

Table 3. Initial treatment of individual patients.

Treatment	Values [number (%)]
Corticosteroid	272 (26.9%)
Steroid combined with tonsillectomy	119 (11.7%)
Tonsillectomy without steroid	15 (1.5%)
Steroid with Immunosuppressing agents	15 (1.5%)
RAS inhibitors	293 (28.9%)
Anti-platelet agents/anti coagulation	600 (59.3%)
EPA	159 (15.7%)
PE/DFPP	3 (0.3%)
No therapy	154 (15.2%)
Unknown	60 (5.9%)

RAS, renin angiotensin system; EPA, eicosapentaenoic acid; PE, plasma exchange; DFPP, double filtration plasmapheresis.

Statistical analysis

Data are presented as means ± standard deviation (SD) and were analyzed using JMP 10.0.1 (SAS Institute, Cary, NC, USA). Cumulative renal survival rates until ESRD were calculated according to the Kaplan–Meier method and compared using the log rank test. Univariate and multivariate Cox regression analysis were used to evaluate the risk of deterioration to ESRD. In univariate analyses, sex (male/female) was regarded as a categorical variable, whereas age, BMI, MAP, interval from onset, eGFR, serum albumin, uric acid, total cholesterol, U-Prot, U-RBC, IgA, IgA/C3 and histological grading were regarded as quantitative variables. Multivariate analysis included the factors differing significantly in univariate analysis. The results of these univariate and multivariate analyses are expressed as hazard ratios (HRs) with 95% confidence intervals (CIs). In all analyses, $P<0.05$ was considered statistically significant.

Results

Clinical findings at the time of renal biopsy

Table 1 shows the clinical characteristics at the time of renal biopsy. Of the 1,012 patients, 40.5% were male. Mean patient age was 32.9±12.0 years, with 41% aged 20–29 years and 25% aged 30–39 years. Mean S-BP was 121.7±17.1 mmHg and mean D-BP was 74.6±12.8 mmHg. Mean MAP was 90.4±12.8 mmHg and 79% of IgAN patients had a MAP below 100 mmHg. Mean interval from IgAN onset to renal biopsy was 7.9±7.1 years. We found that renal biopsies were obtained from 32% of patients within 2 years of IgAN onset and from 21% 10 years after onset.

Table 1 also shows laboratory data at the time of renal biopsy. Mean total protein concentration was 6.69±0.73 g/dl, and mean serum albumin concentration was 3.92±0.53 g/dl. Of these patients, 6% had serum albumin concentrations <3.0 g/dl and 12% had serum albumin concentrations between 3.0 and 3.5 g/dl, with the remainder having serum albumin concentrations over 3.5 g/dl. The mean eGFR was 78.5±26.2 ml/min/1.73m^2, with 46% of patients having eGFR over 80 ml/min/1.73m^2, 30% between 60 and 80 ml/min/1.73m^2, 19% between 40 and 60 ml/min/1.73m^2, and 5% between 20 and 40 ml/min/1.73m^2. Mean serum total cholesterol and triglyceride concentrations were 197.3±48.5 mg/dl and 123.7±82.2 mg/dl, respectively. Mean IgA concentration was 325.1±126.6 mg/dl, with 28% of patients having IgA concentrations between 300 and 400 mg/dl, and 23% >400 mg/dl. Mean U-Prot was 1.19±1.61 g/day, with 62% of patients having less than 1 g/day, 30% between 1 and 3 g/day, and 9% over 3 g/day. Mean U-RBC was 36.6±35.3 counts/high powered field (HPF), with 51% of patients having <25/HPF, 20% having between 25 and 50 counts/HPF, 4% having between 50 and 100 counts/HPF, and 20% having >100 counts/HPF.

Histological findings

Table 2 shows the histological findings in samples taken from patients with IgAN. The mean number of glomeruli per renal biopsy was 16.1±10.4. Over 8 glomeruli were present in biopsy specimens from 858 patients and these samples were used to evaluate glomerular lesions and Oxford classification. Global sclerosis was observed in a mean 15.5±16.6% of samples, segmental sclerosis or adhesion in 13.6±13.7%, cellular or fibrocellular crescents in 6.72±10.5%, and a fibrous crescent in 2.25±5.76%. According to the Oxford classification, 47.6% of samples were classified as M1, 44.3% as E1, 74.6% as S1, 23.0% as T1 and 5.8% as T2.

Initial treatment

Table 3 shows the initial treatment of patients with IgAN. We found that 272 patients (26.9%) received corticosteroids; 119 (11.7%) received corticosteroid therapy combined with tonsillectomy; 15 (1.5%) underwent tonsillectomy alone; 15 (1.5%) received immunosuppressive agents such as cyclophosphamide, mizoribine, and rituximab; 293 (28.9%) received a renin-angiotensin-aldosterone system inhibitor; 600 (59.3%) received an antiplatelet/anticoagulation agent; 159 (15.7%) received eicosapentaenoic acid; 3 (0.3%) underwent plasma exchange or double filtration plasmapheresis; and 169 (16.7%) received no treatment.

Long term outcome of IgA nephropathy

The cumulative 10-, 20- and 30-year renal survival rates, from renal biopsy to ESRD, were 84.3%, 66.6%, and 50.3%, respectively. The 36-year renal survival rate was 46.4% (Figure 1).

Outcome according to initial treatment

The cumulative renal survival rate relative to initial treatment is shown in Figure 2. The 8.5-year cumulative survival rate in patients treated with steroids plus tonsillectomy was 100%, the 17-year survival rate in patients treated with tonsillectomy was 100%, the 20-year survival rate in patients treated with steroids plus an immunosuppressive agent was 57.6%, and the 25-year survival rate in patients treated with steroids was 41.4%. The 35-year renal survival rates in patients treated with conservative therapy (RAS inhibitors and/or anti-platelet agents/anti-coagulation therapy, and/or EPA) and in untreated patients were 42.0% and 64.5%, respectively. The difference among groups was statistically significant (P = 0.0011).

Univariate and multivariate analysis of factors associated with ESRD

Univariate analysis found that male gender, higher age, higher BMI, higher MAP, lower eGFR, lower serum albumin, higher uric acid, higher total cholesterol, higher U-Prot, higher IgA/C3, and higher T level on the Oxford classification were associated with a risk of progression to ESRD. Multivariate Cox regression analysis showed that lower eGFR (HR, 1.93; 95% CI, 1.47–2.56; P<0.0001), higher uric acid concentration (HR, 1.24; 95% CI, 1.054–1.48, P = 0.0176), and higher U-Prot (HR, 1.34; 95% CI 1.07–1.69, P = 0.0116) were independent factors predicting

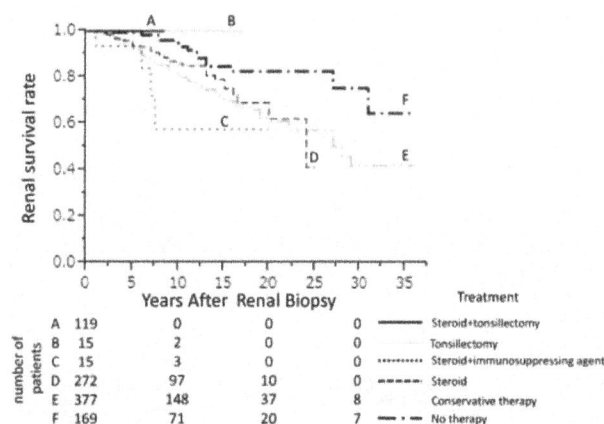

Figure 2. Cumulative renal survival rates in IgAN patients categorized by initial treatment.

Table 4. Univariate and multivariate analysis of risk factors associated with ESRD in patients diagnosed with IgAN.

	HR	95% CI	P value
Univariate Analysis			
male (vs. female)	1.76	1.25–2.49	0.0013
Age (10 year increase)	1.25	1.09–1.44	0.0031
BMI (1 kg/m² increase)	1.10	1.04–1.16	0.0012
MAP (10 mmHg increase)	1.44	1.27–1.65	<0.0001
Interval from onset (1 year increase)	1.02	0.99–1.05	0.0763
eGFR (20ml/min decrease)	2.22	1.86–2.67	<0.0001
Serum Albumin (1 g/dl decrease)	1.99	1.71–2.30	<0.0001
Uric Acid (1 mg/dl increase)	1.57	1.39–1.77	<0.0001
T-Cho (30 mg/dl increase)	1.44	1.26–1.64	<0.0001
U-Prot (1g/day increase)	1.69	1.53–1.86	<0.0001
U-RBC (20/HPF increase)	1.02	0.92–1.13	0.6851
IgA (100 mg/dl increase)	1.09	0.93–1.27	0.2833
IgA/C3 (1 increase)	1.16	1.00–1.35	0.0460
Oxford classification M1(vs. M0)	1.35	0.94–1.97	0.1039
Oxford classification E1 (vs. E0)	1.30	0.89–1.91	0.1733
Oxford classification S1 (vs. S0)	1.23	0.81–1.92	0.3455
Oxford classification T (1 increase)	2.38	1.91–3.20	<0.0001
Multivariate Analysis			
male (vs. female)	1.16	0.72–1.90	0.5390
Age (10 year increase)	0.84	0.67–1.03	0.0992
BMI (1 kg/m² increase)	0.93	0.85–1.01	0.0781
MAP (10 mmHg increase)	1.14	0.94–1.38	0.1755
eGFR (20ml/min decrease)	1.93	1.47–2.56	<0.0001
Alb (1 g/dl decrease)	1.24	0.92–1.66	0.1627
Uric Acid (1 mg/dl increase)	1.24	1.04–1.48	0.0176
T-Cho (30 mg/dl increase)	1.17	0.96–1.42	0.1105
U-Prot (1g/day increase)	1.34	1.07–1.69	0.0116
IgA/C3 (1 increase)	1.17	0.96–1.42	0.1111
Oxford classification T (1 increase)	1.06	0.75–1.50	0.7318

HR, hazard ratio; CI, confidence interval; BMI, body mass index; MAP, mean arterial pressure; eGFR, estimated glomerular filtration rate; T-Cho, total cholesterol; U-Prot, urinary protein excretion; U-RBC, urinary red blood cells; IgA, immunoglobulin A.

progression to ESRD (Table 4). Kaplan–Meier analysis showed that cumulative renal survival rates were significantly higher in patients with higher than lower eGFR (Figure 3a), in patients with lower than higher U-Prot (Figure 3b), and in patients with lower than higher uric acid concentration (Figure 3d; P<0.0001 each). Cumulative survival, however, did not differ significantly according to the degree of hematuria (Figure 3c, P=0.1122). Kaplan–Meier analysis also showed that the cumulative renal survival rate was significantly higher in patients diagnosed with IgAN over the last 20 years than during the previous 20 years (75.2% vs. 59.0 %, P = 0.0002; Figure 4).

Discussion

IgAN is the most common type of chronic glomerulonephritis worldwide [13]. Although slowly progressive over decades, IgAN is not a benign disease. Since IgAN was first described over 40 years ago, patients with this disease have been treated with oral steroids [4,14,15], steroid pulse therapy [5,6], tonsillectomy [7,16,17], renin-angiotensin aldosterone system inhibitors [18–20], eicosa-

pentaenoic acid [21], statins [22] and combinations of these agents [23]. Although these agents were found to improve short and intermediate term renal outcomes, less is known about very long term outcomes in these patients. In this retrospective analysis, we showed that the 10-, 20-, 30-, and 36-year cumulative renal survival rates were 84.3%, 66.6%, 50.3% and 46.4%, respectively, findings similar to those reported previously for up to 20 years. For example, a study of 282 patients in France showed that the cumulative 10- and 20-year renal survival rates from biopsy to S-Cre >1.5 mg/dl were 84% and 64%, respectively [2]. A study of 502 patients in Japan reported that the 10- and 20-year cumulative survival rates from onset of IgAN until ESRD were 85% and 61%, respectively [3], and a study of 1,155 patients in China found that the 10- and 20-year cumulative renal survival rates until eGFR < 15 ml/min/1.73m² were 83% and 64%, respectively [24]. In addition, a study of 1,364 patients in Korea reported that the cumulative 10- and 20-year survival rates from renal biopsy until ESRD or death were 79.8% and 66.9%, respectively [25]. These findings, however, suggested that treatment may not improve

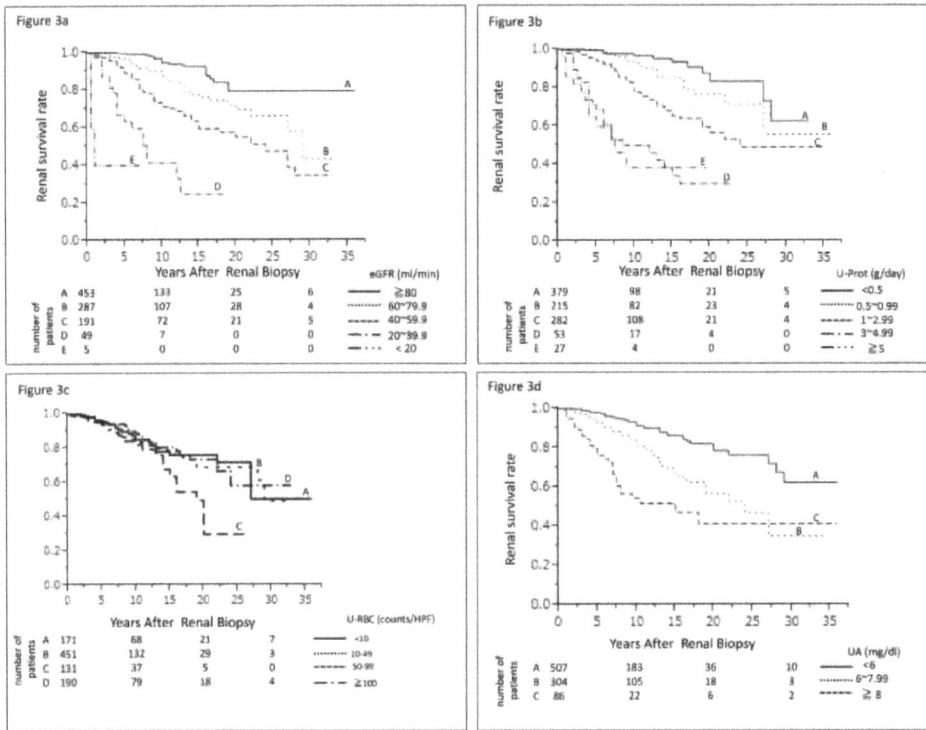

Figure 3. Cumulative renal survival rates in IgAN patients categorized by eGFR, U-Prot, U-RBC and uric acid concentration. (a) The 30-year survival rates of patients with eGFR >80 ml/min/1.73m², between 80 and 60 ml/min/1.73m², and between 60 and 40 ml/min/1.73m² were 80.1%, 43.1%, and 34.6%, respectively. The survival rates of patients with eGFR between 40 and 20 ml/min/1.73m² and <20 ml/min/1.73m² were 24.8% over 18 years and 40.0% over 7 years, respectively. The difference among groups was statistically significant (P<0.0001). (b) The 30-year renal survival rates of patients with U-Prot <0.5 g/day, between 0.5 and 1 g/day, and between 1 and 3 g were 62.6%, 55.6%, and 49.0%, respectively. The survival rates of patients with U-Prot between 3 and 5 g/day and >5 g/day were 29.9% over 20 years and 34.4% over 15 years, respectively. The difference among groups was statistically significant (P<0.0001). (c) The 30-year renal survival rates of patients with U-RBC <10 counts/HF, between 10 and 49 counts/HF, and ≥100 counts/HF were 50.2, 49.0, and 41.7%. The survival rates of patients with U-RBC between 50 and 99 counts/HF was 29.6% over 25 years. The difference among groups was not statistically significant (P = 0.1122). (d) The 30-year renal survival rates of patients with uric acid <6 mg/dl, between 6 and 8 mg/dl, and >8 mg/dl were 62.3, 35.1, and 41.2%, respectively (P<0.0001).

prognosis in patients with IgAN because renal survival rates had not increased dramatically over time. We therefore compared renal survival rates in patients diagnosed with IgAN between 1974 and 1991 and those diagnosed between 1992 and 2011, finding

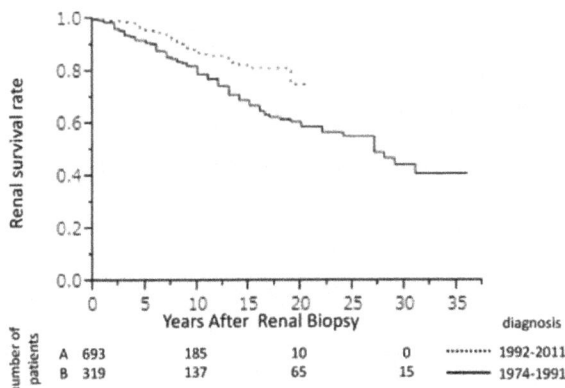

Figure 4. Renal survival rates in IgAN patients diagnosed between 1974 and 1991 and between 1992 and 2001. The 10 year (86.6% vs. 79.1%) and 20 year (75.2% vs. 59.0%) renal survival rates were significantly higher in patients diagnosed between 1992 and 2011 than in between 1974 and 1991 (P = 0.0002).

that the 20-year survival rate was significantly higher in the latter than in the former group (75.2% vs. 59.0%, P = 0.0002). Similar findings were reported previously [23], confirming that treatment of IgAN improved renal outcomes. Beginning in 2004, patients in our institution have been treated with a combination of steroids with tonsillectomy, with none of the 119 patients treated since 2004 progressing to ESRD. This result, indicating that steroid therapy combined with tonsillectomy improves renal outcomes dramatically, was similar to previous findings [7]. In contrast, 169 patients (16.7% of all patients) received no treatment at the time of renal biopsy, because their clinical and histological findings were mild. These patients had a mean eGFR of 80.9±24.7 ml/min/1.73m² and a mean U-Prot of 0.60±0.69 g/day, with 43.3% classified as M1, 23.3% as E1, 54.1% as S1, 15.8% as T1, and 3.3% as T2. Interestingly, their renal survival rate was better than that of the patients who received steroids, immunosuppressive agents, or conservative therapy as initial treatment, although 35.6% progressed to ESRD in 35 years. These results indicate that, despite their mild clinical and histological findings at the time of renal biopsy, some patients with IgAN progressed to ESRD. Furthermore, careful observation of all IgAN patients is needed, regardless of findings at the time of renal biopsy. Moreover, in our cohort, median (interquartile range) U-Prot (0.68 (0.3–1.305) vs. 0.77 (0.225–1.55) g/day, P = 0.0037) and U-RBC (20 (10–50) vs. 30 (10–100) counts/HF, P<0.0001) were significantly lower and eGFR (80.3 (61.7–99.3) vs. 70.9 (58.5–88.3) ml/min/1.73m², P<

0.0001) was significantly higher in patients diagnosed between 1992 and 2011 than in those diagnosed between 1974 and 1991. These findings indicated that more recently diagnosed patients had milder disease at the time of renal biopsy and a better overall prognosis.

In our cohort, about 60% of patients diagnosed as IgAN were female, which contrasts with worldwide findings. We suspected that this may have been due to the name of our institution, Tokyo Women's Medical University, which may have attracted more female than male patients. More women than men were found to undergo underwent renal biopsy [13], with several reports from Japan yielding results similar to ours [8,23,31]. In addition, two reports from Asia, evaluating over 1,000 IgAN patients, found that the gender distribution was even [24,25]. The frequency of IgAN in Japan was similar to that of other nations in East Asia, but different from that of other regions in the world [13]. These results indicated that specific genetic and ethnic backgrounds may be related to gender distribution of this disease. Using the Oxford classification, we found that 47.6% of patients could be classified as M1, 44.3% as E1, 74.6% as S1, 23.0% as T1, and 5.8% as T2, although including criteria different from those of the original Oxford classification. We selected all patients diagnosed with IgAN in our institution, including patients with U-Prot <0.5 g/day or eGFR <30 ml/min/1.74^2, patient not selected by the original Oxford classification. Except for M1, however, the distribution of patients in our cohort was similar to that of the cohort from the original Oxford classification, in which 81% of patients were classified as M1, 42% as E1, 76% as S1, 30% as T1, and 5% as T2 [11,12]. The lower percentage of our patients classified as M1 may have been due to the large percentage of patients with mild IgAN, defined as U-Prot <0.5 g/day.

Multivariate Cox regression analysis showed that risk factors associated with deterioration to ESRD were impaired renal function and severe proteinuria at the time of renal biopsy, findings similar to those of previous reports [2,3,23,24,25]. Kaplan–Meier analysis also indicated that renal function and proteinuria affected renal outcome. Acute deterioration of renal function after 25 years was observed in patients with very low proteinuria (<0.5 g/day). The renal survival rate, which was 83.4% at 25 years after renal biopsy, decreased to 73.0% at 27 years and 62.6% at 28 years. However, only nine patients were available for follow-up after 25 years in patients with low proteinuria, with two of these nine patients progressing to ESRD. One of these two patients had diabetic nephropathy and the other had multiple organ failure with severe infection, suggesting that, in the absence of these complications, their renal function may not have deteriorated after 25 years. Other risk factors reported associated with ESRD included uncontrolled hypertension [3,23,24,25] and severe histological damage [3,23,25], although none of these was significant in our analysis. We also found that age, sex, hematuria, IgA/C3 ratio and serum albumin were not associated with deterioration to ESRD. Kaplan–Meier analysis

also indicated that hematuria did not affect renal outcome. Interestingly, uric acid concentration was a risk factor for progression to ESRD by multivariate Cox regression analysis and Kaplan–Meier analysis. Indeed, higher uric acid concentration has been associated with glomerular damage [26,27], tubulointerstitial change [26,27,28], and vascular damage [26], as well as with poor prognosis [24,26,27,29], and it was independent from renal function [24,27], further suggesting the importance of controlling uric acid concentration in patients with IgAN.

Univariate analysis showed that the only Oxford classification associated with patient prognosis was T grade (HR 2.38, 95% CI 1.91–3.20, P<0.0001), whereas M, E, and S grades were not. Following multivariate analysis, however, T grade was no longer prognostic, whereas clinical factors, such as lower eGFR, higher U-Prot, and higher uric acid were powerful predictors of renal deterioration. Similar findings have been observed in several other studies. For example, Kaplan–Meier analysis showed no significant differences in renal survival rate in patients assorted by M, E, and S grades, with T grade being the only Oxford classification predictive of renal outcome [30]. Another study reported that higher T grade and extracapillary lesions were risk factors for progression to ESRD, as were lower eGFR, higher U-Prot and the absence of steroid treatment, whereas M, E, and S grades were not [31]. Multivariate analysis showed that the most powerful predictor of renal outcome was renal function at biopsy, with eGFR, U-Prot and hypertension being prognostic; in contrast, none of the Oxford classifications was predictive of progression to ESRD [32]. Although Oxford classification is recognized as useful in predicting renal outcomes, these findings suggest that the Oxford classification be evaluated in prospective, large sized, worldwide validation studies.

Our study had several limitations, including the relatively low number of patients followed-up. Of the 1,012 patients who underwent of renal biopsy, only about 30% could be evaluated at 10 years, and only 6% at 20 years. Loss of patients with milder disease to follow-up, with more severely ill patients remaining under observation, may have biased our results towards more severe outcomes. In conclusion, we assessed long term renal survival in patients with IgAN, as well as evaluating factors associated with renal survival. We found that about 50% of patients with IgAN developed ESRD within 30 years. Higher U-Prot, lower eGFR, and higher uric acid were independent risk factors for the development of ESRD.

Author Contributions

Conceived and designed the experiments: TM HK MI TT KU KN. Performed the experiments: TM KT CI YO AO. Analyzed the data: TM KT CI YO AO. Contributed reagents/materials/analysis tools: TM TT KN. Wrote the paper: TM.

References

1. Berger J, Hinglais N (1968) Intercapillary deposits of IgA-IgG. J Urol Nephrol 74: 694–695.
2. Alamartine E, Sabatier JC, Guerin C, Berliet JM, Berthoux F (1991) Prognostic factors in mesangial IgA glomerulonephritis: an extensive study with univariate and multivariate analysis. Am J Kidney Dis 18: 12–19.
3. Koyama A, Igarashi M, Kobayashi M (1997) Coworkers of the research group on progressive renal disease. Natural history and risk factors for immunoglobulin A nephropathy in Japan. Am J Kidney Dis 29: 526–532.
4. Kobayashi Y, Hiki Y, Kokubo T, Tateno S (1996) Steroid therapy during the early stage of progressive IgA nephropathy. A 10-year follow-up study. Nephron 72: 237–242.

5. Pozzi C, Bolasco PG, Fogazzi GB, Andrulli S, Altieri P, et al. (1999) Corticosteroids in IgA nephropathy: a randomized controlled trial. Lancet 353: 883–887.
6. Pozzi C, Andrulli S, Del Vecchio L, Melis P, Fogazzi GB, et al. (2004) Corticosteroid effectiveness in IgA nephropathy: long-term results of a randomized, controlled trial. J Am Soc Nephrol 15: 157–163.
7. Hotta O, Miyazaki M, Furuta T, Tomioka S, Chiba S, et al. (2001) Tonsillectomy and steroid pulse therapy significantly impact on clinical remission in patients with IgA nephropathy. Am J Kidney Dis 38: 736–743.
8. Miura N, Imai H, Kikuchi S, Hayashi S, Endoh M, et al. (2009) Tonsillectomy and steroid pulse (TSP) therapy for patients with IgA nephropathy: a nationwide

survey of TSP therapy in Japan and an analysis of the predictive factors or resistance to TSP therapy. Clin Exp Nephrol 13: 460–466.

9. Matsuzaki K, Suzuki Y, Nakata J, Sakamoto N, Horikoshi S, et al. (2013) Nationwide survey on current treatments for IgA nephropathy in Japan. Clin Exp Nephrol, in press.

10. Matsuo S, Imai E, Horio M, Yasuda Y, Tomita K, et al. (2009) Revised equation for estimated GFR from serum creatinine in Japan: Am J Kidney Dis 53: 982–992.

11. A Working Group of the International IgA Nephropathy Network and the Renal Pathology Society (2009) the Oxford Classification of IgA Nephropathy: rationale, clinicopathological correlations, and classification. Kidney Int 76: 534–545.

12. A Working Group of the International IgA Nephropathy Network and the Renal Pathology Society (2009) the Oxford Classification of IgA Nephropathy: pathology definitions, correlations, and reproducibility. Kidney Int 76: 546–556.

13. Moriyama T, Suzuki K, Sugiura H, Itabashi M, Tsukasa M, et al. (2010) Frequency of renal disease in Japan: An analysis of 2,404 renal biopsies at a single center. Nephron Clin Pract 115: c227–c236.

14. Moriyama T, Honda K, Nitta K, Yumura W, Nihei H (2004) The effectiveness of steroid therapy for patients with advanced IgA nephropathy and impaired renal function: Clin Exp Nephrol 8: 237–242.

15. Moriyama T, Nakayama K, Iwasaki C, Ochi A, Tsuruta Y, et al. (2012) Severity of nephrotic IgA nephropathy according to the Oxford classification: Int Urol Nephrol 44: 1177–1184.

16. Ochi A, Moriyama T, Takei T, Uchida K, Nitta K (2013) Comparison between steroid pulse therapy alone and in combination with tonsillectomy for IgA nephropathy: Int Urol Nephrol 45: 469–476.

17. Kamei D, Moriyama T, Takei T, Wakai S, Nitta S (2013) Comparison between consecutive and intermittent steroid pulse therapy combined with tonsillectomy for clinical remission of IgA nephropathy: Clin Exp Nephrol: In press.

18. Moriyama T, Amamiya N, Ochi A, Tsuruta Y, Shimizu A, et al. (2011) Long-term beneficial effects of angiotensin-converting enzyme inhibitor and angiotensin receptor blocker therapy for patients with advanced immunoglobulin A nephropathy and impaired renal function: Clin Exp Nephrol 15: 700–707.

19. Moriyama T, Amemiya N, Ochi A, Tsuruta S, Shimizu A, et al. (2011) Comparison of steroids and angiotensin receptor blockers for patients with advanced IgA nephropathy and impaired renal function: Am J Nephrol 34: 233–240.

20. Moriyama T, Nakayama K, Ochi A, Amemiya N, Tsuruta Y, et al. (2012) Comparison of inhibitors of renin-angiotensin-aldosterone system (RAS) and combination therapy of steroids plus RAS inhibitors for patients with advanced immunoglobulin A nephropathy and impaired renal function: Clin Exp Nephrol 16: 231–237.

21. Moriyama T, Iwasaki C, Tanaka K, Ochi A, Shimizu A, et al. (2013) Effects of combination therapy with renin-angiotensin system inhibitors and eicosapentaenoic acid on IgA nephropathy: Intern Med 52: 193–199.

22. Moriyama T, Oshima Y, Tanaka K, Iwasaki C, Ochi A, et al. (2013) Statin stabilize the renal function of IgA nephropathy: Ren Fail: In press.

23. Komatsu H, Fujimoto S, Hara S, Fukuda A, Fukudome K, et al. (2009) Recent therapeutic strategies improve renal outcome in patients with IgA nephropathy. Am J Nephrol 30: 19–25.

24. Le W, Liang S, Hu Y, Deng K, Bao H, et al. (2012) Long-term renal survival and related risk factors in patients with IgA nephropathy: results from a cohort of 1155 cases in a Chinese adult population. Nephrol Dial Transplant 27: 1479–1485.

25. Lee H, Kim DK, Oh KH, Joo KW, Kim YS, et al. (2012) Mortality of IgA nephropathy patients: a single center experience over 30 years. PLOS One 7: e51225.

26. Cheng GY, Liu DW, Zhang N, Tang L, Zhao ZZ, et al. (2013) Clinical and prognostic implications of serum uric acid levels on IgA nephropathy: a cohort study of 348 cases with a mean 5-year follow up. Clin Nephrol 80: 40–46.

27. Ohno I, Hosoya T, Gomi H, Ichida K, Okabe H, et al. (2001) Serum uric acid and renal prognosis in patients with IgA nephropathy. Nephron 87: 333–339.

28. Myllmäki J, Honkanen T, Syrjänen J, Helin H, Rantala l, et al. (2005) Uric acid correlates with the severity of histopathological parameters in IgA nephropathy. Nephrol Dial Transplant 20: 89–95.

29. Shi Y, Chen W, Jalal D, Li Z, Chen W, et al. (2012) Clinical outcome of hyperuricemia in IgA nephropathy: A retrospective cohort study and randomized controlled trial. Kidney Blood Press Res 35: 153–160.

30. Yau T, Korbet AM, Schwartz MM, Cimbaluk DJ (2011) The Oxford classification of IgA nephropathy: a retrospective analysis: Am J Nephrol 34: 435–444.

31. Katafuchi R, Ninomiya T, Nagata M, Mitsuki K, Hiraoka H (2011) Validation study of Oxford classification of IgA nephropathy: The significance of extracapillary proliferation: Clin J Am Soc Nephrol 6: 2806–2813.

32. Alamartine E, Sauron C, Laurent B, Sury A, Seffert A, et al. (2011) The use of Oxford Classification of IgA nephropathy to predict renal survival: Clin J Am Soc Nephrol 6: 2384–2388.

29

Association of Heart-Type Fatty Acid-Binding Protein with Cardiovascular Risk Factors and All-Cause Mortality in the General Population

Yoichiro Otaki[1], Tetsu Watanabe[1]*, Hiroki Takahashi[1], Atushi Hirayama[1], Taro Narumi[1], Shinpei Kadowaki[1], Yuki Honda[1], Takanori Arimoto[1], Tetsuro Shishido[1], Takuya Miyamoto[1], Tsuneo Konta[1], Yoko Shibata[1], Akira Fukao[2], Makoto Daimon[3], Yoshiyuki Ueno[2], Takeo Kato[2], Takamasa Kayama[2], Isao Kubota[1]

1 Department of Cardiology, Pulmonology, and Nephrology, Yamagata University School of Medicine, Yamagata, Japan, 2 Global Center of Excellence Program Study Group, Yamagata University School of Medicine, Yamagata, Japan, 3 Department of Endocrinology and Metabolism, Hirosaki University Graduate School of Medicine, Aomori, Japan

Abstract

Background: Despite many recent advances in medicine, preventing the development of cardiovascular diseases remains a challenge. Heart-type fatty acid-binding protein (H-FABP) is a marker of ongoing myocardial damage and has been reported to be a useful indicator for future cardiovascular events. However, it remains to be determined whether H-FABP can predict all-cause and cardiovascular deaths in the general population.

Methods and Results: This longitudinal cohort study included 3,503 subjects who participated in a community-based health checkup with a 7-year follow-up. Serum H-FABP was measured in registered subjects. The results demonstrated that higher H-FABP levels were associated with increasing numbers of cardiovascular risk factors, including hypertension, diabetes mellitus, obesity, and metabolic syndrome. There were 158 deaths during the follow-up period, including 50 cardiovascular deaths. Deceased subjects had higher H-FABP levels compared to surviving subjects. Multivariate Cox proportional hazard regression analysis revealed that H-FABP is an independent predictor of all-cause and cardiovascular deaths after adjustments for confounding factors. Subjects were divided into four quartiles according to H-FABP level, and Kaplan-Meier analysis demonstrated that the highest H-FABP quartile was associated with the greatest risks for all-cause and cardiovascular deaths. Net reclassification index and integrated discrimination index were significantly increased by addition of H-FABP to cardiovascular risk factors.

Conclusions: H-FABP level was increased in association with greater numbers of cardiovascular risk factors and was an independent risk factor for all-cause and cardiovascular deaths. H-FABP could be a useful indicator for the early identification of high-risk subjects in the general population.

Editor: Michael Lipinski, Washington Hospital Center, United States of America

Funding: This study was supported by a grant-in-aid from the 21st 9 Century Center of Excellence (COE) and the Global COE program of the Japan Society for the Promotion of Science. The funders had no role in study design, data collection and analysis, decision to publish, or preparation of the manuscript.

Competing Interests: The authors have declared that no competing interests exist.

* E-mail: tewatana@med.id.yamagata-u.ac.jp

Introduction

Despite technical advances in medicine, chronic heart failure remains a public health problem associated with high all-cause and cardiovascular mortality [1,2]. According to the American College of Cardiology/American Heart Association (ACC/AHA) guide-line, treatment of cardiovascular risk factors, such as hypertension, diabetes mellitus, obesity, and metabolic syndrome are recommended in subjects at high risk for developing stage A heart failure [3]. Therefore, early identification and risk-stratification of high-risk subjects in the general population would be helpful in preventing cardiovascular disease and subsequent premature deaths.

Cardiac biomarkers are generally used for the diagnosis or assessment of heart diseases [4,5,6,7]. Recent studies demonstrated that cardiac biomarkers can predict an increased risk for death in subjects in the general population [8,9]. Heart-type fatty acid-binding protein (H-FABP) is a low molecular weight protein in the cytosol of cardiomyocytes. H-FABP is rapidly released into the circulation from damaged myocardial tissue [10], which makes it a useful marker for ongoing myocardial damage. H-FABP levels can therefore be used to stratify risk for various heart diseases [11,12,13]. However, it remains to be determined whether serum H-FABP levels can predict cardiovascular diseases in the general population.

Table 1. Clinical characteristics of subjects with and without all-cause deaths.

Variables	All subject n = 3503	All-cause deaths(−) n = 3345	All-cause deaths(+) n = 158	P value
Age, years	63±10	62±10	73±8	<0.0001
Men/women, n	1570/1933	1455/1890	115/43	<0.0001
Obesity, n (%)	1035 (30%)	996 (30%)	39 (25%)	0.1704
Previous CVD, n (%)	461 (13%)	427 (13%)	34 (22%)	0.0015
Previous cancer, n (%)	74 (2.1%)	70 (2.1%)	4 (2.5%)	0.7077
Smoking, n (%)	1126 (32%)	1052 (31%)	74 (47%)	<0.0001
Hypertension, n (%)	1285 (37%)	1202 (36%)	83 (53%)	<0.0001
Diabetes mellitus, n (%)	243 (10%)	223 (7%)	20 (13%)	0.0038
Hyperlipidemia, n (%)	1361 (39%)	1301 (39%)	60 (38%)	0.8168
CKD, n (%)	235 (7%)	210 (6%)	25 (16%)	<0.0001
MetS, n (%)	454 (13%)	431 (13%)	23 (15%)	0.5409
Insulin resistance	354 (11%)	333 (11%)	21 (15%)	0.1180
Electrocardiographic LVH, n (%)	143 (4.1%)	135 (4%)	8 (5.1%)	0.5236
AF, n (%)	52 (1.5%)	38 (1.1%)	14 (9%)	<0.0001
Systolic BP, mmHg	134±16	134±16	138±18	0.0019
Diastolic BP, mmHg	80±10	80±10	80±11	0.9799
HbA1c, %	5.7±0.7	5.7±0.7	5.8±0.8	0.0065
FBG, mmol/L	5.27±0.94	5.27±0.94	5.50±0.83	0.0010
eGFR, mL/min/1.73 m^2	82±16	82±16	74±18	<0.0001
Log$_e$ BNP, pg/mL	3.00±0.85	2.97±0.83	3.54±1.11	<0.0001
Log$_e$ H-FABP, ng/mL	1.25±0.43	1.23±0.43	1.52±0.49	<0.0001

Data are expressed as mean ± standard deviation or number (%).
CVD, cardiovascular disease; CKD, chronic kidney disease; MetS, metabolic syndrome; LVH, left ventricular hypertrophy; AF, atrial fibrillation; BP, blood pressure; HbA1c, glycosylated hemoglobin A1c, FBG, fasting blood glucose; eGFR, estimated glomerular filtration rate; BNP, brain natriuretic peptide; H-FABP, heart type fatty acid binding protein.

The purposes of the present study were to study the association of H-FABP levels with the presence of cardiovascular risk factors, and to determine whether H-FABP levels can predict all-cause and cardiovascular mortality in subjects from the general population.

Methods

Ethics Statement and Study population

The institutional ethics committee of Yamagata University School of Medicine approved the study, and all participants provided written informed consent. The procedures were performed in accordance with the Helsinki Declaration.

This study was a part of the ongoing Molecular Epidemiological Study, utilizing the resources of the Regional Characteristics of 21st Century Centers of Excellence (COE) Program and the Global COE in Japan.

This study was based on a community-based annual health check-up of inhabitants from the town of Takahata in northern Japan (total population 26,026). Community members, aged > 40 years were invited to participate. Between June 2004 and November 2007, 3,520 subjects (1,579 men and 1,941 women) were enrolled in the study. Subjects completed a self-reported questionnaire to document their medical history, current medication use, and clinical symptoms. Seventeen subjects were excluded due to incomplete data or study withdrawal.

Measurement

Hypertension was defined as systolic blood pressure (BP) ≥ 140 mmHg, diastolic BP ≥90 mmHg, or antihypertensive medication use. Diabetes mellitus was defined as fasting blood glucose (FBG) ≥7.0 mmol/L, glycosylated hemoglobin A1c ≥ 6.5% (National Glyco hemoglobin Standardization Program), or anti-diabetic medication use. Hyperlipidemia was defined as total cholesterol ≥5.7 mmol/L, triglyceride ≥1.7 mmol/L, or anti-hyperlipidemic drug use. Obesity was defined as body mass index ≥25 kg/m^2 [14]. Metabolic syndrome (Mets) was defined according to the modified National Cholesterol Education Program Adult Treatment Panel III (NCEP-ATP III) criteria, which require fulfilment of at least three of the five following: BMI ≥25 kg/m^2, elevated triglyceride (TG) level (≥1.7 mmol/L), reduced level of high-density lipoprotein cholesterol (HDL-C; <1.03 mmol/L in men and <1.29 mmol/L in women), elevated FBG level (≥6.1 mmol/L) or previously diagnosed diabetes mellitus, and elevated BP (systolic BP ≥130 mmHg and diastolic BP ≥85 mmHg) or anti-hypertensive medication use [15,16]. Chronic kidney disease (CKD) was defined as a reduced glomerular filtration rate (<60 mL/min/1.73m^2) according to Kidney Disease Outcomes Quality Initiative clinical guideline [17,18]. Electrocardiographic left ventricular hypertrophy was diagnosed by a cardiologist according to the Minnesota code (1982 revised edition).

(A)

(B)

(C)

(D)

(E)

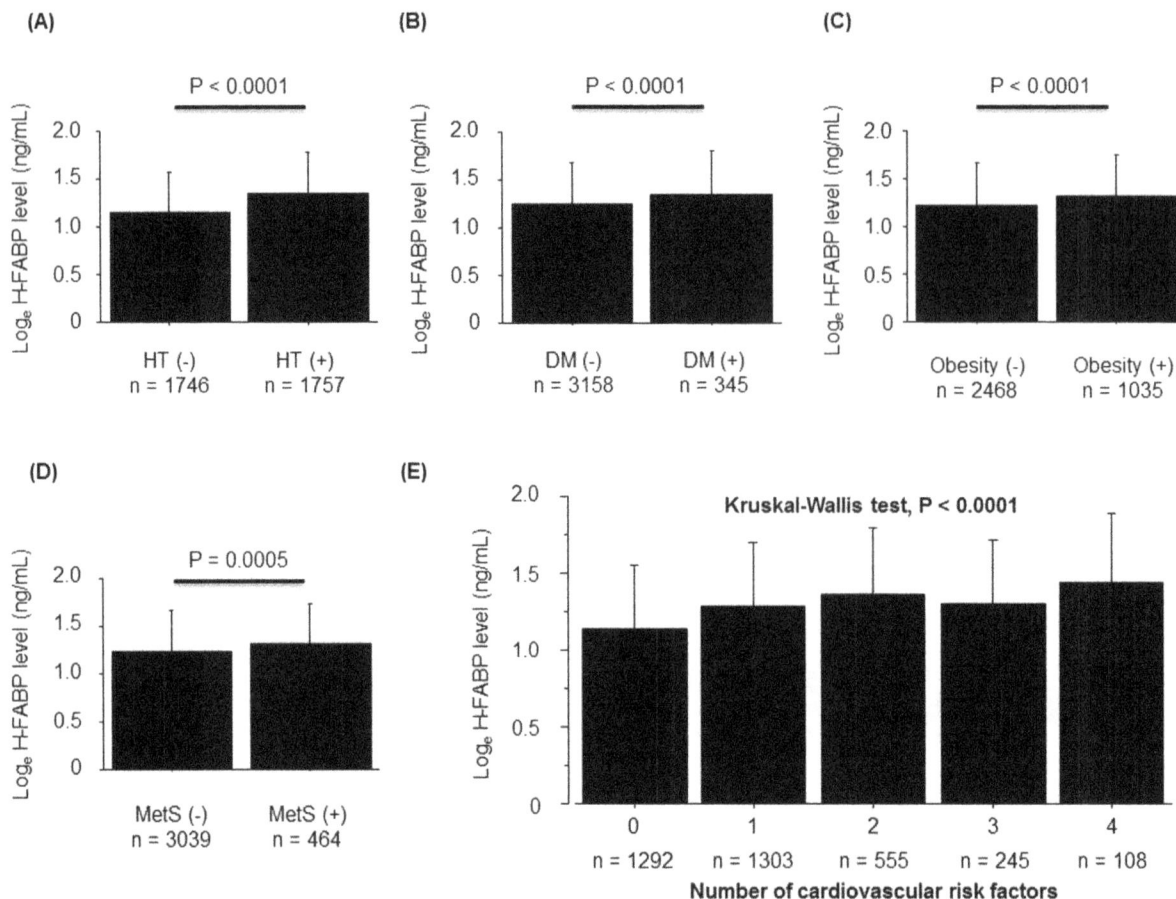

Figure 1. Associations between H-FABP levels and cardiovascular risk factors in the general population. H-FABP levels were higher in subjects with hypertension (**A**), diabetes mellitus (**B**), obesity (**C**), and metabolic syndrome (**D**). (**E**) Higher H-FABP levels were associated with greater numbers of cardiovascular risk factors (Kruskal-Wallis test, P<0.0001). HT, hypertension; DM, diabetes mellitus; MetS, metabolic syndrome.

Biochemical markers

Blood samples for measurements of serum H-FABP concentrations were drawn and centrifuged at 2,500 g for 15 min at 4°C within 30 min of collection, and the obtained serum was stored at −70°C until analysis. H-FABP levels were measured using a two-step sandwich enzyme-linked immunosorbent assay (ELISA) kit (MARKIT-M H-FABP, Dainippon Pharmaceutical Co. Ltd., Tokyo, Japan), as previously described [19]. Detection limit, measurement range, and reference interval of H-FABP were 0–250 ng/mL, 1.0–37, <6.2 ng/mL, respectively.

Blood samples were also obtained for measuring brain natriuretic peptide (BNP). These samples were transferred to chilled tubes containing 4.5 mg ethylenediaminetetraacetic acid disodium salt and aprotinin (500 U/mL), and centrifuged at 1,000 g for 15 minutes at 4°C. The clarified plasma samples were frozen, stored at −70°C, and thawed just before the assay was performed. BNP concentrations were measured using a commercially available radioimmunoassay specific for human BNP (Shiono RIA BNP assay kit, Shionogi Co. Ltd., Tokyo, Japan) [20,21]. Detection limit, measurement range, and reference interval of BNP were 0–2902, 3.4–1392, <18.4 pg/mL, respectively.

Estimated glomerular filtration rate (eGFR) was calculated by the modification of diet in renal disease (MDRD) equation with the Japanese coefficient [22].

Insulin resistance was defined as elevated homeostasis model assessment ratio (>2.5). Homeostasis model assessment ratio was calculated by the following equation: (FBG ×fasting insulin)/405 [23].

Glycosylated hemoglobin A1c, FBG, total cholesterol, TG, and HDL cholesterol, and creatinine were measured by standard method as illustrated in Table S1.

Endpoint and follow-up

All subjects were prospectively followed for a median period of 2,124 days (interquartile range, 1,972–2,343 days). The endpoint was all-cause death, which was also broken down into cancer death, cardiovascular death, lung disease death including pneumonia, and others. Cardiovascular death was defined as death due to coronary artery disease, heart failure, arrhythmia, stroke, and aortic artery disease. The cause of death was determined by reviewing death certificates through the end of 2010. The death code (International Classification of Diseases, 10th Revision) and the data place of death were reviewed.

Statistical analysis

Normality of continuous variables was checked by a Kolmogorov-Smirnov-Lillefors test. Since H-FABP and BNP were not normally distributed, we used log$_e$ H-FABP and log$_e$ BNP for all analyses. All values are expressed as the mean ± standard deviation. Continuous and categorical variables were compared

(A)

(B)

(C)

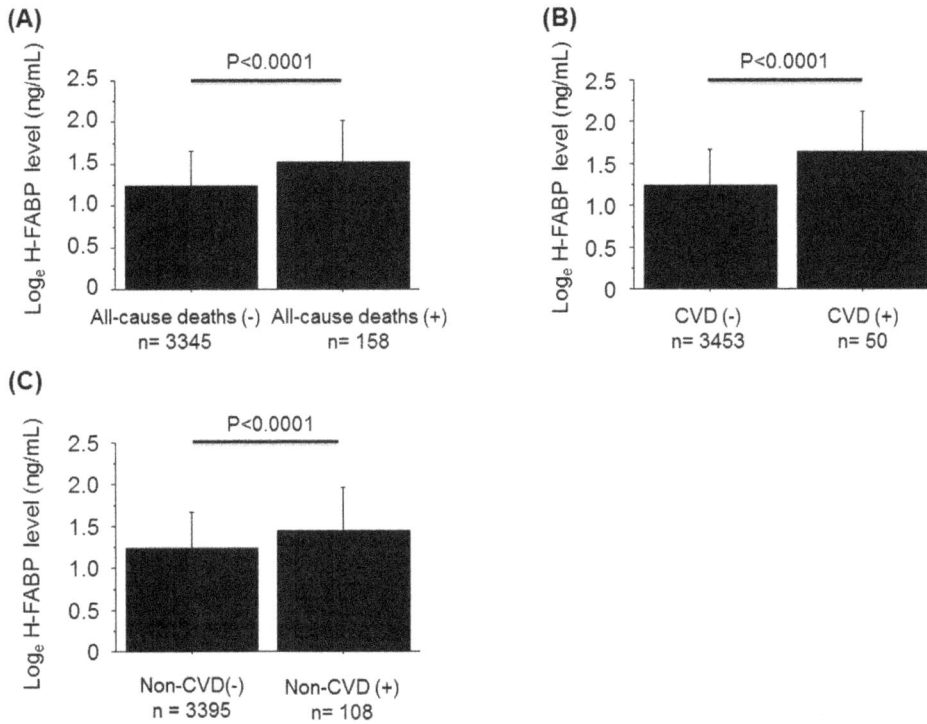

Figure 2. Associations between H-FABP levels and all-cause deaths, cardiovascular deaths, and non-cardiovascular deaths.

with t-tests and chi-square tests, respectively. Kruskal-Wallis test was used to compare cardiovascular risk number with H-FABP levels. A Cox proportional hazard analysis was performed to determine independent predictors for all-cause deaths, and cardiovascular risk factors and significant predictors selected in

the univariate analysis were entered into the multivariate analysis. To determine the independent predictors for cardiovascular deaths, cardiovascular risk factors and significant predictors selected in the univariate analysis were entered into multivariate analysis in a stepwise manner. The receiver operating character-

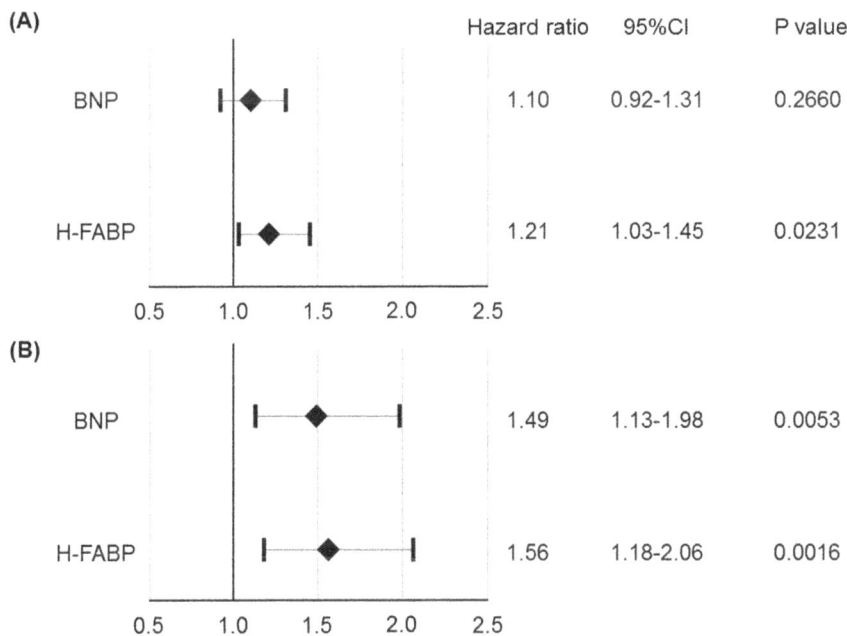

(A)

	Hazard ratio	95%CI	P value
BNP	1.10	0.92-1.31	0.2660
H-FABP	1.21	1.03-1.45	0.0231

(B)

	Hazard ratio	95%CI	P value
BNP	1.49	1.13-1.98	0.0053
H-FABP	1.56	1.18-2.06	0.0016

Figure 3. Multivariate Cox proportional hazard regression analysis for predicting all-cause deaths (A) and cardiovascular deaths (B). (A) Hazard ratios after adjustment for age, gender, smoking, previous cardiovascular disease, obesity, hypertension, diabetes mellitus, metabolic syndrome, chronic kidney disease, atrial fibrillation, and BNP. **(B)** Hazard ratio after adjustment for age, gender, atrial fibrillation and BNP.

Table 2. Univariate Cox proportional hazard analysis for all-cause mortality.

Variables	Hazard ratio	95%CI	P Value
Age	1.13	1.10–1.15	<0.0001
Men/women	3.44	2.43–4.89	<0.0001
Obesity	1.31	0.92–1.89	0.1362
Previous CVD	1.74	1.19–2.54	0.0042
Smoking	1.94	1.42–2.64	<0.0001
Hypertension	1.82	1.33–2.49	0.0002
Diabetes mellitus	1.92	1.20–3.07	0.0063
Hyperlipidemia	1.00	0.73–1.39	0.9805
CKD	2.74	1.79–4.20	<0.0001
MetS	1.13	0.73–1.77	0.5734
Insulin resistance	1.35	0.85–2.15	0.2039
Electrocardiographic LVH	1.30	0.68–2.68	0.4753
AF	7.23	4.17–12.51	<0.0001
Systolic BP	1.02	1.01–1.03	0.0010
Diastolic BP	1.00	0.99–1.02	0.7909
HbA1c	1.28	1.10–1.48	0.0011
FBG	1.01	1.01–1.02	0.0002
eGFR(Per 1-SD increase)	0.59	0.49–0.70	<0.0001
BNP (Per 1-SD increase)	1.71	1.50–1.96	<0.0001
H-FABP (Per 1-SD increase)	1.72	1.51–1.96	<0.0001

CVD, cardiovascular disease; CKD, chronic kidney disease; MetS, metabolic syndrome; LVH, left ventricular hypertrophy; AF, atrial fibrillation; BP, blood pressure; HbA1c, glycosylated hemoglobin A1c; FBG, fasting blood glucose; eGFR, estimated glomerular filtration rate; BNP, brain natriuretic peptide; H-FABP, heart type fatty acid binding protein.

istics (ROC) curves for all-cause deaths were constructed and used as a measure of the predictive accuracy of H-FABP and BNP on all-cause deaths. In addition, we calculated the net reclassification index (NRI) and the integrated discrimination index (IDI) to measure the quality of improvement for the correct reclassification according to the addition of H-FABP to the model. The interaction between H-FABP and BNP levels was analyzed by Cox proportional hazard regression analysis, using H-FABP and BNP cut-off values. Differences among four groups based on H-FABP quartiles were analyzed by analysis of variance (ANOVA) with Scheffe's post hoc tests. Survival curves were constructed with the Kaplan-Meier method and compared using log-rank tests. A value of $P<0.05$ was considered statistically significant. All statistical analyses were performed with a standard program package (JMP version 8; SAS Institute Inc., Cary, NC, USA and R 3.0.2 with additional packages including Rcmdr, Epi, pROC, and PredictABEL).

Results

Comparison of clinical characteristics between surviving and deceased subjects

The subject's baseline characteristics are shown in Table 1. There were 1,570 men and 1,933 women. The mean $\log_e$ H-FABP value was 1.25 ng/mL. Subjects who died during the course of the study were older and had higher prevalence rates of previous cardiovascular diseases, smoking, hypertension, diabetes mellitus, CKD, and atrial fibrillation (AF) than those who survived. The deceased subjects had higher systolic BP, glycosylated hemoglobin A1c, FBG, BNP, and H-FABP levels than those

who did not. eGFR was lower in deceased subjects than in those who survived.

Association between H-FABP levels and cardiovascular risk factors for stage A heart failure

As shown Figure 1, subjects who had each cardiovascular risk factor (hypertension, diabetes mellitus, obesity, and metabolic syndrome) showed higher H-FABP levels compared with those who did not. In addition, H-FABP levels increased with higher numbers of these cardiovascular risk factors, suggesting that subjects at higher risk for stage A heart failure had higher H-FABP levels than those with lower risk.

All-cause and cardiovascular mortality and H-FABP

During the follow-up period, there were 158 all-cause deaths including 50 cardiovascular deaths, 74 cancer deaths, 20 lung disease deaths, and 14 other cause deaths.

As shown in Figure 2, subjects who died during the course of the study had higher H-FABP levels compared to those who did not.

To determine the risk factors for predicting all-cause deaths, we performed univariate and multivariate Cox proportional hazard regression analyses. In the univariate analysis, H-FABP was significantly associated with all-cause mortality (Table 2). Age, male gender, previous cardiovascular disease, smoking, hypertension, diabetes mellitus, CKD, AF, systolic BP, glycosylated hemoglobin A1c, FBG, eGFR, and BNP were also related to all-cause mortality. A multivariate Cox proportional hazard regression analysis demonstrated that H-FABP was an independent predictor of future all-cause mortality after adjusting for age, gender, smoking, previous cardiovascular disease, hypertension,

(A)   **(B)**

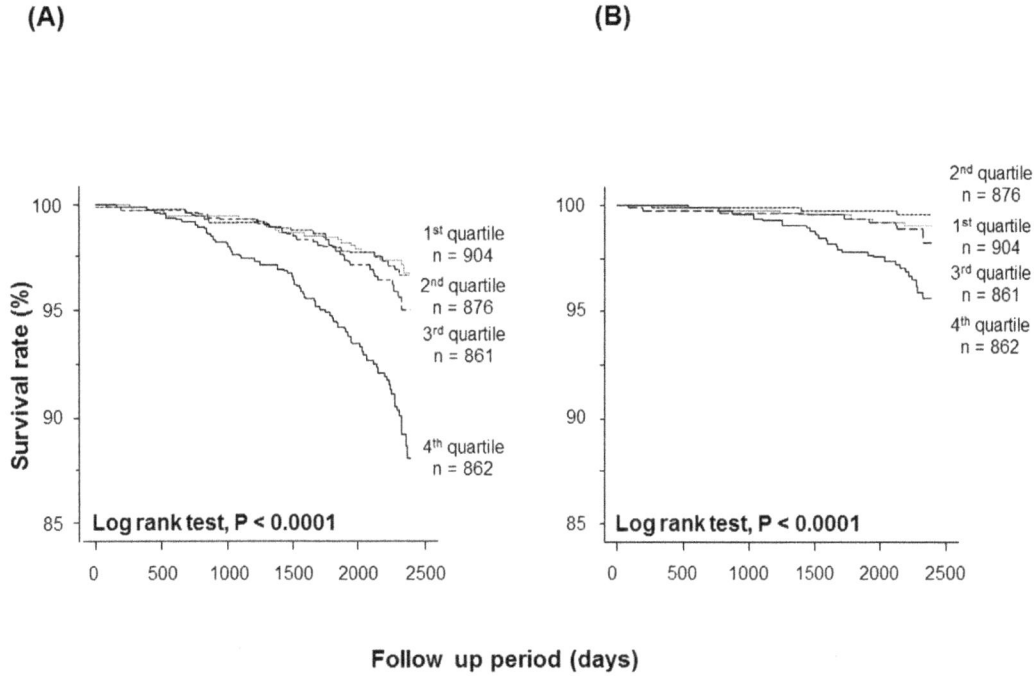

Figure 4. Kaplan-Meier analysis of all-cause deaths (A) and cardiovascular deaths (B) among subjects in all H-FABP quartiles.

Table 3. Clinical characteristics among subjects with 1st to 4th quartile.

Variables	1st quartile n = 904	2nd quartile n = 876	3rd quartile n = 861	4th quartile n = 862
Age, years	57±9	61±10*	65±9*†	69±9*†‡
Men/women, n	348/556	373/503	422/439	427/435§
Obesity, n (%)	203 (22%)	247 (28%)	272 (32%)	313 (36%)§
Previous CVD, n (%)	71 (8%)	94 (11%)	135 (15%)	161 (19%)§
Previous cancer, n (%)	23 (2.5%)	15 (1.7%)	16 (1.9%)	20 (2.3)
Smoking, n (%)	293 (32%)	281 (32%)	271 (32%)	281 (33%)
Hypertension, n (%)	207 (23%)	278 (32%)	356 (41%)	444 (52%)§
Diabetes mellitus, n (%)	54 (6%)	53 (6%)	55 (6%)	81 (9%)§
Hyperlipidemia, n (%)	371 (41%)	369 (42%)	298 (35%)	323 (37%)§
CKD, n (%)	9 (1%)	26 (3%)	47 (6%)	153 (18%)§
MetS, n (%)	87 (10%)	120 (14%)	103 (12%)	144 (32%)§
Insulin resistance	59 (7%)	97 (12%)	93 (12%)	105 (13%)§
Electrocardiographic LVH, n (%)	35 (4%)	27 (3%)	31 (4%)	50 (6%)§
AF, n (%)	3 (0.3%)	12 (1.4%)	17 (2.0%)	20 (2.3%)§
Systolic BP, mmHg	130±16	133±15*	136±15*†	138±16*†‡
Diastolic BP, mmHg	79±10	80±10	80±10	80±10
HbA1c, %	5.6±0.7	5.7±0.7	5.7±0.7*	5.8±0.7*†
FBG, mmol/L	5.16±0.78	5.22±0.99	5.33±0.99*	5.38±0.94*
eGFR, mL/min/1.73 m²	90±16	83±15*	79±14*†	73±16*†‡
Log_e BNP, pg/mL	2.78±0.71	2.91±0.81*	3.05±0.89*†	3.26±0.93*†‡

Data are expressed as mean ± standard deviation or number (%).
CVD, cardiovascular disease; CKD, chronic kidney disease; Mets, metabolic syndrome; LVH, left ventricular hypertrophy; AF, atrial fibrillation; BP, blood pressure; HbA1c, glycosylated hemoglobin A1c; FBG, fasting blood glucose; eGFR, estimated glomerular filtration rate; BNP, brain natriuretic peptide; H-FABP, heart type fatty acid binding protein. *$p<0.05$ vs. 1st quartile, †$p<0.05$ vs. 2nd quartile, ‡$p<0.05$ vs. 3rd quartile by analysis of variance (ANOVA) with Scheffe post hoc test. §$p<0.05$ by chi-square test.

diabetes mellitus, obesity, MetS, CKD, AF, and BNP (hazard ratio, 1.21; 95% confidence interval, 1.03–1.45; P = 0.0231; Figure 3A). A second, age, gender, smoking, previous cardiovascular disease, hypertension, diabetes mellitus, obesity, MetS, CKD, AF, BNP, and H-FABP were entered into the stepwise multivariate Cox proportional hazard regression analysis and it demonstrated that H-FABP was an independent predictor of future cardiovascular mortality (hazard ratio, 1.56; 95% confidence interval, 1.18–2.06; P = 0.0016; Figure 3B).

Risk stratification

All subjects were divided into quartiles according to H-FABP level: first quartile (≤0.96 ng/mL, n = 904), second quartile (0.96–1.22 ng/mL, n = 876), third quartile (1.22–1.50 ng/mL, n = 861), and fourth quartile (>1.50 ng/mL, n = 862). As shown in Table 3, subjects in the highest H-FABP quartile were older and had higher prevalence rates of obesity, previous cardiovascular disease, hypertension, diabetes mellitus, CKD, MetS, insulin resistance, electrocardiographic left ventricular hypertrophy, and AF, compared with the other three groups. Subjects in the highest quartile also showed lower eGFR and higher systolic BP and BNP compared with the other three groups. The mean glycosylated hemoglobin A1c was significantly greater in fourth quartile than in first and second quartiles. FBG was higher in the fourth quartile than in the first quartile. Subjects in the third quartile were older and showed higher systolic BP and lower eGFR than the first and second quartiles. Glycosylated hemoglobin A1c and FBG were higher in the third quartile than in the first quartile. Subjects in the second quartile were older and had higher systolic BP and lower eGFR than the first quartile. Kaplan-Meier analysis demonstrated that both all-cause and cardiovascular mortalities were the highest in fourth quartile compared with other three groups (Figure 4).

Combination of H-FABP and BNP

To examine whether H-FABP improves the prognostic capacity of BNP, ROC analysis were performed. AUC of H-FABP, sensitivity, and specificity were 0.676, 78%, and 49%, respectively. The cut-off value of $\log_e$ H-FABP was 1.59 ng/mL. AUC of BNP, sensitivity, and specificity were 0.645, 76%, and 47%, respectively. The cut-off value of $\log_e$ BNP was 3.6 pg/mL. There was no significant difference in AUC of H-FABP and that of BNP. However, the AUC of BNP was significantly improved by addition of H-FABP (Figure 5A). Also, NRI and IDI were significantly improved in model with H-FABP than those with BNP only (NRI, 0.4498; 95% confidence interval, 0.2925–0.6071; P<0.0001 and IDI, 0.0209; 95% confidence interval, 0.0129–0.0292; P<0.0001). Next, we studied the statistical interaction between H-FABP and BNP. As shown in Figure 5B, multivariate Cox proportional hazard regression analysis demonstrated that subjects with high H-FABP (≥1.59 ng/mL) and high BNP (≥3.6 pg/mL) were at significantly increased risk for all-cause death after adjustments for high H-FABP and high BNP (hazard ratio, 2.39; 95% confidence interval, 1.19–4.37; P = 0.0126).

Improvement of reclassification by addition of H-FABP to predict all-cause mortality

To examine whether model fit and discrimination improve with addition of H-FABP or BNP to the basic predictors such as age, HT, DM, obesity, and MetS, we evaluated the improvement of NRI and IDI. As shown in Table 4, NRI and IDI were significantly improved by addition of H-FABP. On the other

hand, there was no significant difference in NRI by addition of BNP to the basic predictors.

Discussion

Main findings

The results of this study revealed four novel findings: 1) H-FABP was detectable in all subjects and was higher in deceased subjects than in surviving subjects; 2) increased H-FABP values were associated with greater numbers of cardiovascular risk factors; 3) multivariate Cox proportional hazard regression analysis revealed that high H-FABP levels independently predicted future all-cause and cardiovascular mortality; and 4) Kaplan-Meier analysis demonstrated that all-cause and cardiovascular mortality were greatest in subjects in the highest H-FABP quartile.

Latent myocardial damage assessed by H-FABP

Research into cardiac biomarkers has shifted toward identifying subjects in the general population who are at high risk. Previous studies have reported that BNP, troponin I, and troponin T are useful indicators of all-cause deaths and cardiovascular deaths in the general population [5,8,24,25]. Although H-FABP is also a diagnostic marker of myocardial infarction [26], there has been no clinical research to reveal the prognostic value of H-FABP in general population.

Myocardial damage plays a key role in the progression of left ventricular remodeling in heart failure [27,28]. Troponin leakage detected by a highly sensitive assay kit was reported to occur in 20–25% of the general population and 60% of elderly adults [24,25,29]. Importantly, H-FABP was detectable in all subjects who participated in this study. Studies in rats and clinical research with human autopsy cases have shown that H-FABP leakage occurs in the absence of myocyte necrosis [30]. Because H-FABP is a low molecular weight protein, cytosolic H-FABP is easily released into the circulation through the porous membranes of damaged myocardial cells [26]. Therefore, H-FABP is a sensitive marker for detecting latent myocardial damage.

Associations of H-FABP with cardiovascular risk factors

Myocardial damage in an apparently healthy population may result from several chronic disease states such as CKD, subclinical myocardial infarction, coronary artery disease, and heart failure [29,31]. In the present study, myocardial damage assessed by H-FABP was observed in the presence of cardiovascular risk factors, such as hypertension, diabetes mellitus, obesity and metabolic syndrome. The underlying mechanism of latent myocardial damage was reported to be involved in renin-angiotensin-aldosterone system activation, sympathetic nervous activation, and insulin resistance [32,33,34,35,36]. Interestingly, latent myocardial damage was more severe in subjects with higher numbers of cardiovascular risk factors in the present study. These findings suggest that H-FABP is a useful marker for detecting subjects at high risk for developing structural heart diseases (stage B heart failure).

Clinical outcomes and H-FABP in the general population

Increased concentration of cardiac biomarker has been shown to associate with an increased risk for cardiovascular disease and subsequent high mortality in general population [8,24,37]. Similarly, our results show for the first time that H-FABP is a feasible marker for all-cause and cardiovascular deaths in the general population. Given that heart failure caused by HT, DM, and ischemic heart disease was significantly increased in Asian countries [38], it was plausible that H-FABP predicted future

(A)

(B)

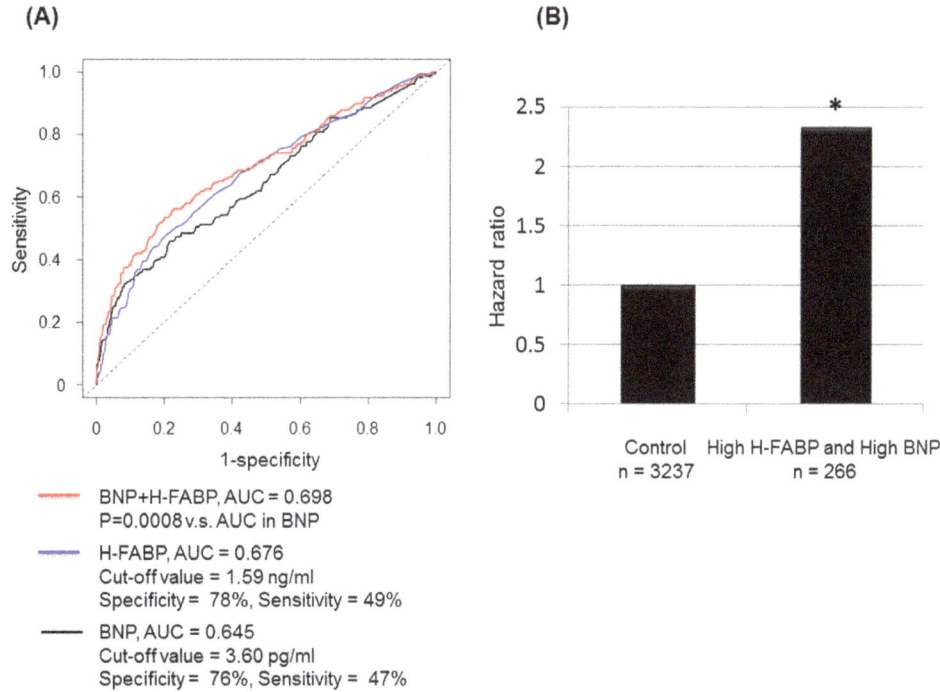

BNP+H-FABP, AUC = 0.698
P=0.0008 v.s. AUC in BNP

H-FABP, AUC = 0.676
Cut-off value = 1.59 ng/ml
Specificity = 78%, Sensitivity = 49%

BNP, AUC = 0.645
Cut-off value = 3.60 pg/ml
Specificity = 76%, Sensitivity = 47%

Figure 5. Combination of H-FABP and BNP. (A) The ROC curves of H-FABP, BNP, and H-FABP+BNP for all-cause deaths. **(B)** The statistical interaction between H-FABP and BNP. Subjects with high $\log_e$ H-FABP ($\geq$1.59 ng/mL) and high $\log_e$ BNP ($\geq$3.6 pg/mL) were at increased risk for all-cause death after adjustments for high H-FABP and high BNP (hazard ratio, 2.39; 95% confidence interval, 1.19–4.37; P = 0.0126).

cardiovascular deaths in general population. Since this was the prospective cohort study, we did not confirm the precise mechanism by which circulating H-FABP level was related to all-cause mortality including cancer deaths. Subjects with elevated H-FABP had higher prevalence of HT, DM, obesity, Mets, and CKD, which are risks for all-cause deaths and cancer deaths [39,40,41]. Renin-angiotensin-aldosterone system activation and insulin resistance were also risks for the development of cancer in addition to worsening myocardial damage [42,43]. These findings contributed to the fact that elevated H-FABP levels were significantly associated with future all-cause mortality as well as cardiovascular deaths.

H-FABP is reportedly a useful indicator of future cardiac prognosis independent of BNP in patients with CHF [20,44]. Similarly, we found a statistically significant interaction between H-FABP and BNP that predicted future all-cause deaths, indicating that the combination of H-FABP and BNP evaluations would be useful in determining risk in the general population. Although 92% of subjects were within the normal range, H-FABP

can be used to risk-stratify subjects in the general population based on their risk for all-cause and cardiovascular death.

Limitation

This study was conducted with a large number of participants and had a long follow-up period, suggesting that results are reliable. However, there are some limitations. First, this study collected baseline information at a single time point. Subsequent medical interventions may have affected serum H-FABP levels. Second, non-fatal diseases were not assessed, which could result in an underestimation of the association between H-FABP levels and clinical outcomes. Third, because structural heart disease was not diagnosed by echocardiogram, we could not confirm the association between H-FABP level and heart disease. Fourth, since H-FABP level is elevated due to disordered elimination of H-FABP in subjects with kidney dysfunction, we could not completely eliminate effect of kidney dysfunction on H-FABP level. However, 93% of subjects had normal eGFR in the present study. Finally, the low rate of cardiovascular mortality observed in

Table 4. Statics for model fit and improvement with the addition of H-FABP on the prediction of all-cause mortality.

	AUC (P value)	NRI (95%CI, P value)	IDI (95%CI, P value)
Age+HT+DM+Obesity+Mets	0.793	Reference	Reference
Age+HT+DM+Obesity+Mets+BNP	0.793 (P = 0.9980)	0.0556 (−0.1053–0.2165, P = 0.4982)	0.0057 (0.0014–0.0100, P = 0.0101)
Age+HT+DM+Obesity+Mets+H-FABP	0.798 (P = 0.3374)	0.1632 (0.0023–0.324, P = 0.0467)	0.0073 (0.0022–0.0125, P = 0.0051)

AUC, area under the curve; 95%CI, 95% confidence interval; NRI, net reclassification index; IDI, integrated discrimination index; HT, hypertension; DM, diabetes mellitus; Mets, metabolic syndrome; BNP, brain natriuretic peptide; H-FABP, heart type fatty acid binding protein.

this study may primarily result from low prevalence of ischemic heart disease in Japan. The prevalence of ischemic heart disease is reportedly markedly lower in Japan compared with the western countries [45]. The rate of cardiovascular mortality in this study is thought to be equivalent to that seen in Japanese population based registry [46].

Conclusions

Serum H-FABP is increased in subjects with increased numbers of cardiovascular risk factors. Notably, H-FABP could predict all-

cause and cardiovascular mortality in subjects in the general population, suggesting that it is a promising marker to risk-stratify apparently healthy general populations.

Author Contributions

Conceived and designed the experiments: YO TW T. Konta YS AF MD YU T. Kato T. Kayama IK. Performed the experiments: YO HT AH TN SK YH. Analyzed the data: YO TW AH. Contributed reagents/materials/analysis tools: YO TW. Wrote the paper: YO TW TA TS TM.

References

1. Chen J, Normand SL, Wang Y, Krumholz HM (2011) National and regional trends in heart failure hospitalization and mortality rates for Medicare beneficiaries, 1998–2008. JAMA 306: 1669–1678.
2. Lloyd-Jones DM, Larson MG, Leip EP, Beiser A, D'Agostino RB, et al. (2002) Lifetime risk for developing congestive heart failure: the Framingham Heart Study. Circulation 106: 3068–3072.
3. Hunt SA, Abraham WT, Chin MH, Feldman AM, Francis GS, et al. (2005) ACC/AHA 2005 Guideline Update for the Diagnosis and Management of Chronic Heart Failure in the Adult: a report of the American College of Cardiology/American Heart Association Task Force on Practice Guidelines (Writing Committee to Update the 2001 Guidelines for the Evaluation and Management of Heart Failure): developed in collaboration with the American College of Chest Physicians and the International Society for Heart and Lung Transplantation: endorsed by the Heart Rhythm Society. Circulation 112: 154–235.
4. Tsutamoto T, Wada A, Maeda K, Hisanaga T, Maeda Y, et al. (1997) Attenuation of compensation of endogenous cardiac natriuretic peptide system in chronic heart failure: prognostic role of plasma brain natriuretic peptide concentration in patients with chronic symptomatic left ventricular dysfunction. Circulation 96: 509–516.
5. Omland T, Pfeffer MA, Solomon SD, de Lemos JA, Rosjo H, et al. (2013) Prognostic value of cardiac troponin I measured with a highly sensitive assay in patients with stable coronary artery disease. J Am Coll Cardiol 61: 1240–1249.
6. Braga JR, Tu JV, Austin PC, Chong A, You JJ, et al. (2013) Outcomes and care of patients with acute heart failure syndromes and cardiac troponin elevation. Circ Heart Fail 6: 193–202.
7. Ahmad T, Fiuzat M, Felker GM, O'Connor C (2012) Novel biomarkers in chronic heart failure. Nat Rev Cardiol 9: 347–359.
8. Eggers KM, Venge P, Lindahl B, Lind L (2013) Cardiac troponin I levels measured with a high-sensitive assay increase over time and are strong predictors of mortality in an elderly population. J Am Coll Cardiol 61: 1906–1913.
9. Leistner DM, Klotsche J, Pieper L, Stalla GK, Lehnert H, et al. (2012) Circulating troponin as measured by a sensitive assay for cardiovascular risk assessment in primary prevention. Clin Chem 58: 200–208.
10. Glatz JF, Paulussen RJ, Veerkamp JH (1985) Fatty acid binding proteins from heart. Chem Phys Lipids 38: 115–129.
11. Daidoji H, Arimoto T, Nitobe J, Tamura H, Kutsuzawa D, et al. (2012) Circulating heart-type fatty acid binding protein levels predict the occurrence of appropriate shocks and cardiac death in patients with implantable cardioverter-defibrillators. J Card Fail 18: 556–563.
12. Matsumoto S, Nakatani D, Sakata Y, Suna S, Shimizu M, et al. (2013) Elevated Serum Heart-Type Fatty Acid-Binding Protein in the Convalescent Stage Predicts Long-Term Outcome in Patients Surviving Acute Myocardial Infarction. Circ J. 77: 1026–1032.
13. Arimoto T, Takeishi Y, Shiga R, Fukui A, Tachibana H, et al. (2005) Prognostic value of elevated circulating heart-type fatty acid binding protein in patients with congestive heart failure. J Card Fail 11: 56–60.
14. Examination Committee of Criteria for 'Obesity' in Japan; Japan Society for the Study of Obesity (2002) New criteria for 'obesity disease' in Japan. Circ J 66: 987–992.
15. Expert Panel on Detection, Evaluation, and Treatment of High Blood Cholesterol in Adults (2001) Executive Summary of The Third Report of The National Cholesterol Education Program (NCEP) Expert Panel on Detection, Evaluation, And Treatment of High Blood Cholesterol In Adults (Adult Treatment Panel III). JAMA 285: 2486–2497.
16. National Cholesterol Education Program (NCEP) Expert Panel on Detection, Evaluation, and Treatment of High Blood Cholesterol in Adults (Adult Treatment Panel III) (2002) Third Report of the National Cholesterol Education Program (NCEP) Expert Panel on Detection, Evaluation, and Treatment of High Blood Cholesterol in Adults (Adult Treatment Panel III) final report. Circulation 106: 3143–3421.
17. Eckardt KU, Berns JS, Rocco MV, Kasiske BL (2009) Definition and classification of CKD: the debate should be about patient prognosis – a position statement from KDOQI and KDIGO. Am J Kidney Dis 53: 915–920.
18. National Kidney Foundation (2002) K/DOQI clinical practice guidelines for chronic kidney disease: evaluation, classification, and stratification. Am J Kidney Dis 39: 1–266.
19. Arimoto T, Takeishi Y, Niizeki T, Nozaki N, Hirono O, et al. (2007) Cardiac sympathetic denervation and ongoing myocardial damage for prognosis in early stages of heart failure. J Card Fail 13: 34–41.
20. Niizeki T, Takeishi Y, Arimoto T, Takahashi T, Okuyama H, et al. (2005) Combination of heart-type fatty acid binding protein and brain natriuretic peptide can reliably risk stratify patients hospitalized for chronic heart failure. Circ J 69: 922–927.
21. Niizeki T, Takeishi Y, Arimoto T, Takabatake N, Nozaki N, et al. (2007) Heart-type fatty acid-binding protein is more sensitive than troponin T to detect the ongoing myocardial damage in chronic heart failure patients. J Card Fail 13: 120–127.
22. Matsuo S, Imai E, Horio M, Yasuda Y, Tomita K, et al. (2009) Revised equations for estimated GFR from serum creatinine in Japan. Am J Kidney Dis 53: 982–992.
23. Matthews DR, Hosker JP, Rudenski AS, Naylor BA, Treacher DF, et al. (1985) Homeostasis model assessment: insulin resistance and beta-cell function from fasting plasma glucose and insulin concentrations in man. Diabetologia 28: 412–419.
24. de Lemos JA, Drazner MH, Omland T, Ayers CR, Khera A, et al. (2010) Association of troponin T detected with a highly sensitive assay and cardiac structure and mortality risk in the general population. JAMA 304: 2503–2512.
25. deFilippi CR, de Lemos JA, Christenson RH, Gottdiener JS, Kop WJ, et al. (2010) Association of serial measures of cardiac troponin T using a sensitive assay with incident heart failure and cardiovascular mortality in older adults. JAMA 304: 2494–2502.
26. Viswanathan K, Kilcullen N, Morrell C, Thistlethwaite SJ, Sivananthan MU, et al. (2010) Heart-type fatty acid-binding protein predicts long-term mortality and re-infarction in consecutive patients with suspected acute coronary syndrome who are troponin-negative. J Am Coll Cardiol 55: 2590–2598.
27. Kostin S, Pool L, Elsasser A, Hein S, Drexler HC, et al. (2003) Myocytes die by multiple mechanisms in failing human hearts. Circ Res 92: 715–724.
28. Olivetti G, Abbi R, Quaini F, Kajstura J, Cheng W, et al. (1997) Apoptosis in the failing human heart. N Engl J Med 336: 1131–1141.
29. Eggers KM, Lind L, Ahlstrom H, Bjerner T, Ebeling Barbier C, et al. (2008) Prevalence and pathophysiological mechanisms of elevated cardiac troponin I levels in a population-based sample of elderly subjects. Eur Heart J 29: 2252–2258.
30. Meng X, Ming M, Wang E (2006) Heart fatty acid binding protein as a marker for postmortem detection of early myocardial damage. Forensic Sci Int 160: 11–16.
31. Mann J, Davies MJ (1999) Mechanisms of progression in native coronary artery disease: role of healed plaque disruption. Heart 82: 265–268.
32. Mervaala E, Muller DN, Park JK, Dechend R, Schmidt F, et al. (2000) Cyclosporin A protects against angiotensin II-induced end-organ damage in double transgenic rats harboring human renin and angiotensinogen genes. Hypertension 35: 360–366.
33. Hernandez AF, Mi X, Hammill BG, Hammill SC, Heidenreich PA, et al. (2012) Associations between aldosterone antagonist therapy and risks of mortality and readmission among patients with heart failure and reduced ejection fraction. JAMA 308: 2097–2107.
34. Chiu YT, Chen YT, Lin NN, Cheng CC, Gong CL, et al. (2005) Sympathetic activity and myocardial damage after stimulation of dorsal medulla and vagotomy in a novel animal model. Int J Cardiol 100: 401–407.
35. Narumi T, Shishido T, Kiribayashi N, Kadowaki S, Nishiyama S, et al. (2012) Impact of insulin resistance on silent and ongoing myocardial damage in normal subjects: the Takahata study. Exp Diabetes Res 2012: 815098.

36. Niizeki T, Takeishi Y, Takabatake N, Shibata Y, Konta T, et al. (2007) Circulating levels of heart-type fatty acid-binding protein in a general Japanese population: effects of age, gender, and physiologic characteristics. Circ J 71: 1452–1457.

37. Saunders JT, Nambi V, de Lemos JA, Chambless LE, Virani SS, et al. (2011) Cardiac troponin T measured by a highly sensitive assay predicts coronary heart disease, heart failure, and mortality in the Atherosclerosis Risk in Communities Study. Circulation 123: 1367–1376.

38. Sakata Y, Shimokawa H (2013) Epidemiology of heart failure in Asia. Circ J 77: 2209–2217.

39. Renehan AG, Tyson M, Egger M, Heller RF, Zwahlen M (2008) Body-mass index and incidence of cancer: a systematic review and meta-analysis of prospective observational studies. Lancet 371: 569–578.

40. Calle EE, Rodriguez C, Walker-Thurmond K, Thun MJ (2003) Overweight, obesity, and mortality from cancer in a prospectively studied cohort of U.S. adults. N Engl J Med 348: 1625–1638.

41. Stengel B (2010) Chronic kidney disease and cancer: a troubling connection. J Nephrol 23: 253–262.

42. George AJ, Thomas WG, Hannan RD (2010) The renin-angiotensin system and cancer: old dog, new tricks. Nat Rev Cancer 10: 745–759.

43. Jee SH, Kim HJ, Lee J (2005) Obesity, insulin resistance and cancer risk. Yonsei Med J 46: 449–455.

44. de Antonio M, Lupon J, Galan A, Vila J, Urrutia A, et al. (2012) Combined use of high-sensitivity cardiac troponin T and N-terminal pro-B type natriuretic peptide improves measurements of performance over established mortality risk factors in chronic heart failure. Am Heart J 163: 821–828.

45. Shiba N, Nochioka K, Miura M, Kohno H, Shimokawa H (2011) Trend of westernization of etiology and clinical characteristics of heart failure patients in Japan – first report from the CHART-2 study. Circ J 75: 823–833.

46. NIPPON DATA80 Research Group (2006) Risk assessment chart for death from cardiovascular disease based on a 19-year follow-up study of a Japanese representative population. Circ J 70: 1249–1255.

Permissions

All chapters in this book were first published in PLOS ONE, by The Public Library of Science; hereby published with permission under the Creative Commons Attribution License or equivalent. Every chapter published in this book has been scrutinized by our experts. Their significance has been extensively debated. The topics covered herein carry significant findings which will fuel the growth of the discipline. They may even be implemented as practical applications or may be referred to as a beginning point for another development.

The contributors of this book come from diverse backgrounds, making this book a truly international effort. This book will bring forth new frontiers with its revolutionizing research information and detailed analysis of the nascent developments around the world.

We would like to thank all the contributing authors for lending their expertise to make the book truly unique. They have played a crucial role in the development of this book. Without their invaluable contributions this book wouldn't have been possible. They have made vital efforts to compile up to date information on the varied aspects of this subject to make this book a valuable addition to the collection of many professionals and students.

This book was conceptualized with the vision of imparting up-to-date information and advanced data in this field. To ensure the same, a matchless editorial board was set up. Every individual on the board went through rigorous rounds of assessment to prove their worth. After which they invested a large part of their time researching and compiling the most relevant data for our readers.

The editorial board has been involved in producing this book since its inception. They have spent rigorous hours researching and exploring the diverse topics which have resulted in the successful publishing of this book. They have passed on their knowledge of decades through this book. To expedite this challenging task, the publisher supported the team at every step. A small team of assistant editors was also appointed to further simplify the editing procedure and attain best results for the readers.

Apart from the editorial board, the designing team has also invested a significant amount of their time in understanding the subject and creating the most relevant covers. They scrutinized every image to scout for the most suitable representation of the subject and create an appropriate cover for the book.

The publishing team has been an ardent support to the editorial, designing and production team. Their endless efforts to recruit the best for this project, has resulted in the accomplishment of this book. They are a veteran in the field of academics and their pool of knowledge is as vast as their experience in printing. Their expertise and guidance has proved useful at every step. Their uncompromising quality standards have made this book an exceptional effort. Their encouragement from time to time has been an inspiration for everyone.

The publisher and the editorial board hope that this book will prove to be a valuable piece of knowledge for researchers, students, practitioners and scholars across the globe.

List of Contributors

Hesamoddin Jahanian, Thomas Christen, Michael E. Moseley and Manjula Greg Zaharchuk
Department of Radiology, Stanford University, Stanford, California, United States of America

Akira Fukao, Yoshiyuki Ueno, Takeo Kato and Takamasa Kayama
Global Center of Excellence Program Study Group, Yamagata University School of Medicine, Yamagata, Japan

Makoto Daimon
Department of Endocrinology and Metabolism, Hirosaki University Graduate School of Medicine, Aomori, Japan

Kathy Petoumenos
The Kirby Institute, University of New South Wales, Sydney, Australia

Alan Winston
Department of Medicine, Imperial College, London, England

Wendy W. Ni
Department of Radiology, Stanford University, Stanford, California, United States of America
Department of Electrical Engineering, Stanford University, Stanford, California, Untied States of America

Kurella Tamura
Geriatric Research and Education Clinical Center, Palo Alto Veterans Affairs Health Care System and Division of Nephrology, Stanford University, Stanford, California, United States of America

Chia-Hung Chiang
Division of Cardiology, Department of Medicine, Taipei Veterans General Hospital, Hsinchu Branch, Hsinchu, Taiwan
Division of Cardiology, Taipei Veterans General Hospital, Taipei, Taiwan
Institute of Clinical Medicine, National Yang-Ming University, Taipei, Taiwan
Cardiovascular Research Center, National Yang-Ming University, Taipei, Taiwan

Shing-Jong Lin
Division of Cardiology, Taipei Veterans General Hospital, Taipei, Taiwan
Department of Medical Research and Education, Taipei Veterans General Hospital, Taipei, Taiwan
Institute of Clinical Medicine, National Yang-Ming University, Taipei, Taiwan
Cardiovascular Research Center, National Yang-Ming University, Taipei, Taiwan

Hsin-Bang Leu
Division of Cardiology, Taipei Veterans General Hospital, Taipei, Taiwan
Healthcare and Management Center, Taipei Veterans General Hospital, Taipei, Taiwan
Institute of Clinical Medicine, National Yang-Ming University, Taipei, Taiwan
Cardiovascular Research Center, National Yang-Ming University, Taipei, Taiwan

Po-Hsun Huang
Division of Cardiology, Taipei Veterans General Hospital, Taipei, Taiwan
Institute of Clinical Medicine, National Yang-Ming University, Taipei, Taiwan
Cardiovascular Research Center, National Yang-Ming University, Taipei, Taiwan

Chun-Chih Chiu and Chien-Yi Hsu
Division of Cardiology, Taipei Veterans General Hospital, Taipei, Taiwan
Cardiovascular Research Center, National Yang-Ming University, Taipei, Taiwan

Chin-Chou Huang and Jaw-Wen Chen
Division of Cardiology, Taipei Veterans General Hospital, Taipei, Taiwan
Department of Medical Research and Education, Taipei Veterans General Hospital, Taipei, Taiwan
Cardiovascular Research Center, National Yang-Ming University, Taipei, Taiwan
Institute and Department of Pharmacology, National Yang-Ming University, Taipei, Taiwan

Takahito Moriyama, Kayu Tanaka, Chihiro Iwasaki, Yasuko Oshima, Ayami Ochi, Hiroshi Kataoka, Mitsuyo Itabashi, Takashi Takei, Keiko Uchida and Kosaku Nitta
Department of Medicine, Kidney Center, Tokyo Women's Medical University, Tokyo, Japan

Yongqiang Li, Chaomin Zhou, Xiaofei Shao, Xinyu Liu, Jia Guo, Ying Zhang, Honglei Wang, Xiaohong Wang, Bin Li, Kangping Deng, Qin Liu and Hequn Zou
Department of Nephrology, Third Affiliated Hospital of Southern Medical University, Guangzhou, Guangdong, China

Harry Holthöfer
National Centre for Sensor Research/BioAnalytical
Sciences, Dublin City University, Dublin, Ireland

Lukas Schwingshackl and Georg Hoffmann
University of Vienna, Faculty of Life Sciences,
Department of Nutritional Sciences, Vienna, Austria

Shuo-Chun Weng
Center for Geriatrics and Gerontology, Taichung
Veterans General Hospital, Taichung, Taiwan
Division of Nephrology, Department of Internal
Medicine, Taichung Veterans General Hospital,
Taichung, Taiwan
Institute of Clinical Medicine, National Yang-Ming
University, Taipei, Taiwan

Der-Cherng Tarng
Institute of Clinical Medicine, National Yang-Ming
University, Taipei, Taiwan
Department and Institute of Physiology, National
Yang-Ming University, Taipei, Taiwan
Division of Nephrology, Department of Medicine
and Immunology Research Center, Taipei Veterans
General Hospital

Chyong-Mei Chen
Department of Statistics and Informatics Science,
Providence University, Taichung, Taiwan

Chi-Hung Cheng
Division of Nephrology, Department of Internal
Medicine, Taichung Veterans General Hospital,
Taichung, Taiwan
Department of Biotechnology, HungKuang University,
Taichung, Taiwan

Ming-Ju Wu
Division of Nephrology, Department of Internal
Medicine, Taichung Veterans General Hospital,
Taichung, Taiwan
Institute of Clinical Medicine, National Yang-Ming
University, Taipei, Taiwan
School of Medicine, Chung Shan Medical University,
Taichung, Taiwan
School of Medicine, College of Medicine, China
Medical University, Taichung, Taiwan

Cheng-Hsu Chen
Division of Nephrology, Department of Internal
Medicine, Taichung Veterans General Hospital,
Taichung, Taiwan
School of Medicine, College of Medicine, China
Medical University, Taichung,
Taiwan

Tung-Min Yu
Division of Nephrology, Department of Internal
Medicine, Taichung Veterans General Hospital,
Taichung, Taiwan

Kuo-Hsiung Shu
Division of Nephrology, Department of Internal
Medicine, Taichung Veterans General Hospital,
Taichung, Taiwan, Taipei, Taiwan
School of Medicine, Chung Shan Medical University,
Taichung, Taiwan

**Li-Hao Chen, Suzanne L. Advani, Kerri Thai, M.
Golam Kabir, Darren A. Yuen, Kim A. Connelly,
Philip A. Marsden, Richard E. Gilbert and Andrew
Advani**
Keenan Research Centre for Biomedical Science and
Li Ka Shing Knowledge Institute of St. Michael's
Hospital, Toronto, Ontario, Canada

Manish M. Sood
Ottawa Hospital Research Institute, University of
Ottawa, Ottawa, Ontario, Canada

Ian W. Gibson
Health Sciences Centre, University of Manitoba,
Winnipeg, Manitoba, Canada

Darren J. Kelly
Department of Medicine, St. Vincent's Hospital,
Melbourne, Victoria, Australia

Ashwani K Gupta and Waseem David
Department of Nephrology, University of Florida-
Jacksonville, Jacksonville, Florida, United States of
America

Nihil Chitalia and Debasish Banerjee
Renal and Transplantation Unit, St George's Healthcare
NHS Trust, London, United Kingdom
Cardiovascular Research Centre, St George's, University
of London, London, United Kingdom

Juan Carlos Kaski and Tuan Ismail
Cardiovascular Research Centre, St George's, University
of London, London, United Kingdom

Laura Tooth and Frances Boa
Chemical Pathology, St George's Healthcare NHS
Trust, London, United Kingdom

Geeta Hampson and David Goldsmith
Renal and Clinical Chemistry Departments, Guy's and
St Thomas, NHS Foundation Trust, London, United
Kingdom

Young Ok Kim, Dong Chan Jin, Ho Chul Song, Euy Jin Choi and Chul Woo Yang
Department of Internal Medicine, College of Medicine, The Catholic University of Korea, Seoul, Korea

Hyung Wook Kim
Department of Internal Medicine, College of Medicine, The Catholic University of Korea, Seoul, Korea
St. Vincent's Hospital, Suwon, Korea

Su-Hyun Kim
Department of Internal Medicine, College of Medicine, Chung-Ang University, Seoul, Korea

Yong-Lim Kim
Department of Internal Medicine, Kyungpook National University School of Medicine, Daegu, Korea

Yon-Su Kim
Department of Internal Medicine, College of Medicine, Seoul National University, Seoul, Korea

Shin-Wook Kang
Department of Internal Medicine, College of Medicine, Yonsei University, Seoul, Korea

Nam-Ho Kim
Department of Internal Medicine, Chonnam National University Medical School, Gwangju, Korea

Yong Kyun Kim
Department of Internal Medicine, College of Medicine, The Catholic University of Korea, Seoul, Korea
MRC for Cell Death Disease Research Center, The Catholic University of Korea, Seoul, Korea

Max Plischke, Ammon Handisurya and Martin Haas
Division of Nephrology and Dialysis, Department of Internal Medicine III, Medical University Vienna, Vienna, Austria

Maria Kohl and Georg Heinze
Section for Clinical Biometrics, Center of Medical Statistics, Informatics and Intelligent Systems, Medical University of Vienna, Vienna, Austria

Lise Bankir
INSERM UMRS 1138, Equipe 2, Centre de Recherche des Cordeliers, Paris, France

Sascha Shayganfar
Division of Cardiology, Pulmonology, and Vascular Medicine, Medical Faculty, University Hospital Düsseldorf, Düsseldorf, Germany

Hwee-Yeong Ng
Department of Advanced Medicine for Uremia, Nagoya University Graduate School of Medicine, Nagoya, Japan

Division of Nephrology, Department of Internal Medicine, Kaohsiung Chang Gung Memorial Hospital and Chang Gung University College of Medicine, Kaohsiung, Taiwan

Maimaiti Yisireyili, Shinichi Saito, Yelixiati Adelibieke and Toshimitsu Niwa
Department of Advanced Medicine for Uremia, Nagoya University Graduate School of Medicine, Nagoya, Japan

Chien-Te Lee
Division of Nephrology, Department of Internal Medicine, Kaohsiung Chang Gung Memorial Hospital and Chang Gung University College of Medicine, Kaohsiung, Taiwan

Fuyuhiko Nishijima
Biomedical Research Laboratories, Kureha Co., Tokyo, Japan

Huanhuan Su, Guihua Jiang and Junzhang Tian
Department of Medical Imaging, Guangdong No. 2 Provincial People's Hospital, Guangzhou, PR China

Yingwei Qiu
Department of Medical Imaging, Guangdong No. 2 Provincial People's Hospital, Guangzhou, PR China
Department of Medical Imaging, The First Affiliated Hospital of Gannan Medical University, Ganzhou, PR China

Xiaofei Lv
Departments of Medical Imaging and Interventional Radiology, Cancer Center, Sun Yat-Sen University, Guangzhou, PR China

Cheng Li
Department of Renal Transplantation, Guangdong No. 2 Provincial People's Hospital, Guangzhou, PR China

May E. Montasser, Lawrence C. Shimmin and James E. Hixson
Human Genetics Center, School of Public Health, University of Texas Health Science Center at Houston, Houston, Texas, United States of America

Dongfeng Gu, Jie Cao and Jichun Chen
Cardiovascular Institute and Fu Wai Hospital, Chinese Academy of Medical Sciences, Beijing, China

Jing Chen and Lotuce Lee Hamm
Tulane University School of Medicine, New Orleans, Louisiana, United States of America

Charles Gu, Treva K. Rice and Dabeeru C. Rao
Washington University in School of Medicine, St. Louis, Missouri, United States of America

Tanika N. Kelly, Paul K.Whelton and Jiang He
Tulane University School of Public Health and Tropical Medicine, New Orleans, Louisiana, United States of America

Cashell E. Jaquish
National Heart, Lung and Blood Institute, National Institute of Health, Bethesda, Maryland, United States of America

De-PeLiu
National Laboratory of Medical Molecular Biology, Institute of Basic Medical Sciences, Chinese Academy of Medical Sciences, Beijing, China

John W. Pickering
Department of Medicine, University of Otago Christchurch, Christchurch, New Zealand

Zoltán H. Endre
Department of Nephrology, Prince of Wales Clinical School, University of New
South Wales, Sydney, Australia

Isabelle Six, Hirokazu Okazaki, Priscilla Gross, Joanna Cagnard, Cédric Boudot and Julien Tilman B. Drueke
INSERM Unit 1088, Jules Verne University of Picardie, Amiens, France

Maizel and Ziad A. Massy
INSERM Unit 1088, Jules Verne University of Picardie, Amiens, France
Amiens University Medical Center, Amiens, France

Shih-Cheng Yang, Jen-Chieh Chen, Wei-Chen Tai, Cheng-Kun Wu, Keng-Liang Wu, Yi-Chun Chiu, Jing-Houng Wang, Sheng-Nan Lu and Seng-Kee Chuah
Division of Hepato-gastroenterology, Department of Internal Medicine, Kaohsiung Chang Gung Memorial Hospital and Chang Gung University, College of Medicine, Kaohsiung, Taiwan

Chen-Hsiang Lee
Division of Infectious Disease, Department of Internal Medicine, Kaohsiung Chang Gung Memorial Hospital and Chang Gung University; College of Medicine, Kaohsiung, Taiwan

Se Won Oh
Department of Internal Medicine, Inje University College of Medicine, Goyang City, Gyeonggi-do, Korea

Sejoong Kim
Department of Internal Medicine, Seoul National University Bundang Hopsital, Seong-Nam, Korea

Ki Young Na, Dong-Wan Chae and Ho Jun Chin
Department of Internal Medicine, Seoul National University Bundang Hopsital, Seong-Nam, Korea
Department of Internal Medicine, Seoul National University College of Medicine, Seoul, Korea

Ki Woong Kim
Department of Psychiatry, Seoul National University College of Medicine, Seoul, Korea

Christopher J. Miller, Katherine Huppler Hullsiek, Jacqueline Neuhaus, Deborah Wentworth Julian Wolfson and James D. Neaton
Division of Biostatistics, School of Public Health, University of Minnesota, Minneapolis, Minnesota, United States of America

Alison M. Bormann
Division of Infectious Diseases, University of Minnesota, Minneapolis, Minnesota, United States of America

Jason V. Baker
Division of Infectious Diseases, University of Minnesota, Minneapolis, Minnesota, United States of America
Hennepin County Medical Center, Minneapolis, Minnesota, United States of America

Kristine M. Erlandson
Division of Infectious Diseases, University of Colorado Anschutz Medical Campus, Aurora, Colorado, United States of America

Amy C. Justice
Veterans Affairs Connecticut Healthcare System, West Haven, Connecticut, United States of America
School of Medicine and Public Health, Yale University, New Haven, Connecticut, United States of America

Roger Paredes
irsiCaixa Foundation, Hospital Universitari Germans Trias i Pujol, Universitat Auto´noma de Barcelona, Badalona, Spain
Lluita contra la SIDA Foundation, Badalona, Spain

Fatemeh Saheb Sharif-Askari, Syed Azhar Syed Sulaiman and Narjes Saheb Sharif-Askari
Discipline of Clinical Pharmacy, School of Pharmaceutical Science, Universiti Sains Malaysia, Penang, Malaysia,

Jen-Chieh Liao and Chung-Ching Chio
Department of Neurosurgery, Chi-Mei Medical Center, Tainan, Taiwan

Jhi-Joung Wang
Department of Medical Research, Chi-Mei Medical Center, Tainan, Taiwan

Ali Al Sayed Hussain
Pharmacy Department, Dubai Health Authority, Dubai, United Arab Emirates

Beatriz Grinsztejn, Ruth Khalili Friedman, Cynthia B. Cunha, Lara Esteves Coelho, Paula Mendes Luz, Ronaldo Ismério Moreira, Sandra W. Cardoso and Valdilea G. Veloso
STD/AIDS Clinical Research Laboratory, Instituto de Pesquisa Clínica Evandro Chagas-Fundação Oswaldo Cruz, Rio de Janeiro, Brazil

Patrícia Santiago
STD/AIDS Clinical Research Laboratory, Instituto de Pesquisa Clínica Evandro Chagas-Fundação Oswaldo Cruz, Rio de Janeiro, Brazil
Clinical and Academic Unit of Nephrology, Hospital Universitário Pedro Ernesto, Faculdade de Ciências Médicas, Universidade do Estado do Rio de Janeiro, Rio de Janeiro, Brazil

José H. Rocco Suassuna
Clinical and Academic Unit of Nephrology, Hospital Universitário Pedro Ernesto, Faculdade de Ciências Médicas, Universidade do Estado do Rio de Janeiro, Rio de Janeiro, Brazil

Albanita Viana de Oliveira
Department of Pathology, Faculdade de Ciências Médicas, Universidade do Estado do Rio de Janeiro, Rio de Janeiro, Brazil

Xun Liu, Jinxia Chen, Ming Li and Tanqi Lou
Division of Nephrology, Department of Internal Medicine, The Third Affiliated Hospital of Sun Yat-sen University, Guangzhou, China,

Xiaoliang Gan
Department of Anesthesiology, Zhongshan Ophthalmic Center, Sun Yat-sen University, Guangzhou, China

Linsheng Lv
Operating Room, The Third Affiliated Hospital of Sun Yat-sen University, Guangzhou, China

Menno Pruijm, Marie-Eve Muller, Carole Zweiacker, Isabelle Bassi and Michel Burnier
Department of Nephrology, University Hospital, Lausanne, Switzerland,

Bruno Vogt
Department of Nephrology and Hypertension, Bern University Hospital, Bern, Switzerland,

Maciej Piskunowicz
Department of Radiology, Medical University of Gdansk, Gdansk, Poland

Matthias Stuber
Department of Radiology, University Hospital, Lausanne, Switzerland

Konstantinos Sombolos
Nephrology Clinic, Papanikolaou Hospital, Thessaloniki, Greece

Demitrios Tsakiris
Nephrology Clinic, Papageorgiou Hospital, Thessaloniki, Greece

John Boletis
Nephrology Clinic, Laiko Hospital, Athens, Greece

Demetrios Vlahakos
Nephrology Clinic, ATTIKON University Hospital, Athens, Greece

Kostas C. Siamopoulos
Nephrology Clinic, Ioannina University Hospital, Ioannina, Greece

Vassilios Vargemezis
Nephrology Clinic, Alexandroupoli University Hospital, Alexandroupoli, Greece

Pavlos Nikolaidis
Nephrology Clinic, AHEPA Hospital, Thessaloniki, Greece

Christos Iatrou
Center for Nephrology, G Papadakis, Nikea Hospital, Athens, Greece

Eugene Dafnis
Nephrology Clinic, PE.PA.G.N.I, Crete University Hospital, Iraklio, Greece

Konstantinos Xynos
AbbVie Pharmaceuticals, Chicago, Illinois, United States of America

Christos Argyropoulos
AbbVie Pharmaceuticals SA, Athens, Greece

Zhenjie Wu, Le Qu, Huamao Ye, Bing Liu, Qing Yang, Liang Xiao, Chen Lv, Bo Yang, Xu Gao, Xiaofeng Gao, Chuanliang Xu, Jianguo Hou, Yinghao Sun and Linhui Wang
Department of Urology, Changhai Hospital, Second Military Medical University, Shanghai, P. R. China

Mingmin Li and Jing Sheng
Department of Radiology, Changhai Hospital, Second Military Medical University, Shanghai, P. R. China

Teng Moua and Tobias Peikert
Division of Pulmonary/Critical Care, Mayo Clinic Rochester, Rochester, Minnesota, United States of America

Ladan Zand, Dingxin Qin and Qi Qian
Division of Nephrology, Mayo Clinic Rochester, Rochester, Minnesota, United States of America

Robert P. Hartman and Thomas E. Hartman
Department of Radiology, Mayo Clinic Rochester, Rochester, Minnesota, United States of America

Yuanyuan Xie, Xinghua Shao, Xiajing Che, Weijia Xu, Zhaohui Ni and Shan Mou
Department of Nephrology, Molecular Cell Lab for Kidney Disease, Ren Ji Hospital, School of Medicine, Shanghai Jiao Tong University, Shanghai, P.R. China,

Wei Xue
Department of Urology, Ren Ji Hospital, School of Medicine, Shanghai Jiao Tong University, Shanghai, P.R. China

Morten K. Borg, Emil Brøndum and Christian Aalkjær
Department of Biomedicine, Aarhus University, Aarhus, Denmark,

Per Ivarsen and Johan V. Povlsen
Department of Renal Medicine, Aarhus University Hospital and Department of Clinical Medicine, Faculty of Health, Aarhus University, Aarhus, Denmark

Yong Un Kang, Ha Yeon Kim, Joon Seok Choi, Chang Seong Kim, Eun Hui Bae, Seong Kwon Ma and Soo Wan Kim
Department of Internal Medicine, Chonnam National University Medical School, Gwangju, Korea

Ming-Yen Lin
Division of Nephrology, Department of Internal Medicine, Kaohsiung Medical University Hospital, Kaohsiung Medical University, Kaohsiung, Taiwan

Jiun-Chi Huang
Division of Nephrology, Department of Internal Medicine, Kaohsiung Medical University Hospital, Kaohsiung Medical University, Kaohsiung, Taiwan
Department of Internal Medicine, Kaohsiung Municipal Hsiao-Kang Hospital, Kaohsiung Medical University, Kaohsiung, Taiwan

Szu-Chia Chen
Division of Nephrology, Department of Internal Medicine, Kaohsiung Medical University Hospital, Kaohsiung Medical University, Kaohsiung, Taiwan

Department of Internal Medicine, Kaohsiung Municipal Hsiao-Kang Hospital, Kaohsiung Medical University, Kaohsiung, Taiwan
Faculty of Medicine, Kaohsiung Medical University, Kaohsiung, Taiwan

Jer-Ming Chang
Division of Nephrology, Department of Internal Medicine, Kaohsiung Medical University Hospital, Kaohsiung Medical University, Kaohsiung, Taiwan
Department of Internal Medicine, Kaohsiung Municipal Hsiao-Kang Hospital, Kaohsiung Medical University, Kaohsiung, Taiwan
Faculty of Renal Care, College of Medicine, Kaohsiung Medical University, Kaohsiung, Taiwan

Shang-Jyh Hwang, Jer-Chia Tsai and Hung-Chun Chen
Division of Nephrology, Department of Internal Medicine, Kaohsiung Medical University Hospital, Kaohsiung Medical University, Kaohsiung, Taiwan
Faculty of Renal Care, College of Medicine, Kaohsiung Medical University, Kaohsiung, Taiwan

Chung-Han Ho
Department of Medical Research, Chi-Mei Medical Center, Tainan, Taiwan
Department of Hospital and Health Care Administration, Chia Nan University of Pharmacy and Science, Tainan, Taiwan

Fu-Wen Liang
Institute of Public Health, College of Medicine, National Cheng Kung University, Tainan, Taiwan

Kao-Chang Lin
Department of Medical Research, Chi-Mei Medical Center, Tainan, Taiwan
Department of Biotechnology, Southern Taiwan University of Science and Technology, Tainan, Taiwan

Jinn-Rung Kuo
Department of Neurosurgery, Chi-Mei Medical Center, Tainan, Taiwan
Department of Medical Research, Chi-Mei Medical Center, Tainan, Taiwan
Department of Biotechnology, Southern Taiwan University of Science and Technology, Tainan, Taiwan

Yoichiro Otaki, Tetsu Watanabe, Hiroki Takahashi, Atushi Hirayama, Taro Narumi, Shinpei Kadowaki, Yuki Honda, Takanori Arimoto, Tetsuro Shishido, Takuya Miyamoto, Tsuneo Konta, Yoko Shibata and Isao Kubota
Department of Cardiology, Pulmonology, and Nephrology, Yamagata University School of Medicine, Yamagata, Japan

Index